T0315056

Controversies in Neuroendoscopy

Peter Nakaji, MD
Professor
Director of Minimally Invasive and Endoscopic Neurosurgery
Program Director of the Neurosurgery Residency Program
Department of Neurosurgery
Barrow Neurological Institute
Phoenix, Arizona

Hasan A. Zaidi, MD
Assistant Professor
Co-Director of Adult Spinal Deformity/Scoliosis
Department of Neurosurgery
Harvard Medical School/Brigham and Women's Hospital
Boston, Massachusetts

184 illustrations

Thieme
New York • Stuttgart • Delhi • Rio de Janeiro

Executive Editor: Timothy Hiscock
Managing Editor: Kenneth Schubach
Director, Editorial Services: Mary Jo Casey
Production Editor: Torsten Scheihagen
International Production Director: Andreas Schabert
Editorial Director: Sue Hodgson
International Marketing Director: Fiona Henderson
International Sales Director: Louisa Turrell
Director, Institutional Sales: Adam Bernacki
Senior Vice President and Chief Operating Officer: Sarah Vanderbilt
President: Brian D. Scanlan

Library of Congress Cataloging-in-Publication Data

Names: Nakaji, Peter, editor. | Zaidi, Hasan A., editor.
Title: Controversies in neuroendoscopy / [edited by]
Peter Nakaji, Hasan A. Zaidi.
Description: New York : Thieme, [2019] | Includes
bibliographical references and index. |
Identifiers: LCCN 2019015605 (print) | LCCN 2019016148
(ebook) | ISBN 9781626233539 (hardback) | ISBN
9781626233553 (e-ISBN)
Subjects: | MESH: Neuroendoscopy–methods |
Neuroendoscopy–adverse effects |
Comparative Effectiveness Research | Evaluation Studies
Classification: LCC RD593 (ebook) | LCC RD593 (print) |
NLM WL 141.5.N4 | DDC 617.4/810597–dc23
LC record available at https://lccn.loc.gov/2019015605

The views expressed in this book are those of the author and contributors, and do not reflect the official policy or position of the United States Government, the Department of Defense, Department of the Army or the Department of the Air Force.

© 2019 by Thieme Medical Publishers, Inc.
Thieme Publishers New York
333 Seventh Avenue, New York, NY 10001 USA
+1 800 782 3488, customerservice@thieme.com

Thieme Publishers Stuttgart
Rüdigerstrasse 14, 70469 Stuttgart, Germany
+49 [0]711 8931 421, customerservice@thieme.de

Thieme Publishers Delhi
A-12, Second Floor, Sector-2, Noida-201301
Uttar Pradesh, India
+91 120 45 566 00, customerservice@thieme.in

Thieme Revinter Publicações Ltda.
Rua do Matoso, 170 – Tijuca
Rio de Janeiro RJ 20270-135 - Brasil
+55 21 2563-9702
www.thiemerevinter.com.br

Cover design: Thieme Publishing Group
Cover art created by Michael D. Hickman, BA
Typesetting by DiTech Process Solutions

Printed in the United States of America
by King Printing Co., Inc.   5 4 3 2 1

ISBN 978-1-62623-353-9

Also available as an e-book:
eISBN 978-1-62623-355-3

Important note: Medicine is an ever-changing science undergoing continual development. Research and clinical experience are continually expanding our knowledge, in particular our knowledge of proper treatment and drug therapy. Insofar as this book mentions any dosage or application, readers may rest assured that the authors, editors, and publishers have made every effort to ensure that such references are in accordance with **the state of knowledge at the time of production of the book.**

Nevertheless, this does not involve, imply, or express any guarantee or responsibility on the part of the publishers in respect to any dosage instructions and forms of applications stated in the book. **Every user is requested to examine carefully** the manufacturers' leaflets accompanying each drug and to check, if necessary in consultation with a physician or specialist, whether the dosage schedules mentioned therein or the contraindications stated by the manufacturers differ from the statements made in the present book. Such examination is particularly important with drugs that are either rarely used or have been newly released on the market. Every dosage schedule or every form of application used is entirely at the user's own risk and responsibility. The authors and publishers request every user to report to the publishers any discrepancies or inaccuracies noticed. If errors in this work are found after publication, errata will be posted at www.thieme.com on the product description page.

Some of the product names, patents, and registered designs referred to in this book are in fact registered trademarks or proprietary names even though specific reference to this fact is not always made in the text. Therefore, the appearance of a name without designation as proprietary is not to be construed as a representation by the publisher that it is in the public domain.

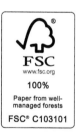

FSC
www.fsc.org
100%
Paper from well-managed forests
FSC® C103101

To our patients who benefit from the controversies we debate on their behalf, our colleagues with whom we deliberate with spirit and ardor, and my family for tolerating so much.

Peter Nakaji, MD

To my family, who have taught me the true meaning of unconditional love.

Hasan A. Zaidi, MD

Contents

Contents

Contents

Foreword

I have always thought of neuroendoscopy as a tool, not a separate discipline in the field of neurosurgery. The introduction of the microscope never spawned a separate society or created a subspecialty. Certainly, there were never books written about or courses dedicated to the use of loupes in neurosurgery, hence my reluctance to support societies and the International Federation of Neuroendoscopy. However, as with any new tool, whether it be a tool to visualize pathology or one with which to eradicate pathology, its utility and applications benefit from a clear definition. Understanding the tools and their precise uses helps us evaluate the value they bring (or don't bring).

Neuroendoscopy offers new ways to accomplish neurosurgical goals for the benefit of patients, but many of the operations that can be done endoscopically have open counterparts, which predate the endoscopic option and are therefore better established. Turning over stones and finding new ways to do things is an essential process in improving any field. But, as with most new ideas, it is not always readily accepted and is often contentious. There are many ways to focus down on the fine distinctions that can help us choose between options—spirited debate between two parties, each defending his or her particular viewpoint, is certainly one of these. This is the format that the editors have chosen for this book.

Nakaji and Zaidi have gathered neurosurgical experts from across the globe who have extensive experience in the use of the microscope and the endoscope, and together they have created the ultimate reference manual for the most practical and effective use of this exceptional visualization tool. The endoscope typically requires a cavity in which it is placed to be maximally effective, so applications in brain surgery, where there are very few cavities, would appear to be limited. However, this excellent book describes multiple different ways cavities might be created to use the endoscope to improve outcomes. The nasal cavity can be expanded to accommodate both endoscopes and instruments. The enhanced illumination and magnification afforded by the endoscope then allow more precise surgery of pathologies of the skull base. When tumors of the cerebrum or cerebellum are removed, the cavity created can be effectively used to accommodate the endoscope, which can, in turn, demonstrate residual pockets of tumor that might be hidden from the direct view of a microscope. The subarachnoid space is a potential medium in which the endoscope becomes an effective tool, and even the carpal tunnel may be better visualized with an endoscope.

As someone who has seen a bit of controversy in his career, I can attest that good can come from embracing controversy instead of avoiding it. This does not mean that it is smooth or enjoyable when you are in it. But being a spectator to this kind of debate can be informative and, at times, even entertaining. I hope you will find some of both in the contents of this book. There is something for everyone here: the diverse chapters cover everything from intraventricular endoscopy to spinal approaches to peripheral nerve. The viewpoints presented here offer a range from the moderate to the extreme.

Peter Nakaji is a former fellow of mine (it seems an age ago) and is now a colleague. His coeditor, Dr. Zaidi, was a resident of his and is now a colleague as well, in practice at the Brigham and Women's Hospital in Boston. Although both are generally regarded as adherents of the school of minimally invasive or "keyhole" surgery, they are, I believe, thoughtful in their adherence and open to measured opinions from both sides. In that spirit, they have produced the book you hold in your hands, with its effort to offer civilized debate about the pros and cons of different endoscopic and open approaches that have arisen from the emergence of endoscopic techniques. All too often, I have witnessed "uncivilized" debate at major meetings and have wanted to stand up and yell to the participants, "Lay down your weapons! We are all on the same side; the enemy is neurological disease!" Eventually, endoscopic approaches will secure their well-deserved position in the neurosurgeon's armamentarium, as have microscopic approaches.

So, I exhort you to buy the book and read it. Whether to be informed or entertained, your patients and your practice will be better for it.

Charles Teo, AM, MBBS, FRACS
Conjoint Professor of Neurosurgery, UNSW
Consulting Professor of Neurosurgery,
Duke Medical College, USA
Yeoh Ghim Seng Visiting Professor, NUH, Singapore
Professor Honoris Causa, Hanoi Medical University, Vietnam
Director, Centre for Minimally Invasive Neurosurgery, Sydney
Founder, Charlie Teo Foundation for Brain Cancer Research

Preface

Why write a book on controversies in neuroendoscopy? Never has the need for spirited but civil debate in the interest of progress been more pressing. As neurosurgery achieves both greater technical refinement and entirely new technologies to deploy in surgery, the options offered to patients must be examined ever more closely. The march of technological progress has brought whole new surgical paradigms into existence that threaten prior management models with competition and even conflict. At times, the separation between open and minimally invasive approaches has become not only incremental but fundamental. When surgeons perform a craniotomy for microsurgical resection of a colloid cyst or neuroendoscopic removal of the cyst, they have similar goals; however, these techniques are not merely versions of each other, and they most definitely are not immediately cross-convertible in terms of the surgeon's skill set. One cannot offer a "blended" approach between them.

Across the spectrum of pathology covered in this book, it is made clear that practitioners of the neurosurgical arts must make stark treatment choices for their patients regarding what they will offer. Seeing all sides in this multifactorial patient-management debate can better inform decisions, further advance the field, and provide the patient with the best options for a good outcome. Patients also have their preferences. While we recognize that the personal values of the patients must be given appropriate weight, ultimately the patient comes to the neurosurgeon because she or he is the expert. In many cases, there are truly two good treatment options; yet in the end, we must recommend one approach. In this book, we have asked each contributor to address the argument in favor of a particular viewpoint to clarify the rationale and evidence for each option. The moderators, meanwhile, provide perspectives on both pro and con viewpoints. The intent is not to provide the legalism of a courtroom but to provide rigorous debate of controversial neuroendoscopy topics. Polemics are neither encouraged or discouraged. We think you will find healthy and occasionally passionate advocacy of a given viewpoint. Martin Luther King Jr. said, "The ultimate measure of a man is not where he stands in moments of comfort and convenience, but where he stands at times of challenge and controversy." Neurosurgeons are in life and death—or function and nonfunction—struggles every day. It is only right and good that they should stand for their patients and share their knowledge as they have done here.

We are proud of the contributions and contributors you will find herein. Read on and enjoy!

Acknowledgments

We thank our colleagues—master surgeons and physicians—who took time from their busy practices to share their knowledge and experience in the chapters they contributed that made this work possible. We also thank the ever-dedicated staff of Neuroscience Publications at Barrow Neurological Institute, including editors Mary Ann Clifft, Paula Higginson, Joseph C. Mills, Dawn Mutchler, and Lynda Orescanin, editorial coordinators Rogena Lake and Samantha Soto, and production editor Cassandra Todd. We thank medical illustrators Peter Lawrence and Joshua Lai as well as Michael Hickman who created the cover art. We thank Thieme Medical Publishers, particularly Tim Hiscock, for seeing the potential in this book, and Kenn Schubach for overseeing its production. Finally, and most importantly, we thank our patients and their families for entrusting us with their lives and for giving us the honor of caring for them.

Contributors

Hussam Abou-Al-Shaar, MD
Department of Neurosurgery
Hofstra Northwell School of
  Medicine—Northwell Health
Manhasset, New York

Nimer Adeeb, MD
Department of Neurosurgery
Louisiana State University—Shreveport
Shreveport, Louisiana

Vijay Agarwal, MD
Department of Neurosurgery
Albert Einstein College of Medicine
Bronx, New York

Syed Hassan Akbari, MD
Department of Neurosurgery
Washington University School of Medicine
St. Louis, Missouri

Brian L. Anderson, MD
Department of Neurosurgery
Pennsylvania State University School of Medicine
Hershey, Pennsylvania

Al-Wala Awad, MD
Department of Neurosurgery
University of Utah School of Medicine
Salt Lake City, Utah

Nicholas C. Bambakidis, MD
Department of Neurological Surgery
Case Western Reserve University
University Hospitals Case Medical Center
Cleveland, Ohio

André Beer-Furlan, MD
Department of Neurological Surgery
Rush University Medical Center
Chicago, Illinois

Ruth E. Bristol, MD
Department of Neurosurgery
Barrow Neurological Institute
Phoenix Children's Hospital
Phoenix, Arizona

Brandon Burroway, MS
Department of Neurological Surgery
University of Miami Miller School of Medicine
Miami, Florida

Margaret Carmody, MD
Department of Neurological Surgery
Case Western Reserve University
University Hospitals Case Medical Center
Cleveland, Ohio

Juanita Celix, MD
Department of Neurosurgery
Aurora Neuroscience Innovation Institute
Aurora St. Luke's Medical Center
Milwaukee, Wisconsin

Srikant Chakravarthi, MD
Department of Neurosurgery
Aurora Neuroscience Innovation Institute
Aurora St. Luke's Medical Center
Milwaukee, Wisconsin

Hsuan-Kan Chang, MD
Department of Neurological Surgery
University of Miami Miller School of Medicine
Miami, Florida

Peng-Yuan Chang, MD
Department of Neurological Surgery
University of Miami Miller School of Medicine
Miami, Florida

Jason Chu, MD
Department of Neurosurgery
Emory University School of Medicine
Atlanta, Georgia

Martin Corsten, MD
Department of Otolaryngology and Head and Neck Surgery
Aurora Neuroscience Innovation Institute
Aurora St. Luke's Medical Center
Milwaukee, Wisconsin

William T. Couldwell, MD
Department of Neurosurgery
University of Utah School of Medicine
Salt Lake City, Utah

Doniel G. Drazin, MD
Department of Neurosurgery
Cedars-Sinai Medical Center
Los Angeles, California

J. Bradley Elder, MD
Department of Neurological Surgery
Ohio State University
Columbus, Ohio

Richard G. Ellenbogen, MD, FACS
Department of Neurological Surgery
University of Washington School of Medicine
Seattle, Washington

Johnathan A. Engh, MD
Department of Neurological Surgery
University of Pittsburgh Medical Center
Pittsburgh, Pennsylvania

Chikezie Eseonu, MD
Department of Neurosurgery
Johns Hopkins Hospital
Baltimore, Maryland

Walid I. Essayed, MD
New York-Presbyterian/Weill Cornell Medical Center
New York, New York

James J. Evans, MD
Department of Neurological Surgery
Jefferson University School of Medicine
Philadelphia, Pennsylvania

Daniel R. Felbaum, MD
Department of Neurosurgery
MedStar Georgetown University Hospital
Washington, D.C.

Juan C. Fernandez-Miranda, MD
Department of Neurological Surgery
University of Pittsburgh Medical Center
University of Pittsburgh School of Medicine
Pittsburgh, Pennsylvania

Richard G. Fessler, MD, PhD
Rush University Medical Center
Chicago, Illinois

Steffen K. Fleck, MD
Department of Neurosurgery
University of Greifswald
Greifswald, Germany

Tatsuhiro Fujii, MD
Department of Neurological Surgery
Keck School of Medicine
Univeristy of Southern California
Los Angeles, California

Melanie Fukui, MD
Department of Neurosurgery
Aurora Neuroscience Innovation Institute, and
Department of Radiology
Aurora St. Luke's Medical Center
Milwaukee, Wisconsin

Paul A. Gardner, MD
Department of Neurological Surgery
University of Pittsburgh Medical Center
University of Pittsburgh School of Medicine
Pittsburgh, Pennsylvania

Samer S. Ghostine, MD
Division of Neurosurgery
University of California, Riverside
Riverside, California

Saksham Gupta, MD
Harvard Medical School
Boston, Massachusetts

Ali S. Haider, MD
Division of Neurosurgery
Hospital for Sick Children
University of Toronto
Toronto, Canada

Douglas A. Hardesty, MD
Department of Neurosurgery
Barrow Neurological Institute
Phoenix, Arizona

Roger Hartl, MD
Weill Cornell Medical School
New York, New York

Tim Heiland, MD
Weill Cornell Medical School
New York, New York

Christopher S. Hong, MD
Department of Neurosurgery
Yale University School of Medicine
New Haven, Connecticut

Mark Iantosca, MD
Department of Neurosurgery
Pennsylvania State University School of Medicine
Hershey, Pennsylvania

Jonathan Jennings, MD
Department of Radiology
Aurora St. Luke's Medical Center
Milwaukee, Wisconsin

J. Patrick Johnson, MD
Department of Neurosurgery
Cedars-Sinai Medical Center
Los Angeles, California

Paul E. Kaloostian, MD
Riverside Community Hospital
Riverside, California

Manish K. Kasliwal, MD, MCh
University Hospitals
Case Western Reserve University
Cleveland, Ohio

Amin Kassam, MD
Department of Neurosurgery
Aurora Neuroscience Innovation Institute
Aurora St. Luke's Medical Center
Milwaukee, Wisconsin

D. Keiner, MD
Department of Neurosurgery
Universität des Saarlandes
Saarbrücken, Germany

Sammy Khalili, MD
Department of Otolaryngology and Head and Neck Surgery
Aurora Neuroscience Innovation Institute
Aurora St. Luke's Medical Center
Milwaukee, Wisconsin

Terrence T. Kim, MD
Department of Orthopedic Surgery
Cedars Sinai Medical Center
Los Angeles, California

Varun R. Kshettry, MD
Department of Neurological Surgery
Jefferson University School of Medicine
Philadelphia, Pennsylvania

Nayan Lamba, BA
Harvard Medical School
Boston, Massachusetts

Edward R. Laws, Jr., MD
Brigham and Women's Hospital
Harvard Medical School
Boston, Massachusetts

Amy Lee, MD
Department of Neurological Surgery
University of Washington School of Medicine
Seattle, Washington

John Y. K. Lee, MD
Department of Neurosurgery
University of Pennsylvania
Philadelphia, Pennsylvania

Andrew S. Little, MD
Department of Neurosurgery
Barrow Neurological Institute
Phoenix, Arizona

Mark A. Mahan, MD
Department of Neurosurgery
University of Utah School of Medicine
Salt Lake City, Utah

Michael W. McDermott, MD
Department of Neurological Surgery
University of California, San Francisco
San Francisco, California

Kevin M. McGrail, MD
Department of Neurosurgery
MedStar Georgetown University Hospital
Washington, D.C.

Justin Moore, MD
Beth Israel Deaconess Medical Center
Harvard Medical School
Boston, Massachusetts

Peter Nakaji, MD
Department of Neurosurgery
Barrow Neurological Institute
Phoenix, Arizona

Rodrigo Navarro-Ramirez, MD
Department of Neurosurgery
Weill Cornell Medical School
New York, New York

Vikram V. Nayar, MD
Department of Neurosurgery
MedStar Georgetown University Hospital
Washington, D.C.

William C. Newman, MD
Department of Neurological Surgery
University of Pittsburgh Medical Center
Pittsburgh, Pennsylvania

Joachim Oertel, MD
Department of Neurosurgery
Universität des Saarlandes
Saarbrücken, Germany

Christopher S. Ogilvy, MD
Division of Neurosurgery
Beth Israel Deaconess Medical Center
Harvard Medical School
Boston, Massachusetts

Joseph A. Osorio, MD, PhD
Department of Neurological Surgery
University of California, San Francisco
San Francisco, California

Nelson Oyesiku, MD, PhD
Department of Neurosurgery
Emory University School of Medicine
Atlanta, Georgia

Sheri K. Palejwala, MD
Department of Neurosurgery
University of Arizona
Tucson, Arizona

Kamlesh Patel, MD
Department of Neurosurgery
Washington University School of Medicine
St. Louis, Missouri

Daniel M. Prevedello, MD
Department of Neurological Surgery
Ohio State University
Columbus, Ohio

Helen Quach, MD
Centre for Minimally Invasive Neurosurgery
New South Wales, Australia

Alfredo Quinones-Hinojosa, MD
Departments of Neurosurgery and Oncology
Johns Hopkins Hospital
Baltimore, Maryland

Amol Raheja, MD
Departments of Neurosurgery
University of Utah School of Medicine
Salt Lake City, Utah

Leonardo Rangel-Castilla, MD
Department of Neurosurgery
Mayo Clinic
Rochester, Minnesota

Jordina Rincon-Torroella, MD
Department of Neurosurgery
The Johns Hopkins University
Baltimore, Maryland

Richard Rovin, MD
Department of Neurosurgery
Aurora Neuroscience Innovation Institute
Aurora St. Luke's Medical Center
Milwaukee, Wisconsin

James T. Rutka, MD
Division of Neurosurgery
Hospital for Sick Children
University of Toronto
Toronto, Canada

Henry W. S. Schroeder, MD, PhD
Department of Neurosurgery
University of Greifswald
Greifswald, Germany

Theodore H. Schwartz, MD
Stanford University School of Medicine
Stanford, California

K. Schwerdtfeger, MD
Department of Neurosurgery
Universität des Saarlandes
Saarbrücken, Germany

Justin Singer, MD
Department of Neurological Surgery
University Hospitals Case Medical Center
Cleveland, Ohio

Harminder Singh, MD
Stanford University School of Medicine
Stanford, California, and
New York-Presbyterian/Weill Cornell Medical Center
New York, New York

Matthew D. Smyth, MD
Department of Neurosurgery
Washington University School of Medicine
St. Louis, Missouri

Carl H. Snyderman, MD
Department of Otolaryngology
University of Pittsburgh Medical Center
University of Pittsburgh School of Medicine
Pittsburgh, Pennsylvania

Robert F. Spetzler, MD
Department of Neurosurgery
Barrow Neurological Institute
University of Arizona College of Medicine
Phoenix, Arizona

Charles Teo, AM, MBBS, FRACS
Centre for Minimally Invasive Neurosurgery
New South Wales, Australia

Philip V. Theodosopoulos, MD
Department of Neurological Surgery
University of California, San Francisco
San Francisco, California

Ajith J. Thomas, MD
Division of Neurosurgery
Beth Israel Deaconess Medical Center
Harvard Medical School
Boston, Massachusetts

Luis M. Tumialán, MD
Department of Neurosurgery
Barrow Neurological Institute
Phoenix, Arizona

Francisco Vaz-Guimaraes, MD
Department of Neurological Surgery
University of Pittsburgh Medical Center
University of Pittsburgh School of Medicine
Pittsburgh, Pennsylvania

Eric W. Wang, MD
Department of Neurological Surgery
University of Pittsburgh Medical Center
University of Pittsburgh School of Medicine
Pittsburgh, Pennsylvania

Michael Y. Wang, MD
Department of Neurological Surgery and
Department of Rehabilitation Medicine
University of Miami Miller School of Medicine
Miami, Florida

Wei-Hsin Wang, MD
Department of Neurological Surgery
University of Pittsburgh School of Medicine
University of Pittsburgh Medical Center
Pittsburgh, Pennsylvania, and
Department of Neurosurgery
Neurological Institute
Taipei Veterans General Hospital
National Yang-Ming University School of Medicine
Taipei, Taiwan

Andrew I. Yang, MD
Department of Neurosurgery
University of Pennsylvania
Philadelphia, Pennsylvania

Brad E. Zacharia, MD
Department of Neurosurgery
Pennsylvania State University School of Medicine
Hershey, Pennsylvania

Gabriel Zada, MD
Department of Neurological Surgery
Keck School of Medicine
University of Southern California
Los Angeles, California

Hasan A. Zaidi, MD
Department of Neurosurgery
Harvard Medical School/Brigham and Women's Hospital
Boston, Massachusetts

Part I

History and Evolution of Neuroendoscopy

1 History and Evolution of Neuroendoscopy

Hasan A. Zaidi and Peter Nakaji

Summary

The evolution of neuroendoscopy originated with tools developed by the ancient Egyptians for use in burial rites, as well as with Jewish, Greek, and Arab medical instruments such as the speculum. After the development of the lichtleiter in the early 1800s came Max Nitze's development of lens magnification and internal illumination. With the subsequent discovery of electricity, the endoscope soon became an integral part of the surgeon's armamentarium. Surgeons in medical specialties such as otorhinolaryngology adapted the technology to produce better cystoscopes, and neurosurgeon Walter Dandy popularized the use of the endoscope for choroid plexectomy. The poor optical fidelity limiting its use to intraventricular pathology was overcome by the Storz–Hopkins endoscopes, which are in wide use today. The collaboration between Harold Hopkins, who invented the rod-lens system in 1960, and Karl Storz, who patented fiberoptic external cold-light transmission, resulted in a small-diameter endoscope allowing wide viewing angles, better illumination, and video-image transmission. In the decades since then, the neuroendoscope has been used in traditional microsurgical transsphenoidal approaches to pituitary lesions and in resecting parasellar lesions and lesions involving the petrous internal carotid artery, the middle cranial fossa, the infratemporal fossa, and the odontoid process. In the late 1980s, neuroendoscopes began to be used to facilitate peripheral nerve neuroendoscopy for ulnar nerve decompression. They were subsequently used for lumbar discectomy, thoracic discectomy, and kyphoscoliotic release, and to correct sagittal craniosynostosis and to aid endonasal surgery. Expanded uses of the neuroendoscope can be expected in the future.

Keywords: development, endonasal, history, neuroendoscopy, optics, skull base, spine

1.1 Introduction

The endoscope is a versatile tool that has fundamentally reshaped modern neurosurgery. Its small profile, improved light penetration, and panoramic visualization have left an indelible mark on endonasal skull base surgery, intraventricular surgery, spine surgery, and vascular neurosurgery. In some cases, the endoscope has usurped the role of the traditional operating microscope. In others, the endoscope has expanded the scope of practice to enable surgeons to treat lesions that were previously considered inoperable. If anything, the endoscope remains in its ascendancy and continues to expand in popularity. Although the endoscope appears to have created a quantum leap facilitated by modern technological innovations, this tool and its applications in neurosurgery did not appear overnight. Rather, one can trace the roots of neuroendoscopy to a myriad of scientists, inventors, physicians, and scholars who contributed to its development for well over a millennium. Understanding the development and evolution of the neuroendoscope provides a historical framework for how this tool is used today, and it also sheds light on opportunities and challenges for neuroendoscopy as the field moves forward.

1.2 Ancient Civilizations and the Age of the Speculum: 2000 BC to AD 1800

The earliest known tools resembling endoscopes were shaped by the complicated religious practices of the ancient Egyptians. As early as 2000 BC, the Egyptians believed that by removing the contents of the skull during burial, the soul would be able to reunite with the body in the afterlife.[1] They paid special attention during burial ceremonies to avoid disfiguring the face, and recent analysis using computed tomography has revealed that excerebration was performed using hook-shaped rods via an endonasal transethmoidal corridor.[2] In 1300 BC, Jewish religious scripture described instruments used to examine female genitals to confirm a woman's purity, drawing parallels to today's modern obstetric specula. Ancient Greeks, starting with Hippocrates (460–370 BC), were known to use specula to remove anogenital warts, with recent archeological excavations demonstrating instruments startlingly similar to the specula used today (► Fig. 1.1).[2] The Romans also developed minimally invasive tools for medical purposes, believing that bad humors causing disease could be removed by placing trocarlike instruments in the abdomen using minimally invasive incisions. Arab physicians, such as Albukasim (AD 936–1013), built on this knowledge by using reflected light in combination with a speculum to aid in visualization of hollow organs.[3] Similarly, in 1585, Tulio Caesare Aranzi redirected sunlight using a glass of water to examine the nasal cavity.[3]

1.3 Victorian Era and the Development of the First Endoscope: 1806 to 1910

Philipp Bozzini (1773–1809), a German–Italian physician, developed the first tool that remotely resembles the modern endoscope. In 1806, he demonstrated the use of his "lichtleiter" to the Academy of Medicine of Vienna; this instrument consisted of a long hollow tube with an eyepiece on one end, along with a small container with a mirror to reflect light generated from candles (► Fig. 1.2). Clinical application of this instrument was often limited because of excruciating discomfort for the patient, and it proved to be of little diagnostic value because of its rudimentary design. Despite its limited utility, the basic design developed by Bozzini was further refined by later generations to create the modern endoscope.

Technological innovation in the development of the endoscope over the next few decades was driven largely by specialists who focused on diseases of various hollow organs. The natural cavities provided by these organs proved to be a fertile

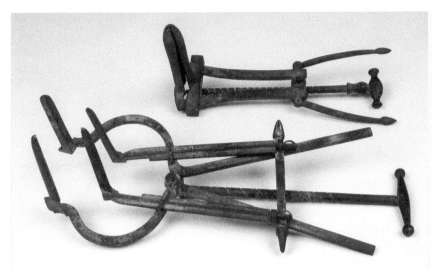

Fig. 1.1 Photograph of a reproduction of the original specula used by the ancient Greeks circa AD 70. (Reproduced with permission from the Milwaukee Public Museum, Milwaukee, WI, Catalog No. 2385.)

testing ground for low-profile endoscopes. One could maneuver endoscopes into a natural working corridor and provide diagnostic information while minimizing tissue trauma. Inspired by Bozzini's lichtleiter, the German urologist Max Nitze (1849–1906) introduced two fundamental concepts still in use in modern endoscopic design: lens magnification and internal illumination. He placed a series of lenses within a hollow metallic tube to magnify the projected image. He combined the tube of lenses with bulky water-cooled platinum wires opposite the eyepiece to illuminate organs from within, thereby increasing light penetration (▶ Fig. 1.3). Although heat from the light source often resulted in thermal tissue damage, this limitation was eliminated by the invention in 1879 of the incandescent light bulb by Thomas Edison. Nitze, a quintessential pioneer, is also credited with taking photographs from endoscopic projections to aid in diagnosis and medical education.

Once the potential of the endoscope was realized by the medical community, it was quickly adopted by other surgical specialties. In 1901, the German otorhinolaryngologist Alfred Hirschmann improved on previous designs of cystoscopes and applied this technology to the inspection of paranasal sinuses. He was the first to generate interest in this tool, which singlehandedly transformed the field of otorhinolaryngology surgery. Shortly thereafter, in 1910, the American urologist Victor Darwin Lespinasse (1878–1946) modified a cystoscope to cauterize choroid plexus in children with hydrocephalus using a transcortical intraventricular approach. Interdisciplinary regard and use led to an explosion of interest by the neurosurgical community and marked the dawn of neuroendoscopy.

1.4 The Dawn of Neuroendoscopy: 1911 to 1969

Johns Hopkins neurosurgeon Walter Dandy (1886–1946) popularized the use of endoscopes within the neurosurgical community, and he was the first to demonstrate its superiority over traditional approaches. One of Dandy's many contributions to the field was an understanding of cerebrospinal fluid dynamics and the development of hydrocephalus. In 1918, he described an open craniotomy for choroid plexectomy as a treatment for hydrocephalus,[1] with low efficacy and high mortality rates. After observing the feasibility of endoscopic approaches pioneered by Lespinasse, Dandy unsuccessfully attempted endoscopic choroid plexectomy in 1922 in a child with communicating hydrocephalus. With persistence and gradual technical improvements (▶ Fig. 1.4), he reported in 1932 that endoscopic plexectomy provided rates of success equal to those of the then-established open craniotomy techniques. With surgical endoscopy in its nascency, Dandy provided the boost necessary to legitimize the endoscope as a viable tool in the treatment of neurosurgical pathology, and he proved that in certain situations it could supersede previously established methods. Thus, he is widely considered to be the father of neuroendoscopy.

Despite early successes, the application of neuroendoscopes was largely limited to intraventricular pathology because of their poor optical fidelity. Unlike intraventricular pathology, the types of pathology requiring skull base approaches necessitate pristine visualization of the operative corridor that rivals or exceeds that of the traditional microsurgical approaches popular at the time. Prior to 1965, the endoscopes of this period remained fundamentally similar to Nitze's lens system, with limited image quality and magnification. When the endoscopes were used in treating neurosurgical lesions outside the ventricular system, surgeons found that this generation of endoscopes provided little helpful information. For example, Gerard Guiot (1912–1998) was the first to report the use of the endoscope as an adjunct for microsurgical approaches for sellar lesions in 1961. He would insert the endoscope to inspect the resection cavity after traditional microscopic transsphenoidal surgery. In his early publications, Guiot continued to use the archaic Nitze-designed endoscopes, but he found the image quality to be too poor to provide much of clinical value, and he ultimately abandoned endoscopic transsphenoidal surgery.

The field of neuroendoscopy remained stagnant in the mid-20th century, and it was not until endoscopic technology caught up with surgical innovation that the field finally progressed. The ability to transmit images through flexible glass cables was developed in 1926, which inspired Harold H. Hopkins, a professor of physics, to develop the rod-lens system in 1960. This development marked a turning point in the field

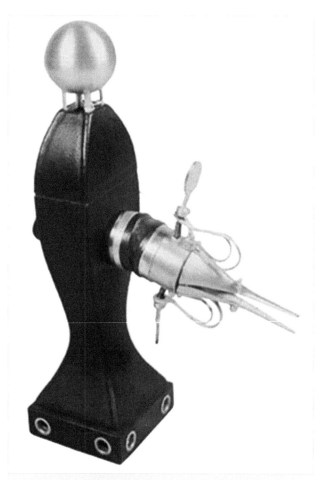

Fig. 1.2 Philipp Bozzini's original design of his "lichtleiter." (Reproduced with permission from Abd-El-Barr and Cohen.[1])

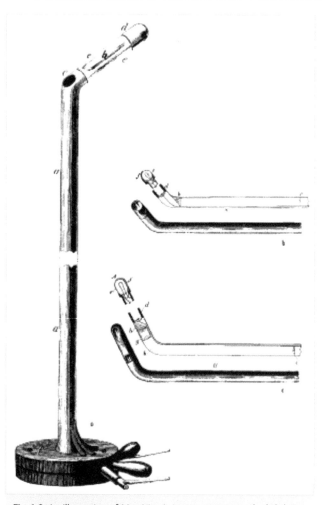

Fig. 1.3 An illustration of Max Nitze's improvements on the lichtleiter, which introduced the concepts of lens magnification and internal illumination. (Illustration is in the public domain.)

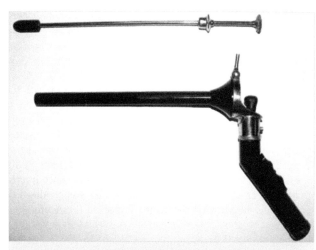

Fig. 1.4 Original funnel-shaped endoscope used by Walter Dandy to access intraventricular lesions. (Photograph courtesy of Dr. Edward R. Laws Jr.)

of neuroendoscopy. Hopkins modified traditional endoscopes by placing a series of glass lenses interspersed with neutral glass instead of air (▶ Fig. 1.5). This format dramatically improved optical efficiency by lowering the refractive index, thereby increasing the functional diameter of the lenses. Furthermore, improving light transmission and image quality within a system with an overall smaller diameter yielded a wider field of view. Nearly simultaneously, American gastroenterologist Basil Hirschowitz (1925–2013) developed endoscopes that could transmit images using flexible glass-coated fibers. A German entrepreneur by the name of Karl Storz (1911–1996) recognized that this technology could also be used to transmit light, and he patented the idea of fiberoptic external cold-light transmission. He brought his invention to Hopkins, and together they began production of the Storz–Hopkins endoscopes that are widely used today by the neurosurgical community. This system allowed for wide viewing

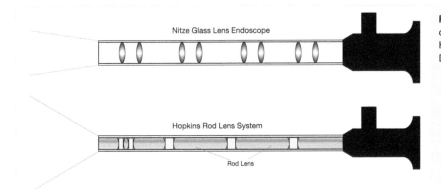

Fig. 1.5 Photograph of an illustration of Nitze's conventional glass-lens endoscope compared to Hopkins' rod-lens system. (Illustration courtesy of Dr. Edward R. Laws Jr.)

angles, better illumination, and video-image transmission with high fidelity, all within a small-diameter endoscope. With the advent and popularization of this new generation of endoscopes, the field of neuroendoscopy began rapidly expanding its applications across neurosurgical subspecialties.

1.5 Rapidly Expanding Indications for Neuroendoscopic Surgery: 1970 to Present

The late 20th century marked a time of rapid transformation, expanding indications, and wider adoption of the neuroendoscope by the neurosurgical community. Michael Apuzzo demonstrated in 1977 that endoscopes could reliably assist traditional microsurgical transsphenoidal approaches for pituitary lesions, and that they could improve visualization of anatomical landmarks and aid assessment of the presence of residual disease.[6] In 1992, Roger Jankowski of France reported three successful cases of endoscopic transsphenoidal resection of pituitary adenomas without the aid of the operating microscope.[7] Others caught on to a "pure" endoscopic approach for skull base lesions, with Drahambir Sethi and Prem Pillay from Singapore reporting successful treatment of 38 patients with pituitary adenoma and 2 patients with craniopharyngioma without the assistance of the operating microscope.[8] Similarly, in 1997, Hae Dong Jho and Ricardo Carrau introduced the purely endoscopic approach to the United States when they reported on 46 patients with pituitary lesions who were successfully treated using endoscope visualization alone.[9] With an international following, increased confidence, and burgeoning expertise with endoscopic endonasal surgery, Italian pioneers, such as Paolo Cappabianca, Enrico de Divitiis, Giorgio Frank, and Ernesto Pasquini, expanded the indications further by resecting parasellar lesions, such as cavernous sinus tumors and planum sphenoidale tumors.[10] In the early 2000s, Amin Kassam and Ricardo Carrau advanced the use of the technology further by reporting successful resection of lesions involving the petrous internal carotid artery, the middle cranial fossa, the infratemporal fossa, and the odontoid process.[11]

The rapid adoption of neuroendoscopic approaches was not simply limited to endonasal skull base surgery. In 1989, Okutsu et al[12] reported the use of the endoscope for carpal tunnel syndrome, which gained rapid popularity among peripheral nerve surgeons. In 1995, Tsai et al[13] applied peripheral nerve neuroendoscopy to perform ulnar nerve decompressions. After the early application of endoscopes in the lumbar spine for diagnostic purposes by Pool,[14] Cloyd and Obenchain[15] described laparoscopic approaches for lumbar discectomy in 1991. A short 4 years later in 1995, Mack et al[16] applied thoracoscopic techniques developed for cardiothoracic indications to treat complex spine pathology, including thoracic discectomies and kyphoscoliotic release. In 1998, Jimenez and Barone[17] described the use of endoscopes to correct sagittal craniosynostosis. In 2007, Kassam et al[18] reported the clipping of a superior hypophyseal aneurysm using an endoscopic endonasal route.

1.6 Conclusion

During the past 200 years, the endoscope has evolved from a candlelit rudimentary tube to a sophisticated and multifaceted tool that has been used in nearly every subspecialty within neurosurgery. In certain cases, the endoscope has replaced traditional approaches with high-quality data supporting its efficacy. In other cases, the endoscope is an untested contender awaiting the opportunity to make an impact. A growing controversy exists within the neurosurgical community regarding whether this tool represents a panacea destined to replace the operating microscope, or whether this tool, like any other tool, has its proper place and time. In this book, we set out to identify the subspecialty procedures within neurosurgery in which the endoscope has been introduced. By developing a discourse among surgeons who promote the conventional route and neuroendoscopists, we hope that this book will create a better understanding of the arguments for and against the use of endoscopy for any given indication. Thus, it summarizes where the field of neuroendoscopy stands today and, most importantly, indicates the directions it should be going. Although only time will tell what the lasting impact of the neuroendoscope will be, this book should serve as a guide to experts and novices alike on the advantages and limitations of this exciting technology.

References

[1] Abd-El-Barr MM, Cohen AR. The origin and evolution of neuroendoscopy. Childs Nerv Syst. 2013; 29(5):727–737

[2] Fanous AA, Couldwell WT. Transnasal excerebration surgery in ancient Egypt. J Neurosurg. 2012; 116(4):743–748

[3] Spaner SJ, Warnock GL. A brief history of endoscopy, laparoscopy, and laparoscopic surgery. J Laparoendosc Adv Surg Tech A. 1997; 7(6):369–373

[4] Nitze M. Lehrbuch der Kystoskopie: ihre Technik und klinische Bedeutung. Wiesbaden: J. F. Bergmann; 1889

[5] Prevedello DM, Doglietto F, Jane JA, Jr, Jagannathan J, Han J, Laws ER, Jr. History of endoscopic skull base surgery: its evolution and current reality. J Neurosurg. 2007; 107(1):206–213

[6] Apuzzo ML, Heifetz MD, Weiss MH, Kurze T. Neurosurgical endoscopy using the side-viewing telescope. J Neurosurg. 1977; 46(3):398–400

[7] Jankowski R, Auque J, Simon C, Marchal JC, Hepner H, Wayoff M. Endoscopic pituitary tumor surgery. Laryngoscope. 1992; 102(2):198–202

[8] Sethi DS, Pillay PK. Endoscopic management of lesions of the sella turcica. J Laryngol Otol. 1995; 109(10):956–962

[9] Carrau RL, Jho HD, Ko Y. Transnasal-transsphenoidal endoscopic surgery of the pituitary gland. Laryngoscope. 1996; 106(7):914–918

[10] Cappabianca P, Alfieri A, Thermes S, Buonamassa S, de Divitiis E. Instruments for endoscopic endonasal transsphenoidal surgery. Neurosurgery. 1999; 45 (2):392–395, discussion 395–396

[11] Kassam A, Snyderman CH, Mintz A, Gardner P, Carrau RL. Expanded endonasal approach: the rostrocaudal axis. Part I. Crista galli to the sella turcica. Neurosurg Focus. 2005; 19(1):E3

[12] Okutsu I, Ninomiya S, Takatori Y, Ugawa Y. Endoscopic management of carpal tunnel syndrome. Arthroscopy. 1989; 5(1):11–18

[13] Tsai TM, Bonczar M, Tsuruta T, Syed SA. A new operative technique: cubital tunnel decompression with endoscopic assistance. Hand Clin. 1995; 11 (1):71–80

[14] Pool J. Direct visualization of dorsal nerve roots of the cauda equina by means of a myeloscope. Arch Neurol Psychiatry. 1938; 39(6):1308–1312

[15] Cloyd DW, Obenchain TG. Laparoscopic lumbar discectomy. Semin Laparosc Surg. 1996; 3(2):95–102

[16] Mack MJ, Regan JJ, McAfee PC, Picetti G, Ben-Yishay A, Acuff TE. Video-assisted thoracic surgery for the anterior approach to the thoracic spine. Ann Thorac Surg. 1995; 59(5):1100–1106

[17] Jimenez DF, Barone CM. Endoscopic craniectomy for early surgical correction of sagittal craniosynostosis. J Neurosurg. 1998; 88(1):77–81

[18] Kassam AB, Gardner PA, Mintz A, Snyderman CH, Carrau RL, Horowitz M. Endoscopic endonasal clipping of an unsecured superior hypophyseal artery aneurysm. Technical note. J Neurosurg. 2007; 107(5):1047–1052

Part II

Skull Base Surgery

2 Microscopic versus Endoscopic Nasal Morbidity and Quality of Life after Skull Base Surgery

Douglas A. Hardesty and Andrew S. Little

Summary

Nasal morbidity after skull base surgery is an important consideration when using either endoscopic or microscopic transsphenoidal approaches. Over the past two decades, numerous metrics have been validated to quantify and study sinonasal-related quality of life and postoperative morbidity in this patient population. Herein, we summarize these available metrics and their individual advantages and disadvantages in quality-of-life research. The normal recovery period after transsphenoidal surgery is reviewed. We also explore the differences between endoscopic endonasal transsphenoidal approaches and microscopic transsphenoidal approaches on patient quality-of-life outcomes.

Keywords: endoscopic endonasal approach, microsurgical transsphenoidal approach, nasoseptal flap, quality of life, sinonasal morbidity, skull base surgery

2.1 Introduction

Endonasal approaches to the skull base with either an endoscope or the surgical microscope use natural sinus corridors to approach myriad lesions. Even large, complex tumors may be resected without the approach-related morbidity associated with anterior fossa transbasal approaches. Because endonasal approaches exploit the paranasal sinuses, they may result in decreased nasal function due to nasal obstruction, crusting, sinusitis, and epistaxis. Nevertheless, the use of these natural corridors to the skull base comes with sinonasal morbidity. Damage to the sinonasal passages during endonasal skull base surgery can lead to a host of patient symptoms of varying severity (▶ Table 2.1) as well as sinonasal complications (▶ Table 2.2). Endonasal surgery disrupts normal airflow, nasal mucosa structure, and physiological mucociliary clearance with varying effects on the patient.[1,2,3] Herein, we review the standardized assessment metrics of sinonasal morbidity and approach-related quality of life (QOL), and compare the outcomes for the canonical microscopic open and endonasal techniques to those of the newer endoscopic endonasal approach.

2.2 Measuring Sinonasal Morbidity

The study of sinonasal morbidity must include standardized and validated patient-centered metrics to assess subjective symptoms and their relative impact on patient QOL. The term *approach-related QOL* refers to a narrow domain of QOL affected by the approach to a surgical lesion. Metrics that measure approach-related QOL are the best tools by which to compare different surgical techniques relative to sinonasal morbidity. An ideal scale is reproducible, useful at multiple time points postoperatively, and literature-validated in the patient population of interest.

Table 2.1 Common patient subjective symptoms after skull base surgery affecting approach-related quality of life

Symptom
Worsened sense of smell
Worsened sense of taste
Urge to blow nose
Trouble breathing
Postnasal discharge
Thick nasal discharge
Dried nasal material
Trouble breathing at night
Facial pain and pressure
Nasal whistling
Foul nasal cavity smell

Table 2.2 Sinonasal complications after endonasal microsurgery or endonasal endoscopy

Complication
Sinusitis
Anosmia
Cerebrospinal fluid leak
Nasal obstruction
Synechiae (adhesions)
Nasal bridge deformity
Epistaxis

Note: Incidence varies, depending on the exact procedure performed and patient characteristics.

2.2.1 Sino-Nasal Outcome Test

The Sino-Nasal Outcome Test (SNOT-20 or SNOT-22) is a self-reported metric of sinonasal symptoms and related concerns, such as emotional status, that was originally validated for otorhinolaryngology patients with chronic rhinosinusitis.[4,5] Symptom frequency and severity are subjectively combined to rate individual questions from 0 (not a problem) to 5 (severe problem). Higher scores portent worse sinonasal function. The SNOT-20 or SNOT-22 scale is used frequently in endonasal skull base surgery, but some items are not applicable to postoperative patients (e.g., ear pain, cough) because the scale was originally used for chronic rhinosinusitis and not validated in endonasal skull base surgery. Nevertheless, it is a valuable addition to other metrics, and it is probably the most commonly used sinonasal QOL instrument in endonasal skull base surgery.

2.2.2 Anterior Skull Base Questionnaire

The Anterior Skull Base Questionnaire (ASBQ) is a commonly used tool for anterior skull base surgery QOL assessment.[6,7,8] The ASBQ was developed to study multidimensional QOL in patients with anterior skull base malignancy. The ASBQ is multidimensional and provides a more global assessment than it does an assessment of approach-related sinonasal morbidity. However, the metric does include nasal secretions, olfaction, and taste questions. The ASBQ has been used successfully in patients undergoing open transcranial, microscopic endonasal, and endoscopic endonasal approaches to the anterior fossa. This patient-reported scale consists of 35 questions rated on a scale from 1 to 5. This instrument is a de facto standard in skull base QOL assessment.

2.2.3 Rhinosinusitis Disability Index

The Rhinosinusitis Disability Index (RSDI) was originally purposed to assess sinonasal QOL in both operative and nonoperative rhinology patients,[9] including chronic rhinosinusitis. The RSDI is multidimensional and includes items on emotional well-being, social interaction, activity level, and more specific sinonasal symptoms of sinonasal discharge, taste, and smell. The RSDI has been used more extensively in the otolaryngology literature than in the neurosurgical literature, and it has been most extensively validated in nonneurosurgical populations. However, the RSDI has been used by at least one group in studying approach-related morbidity and QOL before and after endoscopic endonasal transsphenoidal surgery.[10]

2.2.4 Anterior Skull Base Nasal Inventory

The Anterior Skull Base Nasal Inventory (ASK Nasal-12) was designed by the senior author (A.S.L) and colleagues to assess sinonasal symptoms such as ease of breathing and crusting in postoperative endonasal patients based on 12 self-reported items.[11,12] As with the SNOT-22, a higher score on the ASK Nasal-12 portends worse symptoms. The current ASK Nasal-12 questions are scored on a 6-point system (0–5) based on symptom severity. The ASK Nasal-12 is the only scale currently validated for the assessment of sinonasal morbidity after endoscopic endonasal surgery and thus is considered the most applicable of the three QOL metrics discussed. The instrument was validated prospectively in a multicenter QOL study.[12]

2.3 Endonasal Approaches: Normal Postoperative Recovery and General Principles

Multiple studies have analyzed the routine postoperative sinonasal recovery time after endonasal transsphenoidal surgery. As expected, the immediate postoperative sinonasal approach–related QOL decreases as measured by metrics such as SNOT-22 and ASK Nasal-12. A return to preoperative sinonasal QOL baseline is expected 6 to 12 weeks after surgery.[13,14] Our group at Barrow Neurological Institute has identified the patient factor of advanced age, and the use of nasal packing or nasal splits, to be associated with reduced immediate postoperative approach-related QOL.[15] The University of California, Los Angeles group has also identified reduced soft-tissue manipulation with improved approach-related QOL postoperatively.[13,16] Additional work from Korea has demonstrated improved QOL with modifications to

the canonical endoscopic endonasal approach, again with an emphasis on reduction of mucosal damage.[17] This finding argues for judicious exposure (perhaps limiting turbinate resection) customized to the surgical pathology of the individual patient, rather than a one-size-fits-all maximal endonasal exposure in all cases.

The use of nasoseptal mucosal flaps in the endoscopic approach may also result in additional sinonasal morbidity. The advent of the vascularized mucosal graft has dramatically decreased the rate of postoperative cerebrospinal fluid leaks in endoscopic endonasal surgery.[18,19] However, the harvest of a mucosal graft, by definition, significantly disrupts the normal sinonasal mucosa along the nasal septum. Multiple institutional series have demonstrated worsened sinonasal QOL with the use of a vascularized mucosal graft, especially in the realm of nasal crusting and discharge.[20,21] However, other groups have reported no significant differences between patients with and without nasoseptal flaps.[8,22] One group even showed postoperative sinonasal QOL improvement after nasoseptal flap use, although there was no control group without a flap.[23] Our experience suggests that nasal crusting and mucopurulence can persist along the denuded septum for several months after surgery and may require occasional nasal debridement. As with turbinate resection, we therefore recommend the use of a nasoseptal flap not as a matter of routine, but only when required by the pathology at hand.

Postoperatively, various regimens have been suggested to improve sinonasal symptoms of patients, therefore improving approach-related sinonasal QOL. These include nasal sprays, prophylactic antibiotics, and outpatient sinus debridement. General themes emerge in the postoperative nasal care recommendations of numerous treatment centers. Postoperative nasal debridements are recommended 1 to 2 weeks after surgery or in patients with persistent sinonasal symptoms. The purpose of debridement is to clean the nasal passages, remove blood and crusting, and restore function. Most teams also recommend nasal irrigation with saline spray or saline rinses several times per day. One randomized trial examining the use of surfactant-based irrigation versus hypertonic saline in postoperative endoscopic endonasal patients demonstrated relatively poor tolerance of surfactant-based irrigation.[24] More than 50% of patients treated with surfactant reported side effects, and 20% stopped the treatment, despite similar QOL improvements in both groups on the SNOT-22. This may suggest that hypertonic saline is preferable in this patient population. There are no data regarding postoperative antibiotic use after transsphenoidal surgery, although 7 to 10 days of oral antibiotics is common practice. Antibiotics are commonly used despite the lack of support for it in functional endoscopic sinus surgery, the closest correlate to transsphenoidal surgery.[25] Postoperative nasal care is an area suitable for future study.

2.4 Endoscopic versus Microscopic Endonasal Approaches and Sinonasal QOL

Numerous variations of the transsphenoidal approach are used, including the uni-nostril or bi-nostril endoscopic endonasal approach, the sublabial endonasal microscopic approach, and the endonasal microscopic approach. The canonical standard for endonasal surgery is the microscopic, uni-nostril approach. A nasal speculum is placed, out-fracturing the turbinates, and a standard bimanual microneurosurgical technique is performed through the speculum. In comparison, the endoscopic approach most often uses a bi-nostril approach, with variable soft-tissue resection and no fixed speculum. As discussed above, both of these techniques have a temporary negative effect on sinonasal QOL postoperatively. However, a multicenter prospective cohort study led by our institution demonstrated no significant approach-related sinonasal QOL differences (as measured by ASK Nasal-12) postoperatively between the endoscopic and microscopic endonasal techniques at most time points.[15] No differences were found preoperatively, at 2 weeks or at 6 months postoperatively; a small difference favoring QOL in the endoscopic group at 3 months postoperatively was of limited clinical relevance. In this same cohort study, more than 75% of patients undergoing the endoscopic endonasal approach required sinonasal debridement in the outpatient setting postoperatively, compared to only 6% in the microscopic group. More aggressive postoperative debridement may partly reflect the increased involvement by otolaryngology colleagues in the endoscopic approach. Regardless, patient sinonasal QOL was not adversely affected. However, other groups have found worse sinonasal morbidity with the use of the endoscopic endonasal approach. Hong et al[26] retrospectively reviewed a prospectively maintained patient database of 55 patients and identified worse sinonasal QOL postoperatively as measured by a modified ASK Nasal inventory. This finding held true at 1 and 3 months postoperatively, and was most significant in the domains of nasal crusting and nose-blowing. Differences in surgical technique may explain the incongruous findings of Little et al[14] and Hong et al.[26] For example, Little et al used nasoseptal flaps in only 5% of cases and rarely used nasal packing; in comparison, Hong et al routinely used vascularized mucosal flaps and Silastic (Dow Corning Corp.) nasal splints. In addition, Little et al[14] report that absorbable nasal packing has been shown to negatively affect sinonasal QOL. Most studies contrasting the endoscopic endonasal approach to a microsurgical approach use the endonasal microsurgical approach as the comparison. However, the microscopic sublabial transsphenoidal approach has also been used with excellent results, and at least one group has studied patient QOL after the use of this technique. Pledger et al[27] examined the University of Virginia experience using either endonasal endoscopic transsphenoidal surgery or microscopic sublabial transsphenoidal surgery for nonfunctional pituitary adenomas. Both groups were evaluated with the SNOT-20 and other QOL metrics at time points up to 1 year postoperatively and found no significant differences between techniques in approach-related sinonasal or overall patient QOL. However, early time points of 24 hours to 8 weeks favored the endoscopic approach over the microsurgical approach for approach-related sinonasal morbidity, but not for overall QOL.[27]

2.5 Endoscopic versus Microscopic Endonasal Approaches: Olfaction

Olfaction is a major factor in QOL for patients with anterior fossa skull base lesions. Temporary impairment or loss of olfaction can arise from postoperative nasal obstruction and

rhinosinusitis, whereas permanent anosmia is usually due to thermal or mechanical damage to the olfactory mucosa. Several studies have implicated the endoscopic endonasal approach, specifically the use of nasoseptal flaps, in the loss of olfaction, leading to worse approach-related QOL.[28,29] However, not all publications demonstrate worsened olfactory function after endoscopic approaches, and different authors have reported conflicting results in this realm (▶ Table 2.3, ▶ Table 2.4).[15,22,26,28,29,30,31,32,33]

The University of Alabama Birmingham group prospectively enrolled 18 patients to undergo standardized and objective olfaction assessments preoperatively and postoperatively. They found that olfaction was largely preserved and that the use of nasoseptal flaps was not associated with anosmia.[32] Similar results showing excellent preservation of olfaction even in reoperative endoscopic endonasal surgery were reported in 2014 by another North American group.[30] However, contradictory results were published that same year in a large Korean series demonstrating that a significant proportion of endoscopic endonasal patients experienced dysfunctional postoperative olfaction.[31] Overall, the literature on postoperative olfaction and endoscopic approaches is limited by considerable differences in surgical technique, patient characteristics, and heterogeneous olfaction assessments. Comparisons of olfaction outcomes are sparse for the microscopic and endoscopic approaches. In two large 2015 cohort publications, Little et al[15] and Hong et al[26] assessed QOL after microscopic versus endoscopic approaches and found no olfactory differences between the two techniques as assessed by the ASK Nasal inventory and as assessed by the cross-cultural smell identification test and the butanol threshold test, respectively. In summary, they concluded that there is insufficient evidence at present to recommend either the endoscopic technique or the microscopic technique over the other for olfactory preservation. If an endoscopic approach is chosen and a nasoseptal mucosal flap is harvested, we recommend (as do other groups) using caution at the superior limb of the flap near the olfactory epithelium and leaving a margin of at least 1 to 2 cm below the superior aspect of the septum to avoid injury.[30]

2.6 Endoscopic versus Microscopic Endonasal Approaches: Extent of Resection Related to QOL

The extent of resection (EOR) is an independent variable affecting overall patient QOL after resection of both secreting and nonsecreting pituitary adenomas.[34] These findings were demonstrated in a broader QOL metric (the ASBQ), rather than one specific to sinonasal symptoms, but it emphasizes the importance of EOR on the overall patient experience. Therefore, if either the endoscopic or microscopic approach to pituitary adenomas led to better EOR, or if a variation of either approach improved EOR, it would support the use of the technique both for tumor outcomes and for improved patient QOL. Our group at Barrow Neurological Institute recently examined the EOR outcomes of a fully endoscopic approach and a fully microscopic approach and found no difference in volumetric tumor resection, rates of gross total resection, or residual tumor volume.[35] Thus, surgeons should use the technique with which they can safely achieve the best tumor outcome, which should lead to long-term improved patient QOL.

Table 2.3 Selected reports of olfactory outcomes in microscopic and endoscopic transsphenoidal surgery

Authors	Year	Patients (N)	Metric(s) used	Comparison group(s)	Olfaction outcomes
Cohort studies					
Zada et al[28]	2003	100	Subjective assessment	EEA cohort study	Subjectively "no problems with smell" in 73% of patients
Rotenberg et al[29]	2011	17	UPSIT, subjective assessment	EEA cohort study	Significant decrease in UPSIT postoperatively; 100% subjective problems with smell
Griffiths et al[30]	2014	35	BSIT	EEA cohort study	No significant change in BSIT scores pre- and postoperatively in 97% of patients
Kim et al[31]	2014	226	VAS, CCCRC, CCSIT	EEA cohort study, two mucosal flap techniques	Significant postoperative decrease in olfactory assessments with either EEA technique, worse in patients over age 30 years
Chaaban et al[32]	2015	18	UPSIT	EEA cohort study	No significant change in UPSIT scores pre- and postoperatively in 100% of patients
Harvey et al[22]	2015	98	BSIT	EEA cohort study	No significant difference in olfaction outcomes pre- and postoperatively
Rioja et al[33]	2016	55	VAS, BAST-24, MCT, SF-36	Limited EEA or expanded EEA cohorts	Subjective smell impairment in both groups at 12 months postoperatively, no change in postoperative objective olfactometry

Abbreviations: BAST-24, Barcelona Smell Test 24; BSIT, Brief Smell Identification Test; CCCRC, Connecticut Chemosensory Clinical Research Center Test; CCSIT, Cross-Cultural Smell Identification Test; EEA, expanded endonasal approach; MCT, mucociliary clearance time (saccharin test); SF-36, 36-Item Short Form Health Survey; UPSIT, University of Pennsylvania Smell Identification Test; VAS, visual analog scale.

Table 2.4 Comparison studies of olfactory outcomes in microscopic and endoscopic transsphenoidal surgery

Authors	Year	Patients (N)	Metric(s) used	Comparison group(s)	Olfaction outcomes
Little et al[15]	2015	218	ASK Nasal-12	EEA vs. microscopic endonasal	No difference in olfactory outcomes between endoscopic and microscopic groups at 6 months (EEA olfactory outcomes mildly superior at 3 months)
Hong et al[26]	2015	55	ASK Nasal-12, CCSIT, BTT	EEA vs. microscopic endonasal	No difference in olfactory outcomes between endoscopic and microscopic groups at 3 months

Abbreviations: ASK Nasal-12, Anterior Skull Base Nasal Inventory; BTT, butanol threshold test; CCSIT, Cross-Cultural Smell Identification Test; EEA, expanded endonasal approach.

2.7 Conclusion

The endoscopic endonasal approach to the anterior skull base is increasingly used instead of the traditional microscopic endonasal approach. Both approaches temporarily reduce sinonasal QOL because of intraoperative soft-tissue trauma. However, patients undergoing either technique usually return to preoperative baselines within 6 to 12 weeks after surgery. Although the nasoseptal flap has also been implicated in the loss of olfaction, several modern publications have found no difference between the endoscopic and microscopic techniques regarding postoperative olfactory function with or without a vascularized mucosal graft. Whenever possible, the meticulous preservation of mucosa and limited soft-tissue resection are key to maximizing sinonasal function and reducing approach-related perioperative morbidity. Because the long-term nasal outcomes are similar for the microscopic approach and the endoscopic approach, surgeons should choose the approach that gives them the best tumor outcomes for their patients rather than focus on minor differences in short-term sinonasal QOL. Postoperative nasal care standards have not been determined definitively because of the absence of objective comparative data, but such care may include the use of sinus rinses and nasal debridement.

References

[1] Cappabianca P, Cavallo LM, Colao A, de Divitiis E. Surgical complications associated with the endoscopic endonasal transsphenoidal approach for pituitary adenomas. J Neurosurg. 2002; 97(2):293–298

[2] Dusick JR, Esposito F, Mattozo CA, Chaloner C, McArthur DL, Kelly DF. Endonasal transsphenoidal surgery: the patient's perspective-survey results from 259 patients. Surg Neurol. 2006; 65(4):332–341, discussion 341–342

[3] de Almeida JR, Snyderman CH, Gardner PA, Carrau RL, Vescan AD. Nasal morbidity following endoscopic skull base surgery: a prospective cohort study. Head Neck. 2011; 33(4):547–551

[4] Piccirillo JF, Merritt MG, Jr, Richards ML. Psychometric and clinimetric validity of the 20-Item Sino-Nasal Outcome Test (SNOT-20). Otolaryngol Head Neck Surg. 2002; 126(1):41–47

[5] Hopkins C, Gillett S, Slack R, Lund VJ, Browne JP. Psychometric validity of the 22-item Sinonasal Outcome Test. Clin Otolaryngol. 2009; 34(5):447–454

[6] Gil Z, Abergel A, Spektor S, et al. Quality of life following surgery for anterior skull base tumors. Arch Otolaryngol Head Neck Surg. 2003; 129(12):1303–1309

[7] Gil Z, Abergel A, Spektor S, Shabtai E, Khafif A, Fliss DM. Development of a cancer-specific anterior skull base quality-of-life questionnaire. J Neurosurg. 2004; 100(5):813–819

[8] McCoul ED, Anand VK, Schwartz TH. Improvements in site-specific quality of life 6 months after endoscopic anterior skull base surgery: a prospective study. J Neurosurg. 2012; 117(3):498–506

[9] Benninger MS, Senior BA. The development of the Rhinosinusitis Disability Index. Arch Otolaryngol Head Neck Surg. 1997; 123(11):1175–1179

[10] Suberman TA, Zanation AM, Ewend MG, Senior BA, Ebert CS, Jr. Sinonasal quality-of-life before and after endoscopic, endonasal, minimally invasive pituitary surgery. Int Forum Allergy Rhinol. 2011; 1(3):161–166

[11] Little AS, Jahnke H, Nakaji P, Milligan J, Chapple K, White WL. The anterior skull base nasal inventory (ASK nasal inventory): a clinical tool for evaluating rhinological outcomes after endonasal surgery for pituitary and cranial base lesions. Pituitary. 2012; 15(4):513–517

[12] Little AS, Kelly D, Milligan J, et al. Prospective validation of a patient-reported nasal quality-of-life tool for endonasal skull base surgery: The Anterior Skull Base Nasal Inventory-12. J Neurosurg. 2013; 119(4):1068–1074

[13] Thompson CF, Suh JD, Liu Y, Bergsneider M, Wang MB. Modifications to the endoscopic approach for anterior skull base lesions improve postoperative sinonasal symptoms. J Neurol Surg B Skull Base. 2014; 75(1):65–72

[14] Little AS, Kelly D, Milligan J, et al. Predictors of sinonasal quality of life and nasal morbidity after fully endoscopic transsphenoidal surgery. J Neurosurg. 2015; 122(6):1458–1465

[15] Little AS, Kelly DF, Milligan J, et al. Comparison of sinonasal quality of life and health status in patients undergoing microscopic and endoscopic transsphenoidal surgery for pituitary lesions: a prospective cohort study. J Neurosurg. 2015; 123(3):799–807

[16] Balaker AE, Bergsneider M, Martin NA, Wang MB. Evolution of sinonasal symptoms following endoscopic anterior skull base surgery. Skull Base. 2010; 20(4):245–251

[17] Hong SD, Nam DH, Kong DS, Kim HY, Chung SK, Dhong HJ. Endoscopic modified transseptal transsphenoidal approach for maximal preservation of sinonasal quality of life and olfaction. World Neurosurg. 2016; 87:162–169

[18] Hadad G, Bassagasteguy L, Carrau RL, et al. A novel reconstructive technique after endoscopic expanded endonasal approaches: vascular pedicle nasoseptal flap. Laryngoscope. 2006; 116(10):1882–1886

[19] Kassam AB, Prevedello DM, Carrau RL, et al. Endoscopic endonasal skull base surgery: analysis of complications in the authors' initial 800 patients. J Neurosurg. 2011; 114(6):1544–1568

[20] Jalessi M, Jahanbakhshi A, Amini E, Kamrava SK, Farhadi M. Impact of nasoseptal flap elevation on sinonasal quality of life in endoscopic endonasal approach to pituitary adenomas. Eur Arch Otorhinolaryngol. 2016; 273 (5):1199–1205

[21] Alobid I, Enseñat J, Mariño-Sánchez F, et al. Expanded endonasal approach using vascularized septal flap reconstruction for skull base tumors has a negative impact on sinonasal symptoms and quality of life. Am J Rhinol Allergy. 2013; 27(5):426–431

[22] Harvey RJ, Malek J, Winder M, et al. Sinonasal morbidity following tumour resection with and without nasoseptal flap reconstruction. Rhinology. 2015; 53(2):122–128

[23] Hanson M, Patel PM, Betz C, Olson S, Panizza B, Wallwork B. Sinonasal outcomes following endoscopic anterior skull base surgery with nasoseptal flap reconstruction: a prospective study. J Laryngol Otol. 2015; 129 Suppl 3: S41–S46

[24] Farag AA, Deal AM, McKinney KA, et al. Single-blind randomized controlled trial of surfactant vs hypertonic saline irrigation following endoscopic endonasal surgery. Int Forum Allergy Rhinol. 2013; 3(4):276–280

[25] Saleh AM, Torres KM, Murad MH, Erwin PJ, Driscoll CL. Prophylactic perioperative antibiotic use in endoscopic sinus surgery: a systematic review and meta-analysis. Otolaryngol Head Neck Surg. 2012; 146(4):533–538

[26] Hong SD, Nam DH, Seol HJ, et al. Endoscopic binostril versus transnasal transseptal microscopic pituitary surgery: sinonasal quality of life and olfactory function. Am J Rhinol Allergy. 2015; 29(3):221–225

[27] Pledger CL, Elzoghby MA, Oldfield EH, et al. Prospective comparison of sinonasal outcomes after microscopic sublabial or endoscopic endonasal transsphenoidal surgery for nonfunctioning pituitary adenomas. J Neurosurg. 2016; 125(2):323–333

[28] Zada G, Kelly DF, Cohan P, Wang C, Swerdloff R. Endonasal transsphenoidal approach for pituitary adenomas and other sellar lesions: an assessment of efficacy, safety, and patient impressions. J Neurosurg. 2003; 98(2):350–358

[29] Rotenberg BW, Saunders S, Duggal N. Olfactory outcomes after endoscopic transsphenoidal pituitary surgery. Laryngoscope. 2011; 121(8):1611–1613

[30] Griffiths CF, Cutler AR, Duong HT, et al. Avoidance of postoperative epistaxis and anosmia in endonasal endoscopic skull base surgery: a technical note. Acta Neurochir (Wien). 2014; 156(7):1393–1401

[31] Kim BY, Kang SG, Kim SW, et al. Olfactory changes after endoscopic endonasal transsphenoidal approach for skull base tumors. Laryngoscope. 2014; 124(11):2470–2475

[32] Chaaban MR, Chaudhry AL, Riley KO, Woodworth BA. Objective assessment of olfaction after transsphenoidal pituitary surgery. Am J Rhinol Allergy. 2015; 29(5):365–368

[33] Rioja E, Bernal-Sprekelsen M, Enriquez K, et al. Long-term outcomes of endoscopic endonasal approach for skull base surgery: a prospective study. Eur Arch Otorhinolaryngol. 2016; 273(7):1809–1817

[34] McCoul ED, Bedrosian JC, Akselrod O, Anand VK, Schwartz TH. Preservation of multidimensional quality of life after endoscopic pituitary adenoma resection. J Neurosurg. 2015; 123(3):813–820

[35] Zaidi HA, Awad AW, Bohl MA, et al. Comparison of outcomes between a less experienced surgeon using a fully endoscopic technique and a very experienced surgeon using a microscopic transsphenoidal technique for pituitary adenoma. J Neurosurg. 2016; 124(3):596–604

3 Pituitary Tumor Surgery: Endoscope versus Microscope— Moderator

Varun R. Kshettry and James J. Evans

Summary

Pituitary tumors are medically and surgically complex pathologies to treat. Although the endonasal approach has been described for well over 100 years, controversy exists today regarding the ideal visualization modality to work with in the crowded surgical corridor. In this chapter, we discuss the natural history of pituitary tumors, the history of pituitary tumor surgery, the traditional microscopic visualization techniques employed today, and the novel endoscopic endonasal approaches.

Keywords: endoscopic endonasal approaches, microsurgical transsphenoidal approaches, skull base surgery, pituitary tumors

3.1 Moderator

3.1.1 Pituitary Adenomas: Epidemiology, Presentation, and Management

Pituitary adenomas are neoplastic lesions arising from cells of the adenohypophysis (Fig. 3.1). Typically, they are benign, slow-growing lesions.[1,2] The incidence of pituitary adenomas is approximately 3.13 per 100,000 population.[3] Pituitary adenomas are almost twice as common in African Americans compared to whites.[3,4] The incidence increases with age, from approximately 1.56 per 100,000 from ages 15 to 24 years to approximately 6.39 per 100,000 from ages 65 to 74 years.[3] In the last two decades, the incidence appears to be increasing.[3,5,6] This phenomenon is in part due to the increased detection of incidental pituitary adenomas (incidentalomas) due to the increased sensitivity and utilization of diagnostic magnetic resonance imaging (MRI) and computed tomography (CT) for indications such as headache, sinusitis, and trauma.[2,7]

While some pituitary tumors are asymptomatic, others can result in headaches, vision loss, and hormonal disturbances resulting from either hypersecretion or pituitary insufficiency. This can result in a wide array of clinical symptoms and disorders such as fatigue, memory loss, menstrual irregularities, sexual dysfunction, infertility, urinary abnormalities, obesity, hypertension, diabetes, and heart disease.

Clinical evaluation requires thorough history and comprehensive physical examination to evaluate for both neurological deficits and systemic features of hormonal disturbances. A full baseline endocrinological evaluation includes AM (ante meridiem) serum cortisol or adrenocorticotropin hormone (ACTH) stimulation test, AM ACTH, growth hormone (GH), insulin-like growth factor-1, prolactin, thyroid-stimulating hormone, free T4, luteinizing hormone, follicle-stimulating hormone, and estradiol and/or free and total testosterone depending on gender. Additional testing may be required if a secretory pituitary adenoma is suspected. A full ophthalmologic assessment is performed including formal visual field testing with either Humphrey or Goldmann perimetry visual field test.

Management options for pituitary adenoma include observation, medical therapy in select cases, radiotherapy, and surgical resection. Nonfunctioning adenomas that do not cause neurologic deficits, visual compromise referable to the lesion, or even radiographic chiasmal compression can be observed. While natural history data are somewhat limited for pituitary adenomas, studies suggest that most macroadenomas remain stable in size over a median follow-up period of 4.3 years and approximately 10% may actually decrease in size.[2] A little more than 20% will grow during this time period. Conversely, 80% of microadenomas will remain unchanged in size, 10% will decrease in size, and 10% will increase in size.[2] Tumors that result in visual compromise or other neurologic deficits, observed lesions that demonstrate growth over time, and secretory adenomas all represent indications for treatment. In addition, lesions without

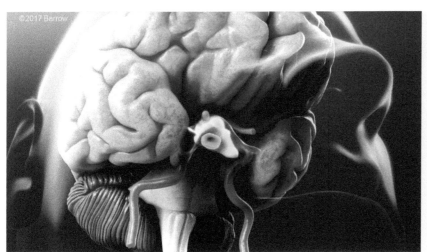

Fig. 3.1 Illustration showing the deep-seated location of the pituitary gland and sella. (Used with permission from Barrow Neurological Institute.)

visual loss but with radiographic chiasmal compression may also be considered for intervention in patients of young age. Secretory adenomas are treated not only to alleviate symptoms, but also to prolong survival in GH- and ACTH-secreting tumors.[8,9] Surgical resection is generally performed via a transnasal transsphenoidal route. While controversy exists whether a microscopic or endoscopic approach is more advantageous, understanding the evolution of these techniques can help inform the debate.

3.1.2 A Brief History of the Evolution of Transsphenoidal Surgery

The first attempted resection of a pituitary tumor using a transnasal route was credited to Hermann Schloffer in Austria in 1907.[10] In this initial operation, Schloffer used a lateral rhinotomy incision to perform a superior nasal approach to the sella. Several others including Allen Kanavel, Theodor Kocher, and Harvey Cushing began to perform transnasal operations for pituitary tumors. Cushing primarily used a sublabial approach, and by 1929, he had performed 272 transsphenoidal operations.[11,12] Simultaneously, an otolaryngologist in Vienna, Oskar Hirsch, developed and championed the endonasal transseptal transsphenoidal approach.[13] The transsphenoidal approach to the sella unfortunately did not gather widespread acceptance and was nearly abandoned. One of Cushing's students, Norman Dott, carried his experiences with Cushing to Scotland and continued to perform transsphenoidal operations, further refining the technique by way of introducing a lighted speculum.[14] However, the transsphenoidal route still did not garner significant acceptance and utilization. Gerard Guiot, a neurosurgeon from France, truly reinvigorated interest in the transsphenoidal approach and was the first to develop the use of fluoroscopy for image guidance in his transsphenoidal operations.[12] After performing over 1000 transsphenoidal operations for pituitary tumors, Guiot demonstrated with objective evidence that this approach achieved superior outcomes as compared with the transcranial route for the majority of cases.[15] One of his fellows, Jules Hardy, returned to Montreal and expanded on Guiot's revival of the transsphenoidal operation. Using the intraoperative microscope and microsurgical techniques, Hardy was able to refine the operation and describe the technique of selective adenomectomy.[16]

One of the major challenges in the history of transsphenoidal surgery was obtaining adequate illumination and visualization. Variations in headlights, lighted speculums, and microscope lights were used to increase illumination. Visualization was advanced through operative loupes, followed by the microscope. In fact, Hardy posited that he was only able to refine the transsphenoidal technique because of the improved visualization provided by the operative microscope, which enabled the surgeon to differentiate between tumor and normal gland.

One of the primary drivers of renewed interest in endoscopic transsphenoidal surgery has been related to the possibility of increased illumination through focused light delivered closer to the target, and enhanced visualization by directing the eye deep into the surgical field. The German physician Philipp Bozzini was the first to propose the concept of utilizing natural body cavities in combination with a directed light source and mirrors for internal visualization. In 1806, he revealed the first rudimentary endoscope, the *lichtleiter*, which was composed of an eyepiece, an opening for a candle, and a mirror to reflect the light through a tube.[17] In 1877, Max Nitze further advanced Bozzini's concept with the addition of a lens to produce image magnification, and he essentially developed the first cystoscope to remove urinary calculi.[18] However, it was in the 1960s that Harold Hopkins and Karl Storz revolutionized endoscopic technology by developing the rod-lens and fiberoptic light bundles, respectively.[17,19,20] Following the adoption of endoscopic technology for surgery of the paranasal sinuses, several key figures expanded its use to pure endoscope pituitary surgery.[21,22,23,24,25]

3.1.3 Microscope versus Endoscope: Why the Controversy?

When comparing alternative technologies, one must first make clear what the goals of surgery are. For pituitary surgery, there are primary neurologic, endocrinologic, rhinologic, and oncologic goals. The primary neurologic, endocrinologic, and rhinologic goals are to preserve and restore, when possible, neurologic/visual, pituitary gland, and nasal function, respectively. The oncologic goal is to safely maximize the extent of tumor resection. One must also consider patient satisfaction, with the goal to minimize operative time, blood loss, length of stay, and pain. Finally, from the perspective of the payer, one must maximize these quality end points while minimizing cost. Therefore, a thorough comparison of these technologies must factor all these important outcomes. In the forthcoming chapters, experts with unparalleled experience in both microscopic and endoscopic transsphenoidal approaches will present the advantages and disadvantages of each approach, patient selection, technical nuances, surgical outcomes, and complication avoidance.

3.1.4 Final Thoughts/Expert Recommendation

Both authors nicely elucidate the advantages and limitations for both microscopic and endoscopic technologies. The microscopic technique may be faster in the nasal approach, requires less startup equipment, provides more familiarity to the neurosurgeon not trained in endoscopy, provides 3D depth perception, and avoids dealing with blood or debris obscuring visualization. Endoscopy provides superior visualization and the ability to expand the working space with the use of angled endoscopes. Although the authors believe endoscopy provides better visualization of both the gland–tumor and tumor–diaphragma interface and is especially useful in functional microadenomas, for strictly sellar pathology, studies do not report a significant advantage of either approach when comparing experts in each of these techniques. As both authors note, endoscopy provides an indubitable benefit in pituitary adenomas with significant suprasellar or parasellar extension. Expanded endoscopic techniques have allowed safe tumor resection in these areas, which was previously not feasible with microscopic techniques. Finally, to build and refine the skills to perform these more difficult expanded approaches, the authors believe that building experience in performing endoscopic pituitary surgeries is invaluable.

References

[1] Fernández-Balsells MM, Murad MH, Barwise A, et al. Natural history of non-functioning pituitary adenomas and incidentalomas: a systematic review and metaanalysis. J Clin Endocrinol Metab. 2011; 96(4):905–912

[2] Orija IB, Weil RJ, Hamrahian AH. Pituitary incidentaloma. Best Pract Res Clin Endocrinol Metab. 2012; 26(1):47–68

[3] Gittleman H, Ostrom QT, Farah PD, et al. Descriptive epidemiology of pituitary tumors in the United States, 2004–2009. J Neurosurg. 2014; 121 (3):527–535

[4] McDowell BD, Wallace RB, Carnahan RM, Chrischilles EA, Lynch CF, Schlechte JA. Demographic differences in incidence for pituitary adenoma. Pituitary. 2011; 14(1):23–30

[5] Raappana A, Koivukangas J, Ebeling T, Pirilä T. Incidence of pituitary adenomas in Northern Finland in 1992–2007. J Clin Endocrinol Metab. 2010; 95 (9):4268–4275

[6] Nilsson B, Gustavasson-Kadaka E, Bengtsson BA, Jonsson B. Pituitary adenomas in Sweden between 1958 and 1991: incidence, survival, and mortality. J Clin Endocrinol Metab. 2000; 85(4):1420–1425

[7] Brenner DJ, Hall EJ. Computed tomography–an increasing source of radiation exposure. N Engl J Med. 2007; 357(22):2277–2284

[8] Graversen D, Vestergaard P, Stochholm K, Gravholt CH, Jørgensen JO. Mortality in Cushing's syndrome: a systematic review and meta-analysis. Eur J Intern Med. 2012; 23(3):278–282

[9] Swearingen B, Barker FG, II, Katznelson L, et al. Long-term mortality after transsphenoidal surgery and adjunctive therapy for acromegaly. J Clin Endocrinol Metab. 1998; 83(10):3419–3426

[10] Schmidt RF, Choudhry OJ, Takkellapati R, Eloy JA, Couldwell WT, Liu JK. Hermann Schloffer and the origin of transsphenoidal pituitary surgery. Neurosurg Focus. 2012; 33(2):E5

[11] Rosegay H. Cushing's legacy to transsphenoidal surgery. J Neurosurg. 1981; 54(4):448–454

[12] Patel SK, Husain Q, Eloy JA, Couldwell WT, Liu JK. Norman Dott, Gerard Guiot, and Jules Hardy: key players in the resurrection and preservation of transsphenoidal surgery. Neurosurg Focus. 2012; 33(2):E6

[13] Hirsch O. Endonasal method of removal of hypophyseal tumors with report of two successful cases. JAMA. 1910; 55:772–774

[14] Lanzino G, Laws ER, Jr. Pioneers in the development of transsphenoidal surgery: Theodor Kocher, Oskar Hirsch, and Norman Dott. J Neurosurg. 2001; 95 (6):1097–1103

[15] Hardy J. Neurosurgeon of the year. Gerard Guiot. Surg Neurol. 1979; 11(1): 1–2

[16] Hardy J, Ciric IS. Selective anterior hypophysectomy in the treatment of diabetic retinopathy. A transsphenoidal microsurgical technique. JAMA. 1968; 203(2):73–78

[17] Doglietto F, Prevedello DM, Jane JA, Jr, Han J, Laws ER, Jr. Brief history of endoscopic transsphenoidal surgery–from Philipp Bozzini to the First World Congress of Endoscopic Skull Base Surgery. Neurosurg Focus. 2005; 19(6):E3

[18] Mouton WG, Bessell JR, Maddern GJ. Looking back to the advent of modern endoscopy: 150th birthday of Maximilian Nitze. World J Surg. 1998; 22 (12):1256–1258

[19] Cockett WS, Cockett AT. The Hopkins rod-lens system and the Storz cold light illumination system. Urology. 1998; 51(5A) Suppl:1–2

[20] Linder TE, Simmen D, Stool SE. Revolutionary inventions in the 20th century. The history of endoscopy. Arch Otolaryngol Head Neck Surg. 1997; 123 (11):1161–1163

[21] Cappabianca P, Alfieri A, de Divitiis E. Endoscopic endonasal transsphenoidal approach to the sella: towards functional endoscopic pituitary surgery (FEPS). Minim Invasive Neurosurg. 1998; 41(2):66–73

[22] Carrau RL, Jho HD, Ko Y. Transnasal-transsphenoidal endoscopic surgery of the pituitary gland. Laryngoscope. 1996; 106(7):914–918

[23] Jankowski R, Auque J, Simon C, Marchal JC, Hepner H, Wayoff M. Endoscopic pituitary tumor surgery. Laryngoscope. 1992; 102(2):198–202

[24] Rodziewicz GS, Kelley RT, Kellman RM, Smith MV. Transnasal endoscopic surgery of the pituitary gland: technical note. Neurosurgery. 1996; 39 (1):189–192, discussion 192–193

[25] Sethi DS, Pillay PK. Endoscopic management of lesions of the sella turcica. J Laryngol Otol. 1995; 109(10):956–962

4 Pituitary Tumor Surgery: Endoscope versus Microscope— Microscope

Al-Wala Awad, Amol Raheja, and William T. Couldwell

Summary

The transnasal transsphenoidal approach has been an important operative corridor for the treatment of sellar lesions. For several decades, this approach had undergone numerous iterations and, when coupled with the use of the operative microscope, it has provided a safe and effect treatment tool for a wide range of pathologies. The advent of the endoscope has added yet another chapter in the saga of this evolving approach, and it has gained wide favor among newly trained neurosurgeons. In this chapter, we explore the limitations of the endoscopic technique and highlight the advantages of the traditional microscope approach. In the end, we find that both methods have important limitations and benefits depending on the specific clinical application and neither technique produces a superior clinical outcome over the other.

Keywords: endoscopic endonasal approaches, microsurgical transsphenoidal approaches, skull base surgery, pituitary tumors

4.1 Microscopic Surgical Management

4.1.1 Introduction

Sellar lesions—pituitary adenomas, Rathke's cleft cysts, meningiomas, and craniopharyngiomas—can now be conveniently accessed through a transsphenoidal corridor, although, historically, accessing the sella turcica safely was challenging. Early attempts were made to utilize various surgical approaches including the lateral subtemporal and fronto-orbital approaches.[1] As early as 1907, Schloffer reported the first successful transnasal transsphenoidal resection of a pituitary adenoma.[2] Although a landmark achievement, this procedure was marred by high mortality and morbidity and often was associated with poor cosmetic outcome.[1] This initial approach underwent numerous revisions by leading experts that were ultimately combined by Cushing in a procedure that used a submucosal dissection instead of the invasive rhinotomy.[3] Cushing's technique was very similar to the transsphenoidal technique that is in use today, but it was Hardy who first introduced the use of the operative microscope in this procedure in the operative technique adopted by modern-day neurosurgeons.[4]

After years of safe and effective use of the microscopic transsphenoidal technique to access the contents of the sella, the advent of the endoscope has led to a steady shift away from the microscope to the widely accepted endoscopic variation of the technique.[5] Each of these methods has particular advantages and disadvantages. Here, we discuss the advantages of the more traditional microscopic approach and the limitations of the endoscopic approach.

4.1.2 Case Example

History

A 58-year-old woman with hypertension and type 2 diabetes was referred to the neurosurgery clinic after presenting to her primary care physician concerned about steady and progressive growth of her hands and feet over the course of 2 years. The patient noted that her wedding ring would no longer fit around her finger, and she had had a 40-pound weight gain during this time period. She denied any changes to her vision or headaches, and she had been amenorrheic since menopause. The patient was evaluated by an endocrinologist and was found to have a serum growth hormone (GH) level of 29 ng/mL (normal, 0.05–8 ng/mL) and a serum insulinlike growth factor 1 (IGF-1) level of 1,041 ng/mL (normal, 71–290 ng/mL). Her symptoms and lab test were consistent with a diagnosis of acromegaly. Magnetic resonance imaging (MRI) of the brain with and without gadolinium contrast demonstrated a moderately large macroadenoma (16 × 18 × 22 mm) with suprasellar extension (▶ Fig. 4.1**a,b**) and evidence of chiasmatic compression. On the basis of her symptoms, GH and IGF-1 levels, and imaging findings, the patient was diagnosed with a GH-secreting pituitary adenoma, for which we recommended a microscopic transsphenoidal surgical resection.

Surgical Technique

For the microscopic removal of pituitary tumors in adult patients, the authors use modifications of the technique described by Griffith and Veerapen.[6] The patient was positioned supine with her head positioned 15 degrees to the right and fixed using a Mayfield three-point fixation device. A small abdominal incision was also surgically prepped for possible fat/fascia harvesting. In this technique, the operative microscope is used to follow the middle turbinate posteriorly and identify the rostrum of the sphenoid sinus. The Cottle elevator is used to incise the mucosa at the junction of the perpendicular plate with the rostrum of the sphenoid sinus, and the septum at this location is mobilized laterally. The rostrum of the sphenoid sinus is then removed using Takahashi and Kerrison rongeurs. The base of the sella is also identified and bone overlying this is removed using Kerrison rongeurs. Next, angled Hardy curettes are used to systematically resect the tumor in all directions. Using tactile feedback and direct visualization through the operating microscope, in this case, we ensured that the tumor had been maximally resected. A cerebrospinal fluid (CSF) leak was noted intraoperatively, and an abdominal fat fascial graft was placed at the sellar opening and within the sphenoid to seal the dural defect. Electrocautery was used to obtain hemostasis along the surrounding mucosa, the speculum was removed, and the middle turbinate was repositioned into its normal anatomic location. Nasal packings were then positioned into each nostril.

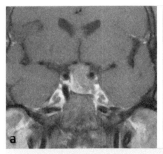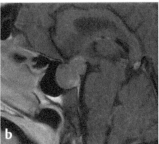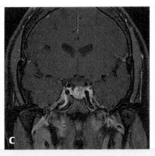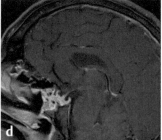

Fig. 4.1 Preoperative coronal **(a)** and sagittal **(b)** MRI of the brain with contrast demonstrating a GH-secreting pituitary macroadenoma with suprasellar extension and optic nerve compression. Coronal **(c)** and sagittal **(d)** MRI of the brain with contrast obtained 6 months postoperatively demonstrating a gross total resection of the GH-secreting pituitary macroadenoma with enhancement of the fat and fascial graft.

Postoperative Outcome

Postoperatively, the patient had an uneventful recovery. On postoperative day 1, her GH and serum IGF-1 levels were 1.93 and 710 ng/mL, respectively. On postoperative day 3, she had no evidence of any endocrinologic abnormalities or CSF rhinorrhea, and she was discharged home. One week after her procedure, she no longer needed insulin injections for management of her diabetes mellitus and was maintained on oral metformin therapy. At a 6-month follow-up examination, her serum GH level was 0.4 ng/mL and the IGF-1 level was 198 ng/mL. A repeat MRI demonstrated no evidence of residual tumor (▶ Fig. 4.1**c,d**).

4.1.3 Advantages of Microscopic Pituitary Resection

The traditional microscopic transsphenoidal resection of pituitary adenomas has been used for nearly 50 years to safely and effectively excise these suprasellar tumors.[4] Avoiding the need for specialized equipment, this approach utilizes the familiar operative microscope, a reliable and integral instrument for any experienced neurosurgeon. The absence of additional specialized equipment is an important advantage that helps limit the cost, training, and learning curve of the procedure and avoids the problem of limited endoscopic availability at some institutions. Additionally, the surgeon is operating in a familiar stance and is free to utilize both hands as in any other procedure, without the need for additional stabilizing equipment.

The anatomy surrounding the sella and cavernous sinus is a considerably complex cross-section of vascular, cranial nerve, and endocrinological elements.[7,8] Although the microscope does not offer the panoramic view offered by the endoscope, the stereoscopic vision it provides is vital to fully appreciate the three-dimensional relationships among adjacent structures. The ability to preserve the most accurate representation of the surgical anatomy may be one reason for the lower incidence of vascular injuries associated with this technique.[9] Like other authors, we find the microscope better suited for controlling intraoperative bleeding because of the larger working area and the lack of optical fogging and obstruction with blood or debris that can occur with endoscopy.[10] Similarly, the ability to independently utilize both hands without the need to coordinate with a second surgeon facilitates the precise surgical dexterity needed to contain acute situations, negotiate challenging anatomy, and avoid injuries.

In practice, the use of the endonasal microscope as described in this chapter is a rapid, efficient method to expose the sella. It tends to be quicker than an endoscopic approach, and when the retractor is placed, there is less bleeding during the tumor resection from the surrounding mucosa.

4.1.4 Disadvantages of Endoscopy

The endoscope was successfully used for transsphenoidal surgery over 50 years ago,[11] and although early adoption was slow, over the last decade its use has steadily increased as the technology and its application became more refined.[5,11] Using the endoscope effectively and safely requires additional training and has a learning curve even for those previously trained in microscopic resections.[12,13,14] The endoscope is dependent on several additional technologies to function properly, including a light source, display monitor, and specialized instrumentation, which add to the greater cost of use. This additional equipment is also a potential source of hardware failure, as the components are wired in series so a failure in one component will disable the entire apparatus. Although we have found the view provided by the endoscope to be larger and more panoramic, there are important drawbacks that should be considered.[15,16] Until recently, the endoscopic perspective has been two-dimensional, which can drastically alter perceptions of critical adjacent structures.[14,17,18] As newer three-dimensional endoscopes are introduced into the operating room, some of these issues will be resolved.

A consequence of having the viewing optic within the operative field is that it necessarily occupies an already limited space, which reduces working room for operating instruments, and there is a constant need to keep the lens clean of blood or debris, which can be challenging when controlling active bleeding. Removing the endoscope for cleaning during critical moments of the case generally requires removing existing instrumentation or risking having an instrument blindly in the field. This dilemma may hinder efforts to control acute situations. A further disadvantage is the need to use either multiple surgeons or additional equipment to stabilize the endoscope or a retractor. More mucosal dissection and removal is performed within the nasal cavity, and more bleeding is encountered with the exposure. Finally, using an endoscope and its additional hardware does not necessarily displace the need for the operative microscope, as many surgeons have reported needing to convert from endoscopic to microscopic resection when encountering difficult anatomy or intraoperative complications.[19,20]

4.1.5 Clinical Pearls and Patient Selection for Transsphenoidal Surgery

Pituitary Apoplexy

Selecting the appropriate surgical candidates for transsphenoidal surgery is of utmost importance in prevalent conditions such as pituitary adenomas. Although each patient presentation is unique, following these general principles can minimize unnecessary harm to patients. The first and simplest category of patient presentation is acute symptomatic pituitary apoplexy. This condition is generally considered a surgical emergency and can result in permanent visual loss, ophthalmoparesis, endocrine deficiencies, and even sudden loss of consciousness. The exact mechanism underlying apoplexy of the gland is unknown, but there are two leading theories. The first is that direct mechanical compression of the supplying vasculature against the diaphragm sella leads to ischemic and subsequent hemorrhagic infarct; alternatively, others theorize that the rapidly growing pituitary adenoma outgrows its blood supply, leading to acute infarct and hemorrhage.[21,22] In rare instances, apoplexy can also occur in nonneoplastic conditions, such as Sheehan's syndrome, with Rathke's cleft cysts, and severe hypotension.[23,24]

In most patients, pituitary apoplexy is easily identifiable by the acute onset of headaches, visual disturbances, or other cranial nerve deficits in the setting of acute hemorrhage on MRI or computed tomography (CT).[25] We treat the majority of these patients with emergent surgical decompression, as early intervention has been associated with improved recovery of normal cranial nerve and pituitary function.[26] Pituitary apoplexy should not be confused with incidental hemorrhage within a preexisting pituitary adenoma discovered during the work-up of chronic symptoms. Apoplexy is more common in patients with pituitary macroadenomas, and in most cases, patients are previously unaware of their underlying lesion.[25] Surgical decompression in apoplectic patients serves two main purposes—namely, rapid decompression of the sella to protect the normal physiologic function of the pituitary gland and the surrounding structures from the mass effect of the acute hemorrhage, and treatment of the underlying pituitary macroadenoma that is generally associated with this condition.

Nonfunctioning Pituitary Adenomas

In the case of nonapoplectic patients, surgical indications are dependent on tumor type but generally include clinically significant endocrinopathies, visual abnormalities, and headaches. The most common pituitary adenomas are nonfunctioning adenomas, which do not secrete any clinically significant hormone. Although they are nonsecretory, they will commonly induce endocrine abnormalities because of their mass effect on the surrounding normal hypophysis. Mass effect can also induce compression of the pituitary stalk, hindering the delivery of dopamine, which removes the physiologic inhibition of the tonic release of prolactin, a phenomenon known as the stalk effect. This ultimately results in an elevated prolactin level, although the prolactin level rarely exceeds 150 ng/mL.[27] This is an important consideration as it can lead to a misdiagnosis of a prolactinoma, which has a different treatment algorithm. Because nonfunctional adenomas do not respond to medical therapy, their mass effect can only be effectively alleviated by surgical decompression. This is an important consideration because as lesions continue to enlarge, the greater risk of cavernous invasion makes them less amenable to surgical intervention alone. In extreme cases, giant adenomas can cause acute hydrocephalus, necessitating immediate decompression and/or CSF diversion.[28,29]

Prolactin-Secreting Pituitary Adenomas

Prolactinomas are the most common secretory pituitary adenomas. Elevated serum prolactin levels can cause symptomatic galactorrhea and can have an inhibitory effect on gonadotropic hormones, leading to hypogonadism. In women, this reduction in gonadotropins predisposes to osteoporosis and anovulation, and in men it can lead to impotence.[30] Serum prolactin levels correlate with tumor size, but it is important to consider other causes of elevated prolactin levels including stalk effect, hypothyroidism, or drug effect. It is important to rule out these other causes, and if a drug effect is suspected, the offending agent should be stopped for at least 72 hours and prolactin levels retested. In the case of true prolactinomas, a serum prolactin level greater than 150 μL/L is generally considered diagnostic.[31] In some cases, patients with large adenomas may have surprisingly low serum prolactin test results due to a phenomenon known as the hook effect.[32] This false reading is due to the saturation of antibodies on the detection assay as a result of excessively high serum prolactin levels.[32] A hook effect should be suspected in patients with clinical or radiographic evidence of a large prolactinoma but lower than expected serum prolactin level. In such a scenario, serial dilutions of patient serum samples should be tested to ensure accurate test reporting.

Unlike nonsecretory adenomas, prolactinomas are highly susceptible to dopamine agonists, and medical therapy is the first-line treatment for both macro- and microadenomas.[33] Treatment with a dopamine agonist not only reduces tumor size but also helps to restore prolactin levels to normal and can correct abnormalities in gonadotropin levels.[33] Prolactin-secreting microadenomas rarely progress to larger macroadenomas; thus, the treatment goal is mainly symptom management from hypersecretion.[34] Medical management alone is generally sufficient to normalize serum prolactin, and in many instances, long-term treatment can shrink lesions to the point that they are no longer detectable on MRI.[35] Patients on medical therapy should be regularly monitored by their endocrinologist to ensure treatment response; a minority of these tumors with inadequate response or evidence of progressive lesion growth (occurs in some tumors with dopamine agonist resistance) should be treated surgically.

Patients who have macroadenomas with evidence of chiasmatic compression on MRI are at risk of permanent visual field deficits. Before initiating therapy, we obtain formal visual field testing, and patients are monitored for improvement of visual symptoms over a 4- to 6-week period. If visual symptoms do not improve in that time, we treat these patients with surgical decompression, if there is no radiographic evidence of reduction of tumor size. Patients with cystic prolactinomas are less likely to benefit from medical therapy alone, because the cystic portions of the lesion do not respond to the dopamine agonist therapy and therefore often require surgical decompression. Other indications for surgical intervention in prolactinoma tumors include intolerance to medical management, drug resistance with tumor progression, or an apoplectic event with discrete cranial nerve deficits attributable to the tumor hemorrhage. In rare instances, spontaneous CSF leak can develop after the patient starts medical management (more common in dural invasive tumors); this is an indication to surgically decompress the mass and correct the dural defect.[36]

GH-Secreting Pituitary Adenomas

GH-secreting pituitary adenomas present with symptoms of either gigantism or acromegaly, depending on the age of onset. In children and adolescents, GH excess leads to gigantism until the point of epiphyseal fusion of long bones. In adults, GH excess leads to acromegaly, which affects not only the bones of hands, feet, and face but also the soft tissues of multiple organs and can even lead to life-threatening cardiomegaly. GH-secreting pituitary adenomas are known for their rapid growth and often present as macroadenomas that commonly extended beyond the sella.[37,38] A serum GH concentration > 1 μg/L after a 75-g oral suppression test is considered diagnostic for GH excess. With elevated GH levels, it is important also to assess serum IGF-1 levels (normalized for age and sex) to rule out confounding factors that may be responsible for the elevated GH levels.

The latest guidelines for assessing surgical cure require a postoperative random GH serum level < 1 μg/L and a normal serum IGF-1 level.[39] As testing assays have increased in sensitivity, cutoffs have become more stringent, which has decreased reported success rates following surgical treatment. Even with these new standards, however, surgical resection continues to be a fast and effective way of achieving normal serum GH levels.[39,40,41] Patients with microadenomas tend to have better surgical cure rates than those with the more common macroadenoma. Macroadenomas have a higher rate of structural invasion and higher presurgical GH levels, which have been found to correlate with recurrence and failure of operative cure.[37] Endocrinological cure rates after surgical resection of microadenomas have been reported to be as high as 75 to 87%.[37,41,42] These high cure rates are likely a direct result of the lack of invasion of the surrounding sella, and in some instances, similar cure rates have been achieved in noninvasive macroadenomas.[37] Endocrinologic cure rates in patients with invasive macroadenomas are significantly lower (ranging from 42 to 50%), and adjuvant therapies are generally needed.[37,40] Although complete surgical cure cannot always be achieved, we still consider surgical treatment to be the first-line treatment option in most patients because it reduces tumor burden and rapidly treats the mass effect associated with the lesion.

Pharmacotherapy with somatostatin analogs should be used in patients with continued elevated GH or IGF-1 levels after surgical resection. Although there have been reports of the use of presurgical treatment of GH-secreting tumors with somatostatin analogs to reduce tumor size and make them more amenable to resection, the results of this practice were found to be insignificant in larger series.[43,44] In our practice, we do not commonly pretreat patients with somatostatin analogs, because,

in addition to being less effective than surgical intervention, pretreatment adds an unnecessary cost to the patient and delays surgery, which is likely to result in a more dramatic reduction in GH level.

We reserve radiation therapy for cases refractory to medical management after surgical resection. Radiotherapy and stereotactic radiosurgery can help reduce tumor size and normalize serum GH levels after surgical resection.[45,46] Unlike surgery, the effects of such treatment can take up to 5 years to appreciate, but long-term cure can ultimately be achieved.[45,47] An important consideration, however, is the risk of panhypopituitarism after radiation treatment, which has been reported in as many as 30 to 51% of patients, depending on the treatment modality.[45,46]

ACTH-Secreting Pituitary Adenomas

The hypersecretion of cortisol from the overproduction of adrenocorticotropic hormone (ACTH) leads to Cushing's disease. The classical presentation of patients with Cushing's disease consists of central obesity, "moon" facies, and proximal muscle wasting. Other common associated findings include easy bruisability, abdominal striae, buffalo hump, and increased risk of osteoporosis.[48] Most ACTH-secreting lesions are microadenomas, which have higher surgical cure rates compared with macroadenomas, in which an endocrinologic cure is rarely achieved after surgery alone.[49] Several methods have been described to diagnose the condition; the most commonly utilized is the low-dose dexamethasone suppression test, in which a dose of 1 mg of dexamethasone is given the night before 8 AM fasting serum ACTH and cortisol levels are remeasured. A serum ACTH > 140 nmol/L indicates a positive result, and surgical resection is indicated in these patients.[50] In addition to the dexamethasone suppression test, 24-hour urinary cortisol or two consecutive midnight salivary cortisol values help confirm the overproduction of cortisol.[50]

Unlike other microadenomas, ACTH-secreting pituitary microadenomas can be notoriously difficult to localize on MRI. As many as 40% of lesions are radiographically occult but have histologically been found to have ACTH overproduction.[51,52] Several strategies have been used to solve this dilemma, including intraoperative ultrasound, sinus sampling, and direct visualization through transsphenoidal surgery.[51] Preoperative bilateral inferior petrosal sinus sampling can localize the laterality of unseen adenomas in the majority but not all cases. This technique can produce remission rates and histological proof of disease at rates similar to those achieved in patients with visible radiographic lesions.[53] In our practice, we prefer to visually explore the sella if a tumor is identified on preoperative imaging. Petrosal venous sampling is always performed in patients whose MRI studies do not demonstrate a tumor. If the petrosal venous sampling does indicate a parasellar ACTH source, the gland is explored with transnasal surgery; if no tumor is found, we perform a partial hypophysectomy (as guided by the laterality of the petrosal venous sampling study) and monitor for an appropriate drop in ACTH levels postoperatively.

Overall, microadenomas contained within the sella have reported cure rates of 86% and relatively high longer-term cure rates. Only 9% of patients who achieve early (6 months postoperatively) remission have recurrence of the microadenoma within 10 years.[54] Macroadenomas have remission rates of 71% when no cavernous sinus invasion is present. When the lesion has invaded the surrounding sellar structures, remission rates can be as low as 50%.[55] Dural invasion is a challenging feature and is directly related to the tumor size. When invasion is present, it preferentially occurs in the lateral walls of the sella and can be difficult to identify on MRI.[55,56,57] For recurrent macro- and microadenomas with radiographically identifiable lesions, we will generally offer repeat surgery. As many as 50% of patients who undergo repeat surgery and adjuvant radiation or adrenolytic therapies can enter remission.[54] In cases in which invasion into the surrounding cavernous sinus is present, we refer the patient for either adjuvant radiation therapy or adrenolytic therapies.

Incidental Pituitary Adenomas

With the increased use of radiographic imaging, the identification of incidental pituitary adenomas has grown and with it the need for management strategies. We advocate for testing of baseline pituitary function at the time of the discovery to serve as historical baseline for monitoring the patient's long-term management. Importantly, screening patients in this way has led to the discovery of endocrinopathies in asymptomatic patients, especially those with macroadenomas. In these patients, surgical intervention may be required if the lesion continues to grow. Additionally, annual visual field testing is an important objective method of discovering visual deficits that are commonly unnoticed by patients with slow-growing lesions.[58] Lastly, it is important to counsel patients on the risk of pituitary apoplexy, which most often presents in the setting of an unknown pituitary adenoma.[25] In cases in which patients have no clinical symptoms of disease, we monitor with imaging every 1 to 2 years, depending on the properties of the initially discovered lesion, including proximity to cranial nerves, carotid arteries, and the surrounding cavernous sinus. Once growth rate characteristics are established, serial imaging time frames can be instituted on an individual basis. We monitor many incidentally diagnosed nonfunctioning microadenomas in this way, especially in elderly patients or those with medical comorbidities that would make them poor surgical candidates.

4.1.6 Technical Nuances and Complication Avoidance

The endonasal microsurgical approach for pituitary tumors is divided into three stages: nasal, sphenoidal, and sellar. It is of paramount importance to understand the pertinent technical nuances and methods of complication avoidance relevant to each stage of surgery.

Nasal Stage

Compared with the predominantly bi-nostril endoscopic endonasal approach, the microscopic endonasal approach as commonly used by the senior authors is essentially uni-nostril. Surgeon preference and handedness, prior transnasal surgical routes used in case of recurrent/residual tumors, and location/extension/pattern of pituitary tumor growth govern which nostril is used to access pituitary tumors. It may be easier to access the tumor in a cross-court fashion because there is often more limited visibility and access to the ipsilateral part of the tumor. To ensure an adequate working corridor and avoid tearing the nasal orifice (especially in patients with small nasal apertures), it may be helpful to make a small episiotomy incision along the inferior aspect of the mucosal ring just inside the nasal vestibule. The next step in augmenting the working space is to fracture and move the root of middle turbinate laterally. Dislocating the bony–cartilaginous junction of the nasal septum adequately and deviating the nasal septum toward the contralateral nasal cavity further facilitates the insertion of a bivalve nasal speculum. Correct placement of the speculum on either side of the keel of the vomer is pivotal because it is easy to stray toward either side if midline anatomical cues are not followed. The correct surgical trajectory to the sphenoid sinus is confirmed using visual cues and stereotactic neuronavigation so as not to enter the ethmoid sinus accidentally. At the end of the procedure, it is essential to move the middle turbinates medially to prevent blockage of the maxillary sinus opening and consequent sinusitis and to align the nasal septum back to midline to prevent sinonasal symptoms arising from an iatrogenically deviated nasal septum.

Sphenoidal Stage

The bilateral sphenoid ostia mark the upper limit of the sphenoid sinus opening. Inferiorly, the rostrum of sphenoid should be adequately removed to visualize the floor of sella turcica and clival recess to allow easy maneuverability of surgical instruments in a tight operative corridor. Careful preoperative evaluation of the septal anatomy within the sphenoid sinus ensures adequate exposure of the sellar margins. Because the paramedian bony septa may end in the carotid protuberances, care should be taken while removing them; otherwise, an overzealous pull on the septum can extend the fracture line toward the carotid artery and cause vascular injury. Care must be taken while removing the superior aspect of the sphenoid rostrum to avoid entering the anterior skull base and causing a CSF leak. Adequate sellar margin exposure can be confirmed using stereotactic neuronavigation.

Sellar Stage

To ensure wide opening of the sella turcica, the bony sellar floor is removed adequately to expose the medial aspect of the bilateral cavernous sinuses and the intercavernous communications superiorly and inferiorly. Both the anterior and the inferior walls of the sella should be opened to facilitate gravity-assisted tumor decompression and easy maneuverability of surgical instruments. The dura is incised in an X-manner, with the limbs of the incisions toward each corner. The inferior (floor) of the pituitary tumor is evacuated first by using ring curettes. Then, the bilateral aspects and finally the anterior/superior aspect of the tumor are addressed to avoid early descent of the arachnoid and suprasellar tumor. The basic principle behind surgical maneuverability for pituitary tumor removal is freeing the floor, back wall, and side gutters of the sellar cavity to allow easy delivery of the tumor. Adequacy of the tumor decompression is marked by the smooth arachnoid bulge with the absence of multiple arachnoidal folds, although one small arachnoid fold can be seen along the pituitary stalk. In the case of firm and large tumors, arachnoid descent may be facilitated by applying a careful Valsalva's maneuver or careful bilateral jugular vein compression. Visual and tactile cues to differentiate tumor from normal pituitary gland should be utilized to avoid inadvertent hypophysectomy along with tumor decompression. In cases of arachnoid breach or a large tumor resection cavity, fat/fascia should be gently packed to plug the dural defect. The sphenoid is then gently packed with fat to bolster the closure; however, overaggressive sellar packing with fat is not advisable because it can increase the mass effect on the overlying optic chiasm, leading to paradoxical decline in visual acuity after surgery. Autologous fascia is used for patching larger arachnoid tears with florid CSF leak. In some cases with extensive arachnoid opening after tumor removal, a lumbar puncture or placement of a lumbar drain may be used to divert CSF transiently to augment healing and reduce postoperative CSF leakage. For routine pituitary tumor removal, the senior author (W.T.C.) does not employ a nasoseptal flap to augment closure. In microadenomas and smaller macroadenomas, if there is no CSF leak, we do not routinely use fat or fascia in closure.[59]

4.1.7 Limitations of Microscopic Transsphenoidal Surgery

Tubular/tunnel vision through the bulky Hardy nasal speculum compared with the panoramic view provided by the endoscope is the primary limitation of microscopic transsphenoidal surgery. The incidence of nasal orifice tear is higher with the microscope than with the endoscope because of placement of the Hardy nasal speculum. Another limitation is the distance of the illumination source (the microscope) from the target tissues, which makes delineation of anatomical details more difficult than with endoscopic visualization. Lastly, the inability to visualize subfrontal, large suprasellar, and parasellar extensions of the tumor into the anterior cranial fossa, third ventricle, and cavernous sinus, respectively, limits the extent of tumor resection that can be achieved using the microscopic transsphenoidal approach. Use of the endoscope or choosing a transcranial approach first in such cases may be justified. In practice, the senior author will use a unilateral transnasal microscopic approach for lesions confined to the sella because it is more rapidly performed and requires less mucosal dissection and removal. For lesions beyond the sella, the panoramic view obtained with the endoscopic approach is extremely valuable and the endoscope is used for the procedure.

In children, the unilateral nasal exposure described here may be too small to provide an adequate working channel; in such cases, a sublabial approach with a wider bilateral nasal passage corridor will enhance exposure.

4.1.8 Review of Literature

To better understand the differences between microscopic and endoscopic transsphenoidal resection, we used RevMan (v5.3) to conduct a literature review and meta-analysis of publications during the past decade (January 2005 to December 2016) to gauge differences in endocrinologic outcomes and complications. Our reasoning for this time frame was to limit the effect of "learning curve" data associated with new techniques and rapidly changing endoscopic hardware. Using the search terms "transsphenoidal pituitary adenoma," "microscopic transsphenoidal," and "endoscopic transsphenoidal" to identify papers and finding additional resources in their reference sections, we identified 29 studies with 6,769 patient outcomes (endoscopic: $n = 3,335$; microscopic: $n = 3,434$). Studies were compared for their endocrinologic cure and complication rates (CSF leak, epistaxis, vascular injury, permanent diabetes insipidus, worsening postoperative vision, meningitis). To accurately compare studies in our meta-analysis, we only considered comparative studies that reported outcomes based on their experience of both endoscopic and microscopic transsphenoidal resection. This limited the 29 studies initially identified to 12 studies (total: $n = 1,644$; endoscopic: $n = 817$; microscopic: $n = 827$) published after January 2005. Not all studies reported relevant data for each comparison made, i.e., some studies only reported complication data but no cure data. To better estimate the comparative outcomes, a weighted analysis was used to give larger studies a greater effect on the overall calculated estimated effect.

Results

Reported cure rates after surgical resection prior to adjuvant therapies are summarized in ▶ Fig. 4.2. The estimated cure rate of the endoscopic approach was 57%, and the cure rate for the microscopic approach was 54%. Although the estimated cure rate was slightly in favor of the endoscopic approach, the overall odds ratio (1.16 [0.78–1.71]; $p = 0.46$) was statistically insignificant. The rates of the complications between the two approaches are also summarized in ▶ Table 4.1. The endoscopic approach was associated with higher rates of epistaxis when compared with microscopic transsphenoidal resections (▶ Fig. 4.3), with an odds ratio of 2.73 (range, 1.01–7.33; $p = 0.05$). There were no statistically significant differences in the rates of other complications (e.g., vascular injury, CSF leak, permanent diabetes insipidus, worsening vision, meningitis) between the two surgical approaches (▶ Fig. 4.4, ▶ Fig. 4.5, ▶ Fig. 4.6, ▶ Fig. 4.7, ▶ Fig. 4.8).

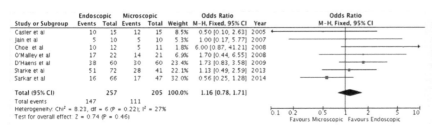

Fig. 4.2 Forest plot of comparison of overall cure rate of endoscopic and microscopic transsphenoidal pituitary adenoma resections. This difference was not statistically significant ($p = 0.46$).

Table 4.1 Summary of meta-analysis results comparing proportion of complications between endoscopic and microscopic transsphenoidal approaches

Complication	No. of patients	Odds ratio	p
Vascular injury	1,260	0.72 [0.17, 2.97]	0.64
Cerebrospinal fluid leak	1,586	1.25 [0.81, 1.94]	0.31
Epistaxis	772	2.73 [1.01, 7.33]	0.05
Permanent diabetes insipidus	1,138	0.81 [0.42, 1.56]	0.52
Worsening vision	1,578	1.19 [0.50, 2.80]	0.69
Meningitis	1,614	1.16 [0.57, 2.35]	0.68

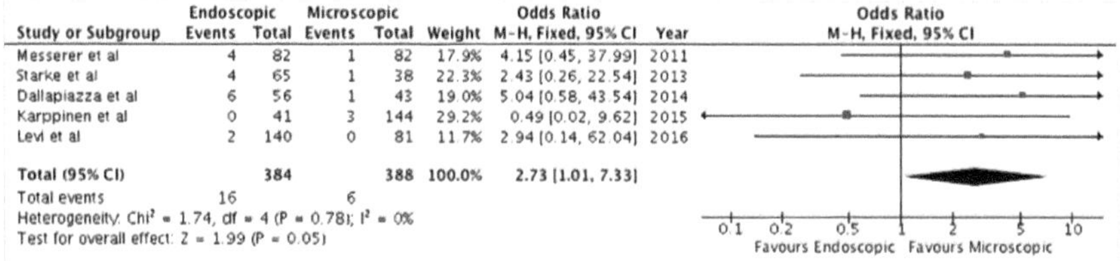

Fig. 4.3 Forest plot of comparison of incidence of epistaxis between endoscopic and microscopic (4.2 vs. 1.5%, respectively, p = 0.05) transsphenoidal approaches.

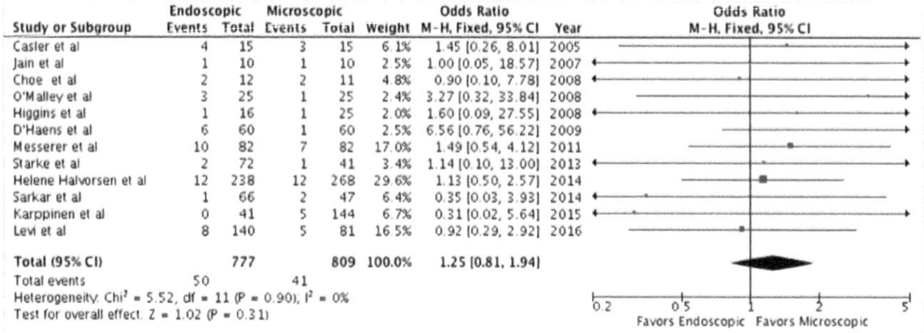

Fig. 4.4 Forest plot of comparison of incidence of CSF leak between endoscopic and microscopic (6.4 vs. 5.1%, respectively, p = 0.31) transsphenoidal approaches.

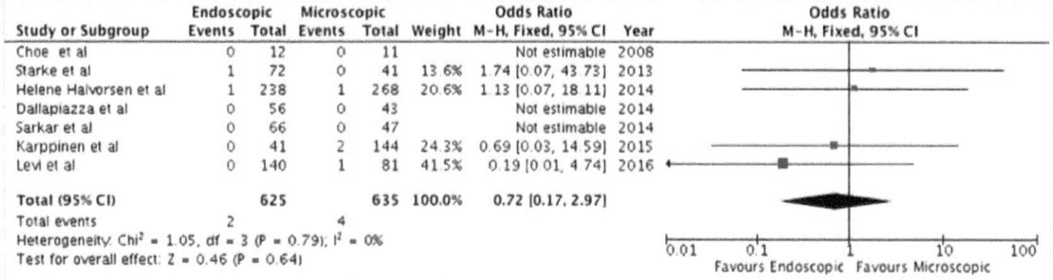

Fig. 4.5 Forest plot of comparison of incidence of vascular injuries between endoscopic and microscopic (0.4 vs. 0.6%, respectively, p = 0.64) transsphenoidal approaches.

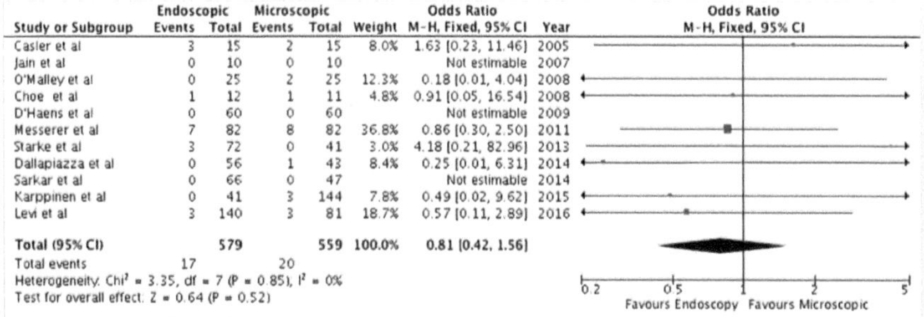

Fig. 4.6 Forest plot of comparison of incidence of permanent diabetes insipidus after endoscopic and microscopic (2.9 vs. 3.6%, respectively, p = 0.52) transsphenoidal approaches.

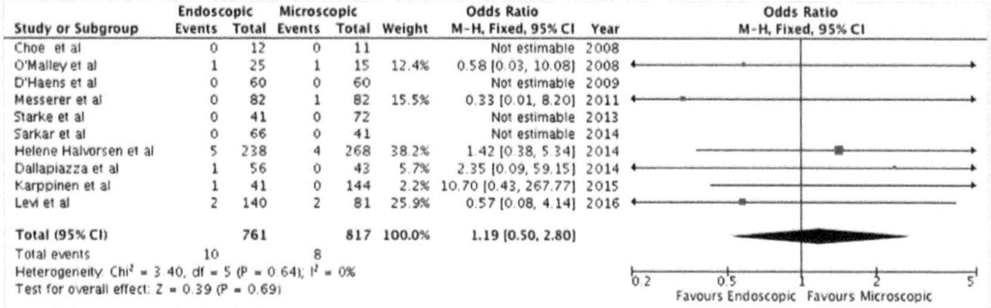

Fig. 4.7 Forest plot of comparison of incidence of worsening vision after endoscopic and microscopic (1.3 vs. 0.98%, respectively, p = 0.69) transsphenoidal approaches.

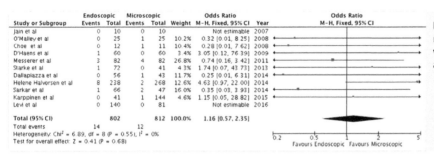

Study or Subgroup	Endoscopic Events	Total	Microscopic Events	Total	Weight	Odds Ratio M–H, Fixed, 95% CI	Year	Odds Ratio M–H, Fixed, 95% CI
Jain et al	0	10	0	10		Not estimable	2007	
O'Malley et al	0	25	1	25	10.2%	0.32 [0.01, 8.25]	2008	
Choe et al	0	12	1	11	10.4%	0.28 [0.01, 7.62]	2008	
D'Haens et al	1	60	0	60	3.4%	3.05 [0.12, 76.39]	2009	
Messerer et al	3	82	4	82	26.8%	0.74 [0.16, 3.42]	2011	
Starke et al	1	72	1	41	4.3%	1.74 [0.07, 43.73]	2013	
Dallapiazza et al	0	56	1	43	11.7%	0.25 [0.01, 6.31]	2014	
Helene Halvorsen et al	8	238	2	268	12.6%	4.63 [0.97, 22.00]	2014	
Sarkar et al	1	66	2	47	16.0%	0.35 [0.03, 3.93]	2014	
Karppinen et al	0	41	1	144	4.6%	1.15 [0.05, 28.82]	2015	
Levi et al	0	140	0	81		Not estimable	2016	
Total (95% CI)		802		812	100.0%	1.16 [0.57, 2.35]		
Total events	14		12					

Heterogeneity: Chi² = 6.89, df = 8 (P = 0.55), I² = 0%
Test for overall effect: Z = 0.41 (P = 0.68)

Favours Endoscopic   Favours Microscopic

Fig. 4.8 Forest plot of comparison of incidence of meningitis after endoscopic and microscopic (1.7 vs. 1.5%, respectively, $p = 0.68$) transsphenoidal approaches.

Discussion

The findings of our analysis were consistent with those reported by others. Ammirati et al[9] completed a robust meta-analysis of the published literature and found there was no difference in incidence of endocrinologic cure rate between the two techniques. For functional adenomas, there appears to be no cure rate or extent of resection advantage between the endoscopic and microscopic approaches. Goudakos et al[60] reached the same conclusion in their meta-analysis, although they also included studies that included nonpituitary adenoma lesions.[61]

In our review, we found the incidence of epistaxis significantly higher among endoscopic resections compared with microscopic approaches. Epistaxis can occur as early as a few hours after surgery or can be delayed up to 3 weeks postsurgery, and in larger dedicated series, the incidence has been reported to range from 0.6 to 2.5% of cases.[62,63,64] In most instances, epistaxis can be treated conservatively with nasal packing, but persistent cases may require coagulation of the sphenopalatine artery.[62,63,64] Ammirati et al[9] found a higher proportion of vascular complications among endoscopically resected lesions (1.58 vs. 0.50%, $p < 0.0001$). Injury to the parasellar carotids can cause serious sequelae, including life-threatening postoperative hematomas or the formation of pseudoaneurysms requiring further treatment.[62,63,64,65] The reasons for this are not entirely clear, but ironically, the superior visual perspective offered by the endoscope may have allowed surgeons to take on more aggressive resections, even when encasement of the carotid arteries was present or when lesions invaded the cavernous sinus. It has been hypothesized that these portions of tumors might have been left for adjuvant therapy if a microscopic resection had been used.

Unsurprisingly, results from other meta-analyses reach varying conclusions depending on the extent of their review and variables considered. Gao et al[66] analyzed comparative series dating back to the late 1990s and found that endoscopy was associated with a statistically significantly greater extent of resection and low incidence of septal perforations, reduced hospital stay, and shorter surgery. Another study by Rotenberg et al[67] during a similar time period found no difference between the extent of gross total resection between endoscopic and microscopic approaches; however, there was increased incidence of postoperative diabetes insipidus and rhinologic complications as well as greater length of stay and operative time in the microsurgical group and decreased need for lumbar drains in the endoscopic group. Although these findings were statistically significant, it is difficult to appreciate their clinical significance. For example, we believe a more clinically relevant measure would be the incidence of permanent as opposed to transient diabetes insipidus, which would have a great impact on patient outcomes. Similarly, in the study by Rotenberg et al,[67] the term *rhinologic complications* encompassed several complications, including postoperative epistaxis, sinusitis, and septal defects, although the impact of each of these on a patient's clinical course will vary.[67] More importantly, it is unlikely these complications would have achieved a statistically significant difference had they been quantified individually.

4.2 Conclusion

Only after weighing the advantages and limitations of the endoscopic and microscopic surgical approaches and considering the individual requirements related to the size, extent, and pattern of tumor growth as well as surgeon preference can the appropriate technique and instruments be chosen. In our experience, despite the advances associated with the endoscopic technique, the traditional microscopic approach is appropriate for use in many patients with the opportunity for excellent outcome. The results from previous meta-analyses are often highly sensitive to study design and inconsistent depending on the time period studied, the experience with each technique, and the extent of tumor size between groups. In our review, we demonstrate that both techniques have comparable treatment outcomes, with the added benefit of reduced rates of epistaxis with microscopic transsphenoidal approach.

References

[1] Liu JK, Das K, Weiss MH, Laws ER, Jr, Couldwell WT. The history and evolution of transsphenoidal surgery. J Neurosurg. 2001; 95(6):1083–1096

[2] Schloffer H. Erfolgreiche Operation eines Hypophysentumors auf nasalem Wege. Wien Klin Wochenschr. 1907; 20:621–624

[3] Cushing H. The Pituitary Body and Its Disorders: Clinical States Produced by Disorders of the Hypophysis Cerebri. Philadelphia, PA: JB Lippincott; 1912

[4] Hardy J. Surgery of the pituitary gland, using the trans-sphenoidal approach. Comparative study of 2 technical methods [in French]. Union Med Can. 1967; 96(6):702–712

[5] Rolston JD, Han SJ, Aghi MK. Nationwide shift from microscopic to endoscopic transsphenoidal pituitary surgery. Pituitary. 2016; 19(3):248–250

[6] Griffith HB, Veerapen R. A direct transnasal approach to the sphenoid sinus. Technical note. J Neurosurg. 1987; 66(1):140–142

[7] Doglietto F, Lauretti L, Frank G, et al. Microscopic and endoscopic extracranial approaches to the cavernous sinus: anatomic study. Neurosurgery. 2009; 64 (5) Suppl 2:413–421, discussion 421–422

[8] Solari D, Villa A, De Angelis M, Esposito F, Cavallo LM, Cappabianca P. Anatomy and surgery of the endoscopic endonasal approach to the skull base. Transl Med UniSa. 2012; 2:36–46

[9] Ammirati M, Wei L, Ciric I. Short-term outcome of endoscopic versus microscopic pituitary adenoma surgery: a systematic review and meta-analysis. J Neurol Neurosurg Psychiatry. 2013; 84(8):843–849

[10] Cho DY, Liau WR. Comparison of endonasal endoscopic surgery and sublabial microsurgery for prolactinomas. Surg Neurol. 2002; 58(6):371–375, discussion 375–376

[11] Guiot J, Rougerie J, Fourestier M, et al. Intracranial endoscopic explorations [in French]. Presse Med. 1963; 71:1225–1228

[12] Koc K, Anik I, Ozdamar D, Cabuk B, Keskin G, Ceylan S. The learning curve in endoscopic pituitary surgery and our experience. Neurosurg Rev. 2006; 29 (4):298–305, discussion 305

[13] Jho HD, Alfieri A. Endoscopic transsphenoidal pituitary surgery: various surgical techniques and recommended steps for procedural transition. Br J Neurosurg. 2000; 14(5):432–440

[14] Cappabianca P, Cavallo LM, Esposito F, de Divitiis E. Endoscopic endonasal transsphenoidal surgery: procedure, endoscopic equipment and instrumentation. Childs Nerv Syst. 2004; 20(11)(–)(12):796–801

[15] Spencer WR, Das K, Nwagu C, et al. Approaches to the sellar and parasellar region: anatomic comparison of the microscope versus endoscope. Laryngoscope. 1999; 109(5):791–794

[16] Catapano D, Sloffer CA, Frank G, Pasquini E, D'Angelo VA, Lanzino G. Comparison between the microscope and endoscope in the direct endonasal extended transsphenoidal approach: anatomical study. J Neurosurg. 2006; 104 (3):419–425

[17] Nassimizadeh A, Muzaffar SJ, Nassimizadeh M, Beech T, Ahmed SK. Three-dimensional hand-to-gland combat: the future of endoscopic surgery? J Neurol Surg Rep. 2015; 76(2):e200–e204

[18] Kari E, Oyesiku NM, Dadashev V, Wise SK. Comparison of traditional 2-dimensional endoscopic pituitary surgery with new 3-dimensional endoscopic technology: intraoperative and early postoperative factors. Int Forum Allergy Rhinol. 2012; 2(1):2–8

[19] Laws ER, Parney IF, Huang W, et al. Glioma Outcomes Investigators. Survival following surgery and prognostic factors for recently diagnosed malignant glioma: data from the Glioma Outcomes Project. J Neurosurg. 2003; 99 (3):467–473

[20] Zada G, Governale LS, Laws ER, Jr. Intraoperative conversion from endoscopic to microscopic approach for the management of sellar pathology: incidence and rationale in a contemporary series. World Neurosurg. 2010; 73(4): 334–337

[21] Cardoso ER, Peterson EW. Pituitary apoplexy: a review. Neurosurgery. 1984; 14(3):363–373

[22] Semple PL, Webb MK, de Villiers JC, Laws ER, Jr. Pituitary apoplexy. Neurosurgery. 2005; 56(1):65–72, discussion 72–73

[23] Vance ML. Hypopituitarism. N Engl J Med. 1994; 330(23):1651–1662

[24] Binning MJ, Liu JK, Gannon J, Osborn AG, Couldwell WT. Hemorrhagic and nonhemorrhagic Rathke cleft cysts mimicking pituitary apoplexy. J Neurosurg. 2008; 108(1):3–8

[25] Singh TD, Valizadeh N, Meyer FB, Atkinson JL, Erickson D, Rabinstein AA. Management and outcomes of pituitary apoplexy. J Neurosurg. 2015; 122 (6):1450–1457

[26] Bills DC, Meyer FB, Laws ER, Jr, et al. A retrospective analysis of pituitary apoplexy. Neurosurgery. 1993; 33(4):602–608, discussion 608–609

[27] Karavitaki N, Thanabalasingham G, Shore HC, et al. Do the limits of serum prolactin in disconnection hyperprolactinaemia need re-definition? A study of 226 patients with histologically verified non-functioning pituitary macroadenoma. Clin Endocrinol (Oxf). 2006; 65(4):524–529

[28] Koktekir E, Karabagli H, Ozturk K. Simultaneous transsphenoidal and transventricular endoscopic approaches for giant pituitary adenoma with hydrocephalus. J Craniofac Surg. 2015; 26(1):e39–e42

[29] Verhelst J, Berwaerts J, Abs R, Dua G, Van Den Weyngaert D, Mahler C. Obstructive hydrocephalus as complication of a giant nonfunctioning pituitary adenoma: therapeutical approach. Acta Clin Belg. 1998; 53 (1):47–52

[30] Klibanski A. Clinical practice. Prolactinomas. N Engl J Med. 2010; 362 (13):1219–1226

[31] Casanueva FF, Molitch ME, Schlechte JA, et al. Guidelines of the Pituitary Society for the diagnosis and management of prolactinomas. Clin Endocrinol (Oxf). 2006; 65(2):265–273

[32] St-Jean E, Blain F, Comtois R. High prolactin levels may be missed by immunoradiometric assay in patients with macroprolactinomas. Clin Endocrinol (Oxf). 1996; 44(3):305–309

[33] Verhelst J, Abs R, Maiter D, et al. Cabergoline in the treatment of hyperprolactinemia: a study in 455 patients. J Clin Endocrinol Metab. 1999; 84(7):2518–2522

[34] Colao A, Savastano S. Medical treatment of prolactinomas. Nat Rev Endocrinol. 2011; 7(5):267–278

[35] Cannavò S, Curtò L, Squadrito S, Almoto B, Vieni A, Trimarchi F. Cabergoline: a first-choice treatment in patients with previously untreated prolactin-secreting pituitary adenoma. J Endocrinol Invest. 1999; 22(5):354–359

[36] Lam G, Mehta V, Zada G. Spontaneous and medically induced cerebrospinal fluid leakage in the setting of pituitary adenomas: review of the literature. Neurosurg Focus. 2012; 32(6):E2

[37] Nomikos P, Buchfelder M, Fahlbusch R. The outcome of surgery in 668 patients with acromegaly using current criteria of biochemical 'cure'. Eur J Endocrinol. 2005; 152(3):379–387

[38] Sarkar S, Rajaratnam S, Chacko G, Chacko AG. Endocrinological outcomes following endoscopic and microscopic transsphenoidal surgery in 113 patients with acromegaly. Clin Neurol Neurosurg. 2014; 126:190–195

[39] Giustina A, Chanson P, Bronstein MD, et al. Acromegaly Consensus Group. A consensus on criteria for cure of acromegaly. J Clin Endocrinol Metab. 2010; 95(7):3141–3148

[40] Wang YY, Higham C, Kearney T, Davis JR, Trainer P, Gnanalingham KK. Acromegaly surgery in Manchester revisited—the impact of reducing surgeon numbers and the 2010 consensus guidelines for disease remission. Clin Endocrinol (Oxf). 2012; 76(3):399–406

[41] Jane JA, Jr, Starke RM, Elzoghby MA, et al. Endoscopic transsphenoidal surgery for acromegaly: remission using modern criteria, complications, and predictors of outcome. J Clin Endocrinol Metab. 2011; 96(9):2732–2740

[42] Starke RM, Raper DM, Payne SC, Vance ML, Oldfield EH, Jane JA, Jr. Endoscopic vs microsurgical transsphenoidal surgery for acromegaly: outcomes in a concurrent series of patients using modern criteria for remission. J Clin Endocrinol Metab. 2013; 98(8):3190–3198

[43] Jacob JJ, Bevan JS. Should all patients with acromegaly receive somatostatin analogue therapy before surgery and, if so, for how long? Clin Endocrinol (Oxf). 2014; 81(6):812–817

[44] Plöckinger U, Quabbe HJ. Presurgical octreotide treatment in acromegaly: no improvement of final growth hormone (GH) concentration and pituitary function. A long-term case-control study. Acta Neurochir (Wien). 2005; 147 (5):485–493, discussion 493

[45] Stapleton CJ, Liu CY, Weiss MH. The role of stereotactic radiosurgery in the multimodal management of growth hormone-secreting pituitary adenomas. Neurosurg Focus. 2010; 29(4):E11

[46] Abu Dabrh A, Asi N, Farah W, et al. Radiotherapy vs. radiosurgery in treating patients with acromegaly: systematic review and meta-analysis. Endocr Pract. 2015; 21(8):943–956

[47] Pollock BE, Jacob JT, Brown PD, Nippoldt TB. Radiosurgery of growth hormone-producing pituitary adenomas: factors associated with biochemical remission. J Neurosurg. 2007; 106(5):833–838

[48] Lonser RR, Nieman L, Oldfield EH. Cushing's disease: pathobiology, diagnosis, and management. J Neurosurg. 201 7; 126(2):404–417

[49] Hofmann BM, Hlavac M, Martinez R, Buchfelder M, Müller OA, Fahlbusch R. Long-term results after microsurgery for Cushing disease: experience with 426 primary operations over 35 years. J Neurosurg. 2008; 108(1):9–18

[50] Nieman LK, Biller BM, Findling JW, et al. The diagnosis of Cushing's syndrome: an Endocrine Society Clinical Practice Guideline. J Clin Endocrinol Metab. 2008; 93(5):1526–1540

[51] Jagannathan J, Sheehan JP, Jane JA, Jr. Evaluation and management of Cushing syndrome in cases of negative sellar magnetic resonance imaging. Neurosurg Focus. 2007; 23(3):E3

[52] Salenave S, Gatta B, Pecheur S, et al. Pituitary magnetic resonance imaging findings do not influence surgical outcome in adrenocorticotropin-secreting microadenomas. J Clin Endocrinol Metab. 2004; 89(7):3371–3376

[53] Jehle S, Walsh JE, Freda PU, Post KD. Selective use of bilateral inferior petrosal sinus sampling in patients with adrenocorticotropin-dependent Cushing's syndrome prior to transsphenoidal surgery. J Clin Endocrinol Metab. 2008; 93(12):4624–4632

[54] Hammer GD, Tyrrell JB, Lamborn KR, et al. Transsphenoidal microsurgery for Cushing's disease: initial outcome and long-term results. J Clin Endocrinol Metab. 2004; 89(12):6348–6357

[55] De Tommasi C, Vance ML, Okonkwo DO, Diallo A, Laws ER, Jr. Surgical management of adrenocorticotropic hormone-secreting macroadenomas: outcome and challenges in patients with Cushing's disease or Nelson's syndrome. J Neurosurg. 2005; 103(5):825–830

[56] Blevins LS, Jr, Christy JH, Khajavi M, Tindall GT. Outcomes of therapy for Cushing's disease due to adrenocorticotropin-secreting pituitary macroadenomas. J Clin Endocrinol Metab. 1998; 83(1):63–67

[57] Lonser RR, Ksendzovsky A, Wind JJ, Vortmeyer AO, Oldfield EH. Prospective evaluation of the characteristics and incidence of adenoma-associated dural invasion in Cushing disease. J Neurosurg. 2012; 116(2):272–279

[58] Reincke M, Allolio B, Saeger W, Menzel J, Winkelmann W. The 'incidentaloma' of the pituitary gland. Is neurosurgery required? JAMA. 1990; 263(20):2772–2776

[59] Couldwell WT, Kan P, Weiss MH. Simple closure following transsphenoidal surgery. Technical note. Neurosurg Focus. 2006; 20(3):E11

[60] Goudakos JK, Markou KD, Georgalas C. Endoscopic versus microscopic transsphenoidal pituitary surgery: a systematic review and meta-analysis. Clin Otolaryngol. 2011; 36(3):212–220

[61] Higgins TS, Courtemanche C, Karakla D, et al. Analysis of transnasal endoscopic versus transseptal microscopic approach for excision of pituitary tumors. Am J Rhinol. 2008; 22(6):649–652

[62] Berker M, Hazer DB, Yücel T, et al. Complications of endoscopic surgery of the pituitary adenomas: analysis of 570 patients and review of the literature. Pituitary. 2012; 15(3):288–300

[63] Mamelak AN, Carmichael J, Bonert VH, Cooper O, Melmed S. Single-surgeon fully endoscopic endonasal transsphenoidal surgery: outcomes in three-hundred consecutive cases. Pituitary. 2013; 16(3):393–401

[64] Gondim JA, Almeida JP, Albuquerque LA, et al. Endoscopic endonasal approach for pituitary adenoma: surgical complications in 301 patients. Pituitary. 2011; 14(2):174–183

[65] Halvorsen H, Ramm-Pettersen J, Josefsen R, et al. Surgical complications after transsphenoidal microscopic and endoscopic surgery for pituitary adenoma: a consecutive series of 506 procedures. Acta Neurochir (Wien). 2014; 156 (3):441–449

[66] Gao Y, Zhong C, Wang Y, et al. Endoscopic versus microscopic transsphenoidal pituitary adenoma surgery: a meta-analysis. World J Surg Oncol. 2014; 12:94

[67] Rotenberg B, Tam S, Ryu WH, Duggal N. Microscopic versus endoscopic pituitary surgery: a systematic review. Laryngoscope. 2010; 120(7):1292–1297

5 Pituitary Tumor Surgery: Endoscope versus Microscope—Endoscope

Hasan A. Zaidi and Edward R. Laws, Jr.

Summary

Fully endoscopic pituitary surgery provides enhanced illumination and magnification within a small surgical corridor. Furthermore, angled endoscopes can allow the surgeon to view out of the line of sight of traditional microsurgical approaches, in order to maximize tumor resection and improve surgical safety. In this chapter, we discuss the advantages of endoscopic approaches versus traditional microsurgical approaches for pituitary tumors.

Keywords: endoscopic endonasal approaches, microsurgical transsphenoidal approaches, skull base surgery, pituitary tumors

5.1 Endoscopic Surgical Management

5.1.1 Case Example

A 53-year-old woman physician presented to our clinic complaining of masculinization of her facial features over the last 3 to 5 years. She reports a prominent jaw line, an enlarging nose, and difficulty wearing her wedding ring, in addition to worsening obstructive sleep apnea and severe arthritis. Upon review of symptoms, the patient reports brittle nails, daily headaches, constipation, hypertension, bilateral carpal tunnel syndrome, depression, and a large tongue. She was referred to her local endocrinologist, who performed a full endocrinological panel and magnetic resonance imaging (MRI). She was noted to have an elevated insulinlike growth factor 1 (693 ng/mL), growth hormone (24.0 ng/mL), prolactin (186.6 ng/mL), and HbA1C (6.1%). On physical examination, the patient appeared to have clinical features consistent with acromegaly, including frontal bossing, deep brow furrows, enlarged nose and hands, and macroglossia. She had a history of hypertension and gastroesophageal reflux disease, well controlled with antihypertensives and proton-pump inhibitors. Gadolinium-enhanced MRI of her skull base demonstrated an avidly enhancing sellar mass invading the left cavernous sinus and encasing her left internal carotid artery (▶ Fig. 5.1). Given her abnormal clinical, laboratory, and imaging findings, we recommended surgical intervention.

An endonasal bi-nostril transsphenoidal approach was taken to resect this lesion using a 3D endoscope (VSii; Visionsense, Philadelphia, PA). After exposing the ventral skull base, the left internal carotid artery in the cavernous sinus appeared enlarged and the tumor extended widely within the sellar compartment. The face of the sella was initially opened using Kerrison punches (▶ Fig. 5.2a), and this bony opening was extended to the left petrous bone overlying the left internal carotid artery (▶ Fig. 5.2b). By placing the endoscope deep within the sphenoid sinus, we were able to safely visualize and develop a border between the dura and bone, avoiding exposure-related iatrogenic vascular injury. The endoscope was then retracted and "parked" in the sphenoid sinus, and the dura overlying the sella was inspected and opened in a cruciate fashion (▶ Fig. 5.2c,d). Within the sella, a firm white acromegalic tumor was encountered. The endoscope was advanced deeper into the endonasal corridor to the sellar face in order to closely examine the sellar contents. The high magnification and illumination afforded by the endoscope allowed us to clearly delineate a distinct border between tumor and normal pituitary gland (▶ Fig. 5.2e). Using a combination of ring curettes and blunt dissection, this border between the tumor and the normal gland was developed, and central debulking of the sellar component of the tumor was initially performed. This created working space in order to allow us to place the endoscope within the

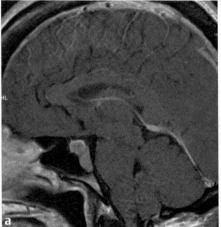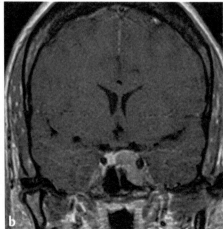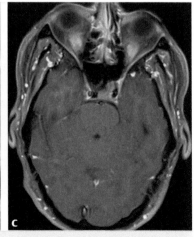

Fig. 5.1 Preoperative **(a)** sagittal, **(b)** coronal, and **(c)** axial T1-weighted gadolinium-enhanced MRI demonstrating a mass in the sella turcica and cavernous sinus circumferentially surrounding the left cavernous carotid artery and displacing the normal pituitary gland to the right.

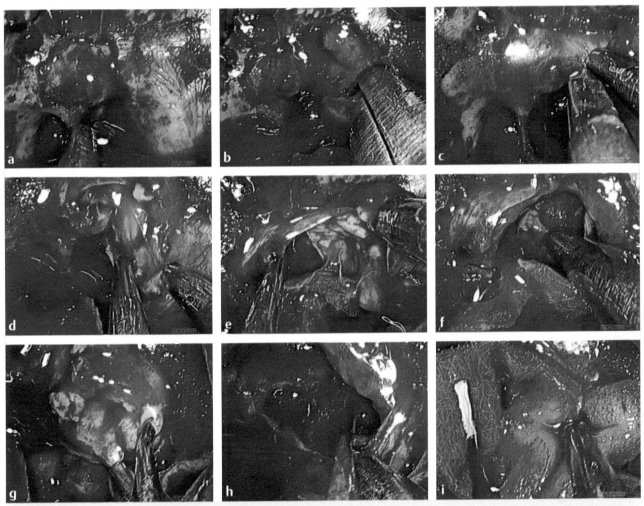

Fig. 5.2 Endoscopic endonasal transsphenoidal view of the ventral skull base **(a)** after opening of the sellar face demonstrated bony expansion of the left petrous carotid artery. **(b)** The petrous bone overlying the left carotid artery is carefully removed by directly visualizing the Kerrison rongeurs in the epidural plane. Angling of the endoscope allows the surgeon to directly visualize instruments in the surgical corridor in order to avoid iatrogenic vascular injury. **(c)** The sellar dura is carefully inspected and opened sharply using an endonasal retractable knife. **(d)** The subdural plane overlying the left carotid artery is developed and carefully opened. The endoscope is parked in the contralateral (right) nare in order to directly visualize the dural opening and to avoid instrument conflict with instruments introduced through the ipsilateral (left) nare. **(e)** The sellar contents are carefully inspected, and the endoscope is advanced close to the sellar opening to identify the border between normal pituitary gland and tumor. This border is further developed, and tumor within the sella is carefully debulked using blunt dissection. **(f)** After debulking of the sellar component of the tumor, angled endoscopes are advanced into the sella to carefully examine the medial cavernous sinus wall and to inspect the field for residual disease. Angled endoscopes allow the surgeon to visualize ventral skull base anatomy outside the direct line of sight. In this view, a small area of residual tumor is identified in the sella, which is not seen in the direct line of sight, and would have been inadvertently left behind with the microscopic transsphenoidal approach. **(g)** Tumor overlying the left petrous carotid artery is carefully removed. Improved magnification and illumination afforded by the endoscope allow the surgeon to directly visualize the ventral skull base during surgical dissection in order to avoid neurovascular injury. **(h)** The cavernous sinus is entered, and tumor is further debulked. **(i)** Gentle tamponade with thrombin-soaked Gelfoam is used to aid in hemostasis.

sella itself to examine and resect tumor within the left cavernous sinus. Using an angled 30-degree endoscope, we were able to look past the dural leaflets to examine the medial cavernous sinus wall, which demonstrated clear invasion of the tumor within this compartment (▸ Fig. 5.2**f**). The tumor was then removed in a piecemeal fashion using a combination of blunt dissection and suction. We were able to moderate the degree of carotid artery manipulation when removing tumor outside the direct line of sight from the within the cavernous sinus and prevent an iatrogenic vascular injury. After achieving hemostasis using thrombin-soaked Gelfoam, the angled endoscope was replaced with a 30-degree endoscope in order to begin debulking tumor lateral to the internal carotid artery

(▸ Fig. 5.2**g**). The contents of the cavernous sinus, including the traversing cranial nerves, were identified intercalating within the tumor (▸ Fig. 5.2**h**). After completely skeletonizing the cavernous carotid artery, we again achieved hemostasis using Gelfoam (▸ Fig. 5.2**i**). Vigorous Valsalva's maneuvers did not indicate a cerebrospinal fluid leak, and no abdominal fat graft was necessary. A MacroPore allograft plate was used to reconstruct the sellar floor and buttress the allograft packing within the sphenoid sinus.

The patient had an uncomplicated postoperative hospital course and was discharged home after 3 days. At her 1-week postoperative visit, she reported that her arthritis and coarse facial features had somewhat regressed. At her 6-week follow-up, her basal growth hormone level had dropped to 1.1 ng/mL and her prolactin had decreased to 20.2 ng/mL. On histopathological analysis, the tumor was confirmed to be a typical pituitary adenoma staining for both human growth hormone and prolactin. There was no evidence of atypical features, and immunohistochemical analysis was negative for luteinizing hormone, follicle stimulating hormone, thyroid stimulating hormone, adrenocorticotropic hormone (ACTH), and alpha subunit. The MIB-1 proliferative index was moderately elevated at 2.5%. An MRI obtained 12 weeks postoperatively demonstrated no residual disease, and she had continued biochemical evidence of remission from her acromegaly.

5.1.2 Advantages of the Endoscope and Disadvantages of the Operating Microscope

Herman Schloffer originally described his direct transnasal transsphenoidal (TNTS) approach for sellar lesions in 1907, and Harvey Cushing subsequently popularized his sublabial TNTS approach during the subsequent decades.[1] The original technique utilized a headlamp with no capacity to assist in magnification of the surgical cavity. This resulted in poor light penetration within a narrow surgical corridor and no magnification of the ventral skull base, frequently resulting in subtotal tumor resection and occasional complications. Harvey Cushing ultimately abandoned the transsphenoidal approach in favor of open transcranial approaches in 1927, largely because of inadequate visualization of critical skull base neurovascular structures, frequent recurrences, and inadequate decompression of the optic chiasm. It was not until Jules Hardy introduced the operating microscope in the 1960s, which dramatically improved illumination and intraoperative magnification, that the transsphenoidal approach was revived as a viable and even preferable method for surgical management of sellar pathology.[2] The microscope provided improved illumination and magnification, and allowed the microscopic TNTS approach to become the gold standard modality in the surgical treatment of pituitary lesions for the next 30 years. Despite these advantages over unassisted visualization techniques, the microscope still had several disadvantages. First, the microscope permitted visualization of a narrow field of vision at a set focal distance, resulting in confined views of the ventral skull base. Second, the light source remained outside the surgical cavity, frequently resulting in poor light penetration within the deep endonasal corridor. Lastly, the microscope only allowed for visualization of structures directly within the line of sight, necessitating that the surgeon had to rely on tactile feedback rather than direct visualization in order to resect residual disease around corners of deep structures.[3]

In 1997, Hae Dong Jho and Ricardo Carrau reported a series of 44 patients who underwent a fully endoscopic transsphenoidal approach for pituitary tumors.[4] Since this initial description, many pituitary centers have adopted a fully endoscopic technique due in large part to the superior visualization afforded by endoscopy. First, endoscopy provides a wider field of view, allowing the surgeon to gain a panoramic understanding of the skull base rather than a small focal point provided by the microscope. Second, angled endoscopes can allow the surgeon to look around corners, outside the direct line of sight. This helps visualize areas of the ventral skull base otherwise obstructed by bone, dura, mucosa, etc. It also allows the surgeon to rely on direct visualization rather than tactile feedback when manipulating critical neurovascular structures of the ventral skull base. Third, the endoscope provides greater magnification of sellar components, allowing one to better differentiate normal gland from adenoma. Finally, the endoscope places the light source directly within the endonasal cavity, allowing for greater light penetration and illumination of ventral skull base structures. Several groups have suggested that the endoscope may allow for safer and more effective resection of sellar pathology. We recently performed a direct comparison of 135 patients harboring pituitary pathology who underwent either an endoscopic or microscopic approach by two different surgeons during a contemporaneous period at the Barrow Neurological Institute.[5] We found that the endoscopic technique allowed for greater pituitary gland preservation and lower complication rates versus traditional microscopic visualization techniques.

Advancements in endoscopic technology in the last two decades have served to improve patient outcomes.[6] In 1998, Paolo Cappabianca and Enrico de Divitiis presented various problems associated with the original endoscopic approaches as compared to traditional microscopic approaches.[1,7] This included potential instrument conflict between the endoscope and dissection tools within a narrow endonasal corridor, increased risk of damage to nasal structures by introduction of instruments into the nostril during the sphenoid and sellar phases of the operation, and loss of stereoscopic visualization utilizing 2D endoscopes. To address these problems, several groups have since developed new instruments specifically dedicated to the endoscopic technique. This includes bent handle instruments to enable simultaneous work with two instruments in the operating field, interchangeable tips for different functions, and the elimination of the previous bayonetlike shape. Furthermore, our group has utilized a novel 3D endoscope to provide stereoscopic visualization in more than 600 cases,[8,9] allowing for improved surgical dexterity by affording the surgeon with depth perception when manipulating tissue and maneuvering the endoscope within the endonasal corridor. Finally, improvements in microchip technology have recently allowed for the development of malleable 3D endoscopes, which can reduce the degree of instrument conflict during surgical dissection of ventral skull base lesions.[9]

5.1.3 Patient Selection and Complication Avoidance

As our collective experience using the endoscope has improved over time, a variety of skull base lesions can now effectively be treated using an endoscopic endonasal approach. Our group recently reviewed our experience using the endoscope for a wide variety of anterior skull base pathologies.[10] The improved panoramic visualization and angled viewing provided by endoscopes can be used in combination with extended and expanded endonasal techniques to treat lesions previously deemed too dangerous for endonasal resection. Patient selection for endoscopic endonasal approaches has expanded drastically not only to include pathologies of the pituitary gland and sellar region (e.g., craniopharyngiomas, Rathke's cleft cysts, arachnoid cysts, pituicytomas) but also for the resection of tumors that have traditionally been treated via more invasive transcranial approaches (e.g., meningiomas, craniopharyngiomas, germinomas).

For the majority of intrasellar microadenomas, the endoscopic view is comparable to the view provided by the microscope. Despite its narrow field of view, the microscope has proven to be safe and effective visualization technique for resection of small intrasellar lesions. Jules Hardy originally described the use of the microscope in transsphenoidal approach in 1962 for the selective removal of an ACTH-secreting microadenoma.[2] In situations with small intrasellar lesions, a panoramic endoscopic view does not prove to be a major advantage for many such cases. One may argue that the higher magnification provided by the endoscope may help novice surgeons to better identify the border between tumor and pituitary gland, allowing for higher rates of normal pituitary gland preservation. Zaidi et al demonstrated that the endoscope may allow for greater preservation of the posterior pituitary gland function, but outcomes were similar for anterior pituitary gland preservation between the two techniques.[5] In our experience, the advantages of the endoscopic technique are most profound for pituitary macroadenomas with extension into the suprasellar or parasellar compartments. In these situations, the panoramic visualization provided by the endoscope allows for safer and more effective resection of these lesions. One can directly visualize the position of the petrous carotid arteries and optic nerve, and avoid iatrogenic injury to these structures. Angled endoscopes help visualize neurovascular structures outside the direct line of sight, allowing surgeons in training to rely on direct visualization rather than experience or tactile feedback to resect residual disease. As demonstrated in our case example, the angled endoscope allowed us to resect tumor located within the cavernous sinus using direct visualization, a feat impossible using the microscope. For these reasons, we recommend that the endoscope be used when removing pituitary macroadenomas with extensive cavernous, parasellar or suprasellar extension in order to avoid complications and to provide a more complete extent of tumor resection.

5.1.4 Conclusion

Technological advances in visualization techniques have largely been responsible for the adoption of the transsphenoidal approach by the greater neurosurgical community.[11] Originally abandoned by Harvey Cushing, who relied solely on headlamps to illuminate the endonasal corridor, the transsphenoidal technique was revived with the advent of operating microscopes, which improved visualization of the ventral skull base. Endoscopes are the latest iteration based on the concept of improving magnification and increasing illumination within a deep and narrow endonasal corridor. The advent of three-dimensional endoscopes as well as malleable endoscopes may serve to incrementally improve the efficacy of transsphenoidal surgical approaches for pituitary adenomas and other types of anterior skull base pathology.

References

[1] Wang AJ, Zaidi HA, Laws ED, Jr. History of endonasal skull base surgery. J Neurosurg Sci. 2016; 60(4):441–453

[2] Hardy J. Transsphenoidal hypophysectomy. 1971. J Neurosurg. 2007; 107(2):458–471

[3] Zaidi HA, De Los Reyes K, Barkhoudarian G, et al. The utility of high-resolution intraoperative MRI in endoscopic transsphenoidal surgery for pituitary macroadenomas: early experience in the Advanced Multimodality Image Guided Operating suite. Neurosurg Focus. 2016; 40(3):E18

[4] Jho HD, Carrau RL. Endoscopic endonasal transsphenoidal surgery: experience with 50 patients. J Neurosurg. 1997; 87(1):44–51

[5] Zaidi HA, Awad AW, Bohl MA, et al. Comparison of outcomes between a less experienced surgeon using a fully endoscopic technique and a very experienced surgeon using a microscopic transsphenoidal technique for pituitary adenoma. J Neurosurg. 2016; 124(3):596–604

[6] Dallapiazza RF, Grober Y, Starke RM, Laws ER, Jr, Jane JA, Jr. Long-term results of endonasal endoscopic transsphenoidal resection of nonfunctioning pituitary macroadenomas. Neurosurgery. 2015; 76(1):42–52, discussion 52–53

[7] Doglietto F, Prevedello DM, Jane JA, Jr, Han J, Laws ER, Jr. Brief history of endoscopic transsphenoidal surgery–from Philipp Bozzini to the First World Congress of Endoscopic Skull Base Surgery. Neurosurg Focus. 2005; 19(6):E3

[8] Barkhoudarian G, Del Carmen Becerra Romero A, Laws ER. Evaluation of the 3-dimensional endoscope in transsphenoidal surgery. Neurosurgery. 2013; 73(1) Suppl Operative:ons74–ons78, discussion ons78–ons79

[9] Zaidi HA, Zehri A, Smith TR, Nakaji P, Laws ER, Jr. Efficacy of three-dimensional endoscopy for ventral skull base pathology: a systematic review of the literature. World Neurosurg. 2016; 86:419–431

[10] Cote DJ, Wiemann R, Smith TR, Dunn IF, Al-Mefty O, Laws ER. The expanding spectrum of disease treated by the transnasal, transsphenoidal microscopic and endoscopic anterior skull base approach: a single-center experience 2008–2015. World Neurosurg. 2015; 84(4):899–905

[11] de Divitiis E, Laws ER, Giani U, Iuliano SL, de Divitiis O, Apuzzo ML. The current status of endoscopy in transsphenoidal surgery: an international survey. World Neurosurg. 2015; 83(4):447–454

6 Endoscopic Approach to the Infratemporal Fossa

Philip V. Theodosopoulos

Summary

The infratemporal fossa is a complex region within the head surrounded by important neurovascular structures. Traditional open microsurgical approaches have demonstrated efficacy in resection of tumors of this region, but carry a significant risk for approach-related morbidity. For certain lesions located in this region, endoscopic endonasal approaches are a viable option and can reduce the risk of approach-related morbidity. We describe in this chapter our treatment algorithm and surgical management strategies for tumors located within the maxillary sinus.

Keywords: endoscopic endonasal approaches, endoscopic transmaxillary approaches, combined open microsurgical approaches, skull base surgery

6.1 Introduction

The infratemporal fossa is a retromaxillary space that borders the middle skull base, where neoplastic lesions can arise primarily or secondarily extending from the nasopharyngeal space, the orbital space, and the intracranial compartment. The borders of the infratemporal fossa are defined medially as the parapharyngeal space and pterygoid buttress, laterally the mandible, anteriorly the posterior wall of the maxillary sinus, and posteriorly the posterior parapharyngeal space. The contents of the fossa include the medial and lateral pterygoid muscles, the internal maxillary artery, and the mandibular division of the trigeminal nerve.[1,2]

There are a variety of tumors that can involve the infratemporal fossa. Schwannomas of the trigeminal nerve and meningiomas of the middle fossa extending through the foramen ovale that is often widened are the most common benign tumors encountered. Malignant tumor can also involve the infratemporal fossa. Lymphoma as well as nasopharyngeal carcinomas can also be found in the area. Finally, pseudotumor, a poorly understood nonneoplastic condition that mimics a tumor, is found in the area as well.

Access into the infratemporal fossa is often required for diagnostic biopsy of a lesion as well as surgical resection. It should be said that given the complex relationships of some of the infiltrative lesions that involve this space as well as the proximity posteriorly to the internal carotid artery (ICA) and the jugular vein that course through the posterior parapharyngeal space, complete resection of any other than the well-encapsulated lesions such as the schwannomas involving the trigeminal nerve is often not possible. The specific goal of treatment should be carefully considered. This is especially important in this difficult-to-access region of the skull base; as for purely tissue diagnosis purposes, computed tomography (CT)-guided biopsy is a good alternative.

Multiple surgical approach corridors have been described for access into the infratemporal fossa (▶ Fig. 6.1a). Approaches described include anterolaterally through an orbitozygomatic craniotomy, laterally through a zygomatic osteotomy and drilling of the floor of the middle fossa, posterolaterally through a Fisch infratemporal type C, or anteriorly through a mandibulotomy (▶ Fig. 6.1b,c). Given the depth of the infratemporal fossa, open approaches involve significant soft tissue and bony removal that confer a certain amount of morbidity, particularly with respect to mastication, facial nerve function, and trigeminal sensation.[3,4,5,6,7,8,9] Several publications have studied the endoscopic approach to the pterygopalatine fossa.[10,11,12,13,14,15,16,17] Our group first described the endoscopic approach to the infratemporal fossa as a minimally invasive alternative to the open approaches in an attempt to minimize the approach-associated morbidity.[2] Since that initial description, multiple other studies have confirmed the effectiveness and safety of the corridor and have expanded on the indications and limitations of the use of endoscopy in approaching lesions in the infratemporal fossa.[18,19,20,21,22,23,24,25,26,27,28,29,30,31,32,33,34,35]

6.2 Endoscopic Technique

The endoscopic approach to the infratemporal fossa can be achieved purely transnasally or in combination with a Caldwell Luc incision. In our experience, anything short of an anteriorly placed lesion within the infratemporal fossa is difficult to safely and comprehensively expose through a pure transnasal approach. The majority of lesions in the area are much better approached through the combination of a transnasal and transmaxillary corridors.

The middle turbinate is frequently removed completely to allow for a wide maxillary antrostomy. Following wide exposure into the maxillary sinus, the posterior wall of the sinus is carefully removed with Kerrison punches. The pterygopalatine ganglion is exposed. The distal branches of the internal maxillary artery are identified within the adipose tissue that fills much of the anterior infratemporal fossa, and the sphenopalatine artery is coagulated and divided. Dissection is carried further back and the medial and lateral pterygoid muscles are identified and divided. Further posterior dissection allows for exposure of the descending mandibular (V3) branch of the trigeminal nerve along the posteromedial aspect of the infratemporal fossa. Dissection here needs to proceed cautiously as the most superior part of the cervical ICA lies immediately behind the trigeminal nerve along the posterior parapharyngeal space. The exposure of the trigeminal nerve often requires drilling of the medial and lateral pterygoid plates along which the medial and lateral pterygoid muscles attach, as, depending on the angle of approach to the nerve, the pterygoid bone can overlay the majority of the nerve as it comes out of the foramen ovale. A purely endonasal approach allows for an exposure whose medial limit is the lateral pterygoid plate, often inadequate for safe exposure of the trigeminal nerve. The Caldwell Luc corridor allows for more medial visualization as well as enough room for drilling of the pterygoid plates.[30,34,36]

For lesions that are predominantly or exclusively extracranial and by default extradural, reconstruction of the skull base is not

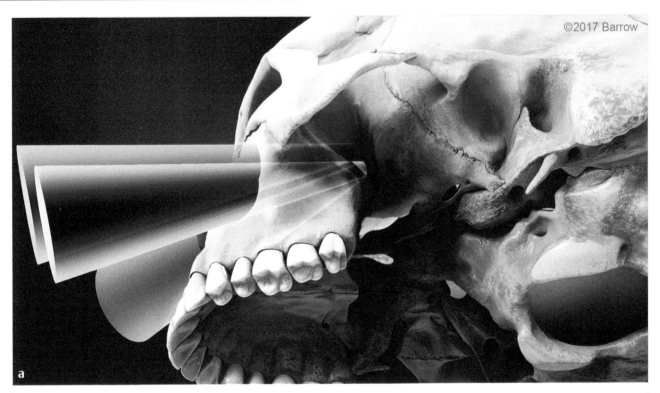

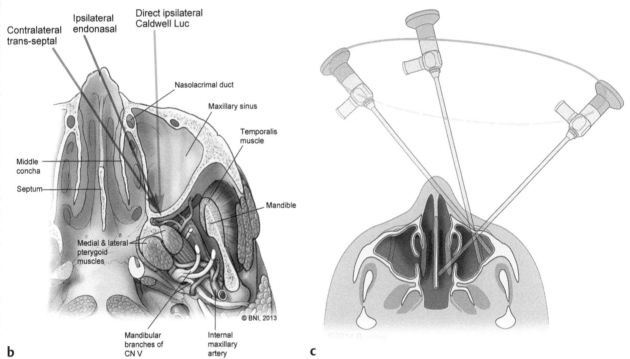

Fig. 6.1 (a) Illustration demonstrating access to the infratemporal fossa and (b) the variety of surgical approaches described to this region. (c) Surgical freedom of endoscopic approaches to the infratemporal fossa can be limited in certain cases. (Used with permission from Barrow Neurological Institute, Phoenix, AZ.)

necessary. However, for lesions that have an intracranial component, obliteration of the "dead space" is crucial and can be achieved with a multilayer technique utilizing fat, muscle, and dural substitute. Pedicled flaps can be used, although, in our experience, they are rarely necessary. It should be noted that any infratemporal fossa lesion with significant extension into

the intracranial space is optimally approached through an open approach or through a staged strategy utilizing a combination of an endoscopic and an open approach. The angle of approach even with the utilization of the Caldwell Luc incision and the depth of the space do not allow for adequate visualization superiorly, the main direction where intracranial extent of lesions involving the space often exhibits (▶ Fig. 6.1c). For such large lesions, an open approach is often the one we would start with, allowing for decompression of the temporal lobe, reconstructing the bottom of the skull base with some artificial dural substitute that is then used as a guide for the depth of exposure during the second endoscopic stage.

6.3 Case Example

An example case can be seen in ▶ Fig. 6.2. A 33-year-old woman presented with tingling and numbness along the V2 distribution of the left trigeminal nerve. Radiographic diagnosis revealed a 3-cm, uniformly enhancing lesion along the infratemporal fossa with the superior extent limited to the area of the foramen ovale. A purely endoscopic approach was utilized and the tumor was resected in a near-total fashion. Intraoperative pictures illustrate the degree of exposure (▶ Fig. 6.3). Histopathological evaluation confirmed this lesion was a schwannoma. The patient recovered well and was discharged home the second postoperative day. Facial sensation postoperatively was somewhat diminished. The only morbidity of the procedure was a first-degree burn of the patient's upper lip from the ultrasonic aspirator that was used to debulk the tumor. This resolved well with local skin care within a couple of weeks.

Other than morbidity associated with the trigeminal nerve, we have observed a risk of denervation of the upper incisors when resecting the bone along the floor of the maxilla. This can lead to significant dental problems and should be avoided. Lesions that are centered or that extend significantly below the floor of the maxilla along the lower aspect of the infratemporal fossa should better be approached through an open corridor. Vascular control of the internal maxillary vessels is of paramount importance during the exposure. Lesions of the area are often fed by internal maxillary branches, which can be significantly enlarged. Direct coagulation is not often adequate and we often opt for utilizing vessel clips followed by coagulation and division in order to ensure durable occlusion. Endovascular obliteration of the feeding arteries is rarely necessary but can also be employed. One should always consider that, following resection of even extradural lesions in the area, postoperative hemorrhage can lead to a symptomatic epidural hematoma by compression along the course of the middle meningeal artery and the foramen ovale.

Injury to the high cervical ICA is a concern when operating in this area. The posterior parapharyngeal space that houses the ICA and internal jugular vein lies posteriorly immediately adjacent to the infratemporal fossa. Extreme caution should be taken when dissecting along the posterior margin of most benign tumors, and in the case of malignancies, dissection along the posterior aspect should be avoided altogether given the potential for invasion into the vessel. Local proximal or distal control of the ICA is not possible, and in cases where any

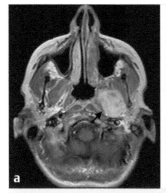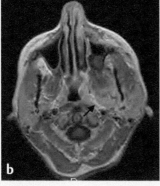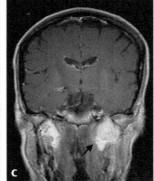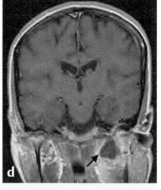

Fig. 6.2 Illustrative case of a 33-year-old woman with a left trigeminal schwannoma. Preoperative **(a,c)** and postoperative **(b,d)** contrast-enhanced T1-weighted images.

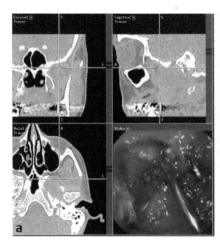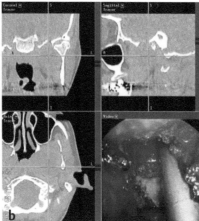

Fig. 6.3 (a,b) Intraoperative images with navigation localization indicating the degree of exposure.

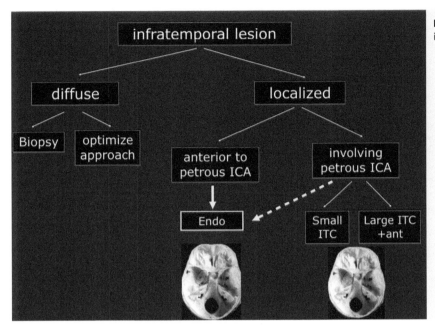

Fig. 6.4 Algorithm for endoscopic treatment of infratemporal lesions.

concern of tumor involvement in the vessel is suspected, ICA exposure in the neck is prudent. In our estimation, however, there is no infratemporal fossa lesion for which even inadvertent sacrifice of the ICA is warranted.

6.4 Conclusion

In conclusion, the endoscopic approach to the infratemporal fossa is effective and less invasive for many benign and malignant lesions that are found in the area. The variety of lesions that involve the area and their extent make direct indications and limitations difficult to define; however, our thinking in treating such lesions has evolved and is best described in the algorithm presented in ▶ Fig. 6.4. Appropriate choice of surgical approach depends on the careful evaluation of the preoperative imaging and determination of the extent of the lesion, particular with respect to the ICA and the skull base. Although an effective approach on its own, combination with an open approach can also be considered in cases of extensive tumors that transgress the skull base in a symmetric fashion.

References

[1] Sennaroglu L, Slattery WH, III. Petrous anatomy for middle fossa approach. Laryngoscope. 2003; 113(2):332–342

[2] Theodosopoulos PV, Guthikonda B, Brescia A, Keller JT, Zimmer LA. Endoscopic approach to the infratemporal fossa: anatomic study. Neurosurgery. 2010; 66(1):196–202, discussion 202–203

[3] Crockett DJ. Surgical approach to the back of the maxilla. Br J Surg. 1963; 50:819–821

[4] Fisch U. Infratemporal fossa approach for glomus tumors of the temporal bone. Ann Otol Rhinol Laryngol. 1982; 91(5, Pt 1):474–479

[5] Fisch U. Infratemporal fossa approach for lesions in the temporal bone and base of the skull. Adv Otorhinolaryngol. 1984; 34:254–266

[6] Fisch U, Fagan P, Valavanis A. The infratemporal fossa approach for the lateral skull base. Otolaryngol Clin North Am. 1984; 17(3):513–552

[7] Fukushima T, Day JD, Hirahara K. Extradural total petrous apex resection with trigeminal translocation for improved exposure of the posterior cavernous sinus and petroclival region. Skull Base Surg. 1996; 6(2):95–103

[8] Sekhar LN, Schramm VL, Jr, Jones NF. Subtemporal-preauricular infratemporal fossa approach to large lateral and posterior cranial base neoplasms. J Neurosurg. 1987; 67(4):488–499

[9] Zhang M, Garvis W, Linder T, Fisch U. Update on the infratemporal fossa approaches to nasopharyngeal angiofibroma. Laryngoscope. 1998; 108(11, Pt 1):1717–1723

[10] Har-El G. Combined endoscopic transmaxillary-transnasal approach to the pterygoid region, lateral sphenoid sinus, and retrobulbar orbit. Ann Otol Rhinol Laryngol. 2005; 114(6):439–442

[11] Hegazy HM, Carrau RL, Snyderman CH, Kassam A, Zweig J. Transnasal endoscopic repair of cerebrospinal fluid rhinorrhea: a meta-analysis. Laryngoscope. 2000; 110(7):1166–1172

[12] Klossek JM, Ferrie JC, Goujon JM, Fontanel JP. Endoscopic approach of the pterygopalatine fossa: report of one case. Rhinology. 1994; 32(4):208–210

[13] Ong BC, Gore PA, Donnellan MB, Kertesz T, Teo C. Endoscopic sublabial transmaxillary approach to the rostral middle fossa. Neurosurgery. 2008; 62(3) Suppl 1:30–36, discussion 37

[14] Pasquini E, Sciarretta V, Farneti G, Ippolito A, Mazzatenta D, Frank G. Endoscopic endonasal approach for the treatment of benign schwannoma of the sinonasal tract and pterygopalatine fossa. Am J Rhinol. 2002; 16(2):113–118

[15] Pasquini E, Sciarretta V, Farneti G, Mazzatenta D, Modugno GC, Frank G. Endoscopic treatment of encephaloceles of the lateral wall of the sphenoid sinus. Minim Invasive Neurosurg. 2004; 47(4):209–213

[16] Schwartz TH, Fraser JF, Brown S, Tabaee A, Kacker A, Anand VK. Endoscopic cranial base surgery: classification of operative approaches. Neurosurgery. 2008; 62(5):991–1002, discussion 1002–1005

[17] DelGaudio JM. Endoscopic transnasal approach to the pterygopalatine fossa. Arch Otolaryngol Head Neck Surg. 2003; 129(4):441–446

[18] Abuzayed B, Tanriover N, Canbaz B, Akar Z, Gazioglu N. Lateral sublabial endoscopic approach to foramen ovale: a novel endoscopic technique to access infratemporal fossa. J Craniofac Surg. 2010; 21(4):1241–1245

[19] Battaglia P, Turri-Zanoni M, Dallan I, et al. Endoscopic endonasal transpterygoid transmaxillary approach to the infratemporal and upper parapharyngeal tumors. Otolaryngol Head Neck Surg. 2014; 150(4):696–702

[20] Chan JY, Li RJ, Lim M, Hinojosa AQ, Boahene KD. Endoscopic transvestibular paramandibular exploration of the infratemporal fossa and parapharyngeal space: a minimally invasive approach to the middle cranial base. Laryngoscope. 2011; 121(10):2075–2080

[21] Dallan I, Fiacchini G, Turri-Zanoni M, et al. Endoscopic-assisted transoral-transpharyngeal approach to parapharyngeal space and infratemporal fossa: focus on feasibility and lessons learned. Eur Arch Otorhinolaryngol. 2016; 273(11):3965–3972

[22] Dallan I, Lenzi R, Bignami M, et al. Endoscopic transnasal anatomy of the infratemporal fossa and upper parapharyngeal regions: correlations with traditional perspectives and surgical implications. Minim Invasive Neurosurg. 2010; 53(5–6):261–269

[23] Devaiah AK, Reiersen D, Hoagland T. Evaluating endoscopic and endoscopic-assisted access to the infratemporal fossa: a novel method for assessment and comparison of approaches. Laryngoscope. 2013; 123(7):1575–1582

[24] Fahmy CE, Carrau R, Kirsch C, et al. Volumetric analysis of endoscopic and traditional surgical approaches to the infratemporal fossa. Laryngoscope. 2014; 124(5):1090–1096

[25] Falcon RT, Rivera-Serrano CM, Miranda JF, et al. Endoscopic endonasal dissection of the infratemporal fossa: Anatomic relationships and importance of eustachian tube in the endoscopic skull base surgery. Laryngoscope. 2011; 121 (1):31–41

[26] Hartnick CJ, Lacy PD, Myer CM, III. Endoscopic evaluation of the infratemporal fossa. Laryngoscope. 2001; 111(2):353–355

[27] Hartnick CJ, Myseros JS, Myer CM, III. Endoscopic access to the infratemporal fossa and skull base: a cadaveric study. Arch Otolaryngol Head Neck Surg. 2001; 127(11):1325–1327

[28] Hofstetter CP, Singh A, Anand VK, Kacker A, Schwartz TH. The endoscopic, endonasal, transmaxillary transpterygoid approach to the pterygopalatine fossa, infratemporal fossa, petrous apex, and the Meckel cave. J Neurosurg. 2010; 113(5):967–974

[29] Jurado-Ramos A, Ropero Romero F, Cantillo Baños E, Salas Molina J. Minimally invasive endoscopic techniques for treating large, benign processes of the nose, paranasal sinus, and pterygomaxillary and infratemporal fossae: solitary fibrous tumour. J Laryngol Otol. 2009; 123(4):457–461

[30] Prosser JD, Figueroa R, Carrau RI, Ong YK, Solares CA. Quantitative analysis of endoscopic endonasal approaches to the infratemporal fossa. Laryngoscope. 2011; 121(8):1601–1605

[31] Sun XC, Li H, Liu ZF, et al. Endoscopic assisted sublabial and buccolabial incision approach for juvenile nasopharyngeal angiofibroma with extensive infratemporal fossa extension. Int J Pediatr Otorhinolaryngol. 2012; 76 (10):1501–1506

[32] Taylor RJ, Patel MR, Wheless SA, et al. Endoscopic endonasal approaches to infratemporal fossa tumors: a classification system and case series. Laryngoscope. 2014; 124(11):2443–2450

[33] Xu F, Sun X, Hu L, et al. Endoscopic surgical treatment of neurogenic tumor in pterygopalatine and infratemporal fossae via extended medial maxillectomy. Acta Otolaryngol. 2011; 131(2):161–165

[34] Youssef A, Carrau RL, Tantawy A, et al. Endoscopic versus open approach to the infratemporal fossa: a cadaver study. J Neurol Surg B Skull Base. 2015; 76 (5):358–364

[35] Zhou B, Huang Q, Shen PH, et al. The intranasal endoscopic removal of schwannoma of the pterygopalatine and infratemporal fossae via the prelacrimal recess approach. J Neurosurg. 2016; 124(4):1068–1073

[36] Upadhyay S, Dolci RL, Buohliqah L, et al. Effect of incremental endoscopic maxillectomy on surgical exposure of the pterygopalatine and infratemporal fossae. J Neurol Surg B Skull Base. 2016; 77(1):66–74

7 Anterior Skull Base Tumors—Microscope

Margaret Carmody, Justin Singer, Nicholas C. Bambakidis

Summary

Anterior skull base lesions have been traditionally treated using microsurgical principles established in the 1970s. With the advent of endoscopic endonasal approaches, a variety of novel techniques and tools have been developed in order to maximize surgical resection of tumors of this region while minimizing approach-related morbidity. In this chapter, we describe the traditional microsurgical approaches to the ventral skull base and compare advantages and disadvantages to novel endoscopic endonasal approaches.

Keywords: anterior skull base, orbitozygomatic, pterional, craniotomy, skull base, tumors, microscope

7.1 Microscopic Perspective

7.1.1 Introduction

Surgical treatment for lesions arising from the skull base has historically been performed via a variety of transcranial approaches. The introduction of and advancements in endoscopic techniques over the past several decades have not only presented surgeons with an alternative method for resection, but also led to controversy and debate regarding the superior approach when treating skull base pathology. Despite the continued progress with endoscopic techniques, at many institutions open transcranial approaches remain the workhorse for skull base procedures. The complex anatomy of the skull base makes the traditional transcranial approaches crucial to ensure the integrity of vital neurovascular structures.

At this institution, all patients who present with cranial base neoplasms undergo extensive workup prior to operative planning. In addition to volumetric magnetic resonance imaging (MRI), noninvasive vascular imaging is often performed. It is subsequently determined if more comprehensive vascular imaging via catheter angiography is necessary to better visualize venous sinuses and/or determine a need for preoperative embolization. Catheter angiography also allows for improved visualization of arterial structures, which often may be encapsulated or displaced by skull base masses.

7.1.2 Case Example

MG is an 85-year-old male with a history of chronic kidney disease, mitral valve prolapse and regurgitation, hypertension, and glaucoma. He initially presented to his primary care physician with a 1-year history of predominantly short-term progressive memory loss. On exam, he was oriented to himself, place, and time. He answered questions appropriately. His cranial nerve function was normal on examination, his strength was 5/5 in all muscle groups, and his sensation was intact to light touch and pinprick. He demonstrated no signs of cerebellar dysfunction and had no perceptible pronator drift on examination. His other organ systems were also normal on examination.

After presenting to his primary care physician with complaints of memory loss, workup included a computed tomography (CT) scan, which revealed what appeared to be a large anterior fossa meningioma with surrounding vasogenic edema. MRI confirmed the presence of a large right-sided planum sphenoidale meningioma with substantial vasogenic edema (▶ Fig. 7.1).

The tumor was not associated with any dural venous sinuses and did not have significant vascular feeders identified on MR angiography; therefore, he did not undergo additional vascular imaging. He was subsequently taken to the operating room (OR) where a modified minipterional was performed for mass excision.

Intraoperative Management

While performing the craniotomy, the patient received 1 g/kg of mannitol and was hyperventilated to improve brain relaxation.

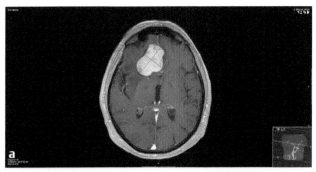
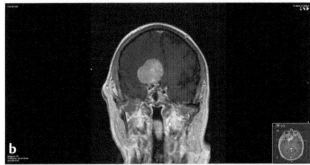
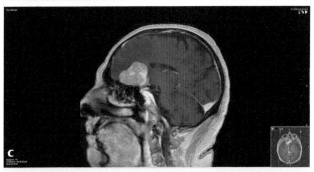

Fig. 7.1 Preoperative imaging of an 85-year-old male with a planum meningioma. Gadolinium-enhanced **(a)** axial, **(b)** coronal, and **(c)** sagittal MRI.

Proceeding with a subfrontal approach, the optic-carotid cistern was identified and fenestrated to allow for cerebrospinal fluid (CSF) egress. Intraoperatively, the tumor was easily visualized via the pterional approach. There was minimal brain retraction necessary after adequate CSF drainage. The optic nerves and anterior cerebral arteries were easily identified posteriorly following internal debulking of the tumor. These structures were easily decompressed with minimal manipulation. Gross total resection was performed with no intraoperative complications.

Postoperative Management

Postoperative imaging showed gross total resection of the tumor (▶ Fig. 7.2). There was no significant retraction injury or infarct identified on imaging. At our institution, we do not routinely perform intraoperative imaging for skull base lesions. The patient remained neurologically intact throughout his hospital stay.

7.1.3 Advantages of the Traditional Approach

The tumor described is a large planum sphenoidale meningioma. Due to the large size and significant lateral extension to the right side of the skull base and lateral extension of the mass beyond the ipsilateral carotid artery, it is a favorable lesion for a transcranial approach. It is difficult to achieve a gross total resection through an endoscopic approach due to both of these features. The pterional approach is superior for allowing an adequate working channel to facilitate good visualization of the tumor and surrounding structures.[1] Utilizing this method allowed for early identification and decompression of both the optic nerves and the anterior cerebral arteries, which were both intimately associated with the lesion (▶ Fig. 7.3). A gross total resection was easily obtained without retraction injury or inadvertent compromise of the surrounding neurovascular structures due to the superior visualization and working corridor provided via the transcranial approach (▶ Fig. 7.4).

7.1.4 Disadvantage of the Endoscope

While endoscopic technique offers a minimally invasive method of tumor resection, there are several potential limitations. Large dural openings often associated with this approach, in addition to the necessity to drill additional bone through the ethmoids and the potential for bony erosion due to tumor growth, lead to a higher risk of CSF leak than what has been reported with microscopic approaches,[2] which subsequently leads to a higher risk of meningitis and often may lead to an extended hospital stay as CSF diversion is required for a prolonged period postoperatively.

Additionally, the potential for rapid CSF egress during endoscopic openings has been reported to cause potentially life-threatening complications. These include subdural hematoma, tension pneumocephalus, and cerebellar hemorrhage.[3] These findings are rare but nonetheless dangerous and often require additional procedures with their concomitant morbidity.

Sinonasal complaints are common after endoscopic surgery and can greatly affect patient satisfaction. Nasal crusting and discharge can be found in 40 to 50% of patients postoperatively.[4] Although these findings typically resolve with time, they can prolong recovery and cause a significant amount of patient discomfort due to frequent and tedious nasal care.

Extent of resection is an important factor in determining rate of recurrence as well as the need for adjuvant treatment for the majority of skull base lesions. Gross total resection is more likely

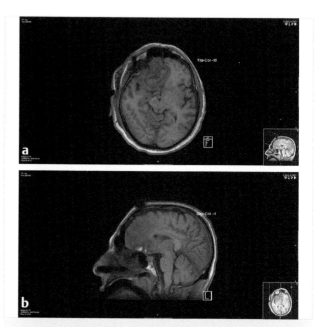

Fig. 7.2 Postoperative MRI. **(a)** Axial and **(b)** sagittal.

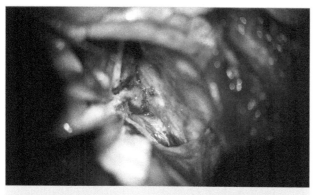

Fig. 7.3 Intraoperative microscopic view containing optic nerve.

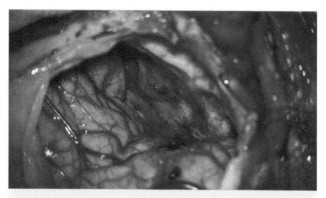

Fig. 7.4 Intraoperative microscopic view following gross total resection.

to be achieved via a transcranial approach when tumor size is large or exhibits lateral extension.[5,6] This is particularly true for lesions that extend lateral to the carotid arteries or optic nerves, or posteriorly to the retrochiasmatic space. Tumors with canalicular extension, particularly those causing visual disturbance, require adequate decompression of the optic nerves. This is difficult to perform safely with an endoscope if the tumor is compressing the nerves superiorly or with a postfixed chiasm.

The ability to navigate an endoscope is a specialized skill. Without additional subspecialty training, most neurosurgeons are unable to perform this task independently. This subsequently creates a need for an additional surgeon to assist with these procedures, a requirement that may be inconvenient or unattainable.

7.1.5 Patient Selection

In the senior author's practice, several factors are taken into account when determining treatment techniques and goals. Initially, tumor size and location are evaluated. Any lesion that is larger than 4 cm in diameter or demonstrating significant calcification is considered for open surgical treatment. The location and proximity of the tumor to neurovascular structures is also considered. Lesions that extend laterally to the carotid artery or superolateral to the optic nerve are treated transcranially. Additionally, cerebral vessels encased by tumor or displaced superiorly by tumor mass are treated via a craniotomy. Doing so allows the surgeon greater control when dissecting these vital structures as well as increased maneuverability, eliminating the restriction of a narrow working channel that is present with an endoscopic approach.

Tumors that are predominantly confined to the sella, with or without extension into the nasal sinuses and without significant suprasellar or lateral extension, or small proximal planum sphenoidale lesions without lateral extension, may be referred for neuroendoscopic resection. In this practice, the vast majority of skull base lesions are treated with an open surgical approach. In our opinion, there is little benefit to using an endoscopic approach over a microscopic approach unless there is significant tumor extension into and destruction of the sinuses.

7.1.6 Complication Avoidance

Thoughtful planning prior to surgery is essential to achieving a successful outcome, and avoids serious complications. Goals of surgery should be addressed prior to the OR, which include consideration of the most likely pathology and extent of resection, tumor location, and proximity to important neurovascular structures.

Delineating vascular supply and use of preoperative embolization can decrease intraoperative blood loss and subsequent need for transfusion.[7] Large, highly vascularized meningiomas should be taken for cerebral angiography to assist with surgical planning by locating vascular supply to the tumor as well as performing preoperative embolization when possible.

Skull base tumors can arise from a number of locations and therefore a variety of craniotomies can be used to approach the skull base. Tumor location as well as proximity to the carotid arteries, cranial nerves, and, if applicable, the craniocervical junction should be taken into account when planning an approach. An exposure that provides the most direct route to the lesion can reduce brain retraction and postoperative edema.

Subfrontal, bifrontal, pterional, and orbitozygomatic craniotomies are the common microscopic transcranial approaches to lesions of the anterior skull base, while posterior fossa tumors are reached with a far-lateral approach (▶ Fig. 7.5). Both the subfrontal and bifrontal interhemispheric approaches have been shown to achieve excellent rates of gross total resection while maintaining low risk of morbidity and mortality when performed by experienced surgeons.[8,9] The far-lateral approach can have high mortality when careful patient selection is not performed. Reserving this method for laterally based tumors or those where only subtotal resection is accomplished (thus leaving the ventromedial aspect of the lesion) can greatly decrease the chance of cranial nerve and sinus injury.[10]

Each cranial approach contains its own risk profile, and all possibilities should be considered during surgical planning. One must keep in mind not only tumor location and goals of surgery but also surgeon expertise, volume, and comfort level.

7.1.7 Technical Nuances

Assuring that all equipment is available and functional prior to incision is vital to a smooth procedure. The assistance of a microscope foot pedal or a mouth-switch when operating the microscope allows for a more efficient surgical performance by allowing the surgeon to keep both hands in the surgical field at all times. It is also beneficial to utilize an ultrasonic aspirator

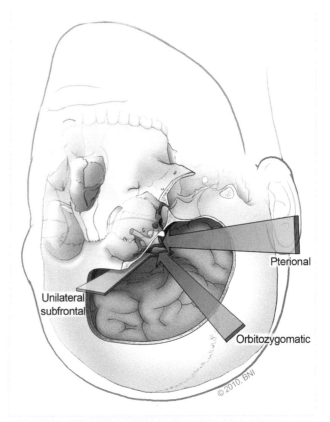

Fig. 7.5 Diagram demonstrating unilateral subfrontal pterional and orbitozygomatic approaches to the skull base. (Used with permission from Barrow Neurological Institute, Phoenix, AZ.)

and dissecting curettes to assist with tumor resection and decrease OR time.

The often larger craniotomies required to expose these complex tumors can require significant bony resection. It is therefore important to remain aware of the potential for related postoperative complications. In addition to meticulous attention to hemostasis, all mastoid air cells that are exposed must be adequately filled with bone wax to prevent CSF leak. Additionally, avoidance of the frontal sinus, if possible, is equally important to avoid CSF leak and meningitis, which should be done by checking anatomic landmarks and with use of intraoperative navigation when it is available.

Additionally, to avert problems with poor cosmetic results, careful placement of incisions and osteotomies should be performed. Visible areas of the cranium such as the forehead should be avoided, if possible.

7.1.8 Clinical Pearls

- Adequate brain relaxation is essential to minimize brain retraction.
- Adequate craniotomy size and drilling of bony ridges around the craniotomy and at the skull base facilitate improved visualization and ample light deep within the surgical field.
- Identification and preservation of neurovascular structures is of paramount importance.
- Adequate presurgical advanced neuroimaging and neurovascular imaging should be performed and reviewed.
- Higher rates of gross total resection are often seen with microscopic approaches.
- Larger masses and masses extending laterally are ideally suited for microscopic resection.

7.1.9 Evidence in Favor of Microscopic Approach

Microscopic surgical approaches have historically been the standard for treating skull base lesions. Despite the advances in technique and the growing body of literature describing endoscopic approaches to these lesions, there remains solid evidence supporting transcranial treatment.

It has been demonstrated in several studies that there is a significantly higher rate of gross total resection with microscopic approaches for meningiomas that originate from the skull base,[5] which is specifically true if the lesion is largely calcified, exhibits significant lateral extension, or is greater than 40 mm in diameter.[11] The extent of resection of meningiomas is inversely proportional to the rate of recurrence; therefore, this evidence supports a transcranial approach for tumors that demonstrate these characteristics.

The increased risk of CSF leak with endoscopic approaches is a persistent concern. Despite advances in closure techniques and nasoseptal flap reconstruction, the risk of postoperative CSF leak remains significantly higher in this patient population and is a persistent problem,[5,11] necessitating careful and meticulous reconstruction and closure of the dural defect by a highly skilled endoscopic surgeon. In our experience, patients who have undergone endoscopic endonasal approaches typically have an increased length of hospital stay due to required lumbar drainage following complex multilayered skull base flap closures.

Patients who present with intact olfaction have a higher chance of postoperative anosmia following endoscopic resection compared with microscopically resected patients.[12,13] Careful evaluation should be performed preoperatively, and individuals found to have this sense intact should preferentially be considered for a microscopic resection. Doing so can significantly impact quality of life and patient satisfaction in the postoperative period.

References

[1] Soni RS, Patel SK, Husain Q, Dahodwala MQ, Eloy JA, Liu JK. From above or below: the controversy and historical evolution of tuberculum sellae meningioma resection from open to endoscopic skull base approaches. J Clin Neurosci. 2014; 21(4):559–568

[2] Cavallo LM, Messina A, Cappabianca P, et al. Endoscopic endonasal surgery of the midline skull base: anatomical study and clinical considerations. Neurosurg Focus. 2005; 19(1):E2

[3] Kerr EE, Prevedello DM, Jamshidi A, Ditzel Filho LF, Otto BA, Carrau RL. Immediate complications associated with high-flow cerebrospinal fluid egress during endoscopic endonasal skull base surgery. Neurosurg Focus. 2014; 37(4):E3

[4] Awad AJ, Mohyeldin A, El-Sayed IH, Aghi MK. Sinonasal morbidity following endoscopic endonasal skull base surgery. Clin Neurol Neurosurg. 2015; 130:162–167

[5] Komotar RJ, Starke RM, Raper DM, Anand VK, Schwartz TH. Endoscopic endonasal versus open transcranial resection of anterior midline skull base meningiomas. World Neurosurg. 2012; 77(5–6):713–724

[6] Abbassy M, Woodard TD, Sindwani R, Recinos PF. An overview of anterior skull base meningiomas and the endoscopic endonasal approach. Otolaryngol Clin North Am. 2016; 49(1):141–152

[7] Borg A, Ekanayake J, Mair R, et al. Preoperative particle and glue embolization of meningiomas: indications, results, and lessons learned from 117 consecutive patients. Neurosurgery. 2013; 73(2) Suppl Operative:ons244–ons251, discussion ons252

[8] Mielke D, Mayfrank L, Psychogios MN, Rohde V. The anterior interhemispheric approach: a safe and effective approach to anterior skull base lesions. Acta Neurochir (Wien). 2014; 156(4):689–696

[9] Pallini R, Fernandez E, Lauretti L, et al. Olfactory groove meningioma: report of 99 cases surgically treated at the Catholic University School of Medicine, Rome. World Neurosurg. 2015; 83(2):219–31.e1, 3

[10] Benet A, Prevedello DM, Carrau RL, et al. Comparative analysis of the transcranial "far lateral" and endoscopic endonasal "far medial" approaches: surgical anatomy and clinical illustration. World Neurosurg. 2014; 81(2):385–396

[11] Koutourousiou M, Fernandez-Miranda JC, Wang EW, Snyderman CH, Gardner PA. Endoscopic endonasal surgery for olfactory groove meningiomas: outcomes and limitations in 50 patients. Neurosurg Focus. 2014; 37(4):E8

[12] Gallagher MJ, Durnford AJ, Wahab SS, Nair S, Rokade A, Mathad N. Patient-reported nasal morbidity following endoscopic endonasal skull base surgery. Br J Neurosurg. 2014; 28(5):622–625

[13] Mortazavi MM, Brito da Silva H, Ferreira M, Jr, Barber JK, Pridgeon JS, Sekhar LN. Planum sphenoidale and tuberculum sellae meningiomas: operative nuances of a modern surgical technique with outcome and proposal of a new classification system. World Neurosurg. 2016; 86:270–286

8 Anterior Skull Base Tumors—Endoscope

Harminder Singh, Walid I. Essayed, Theodore H. Schwartz

Summary

The endoscopic endonasal approach for anterior skull base tumors allows direct visualization of the base of the tumor as well as the ability to decompress the majority of the tumor without traversing the plane of the optic nerves or internal carotid arteries or its branches. Patients with meningiomas of the tuberculum or planum often have visual loss from optic nerve and chiasmal compression as well as from compression of the nerve against the A1 branch, which traverses behind the nerve. The endonasal approach allows the surgeon to first devascularize the tumor, remove any bony invasion, and decompress the chiasm before the nerves are manipulated. This results in improved visual outcomes. The endonasal approach also allows for better control and preservation of the vasa nervorum of the chiasm, decreasing the risk of visual complications. Small, midline anterior skull base lesions without neurovascular encasement are better suited for endoscopic endonasal resection.

Keywords: anterior skull base, meningioma, endoscopic, skull base

8.1 Endoscopic Perspective

8.1.1 Case Example

A 26-year-old, right-handed male presented with a history of headaches, dizziness, and blurry vision, slowly progressing over 4 years, without diplopia or seizures. His physical examination was normal except for decreased vision in the right eye, where he was able to perform finger-counting only. Magnetic resonance imaging (MRI) demonstrated a planum sphenoidale meningioma with sellar extension (▶ Fig. 8.1a,b).

Intraoperative Management

An endoscopic endonasal transplanum approach using the transsphenoidal corridor was performed. After placing a lumbar drain and harvesting a nasoseptal flap, a wide sphenoidotomy was performed. The skull base was drilled out to expose the entire base of the tumor (▶ Fig. 8.2). Anteriorly, the planum sphenoidale was removed just past the anterior extent of the tumor. Laterally, the bone overlying the medial opticocarotid

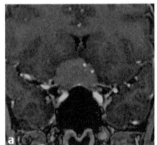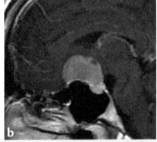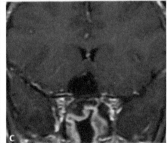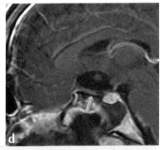

Fig. 8.1 Pre- and postoperative MRI scans. **(a)** Pre-op coronal T1 with gadolinium MRI showing the planum meningioma. **(b)** Pre-op sagittal T1 with gadolinium MRI showing extension of tumor into the tuberculum sella. Post-op **(c)** coronal and **(d)** sagittal T1 MRI with gadolinium showing gross total resection of tumor. *Blue arrow* points to the Medpor graft used for skull base reconstruction, as part of the "gasket seal" technique with fascia lata.

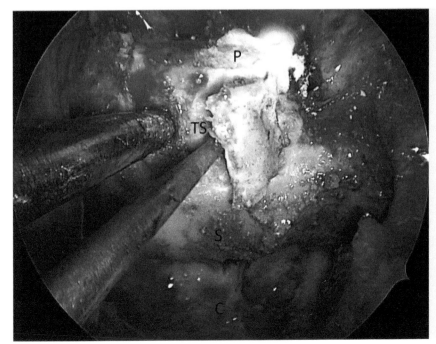

Fig. 8.2 The bone overlying the tuberculum sella (TS) and planum (P) is drilled and removed. C, clivus; S, sella.

recesses was removed, as well as the medial optic canals. Inferiorly, the sella was opened down to the inferior extent of the tumor into the sella using a 3-mm round-diamond drill bit.

The dura was cauterized to devascularize the base of the tumor and opened in a cruciate fashion to expose the base of the tumor. The tumor was internally decompressed using suction, sharp dissection as well as the Elliquence (Innovative Medical Solutions, Baldwin, NY). After internal decompression, the superior aspect of the tumor was rolled off the base of the frontal lobe and dissected free from the A2 branches, anterior communicating artery, and A1 branches above the optic chiasm using sharp and blunt dissection, until the top of the chiasm was visualized (▶ Fig. 8.3**a,b**). Additional internal decompression was pursued if the bulk of the tumor was too large to permit visualization around the capsule of the tumor. The medial optic canals were opened sharply and the tumor was rolled out of the optic canals bilaterally and decompressed. The tumor was sharply dissected off the optic nerves and chiasm if stuck. Finally, the dura above and below the superior intercavernous sinus was opened, and the sinus was cauterized and cut to open the diaphragma sella. The tumor was rolled up off the pituitary gland and sharply dissected off the pituitary stalk. The central remaining bulk of tumor was further decompressed and then dissected off the chiasm.[1,2]

Once the tumor was completely removed, a 45-degree endoscope was advanced into the cavity to inspect the medial optic canal to ensure there was no additional tumor remaining. Autologous fascia lata was harvested and a "gasket seal" closure was performed using Medpor,[3,4] and then covered with a vascularized nasoseptal flap, which was held in place with a layer of DuraSeal (Covidien-Medtronic, Minneapolis, MI) (▶ Fig. 8.4). A lumbar drain was placed preoperatively and continued for 24 hours after surgery, draining at 5 mL/h.

Surgical Outcomes

The postoperative MRI scan showed a gross total resection. Vision was improved in the right eye. There was no postoperative cerebrospinal fluid (CSF) leak.

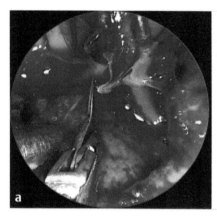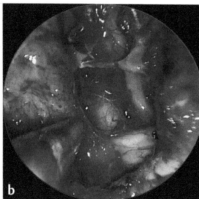

Fig. 8.3 Intraoperative photos. **(a)** Dissection of meningioma from the anterior communicating artery complex. **(b)** Dissection of meningioma from the left optic nerve.

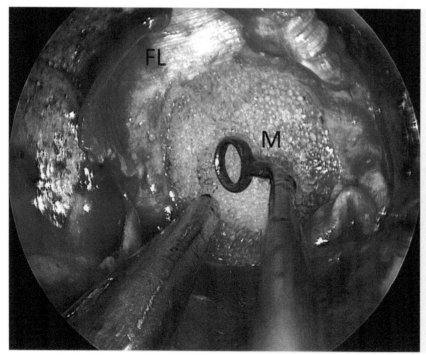

Fig. 8.4 Gasket seal used for skull base reconstruction, using fascia lata (FL) and Medpor (M) graft countersunk into the bony opening. The previously harvested pedicled nasoseptal flap was layered over this closure.

8.1.2 Advantages of Endoscopic Approach

The endoscopic endonasal approach allows direct visualization of the base of the tumor as well as the ability to decompress the majority of the tumor without traversing the plane of the optic nerves or internal carotid arteries or its branches. Patients with meningiomas of the tuberculum or planum often have visual loss from optic nerve and chiasmal compression as well as from compression of the nerve against the A1 branch, which traverses behind the nerve.[5] The endonasal approach allows the surgeon to first devascularize the tumor, remove any bony invasion, and decompress the chiasm before the nerves are manipulated.[2] This advantage results in improved visual outcome and the approach from below lowers the risk of stroke, seizure, or wound infection.[6] The endonasal approach also allows for better control and preservation of the vasa nervorum of the chiasm, decreasing the risk of visual complications.[7]

8.1.3 Disadvantages of the Microscopic Approach

Some degree of frontal lobe retraction is necessary to access the region of the planum. Depending on the extent of retraction, contusion and encephalomalacia can ensue, even if done without retractors, which can lead to postoperative seizures. Frontal lobe retraction also risks iatrogenic injury to the olfactory bulbs and tracts. Performing an orbital osteotomy with orbital roof drilling might decrease the necessity of retraction. However, postoperative discomfort from orbital swelling and approximate aesthetic results can jeopardize the recovery.

The optic nerves and chiasm can be superiorly displaced, particularly when the chiasm is prefixed and the dural tail extends beyond the planum and into the tuberculum. This limits the window for safe resection without optic apparatus manipulation and injury. The anterior clinoid can be removed extra- or intradurally to minimize manipulation, but some degree of optic nerve manipulation still occurs. The anterior communicating artery complex and the A2 s are often draped over the dorsal aspect of the tumor, increasing the risks of inadvertent injury during tumor resection.

The microscopic approach offers limited visualization of the vascularization of the optic apparatus, especially the ipsilateral inferomedial walls of the optic canal.

Tumor devascularization by cauterizing the dura and drilling the planum is usually the last step of the surgery, often slowing the resection, particularly in hemorrhagic lesions. Open surgery offers no control of any eventual nasal extension of the tumor. Extensive coagulation of the skull base can result in postoperative CSF leaks,[8] which are often difficult to diagnose intraoperatively during microscopic surgery. This can lead to secondary open or endoscopic reconstructive surgeries for repairing the leak.

8.1.4 Patient Selection

Although there is no fixed size limit on tumors that can be resected endonasally, small midline tumors are better suited for endoscopic resection. Large tumors not only tend to encase the anterior communicating artery complex and/or the optic nerves, but also can extend laterally over the anterior clinoid or orbital roof, thereby limiting the ability to achieve a complete resection. Careful preoperative anatomical evaluation using MRI and CT angiography (CTA) is important for patient selection.[2] The presence of a cortical cuff is not required as most of these tumors touch the anterior communicating artery complex to some degree.[9,10] In general, as long as the entire basal attachment of the tumor can be exposed, then the superior extent of the tumor can be removed unless the tumor extends laterally beyond the clinoid, ICA bifurcation, or circumferentially around optic nerve or chiasm.

8.1.5 Complication Avoidance and Technical Nuances

The most important step in avoiding a complication is making a large enough bone opening to safely remove the tumor. In order to have the confidence to make a large opening, one must have a proven strategy for closure. In our hands, this means harvesting fascia lata for a gasket seal, harvesting a nasoseptal flap, and placing a lumbar drain preoperatively for 24 hours of postoperative drainage.[11] With this closure protocol, we have achieved less than 2% postoperative CSF leaks.[12] Sometimes, if the skull base opening is odd shaped, it might be challenging to perform a "gasket seal" with Medpor and fascia lata. In those cases, a "bilayer button" closure with two pieces of fascia lata stitched together in the middle can form a simultaneous inlay and onlay closure over the dura and help with the prevention of CSF leaks.[13]

Appropriate instrumentation is necessary, including bipolar and adequate microscissors for bimanual dissection. We prefer bayonetted instruments and two-handed surgery with a scope holder but a second surgeon can also hold the scope if dynamic scope movement is desired. Any blind dissection or pulling should be avoided. Intraoperatively, the micro-Doppler is used to identify encased vessels. A preoperative CTA scan can be helpful if the tumor encases blood vessels, and can be used for intraoperative neuronavigation.

Even partial preservation of the arachnoid plane around the tumor can facilitate safe dissection and resection of the tumor, and decreases the postoperative CSF leak rate. Opening the lumbar drain during surgery can help decrease the outpouching of the arachnoid into the surgical field.

It is important to look for and preserve the superior hypophyseal arteries. Often, there is a branch to the stalk and a branch to the chiasm, but variability exists.

8.1.6 Clinical Pearls

The preoperative visual fields and optical coherence tomography tests can be helpful in advising patients regarding their expected visual improvement after surgery. In addition, asymmetric visual loss raises the suspicion of tumor in the optic canal or compression of the nerve against the A1 branch on that side. A preoperative CT scan can help evaluate for any tumor calcification, variant sinus anatomy, and the integrity of the skull base as well as the thickness and ossification of the planum. A vascular study such as the CTA or MR angiography might be helpful to understand the angioarchitecture around the tumor. Sometimes the chiasm can be difficult to identify on preoperative MRI; in these cases, its position can be approximated from the position of the anterior communicating artery. Patients who are obese or with elevated body mass index benefit more from a lumbar drain and are at higher risk of a CSF leak after surgery.

8.1.7 Literature Review/Evidence in Favor of Endoscopic Approach

As we described earlier, prudent preoperative patient selection is mandatory for a successful postoperative outcome, which introduces an inherent selection bias when comparing the outcomes of microscopic versus endoscopic surgery. Open surgery is more versatile when dealing with extensive paramedian tumor. The question is whether it is superior to endoscopic surgery for specific indications. A literature review of 1,426 patients reported better visual outcome with endoscopic surgery and an equivalent overall morbidity rate, but higher postoperative CSF leak rates with endoscopic procedures.[6] The CSF leak rate is, however, overestimated since the reported literature includes the early phase of the endonasal learning curve, whereas the transcranial approach is at the latter stages of its learning curve. The above-described closure techniques have drastically decreased the CSF leak rates after extended endonasal anterior skull base surgery to less than 5% in recent literature.[12]

References

[1] Kulwin C, Schwartz TH, Cohen-Gadol AA. Endoscopic extended transsphenoidal resection of tuberculum sellae meningiomas: nuances of neurosurgical technique. Neurosurg Focus. 2013; 35(6):E6

[2] Ottenhausen M, Banu MA, Placantonakis DG, et al. Endoscopic endonasal resection of suprasellar meningiomas: the importance of case selection and experience in determining extent of resection, visual improvement, and complications. World Neurosurg. 2014; 82(3–4):442–449

[3] Leng LZ, Brown S, Anand VK, Schwartz TH. "Gasket-seal" watertight closure in minimal-access endoscopic cranial base surgery. Neurosurgery. 2008; 62 (5) Suppl 2:E342–E343, discussion E343

[4] Garcia-Navarro V, Anand VK, Schwartz TH. Gasket seal closure for extended endonasal endoscopic skull base surgery: efficacy in a large case series. World Neurosurg. 2013; 80(5):563–568

[5] Attia M, Kandasamy J, Jakimovski D, et al. The importance and timing of optic canal exploration and decompression during endoscopic endonasal resection of tuberculum sella and planum sphenoidale meningiomas. Neurosurgery. 2012; 71(1) Suppl Operative:58–67

[6] Komotar RJ, Starke RM, Raper DM, Anand VK, Schwartz TH. Endoscopic endonasal versus open transcranial resection of anterior midline skull base meningiomas. World Neurosurg. 2012; 77(5–6):713–724

[7] Schwartz TH. Editorial: Does chiasmatic blood supply dictate endonasal corridors? J Neurosurg. 2015; 122(5):1163–1164

[8] Fahlbusch R, Schott W. Pterional surgery of meningiomas of the tuberculum sellae and planum sphenoidale: surgical results with special consideration of ophthalmological and endocrinological outcomes. J Neurosurg. 2002; 96 (2):235–243

[9] Dhandapani S, Negm HM, Cohen S, Anand VK, Schwartz TH. Endonasal endoscopic transsphenoidal resection of tuberculum sella meningioma with anterior cerebral artery encasement. Cureus. 2015; 7(8):e311

[10] Khan OH, Anand VK, Schwartz TH. Endoscopic endonasal resection of skull base meningiomas: the significance of a "cortical cuff" and brain edema compared with careful case selection and surgical experience in predicting morbidity and extent of resection. Neurosurg Focus. 2014; 37(4):E7

[11] Raza SM, Schwartz TH. Multi-layer reconstruction during endoscopic endonasal surgery: how much is necessary? World Neurosurg. 2015; 83 (2):138–139

[12] Mascarenhas L, Moshel YA, Bayad F, et al. The transplanum transtuberculum approaches for suprasellar and sellar-suprasellar lesions: avoidance of cerebrospinal fluid leak and lessons learned. World Neurosurg. 2014; 82(1–2):186–195

[13] Luginbuhl AJ, Campbell PG, Evans J, Rosen M. Endoscopic repair of high-flow cranial base defects using a bilayer button. Laryngoscope. 2010; 120(5): 876–880

9 Endoscopic versus Microscopic Approach to the Craniovertebral Junction—Microscope

Ali S. Haider, James T. Rutka

Summary

The craniovertebral junction is a highly complex region containing a variety of load-bearing joints and important neurovascular structures. Lesions in this region are traditionally approached using microsurgical principles developed in the last few decades. These approaches have been proven to maximize surgical efficacy, but carry a significant degree of approach-related morbidity. The advent of endoscopic endonasal approaches in the last two decades has ushered a new era of minimally invasive approaches. However, traditionalists argue that this comes at the cost of efficacy, and potentially increases the risk of cerebrospinal fluid leak and meningitis. In this chapter, we discuss the advantages and disadvantages of endoscopic versus microsurgical approaches to the craniovertebral junction.

Keywords: microscopic, brainstem, cervicomedullary, pediatric, tumor

9.1 Microscopic Perspective

9.1.1 Introduction

Brainstem tumors are among the most difficult lesions for neurosurgeons to treat in the brain. Typically, these tumors respect neuroanatomical boundaries, confining their localization to a discrete region of the brainstem.[1,2] The classification of brainstem tumors includes midbrain (tectal and tegmental), pontine (dorsally exophytic, diffuse intrinsic, and focal), and cervicomedullary lesions. In this chapter, we will be discussing the microscopic management of a cervicomedullary lesion in a young child.[3] As will be discussed, this tumor can only be addressed at this time using microneurosurgical techniques and select neurosurgical adjunctive tools that are not currently available using the endoscopic approach.

9.1.2 Evolution of Current Surgical Treatment Options for Foramen Magnum Tumors

Tumors of the foramen magnum pose specific challenges to neurosurgeons.[4,5] Given its lateral boundaries, and its anteroposterior extent, the foramen magnum can be approached using one of a number of skull base neurosurgical techniques. In some circumstances, combined skull base approaches are required. Some of these approaches include: retrosigmoid approach via suboccipital craniotomy; presigmoid approach via a lateral skull base approach with drilling of the petrous temporal bone; and far-lateral approach to the occipital condyle and foramen magnum (► Fig. 9.1).

9.1.3 Traditional/Microsurgical Management

History

A 5-year-old female initially presented with a first-time seizure for which a magnetic resonance imaging (MRI) scan was performed. This showed an incidentally discovered intramedullary brainstem lesion at the craniocervical junction (► Fig. 9.2). As the child was otherwise well at initial presentation without focal neurological symptoms or signs, she was observed with serial MRI scans. Over time, these showed progressive growth of the cervicomedullary brainstem lesion (► Fig. 9.3). She developed very mild new-onset left-sided hemiparesis and complained of some decreased sensation in both the left upper and lower extremities. Due to new onset of symptoms and radiographic progression, the decision was made to operate.

Physical Examination

There was left hemiparesis affecting the arm more than the leg. The patient was still able to ambulate, but with a tendency to fall to the left. Deep tendon reflexes were more brisk on the left than the right. There was a left Babinski's reflex.

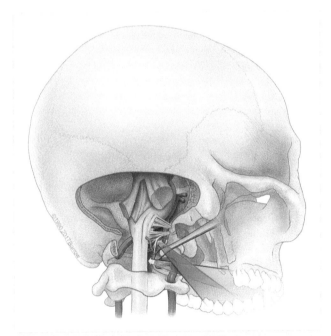

Fig. 9.1 Illustration showing the far-lateral approach to the craniocervical junction. (Used with permission from Barrow Neurological Institute, Phoenix, AZ.)

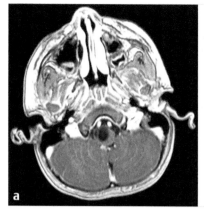
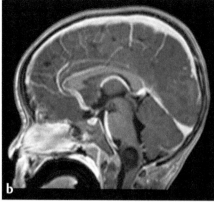

Fig. 9.2 A 5-year-old female with first-time seizures. Preoperative gadolinium-enhanced MRI demonstrated an intramedullary brainstem lesion on **(a)** axial and **(b)** sagittal planes.

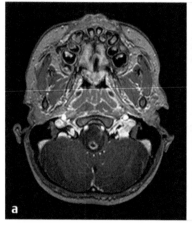
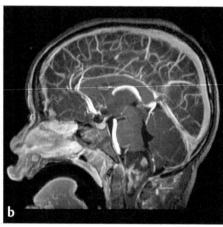

Fig. 9.3 The same patient was managed conservatively, with repeat imaging demonstrating progression of the lesion on gadolinium-enhanced MRI in **(a)** axial and **(b)** sagittal planes.

Intraoperative Management

The patient was taken to the operating room and induced under general anesthetic in the supine position with endotracheal intubation. Intraoperative neurophysiologic monitoring was applied and antibiotics were administered preoperatively. A Sugita head frame was applied in the neutral position and BrainLab system was registered. The patient was subsequently turned to the prone position on bolsters with head fixed in a slightly flexed position while neuromonitoring was being conducted. There were no changes in waveforms. A midline incision was performed spanning approximately the inferior aspect of the spinous process of C2 up toward the inion. The patient was then prepped and draped in the usual fashion. The skin was incised in the midline and dissection proceeded down through the midline raphe to the ligamentum nuchae, to the posterior arch of C1 and the spinous process of C2 including the subocciput.

The posterior arch of C1 was cleared laterally to a width of approximately 1.5 cm on either side and the lamina of C2 was exposed bilaterally. The lateral margins of the foramen magnum were also exposed in the suboccipital region. A curved curette was used to develop the plane posteriorly in the subperiosteal plane at the foramen magnum as well as above and below C1 and above and below C2. Pneumatic drill with craniotome tip was used to create a burr hole in the midline approximately 2.5 cm rostral to the foramen magnum. Two additional burr holes were also placed, one on either side at the level of the foramen magnum, with each being 1.5 cm lateral to the midline.

A dissector was then used to strip below these burr holes and the pneumatic drill with a cutting tip was used to create approximately 4 cm wide × 2.5 cm rostral-caudal craniotomy. The bone flap was then elevated. The matchstick drill bit was used to traverse the lamina of C1 on either side approximately 1.5 cm from the midline. The posterior arch of C1 was then carefully removed. The matchstick drill bit was also used to complete the laminectomy of C2. The craniotomy was preserved for reimplantation at the end of the case.

Intraoperative ultrasound was used to confirm the localization of the lesion and subsequently used at several points throughout the case. The dura was then incised in a Y-shaped fashion with the top ends of the Y over each cerebellar hemisphere and joining approximately at the craniocervical junction and then continuing inferiorly as a single cut toward the base of the exposure. Bleeding from dural edges was cauterized using bipolar cautery. Dural retaining stitches were then used to reflect the dura laterally, and any arachnoid adhesions were removed. At this point, the intraoperative microscope was used to complete the resection.

The arachnoid was opened over the cerebellar hemispheres and inferiorly toward the base of the exposure. A small bulge was noted on the left side of the brainstem at the rostral medulla consistent with a cystic region visualized on the preoperative MRI scan (▸ Fig. 9.4). The left vertebral artery was cleared of any arachnoid adhesions in order to be mobilized superiorly. Intraoperative stimulation was performed in order to determine the midline that was then cauterized using

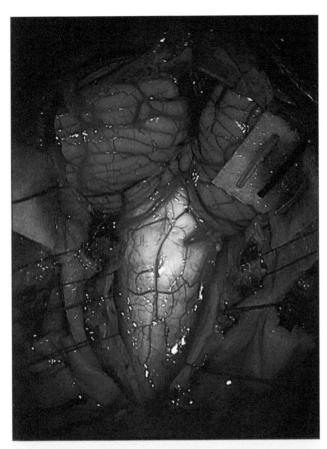

Fig. 9.4 Intraoperative imaging demonstrated a small bulge on the left side of the brainstem at the rostral medulla consistent with a cystic region visualized on preoperative MRI scan.

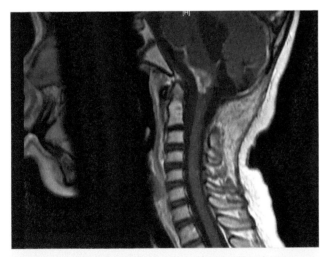

Fig. 9.6 Postoperative gadolinium-enhanced sagittal MRI demonstrates excellent debulking of the tumor.

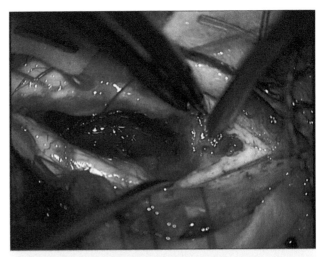

Fig. 9.5 Midline myelotomy was carried for a total distance of approximately 4 cm with the rostral extent near the base of the tonsils, and the caudal extent toward the base of the exposure.

Several small biopsies were taken and sent for quick section. The intraoperative pathological diagnosis was infiltrating astrocytoma. The Cavitron Ultrasonic Surgical Aspirator (CUSA) was then used to complete a subtotal resection of the lesion, with bleeding controlled via bipolar cautery. During the resection, there was a drop in motor evoked potentials in both the right arm and leg. By the end of the case, the right arm returned to 50% of baseline but the right leg remained at 5%. After achieving the decompression and debulking of the lesion and given the intraoperative neuromonitoring changes as well as the intraoperative diagnosis, the procedure was terminated having achieved more than a 50% resection of the tumor. Duraguard was used to complete a duraplasty, creating an enlarged cavity for the purposes of decompression. This was secured in place using several 4–0 Vicryl stitches and closed in a running watertight fashion using running 5–0 Polydioxanone. The lateral aspects of the remaining posterior arch of C1 as well as the lamina of C2 were decorticated and pieces of bone from the operation were placed in an in situ fusion. A large piece of Gelfoam was then placed over the dura. The muscles of the neck were approximated using buried interrupted No. 1 Vicryl sutures and the fascia reapproximated using interrupted No. 1 Vicryl sutures. 3–0 subcutaneous sutures were used in an interrupted fashion to reapproximate the skin followed by running 4–0 Monocryl for skin closure. The wound was then cleaned and dried and dressings applied. The patient was then flipped back to the supine position and the Sugita frame was removed.

Surgical Outcome

The patient's cervicomedullary brainstem tumor was successfully debulked (▶ Fig. 9.6). There was gradual improvement in strength of the upper and lower extremities over a 3-month time period while the child recovered at a rehabilitation hospital. She was much improved in neurological function over the ensuing 2 years. She received maintenance chemotherapy with carboplatin and vinblastine. However, at the age of 7, the patient developed a recurrence of left-sided weakness, and MRI

bipolar cautery and incised using an 11-blade scalpel. The midline myelotomy was carried for a total distance of approximately 4 cm with the rostral extent near the base of the tonsils, and the caudal extent toward the base of the exposure (▶ Fig. 9.5). Below a thin layer of normally appearing brainstem, there was obvious discolored tissue consistent with the tumor.

revealed progressive tumor. In addition, new lesions were found in the lateral ventricles indicative of metastatic disease. For this, she received urgent craniospinal irradiation. A ventriculoperitoneal shunt was also inserted for hydrocephalus. Despite these measures, her tumors progressed, and she died approximately 5 years after initial diagnosis.

9.1.4 Advantages of Traditional/ Microscopic Approach

Intrinsic lesions of the brainstem, especially at the cervicomedullary junction, demand multiple neurosurgical steps that typically require step-by-step exposure of a complex neuroanatomical region.[6] While percutaneous approaches have previously been described for this region (e.g., percutaneous trigeminal tractotomy), the potential spaces that would permit endoscopic approaches are somewhat limited.

In addition, a midline myelotomy and debulking of an intrinsic cervicomedullary brainstem tumor are significantly aided with the use of bipolar cautery, enhanced magnification, and an ability to distinguish infiltrating tumor from normal central nervous system parenchymal planes. Finally, the use of sophisticated intraoperative neuromonitoring strategies is best accomplished with an open exposure that allows placement of subdural electrodes that can be used to identify the h-reflex and the D-waves.

9.1.5 Disadvantage of the Endoscope

The endoscope is best suited when there are large potential spaces for contrast visualization—for example, when performing an endoscopic third ventriculostomy when the endoscope is within the CSF of the ventricular system, or when performing endoscopic endonasal transsphenoidal neurosurgery when there is a well-defined air medium that is separate from the tumor or pituitary gland itself. Unfortunately, the potential space in the subdural compartment at the cervicomedullary junction is rather limited, and will not permit a midline approach with clear visibility especially in the face of a swollen and expanded intrinsic brainstem tumor in this region.

Another limitation of the endoscopic approach here is our relative inability to retract the edges of the myelotomy, which is essential for visualization of the tumor, and differentiation of it from surrounding normal brainstem.

9.1.6 Patient Selection (Author's Experience)

At this time, although lesions at the craniovertebral junction may be approached using endoscopic techniques, intrinsic brainstem tumors will likely still require further advances in endoscopic technologies, optics, magnification, and portals of entry.

9.1.7 Complication Avoidance

For surgery on brainstem tumors at the cervicomedullary junction, the neurosurgical risks can be quite high, with hemiparesis, cranial nerve palsies, and sensory disturbances leading the list. To avoid these complications, we stress the importance of meticulous microneurosurgical techniques, intraoperative neuromonitoring, neuronavigation (on occasion), and, most of all, intraoperative neurosurgical judgment so that decisions on when to stop are informed by experience and direct tumor visualization.

9.1.8 Technical Nuances

The posterior fossa and suboccipital craniotomy, while routinely performed, must be done with precision. Care must be taken not to remove too many posterior cervical spinous processes with the exposure, as this may lead to postoperative kyphosis and cervical instability, and pain. Once the dura is opened and the midline myelotomy is performed, 6–0 pial sutures are used to laterally retract the edges of the myelotomy for optimal visualization of the tumor and for assistance with the delivery of the tumor. The intraoperative cavitron is an essential tool, but the tip of the cavitron should always be visible under the microscope to avoid "core" samples being taken beyond the visibility of the tumor. As these tumors are frequently infiltrative, this latter point is extremely important. Where possible, microneurosurgical dissectors are indispensable for delineating a plane between tumor and normal brainstem. Finally, in the depths of the tumor bed, the bipolar should be used on low power, and extremely sparingly to avoid thermal injury to the descending or ascending neuroanatomical fiber bundles.

9.1.9 Clinical Pearls

Patients with cervicomedullary brainstem tumors may have a clinical presentation pattern that mimics other underlying conditions such as gastrointestinal diseases (recurrent nausea, vomiting, and weight loss), recurrent aspiration pneumonia, and multiple subtle lower cranial nerve palsies. Not infrequently, these patients' diagnoses are delayed for months while several consultants from numerous other specialties review their cases. A plea is made for early neurological examination and clinical pattern recognition so that these patients can come to surgery as soon as possible.

References

[1] Rutka JTDJ, Hoffman HJ. Surgical Disorders of the Fourth Ventricle. Vol. 1. Hoboken, NJ: Blackwell Scientific Publications, Inc.; 1996

[2] Shah NC, Ray A, Bartels U, et al. Diffuse intrinsic brainstem tumors in neonates. Report of two cases. J Neurosurg Pediatr. 2008; 1(5):382–385

[3] Tsai ECRJ. Cervicomedullary gliomas. In: Berger M, Prados M, eds. Textbook of Neuro-Oncology. Vol 1. San Francisco, CA: Elsevier; 2004

[4] Vacchrajani SEM, Rutka JT. Pediatric Brain Tumor Surgery. Vol. 1. New York, NY: Demos Medical; 2011

[5] Weeks AFA, Rutka JT. Posterior Fossa and Brainstem Tumors in Children. Vol. 1. Philadelphia, PA: Elsevier Saunders; 2015

[6] McAbee JH, Modica J, Thompson CJ, et al. Cervicomedullary tumors in children. J Neurosurg Pediatr. 2015; 16(4):357–366

10 Craniovertebral Junction—Endoscope

Wei-Hsin Wang, Juan C. Fernandez-Miranda

Summary

Lesions of the craniovertebral junction have traditionally been approached using a posterior or posterolateral approach. Expanded endonasal approaches now allow for a minimally invasive corridor to approach lesions of the craniovertebral junction. In this chapter, we describe the technical considerations and operative limitations of an expanded endoscopic endonasal approach to lesions of the craniovertebral junction.

Keywords: craniovertebral, skull base, endoscope, expanded endonasal, clival, midline

10.1 Endoscopic Perspective

10.1.1 Case Example

History and Physical Examination

A 46-year-old woman presented with significant neck pain as well as numbness in both arms lasting several months. Preoperative magnetic resonance imaging (MRI) demonstrated an avidly gadolinium-enhancing foramen magnum tumor (▶ Fig. 10.1). Her neurological exam was unremarkable, with no objective findings.

Intraoperative Management

This foramen magnum lesion was approached via an endonasal endoscopic transclival "far-medial" transcondylar and transjugular tubercle approach because of its predominantly ventral location (▶ Fig. 10.2). An extended nasoseptal flap was harvested on the left side. After completing an extended nasopharyngectomy, the inferior clivus was drilled down to the level of the foramen magnum followed by a medial condylectomy bilaterally. The right jugular tubercle was also drilled. The upper aspect of C1 anterior arch and tip of the odontoid were removed without transgressing the C1–odontoid joint and transverse ligament. The dural opening was started from the midline and then extended bilaterally. The tumor was debulked using an ultrasonic aspirator device and the double-suction technique. Meticulous extracapsular microdissection was performed after extensive debulking to remove the tumor from critical neurovascular structures, including vertebral arteries and hypoglossal nerves bilaterally (▶ Fig. 10.3). Reconstruction was completed by a multiple-layer technique, including collagen matrix, fat graft, and nasoseptal flap. A lumbar drain was placed to drain 10 mL of cerebrospinal fluid (CSF) per hour for 3 days.

Surgical Outcome

A near-total resection was achieved with removal of dural attachment and potentially involved bone (▶ Fig. 10.4). A very small residual tumor within the right hypoglossal canal with adhesion of nerve rootlets was left to prevent any nerve injury. She was discharged on postoperative day 5 without any neurological deficits or complications. No CSF leak occurred. Preoperative upper extremities numbness completely disappeared. Gamma Knife radiosurgery for the stable small residual tumor was performed 1 year after surgery. At 3-year follow-up, she was asymptomatic without any tumor growth or craniocervical instability.

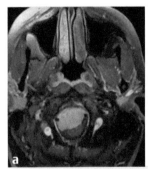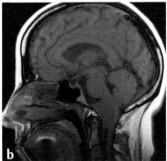

Fig. 10.1 A 46-year-old woman presented with neck pain and arm numbness. A preoperative MRI demonstrated **(a)** an avidly gadolinium-enhancing foramen magnum tumor on axial plane with **(b)** mass effect on the brainstem on non-gadolinium-enhancing sagittal plane.

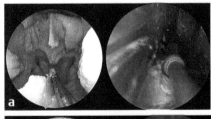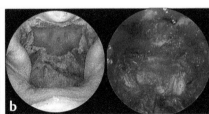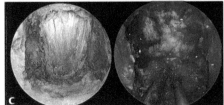

Fig. 10.2 An endonasal endoscopic transclival "far-medial" transcondylar and transjugular tubercle approach. Cadaveric specimen dissection and intraoperative imaging demonstrate approach to this lesion during **(a)** early, **(b)** middle, and **(c)** late phases of approach.

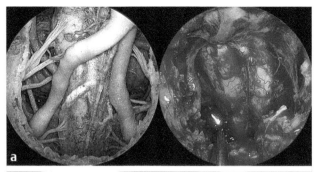

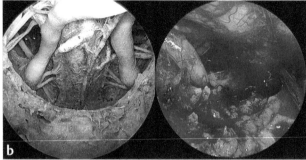

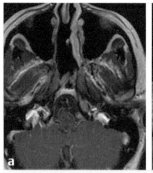

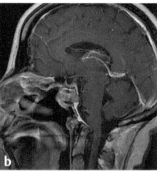

Fig. 10.4 Postoperative imaging. (a) Axial and (b) sagittal gadolinium-enhanced MRIs demonstrate near-total resection of the tumor.

Fig. 10.3 (a,b) Intraoperative and cadaveric specimen dissections demonstrate exposure of the ventral brainstem after resection of the tumor.

10.1.2 Advantages of Endoscopic Approach

The endoscopic endonasal approach (EEA) for predominantly ventral foramen magnum lesions has multiple advantages. When the lesion is located in the midline and there is posterolateral displacement of the neurovascular structures, the EEA provides direct access to the lesion via medial-to-lateral trajectory that may prevent the morbidity related to neurovascular manipulation during a lateral-to-medial approach. This is the main advantage of an endonasal "far-medial" approach over a transcranial far-lateral approach: the lack of manipulation of cerebellum, brainstem, vertebral arteries, anterior spinal artery, hypoglossal nerves, and lower cranial nerves secondary to the direct corridor into the tumor osseous and dural attachment, which allows early devascularization followed by extensive central debulking without even exposing a single posterior fossa neurovascular structure. It is important to remember that even transient and unilateral lower cranial nerves palsies may carry significant morbidity and decrease quality of life with requirement for feeding tubes secondary to dysphagia, and bilateral hypoglossal or lower cranial nerve palsies, although infrequent with transcranial approaches, are devastating for patients. Manipulation of vertebral arteries, especially when dealing with a dominant one, carries the risk of arterial injury, thrombosis, and stroke.

Additional advantages are related to the superior visualization provided by the endoscope and the endonasal route. While getting close to the surface between tumor and normal neurovascular structures, the endoscope provides wide-angle view and great illumination to make microdissection more safely, and the endonasal corridor provides full access to the whole ventral foramen magnum region. This is opposed to the relatively narrow working corridor of the transcranial far-lateral approach (between vertebral artery, medulla, and cranial nerves IX to XII) and the narrow field of view provided by the surgical microscope, which leaves multiple blind spots, in particular on the contralateral side.

There is low approach-related morbidity secondary to the endonasal route because the sinonasal structures are mostly preserved (with the exception of the nasoseptal flap harvesting), the dissection/resection of nasopharyngeal muscles (anterior rectus capitis and longus capitis) carries no functional consequences, and the amount of medial condylectomy required for widening the exposure is less than 20%, which carries virtually no risk of post-op craniocervical instability. This is in comparison with the potential morbidity of posterior cervical musculature contracture and atrophy after far-lateral approaches.

With the endonasal approach, it is possible to achieve a Simpson grade 1 resection, in particular with smaller tumors, which is not feasible with the transcranial route. In the case presented here, we left a very small remnant of tumor within the hypoglossal canal, and therefore it does not qualify as Simpson grade 1 resection; regardless, most of the involved bone and dura were removed.

10.1.3 Disadvantage of the Endonasal Approach

The main disadvantage of the EEA is the higher risk of CSF leakage and subsequent meningitis. The premedullary cistern has a high flow of CSF, which, along with the deep location of the inferior clivus, poses a challenge for reconstruction. Effective reconstruction requires a multilayer technique including, from deep to superficial, inlay DuraGen, onlay AlloDerm or fascia lata, fat grafts to fill up the gap up to the level of the nasopharyngeal posterior wall, and an extended nasoseptal flap to cover everything from the floor of the sphenoid sinus superiorly to the remaining basopharyngeal fascia inferiorly. In comparison, the transcranial far-lateral approach has a higher risk of pseudomeningocele, which is otherwise self-limited and inconsequential for most cases.

10.1.4 Patient Selection

In our experience, the EEA is the preferred choice for extradural lesions originating from the lower clivus or petroclival fissure, such as chordomas and chondrosarcomas, even if they have extensive intradural invasion. The lateral limits of the exposure in these cases are mainly the ventral jugular foramen and the hypoglossal canal. For intradural lesions, such as foramen magnum meningioma, jugular tubercle meningioma, petroclival meningioma, and epidermoid or neuroenteric cysts, we select the EEA when the lesion is predominantly ventral to pons and medulla, being located in between the vertebral arteries, hypoglossal nerves, and lower cranial nerves. For selected lesions that have a large ventral component but extend more laterally beyond the limits of the EEA, we may decide for an EEA in spite of achieving partial or near-total resection when the primary goal is ventral brainstem decompression in symptomatic and perhaps older patients. We may also plan a two-stage procedure, with an initial EEA for tumor resection followed by a transcranial approach. It is important to emphasize that lesions extending below the level of C1 arch should not be approached endonasally because it will require resection of the odontoid body and transverse ligament, causing craniocervical instability. The exception is the treatment of basilar invagination that requires odontoid resection for brainstem decompression and posterior occipital-cervical fusion. For these cases, the EEA has multiple advantages when compared to the transoral approach, including minimal risk of palatal insufficiency. Finally, intraaxial lesions such as brainstem cavernomas, when they have a ventral location within the medulla and pontomedullary junction, may still be candidates for the EEA depending on the displacement of the corticospinal tracts as visualized with fiber tractography.

10.1.5 Complication Avoidance

The nasal cavity should be inspected carefully in the preoperative setting. Sinusitis should be treated before an EEA to avoid post-op infection.

Careful patient selection and proper training and expertise are the key to decrease complications. EEAs to the craniocervical junction for extradural lesions such as basilar invagination or small chordomas are relatively simple procedures with no need for lateral extension or complex reconstruction. Inferior transclival EEA to intradural lesions and those with large volume or lateral extension are, however, highly complex and should only be attempted by well-trained and highly experienced surgical teams. The concept of team approach is essential to endoscopic endonasal surgery as the neurosurgeon and ENT surgeon join their efforts and expertise to achieve the best possible outcome.

It is preferable to indicate a transcranial far-lateral approach for a ventral foramen magnum meningioma by an experienced team, even when there is potentially higher risk of neurovascular complications, than to indicate an EEA for a similar lesion by a not-so-experienced team.

Regardless, contemporary skull base surgeons or teams should master both transcranial microsurgical and endonasal endoscopic approaches to offer patients the most effective and less morbid alternative for every given lesion and patient.

Strict adherence to delicate and gentle microdissection techniques is mandatory for resection of intradural lesions. Extracapsular dissection, however, should only be attempted after extensive intracapsular debulking. It is not recommended to attempt resection of tumors "en bloc" because it jeopardizes proper visualization and dissection of surrounding neurovascular structures, and carries the risk of arterial avulsion and cranial nerve damage.

Familiarity and access to especially designed instruments for endonasal surgery are important in order to adhere to the above-mentioned techniques.

Reconstruction for preventing postoperative CSF leakage is always a challenge for intradural lesions in the area of the craniocervical junction. Particularly challenging are recurrent skull base chordomas with previous surgery and radiation treatment, and intradural extension.

We advocate a multilayer reconstruction technique, as described above, where the key element is a well-designed vascularized nasoseptal flap. The use of a lumbar drain has shown to significantly reduce the incidence of post-op CSF leaks for transclival defects.

As important as preventing complications is to know how to recognize and solve them when they occurred. In the event of postoperative CSF leak at this location, patients not always present with rhinorrhea; given the low location of the skull base defect, they may present with a constant postnasal drip or just with an increase of intracranial pneumocephalus. Once recognized, it is important to perform an MRI to evaluate the vascularization of the flap and assess for other complications, and conduct a lumbar puncture for diagnosis of meningitis. In cases of nasoseptal flap necrosis or absence, an ideal alternative that we have used with success is the combination of fascia lata with a lateral nasal wall/inferior turbinate vascularized flap.

10.1.6 Technical Nuances

The patient's head is fixed with a Mayfield holder in neutral or slightly flexed position. The head is slightly rotated toward the surgeon. The nasal septal flap is elevated from the contralateral side of the main part of the tumor or from the most favorable side if there is prominent septal deviation. The pedicle vessels, posterior nasal artery and branches, should be well protected, and the vascular pedicle should be properly mobilized without narrowing it excessively. The exposure extends from the floor of sphenoid sinus superiorly to the C1 anterior arch inferiorly. The maxillary crest is drilled down to facilitate binarial and inferior maximal access. The mucosal and muscular layers are elevated together from the inferior clivus by a combination of needle-tip cautery for muscle detachment and blunt dissection for muscle elevation. There are two tight muscular insertion lines on the inferior clivus: the superior clival line and inferior clival line. The former correlates with the insertion line of the longus capitis muscle, representing the level of the pharyngeal tubercle; the latter is formed by the insertion line of the rectus capitis anterior muscle, which laterally forms the supracondylar groove representing the level of the hypoglossal canal. These two lines are useful landmarks in the approach and represent the equivalent of the superior and inferior nuchal lines for the suboccipital far-lateral approach. The extension of the bony drilling depends on the lesion at hand. The lateral limits of the inferior clival bone drilling are, from superior to inferior, foramen lacerum, petroclival fissure, jugular tubercle, hypoglossal canal, and occipital condyle. The lateral limit of the medial condylectomy can be estimated superficially by an imaginary line extending inferiorly from the junction of petroclival fissure and foramen lacerum, and deeply by the cortical wall of the hypoglossal canal.

10.1.7 Clinical Pearls

- Extended nasoseptal flap is useful for large clival defects.
- Prep the thigh for fascia lata harvesting and the abdomen for fat graft.
- Maxillary antrostomy is needed to store the flap during the operation away from the surgical field.
- Posterior septectomy can be minimized since most of the binarial work is done posteriorly.
- Drilling the maxillary crest is important to obtain more caudal binarial access.
- Sphenoidotomy is typically not necessary for tumors limited to the inferior clivus.
- It is key to remove the fascia and muscle layers widely to reach the petroclival fissure laterally and to identify the lower aspect of foramen lacerum.
- Drilling should include jugular tubercle and medial condyle following the above-described landmarks.
- Ultrasonic bone curette is useful for laterally oriented drilling in these areas.
- A well-done medial condylectomy provides access to the lateral wall of the foramen magnum, involves less than a quarter of the condylar volume, and carries no risk of craniocervical instability.
- The vertebral artery enters the posterior fossa just behind the condyle and can be accessible after a medial condylectomy.
- Wide dural opening is recommended for meningiomas to facilitate recognition of neurovascular structures and extracapsular dissection.
- Microsurgical-like techniques are used for extracapsular dissection only after extensive intracapsular debulking.
- Angled scopes are beneficial to look around corners and identify residual tumor, especially within the hypoglossal canal.

- Extensive dural resection is performed for meningiomas.
- Multilayer reconstruction: inlay collagen layer, onlay fascial lata graft, fat graft reinforcement, and vascularized extended nasoseptal flap plus nasal packing and postoperative lumbar drain (3 days).

Further Reading

[1] Morera VA, Fernandez-Miranda JC, Prevedello DM, et al. "Far-medial" expanded endonasal approach to the inferior third of the clivus: the transcondylar and transjugular tubercle approaches. Neurosurgery. 2010; 66(6) Suppl Operative:211–219, discussion 219–220

[2] Wang WH, Abhinav K, Wang E, Snyderman CH, Gardner PA, Fernandez-Miranda JC. Endoscopic endonasal transclival transcondylar approach for foramen magnum meningiomas: anatomical considerations and technical note. Neurosurgery. 2015

[3] Fernandez-Miranda JC, Morera VA, Snyderman CH, Gardner P. Endoscopic endonasal transclival approach to the jugular tubercle. Neurosurgery. 2012; 71(1) Suppl Operative:146–158, discussion 158–159

[4] Fernandez-Miranda JC, Gardner PA, Snyderman CH, et al. Clival chordomas: A pathological, surgical, and radiotherapeutic review. Head Neck. 2014; 36 (6):892–906

[5] Peris-Celda M, Pinheiro-Neto CD, Funaki T, et al. The extended nasoseptal flap for skull base reconstruction of the clival region: an anatomical and radiological study. J Neurol Surg B Skull Base. 2013; 74(6) B6:369–385

[6] Vaz-Guimaraes Filho F, Fernandez-Miranda JC, Wang EW, Snyderman CH, Gardner PA. Endoscopic endonasal "far-medial" transclival approach: surgical anatomy and technique. Oper Tech Otolaryngol–Head Neck Surg. 2013; 24 (4):222–228

[7] Kooshkabadi A, Choi PA, Koutourousiou M, et al. Atlanto-occipital instability following endoscopic endonasal approach for lower clival lesions: Experience with 212 cases. Neurosurgery. 2015; 77(6):888–897, discussion 897

[8] Pinheiro-Neto CD, Fernandez-Miranda JC, Rivera-Serrano CM, et al. Endoscopic anatomy of the palatovaginal canal (palatosphenoidal canal): a landmark for dissection of the vidian nerve during endonasal transpterygoid approaches. Laryngoscope. 2012; 122(1):6–12

[9] Zhang X, Wang EW, Wei H, et al. Anatomy of the posterior septal artery with surgical implications on the vascularized pedicled nasoseptal flap. Head Neck. 2015; 37(10):1470–1476

[10] Rastelli MM, Jr, Pinheiro-Neto CD, Fernandez-Miranda JC, Wang EW, Snyderman CH, Gardner PA. Application of ultrasonic bone curette in endoscopic endonasal skull base surgery: technical note. J Neurol Surg B Skull Base. 2014; 75(2):90–95

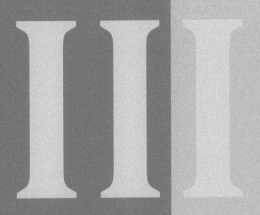

11 Endoscopic Third Ventriculostomy versus Ventriculoperitoneal Shunting

Vijay Agarwal, Helen Quach, Charles Teo

Summary

The treatment of hydrocephalus is complex and potentially fraught with complications. Treatment involves diverting cerebrospinal fluid into natural absorption pathways either cranially or extracranially using shunts. Each carries its own set of advantages and disadvantages. In this chapter, we discuss the utility of cerebrospinal fluid shunting versus endoscopic third ventriculostomy.

Keywords: shunting, ventriculoperitonal, endoscopic third ventriculostomy, cerebrospinal fluid, ventriculostomy

11.1 Introduction

The appropriate treatment of hydrocephalus, in both the pediatric and adult populations, has long plagued neurosurgeons. It is one pathology that unites many disciplines and requires a targeted and comprehensive treatment plan from all involved. Ventriculoperitoneal shunting (VPS) has undergone steady improvements over the decades, including the use of adjustable and magnetic resonance imaging (MRI)-compatible shunts and antibiotic-resistant catheters. Similarly, neuroendoscopy has also improved and benefitted from a technological revolution. From humble beginnings and fringe uses, neuroendoscopy has become a mainstay for specific neurosurgical indications. It is indeed rare nowadays to encounter any major academic center that does not use neuroendoscopy as a mainstay in treatment. However, there exists no widely accepted protocol or consensus on the more appropriate indications of neuroendoscopy versus VPS, especially in terms of oncological management. Our aim is to present the technical nuances, strategic pitfalls, and ideal clinical scenarios for the use of neuroendoscopy versus standard treatment approaches.

11.2 Evolution of Neuroendoscopy

The first neuroendoscopic procedure was performed over a century ago by Victor de L'Éspinasse. Walter Dandy was also a pioneer in the field, having performed the first open and the first endoscopic ventriculostomies.[1,2,3] However, just as it is today, inadequate visualization, poor illumination, and non-versatile instruments impeded functional use. This was until 1936 when Scarff published the results on the use of a versatile endoscope.[4] This modified endoscope was rigged with an irrigation system to maintain the volume of the ventricle. It also featured a moveable mobile cautery tip. Dandy, though the pioneer that he was, surmised that the practice was still limited by difficulty in visualizing and addressing the pathology. It was around this time, in the middle of the 20th century, that ventricular shunting emerged. In 1951, Nulsen and Spitz reported on the diversion of cerebrospinal fluid (CSF) from the ventricles to the jugular vein for communicating hydrocephalus.[5] Due to the rising popularity of ventricular shunting and known problems with neuroendoscopy, endoscopic third ventriculostomy (ETV) would only reemerge

after technological advances to the modern endoscope. These included the development of the self-focusing optic lens, the development of a charge-coupled device allowing for smaller endoscopes, and the introduction of fiberoptic cables. This led to a renaissance of neuroendoscopy and a rising interest in ETV. In 1978, Vries reported on a series of five cases treated with ETV using a fiberoptic endoscope.[6] This report demonstrated the feasibility and the safety of this procedure. The introduction of stereotaxy and familiarity of use led to even greater success rates. More recently, Jones et al helped repopularize ETV with a larger series.[7] Studies have investigated the benefit of ETV over shunting, showing the long-term reliability of ETV.[8]

11.3 Decision-Making Algorithm

11.3.1 Case Example

This is a case of a 24-year-old female administrative assistant who presented with an approximately 10-year history of headaches, nausea, vomiting, and progressive cognitive decline. She reports increased difficulty with concentration while at work. Initial lab workup by her primary care doctor did not reveal any significant abnormalities. On physical exam, she had no focal neurological deficits. An MRI of the brain without contrast revealed increased size of the lateral ventricles and evidence of an infravermian cyst that communicated with the fourth ventricle, suggestive of a Blake's pouch cyst (▸ Fig. 11.1a–c).

The patient was taken to the operating room, and a burr hole was placed on the nondominant side, just anterior to the coronal suture and 3 cm from the midline (▸ Fig. 11.1d, e). In the technique described below, the fornix, the foramen of Monro, and the thalamostriate and septal veins, as well as the choroid plexus passing posteriorly under the roof of the third ventricle, were identified. The floor of the third ventricle was found to be quite thick and double layered. A safe area anterior to the mamillary bodies was identified, and the floor was bluntly entered. Strong, pulsatile flow of CSF was noted after the floor was entered.

Postoperatively, the patient began to have slow improvement in her nausea and general cognitive function.

11.3.2 General Patient Selection

Surgical candidates are chosen on a case-by-case basis, with considerations given to the level of obstruction with noncommunicating hydrocephalus, patient's age, and specific pathology. It is the authors' recommendation to initially consider all patients older than 3 months with noncommunicating hydrocephalus as candidates. The rate of success is very dependent on patient selection. When ETV fails, the primary reason is reduced CSF absorption—specifically, a degree of communicating hydrocephalus. Another common reason for failure is due to closure of the stoma. The vast majority of failures, 60 to 90%, occur in the first few months after treatment; however,

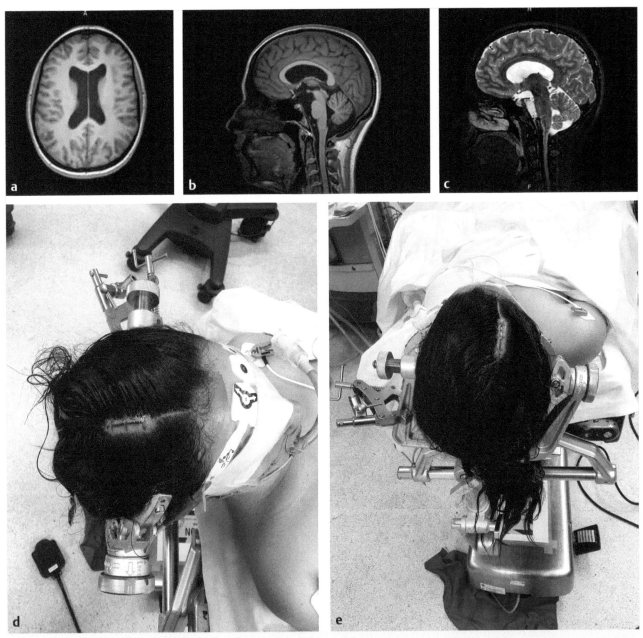

Fig. 11.1 A 24-year-old female presented with headaches, nausea, vomiting, and progressive cognitive decline. Preoperative **(a)** axial and **(b)** sagittal T1 noncontrasted MRI as well as **(c)** sagittal T2 MRI demonstrated ventriculomegaly with an infravermian cyst communicating to the fourth ventricle. Patient was placed in **(d,e)** neutral position.

long-term failures also occur.[9] The mechanism of failure in these long-term cases is unclear. Chances of success have been quantified using the ETV Success Score (ETVSS)[10] (▶ Table 11.1). The ETVSS is derived from three categories: (1) patient age, (2) etiology of hydrocephalus, and (3)

previous shunt score. The total score is calculated as a percentage probability of ETV success. In the authors' experience, positive prognostic factors include a biconvex third ventricle (▶ Fig. 11.2) and a downward bowing of the third ventricular floor (▶ Fig. 11.3).

Table 11.1 Endoscopic third ventriculostomy success scoring system

Score	Age	Etiology	Prior Shunt
0	< 1 mo	Postinfectious	Previous shunt
10	1 mo to < 6 mo		No previous shunt
20		Myelomeningocele, IVH, nontectal brain tumor	
30	6 mo to < 1 y	Aqueductal stenosis, tectal tumor, others	
40	1 y to < 10 y		
50	> 10 y		

Abbreviation: IVH, intraventricular hemorrhage.

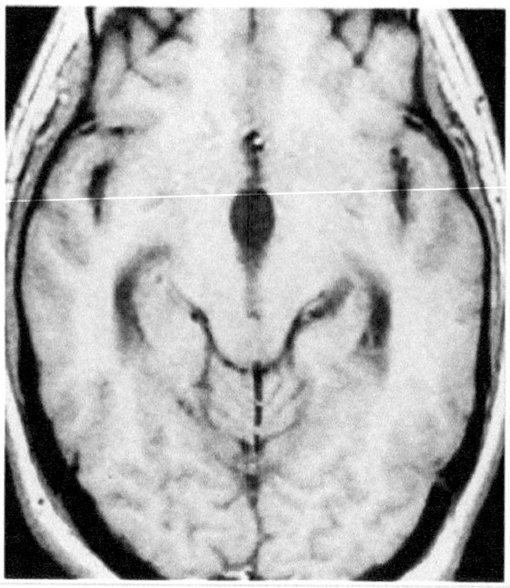

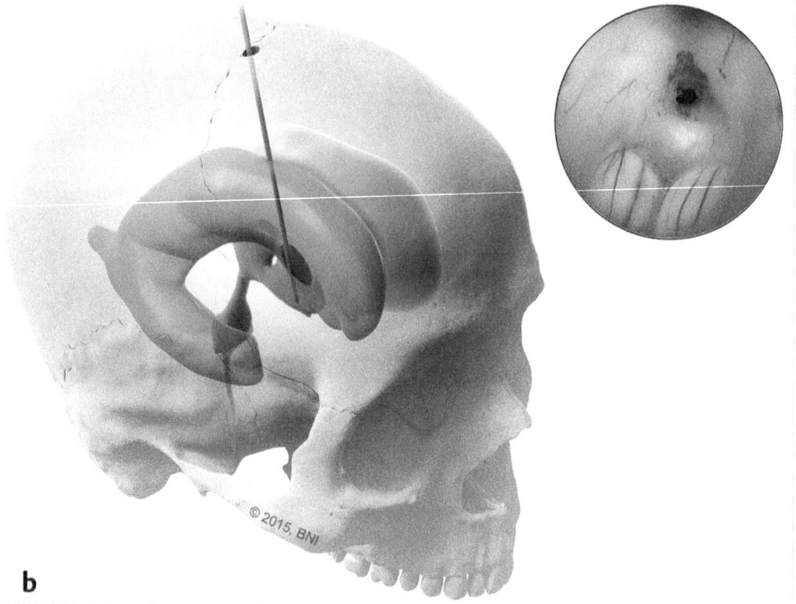

Fig. 11.2 (a) Axial noncontrasted MRI demonstrating a biconvex third ventricle, a positive prognostic indicator. (b) The trajectory for an endoscopic third ventriculostomy and the membrane of Liliequist (inset). (b, Used with permission from Barrow Neurological Institute, Phoenix, AZ.)

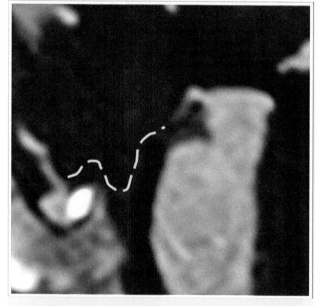

Fig. 11.3 Sagittal MRI demonstrating downward-bowing third ventricle, a positive prognostic indicator.

11.3.3 Etiology

Patients with acquired aqueductal stenosis have traditionally been the most ideal candidates. Their obstruction is distal to the anterior third ventricle, and they clearly have normal absorptive pathways. The impaired flow of CSF from the third to the fourth ventricle in these patients is often best studied via a T2-weighted midsagittal MRI. Specific signs indicative of acquired or congenital aqueductal stenosis include downward bulging of the floor of the third ventricle, enlargement of the suprapineal recess, a flattened mesencephalon, and "funneling" within the upper portion of the aqueduct with a normal-sized fourth ventricle (the "trumpet" sign). Although some authors believe that even patients with communicating hydrocephalus may improve with an ETV, the more commonly held belief is that a patient with true communicating hydrocephalus would be better served with a VPS.

11.3.4 Tumors

The most common cause of acquired noncommunicating hydrocephalus is a tumor obstructing CSF flow at the level of

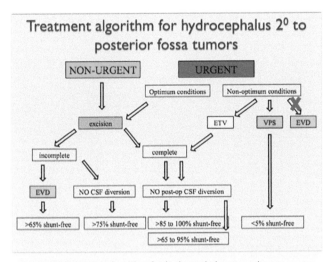

Fig. 11.4 Treatment algorithm for hydrocephalus secondary to posterior fossa tumors.

the cerebral aqueduct. Examples include tectal hamartomas and gliomas, pineal tumors, and other tumors of the posterior fossa. Of course, patients with tumors causing obstruction proximal to the anterior third ventricle such as a colloid cyst are not candidates for ETV. However, the most controversial issue is the role of ETV and VPS in the surgical management of hydrocephalus secondary to a neoplasm. Unfortunately, the literature is ambiguous and surgical algorithms vary from shunting all patients to shunting none. The senior author (C.T.) has been required to place a VPS in only two patients in a 25-year career in pediatric neurosurgical oncology by following the algorithm outlined below.

11.3.5 Surgical Algorithm for the Management of Hydrocephalus Secondary to a Tumor

All patients with asymptomatic hydrocephalus secondary to a tumor are scheduled electively for tumor removal. Steroids are commenced 48 hours before surgery. All patients who present with symptomatic hydrocephalus secondary to a tumor are admitted to the hospital and taken to the operating room for definitive removal of the tumor as soon as possible (▸ Fig. 11.4,

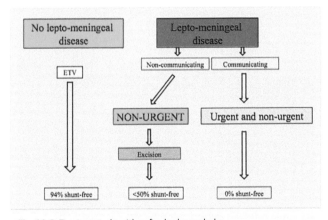

Fig. 11.6 Treatment algorithm for hydrocephalus.

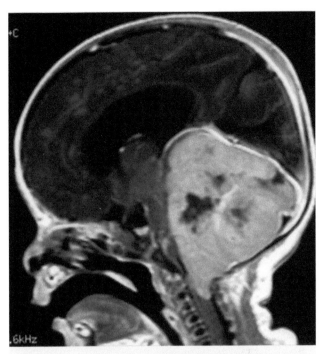

Fig. 11.5 Sagittal gadolinium-enhanced MRI demonstrating a large posterior fossa mass with resultant obstructive hydrocephalus.

▸ Fig. 11.5). Unless the patient is in extremis, he/she is placed on oral or intravenous (IV) steroids, close neurological observation in a high dependency ward or intensive care unit, nil oral intake, reduced IV fluids, absolutely no narcotics, and with the head of the bed 30 degrees to the horizontal plane.

All patients who present in extremis from hydrocephalus and who have a tumor that is relatively uncomplicated and not requiring further preoperative evaluation are taken to the operating room urgently for tumor removal. An example of this would be a small colloid cyst. Any other patient in extremis is taken to the operating room urgently for immediate CSF diversion, either an urgent ETV or an urgent placement of a ventricular drain (▸ Fig. 11.6). An example of when we would recommend an urgent ETV would be a child with a posterior fossa medulloblastoma requiring a preoperative spinal MRI or a difficult pineal tumor that should not be done at 2 am. An example of when we would recommend an urgent ventricular drain would be an intra-axial tumor filling the anterior third ventricle or a huge posterior fossa tumor that obliterates the interpeduncular cistern and prevents an ETV.

Some series demonstrate a significantly higher rate of shunt dependency in patients with tumor-related hydrocephalus. Possible explanations include the following:

- Diverting CSF before definitive tumor removal may increase the incidence of permanent aqueductal obstruction (the concept of secondary aqueductal stenosis).
- Incomplete tumor resection may not reestablish CSF pathways.
- Leaving an external ventricular drain in the ventricle after tumor resection effectively drains the CSF, which deflects CSF from flowing along the normal pathways and allows scar tissue/gliosis to create permanent obstruction.
- In many developing countries, patients present late in their disease with secondary meningeal involvement resulting in an absorptive problem.

- Other reasons for the patient to have a communicating hydrocephalus include chronic raised intracranial pressure (ICP), radiation, multiple craniotomies, infection, or protein-secreting tumors.
- Some tumors cause an overproduction of CSF, such as a choroid plexus papilloma and carcinoma.

11.3.6 Chiari Malformation

Hydrocephalus affects 7 to 10% of those patients with Chiari type 1 malformation. Traditional treatment has included VPS. Recent studies have suggested that ETV is a durable and viable primary treatment modality for this condition).[11,12] In patients with Chiari type 2 malformation associated with myelomeningocele, 80 to 90% will require treatment for hydrocephalus.[13] In selected patients, mostly based on anatomical suitability on imaging, these patients will enjoy a 70% success rate. In those patients deemed unsuitable for ETV, such as those with a large interthalamic adhesion, previous meningitis, and infants younger than 6 months, insertion of a VPS is a reasonable alternative.

11.3.7 Hemorrhage

Subarachnoid and intraventricular hemorrhage (IVH) may result in hydrocephalus. This is due to impaired absorption from the arachnoid granulation tissue and, in rare cases, acquired aqueduct stenosis. ETV has been proposed as a treatment option in this scenario, although results have been variable. Clearly, the mechanism of action is not as simple as bypassing an obstruction, and one of the theories behind its success is that an ETV dampens the pulse pressure. In any case, ETV should be reserved for those patients with triventricular hydrocephalus, diminished CSF spaces over the hemispheres, and downward bowing of the third ventricle.

11.3.8 Postinfectious

The cause of postinfective hydrocephalus is not dissimilar to hemorrhage. In most cases, the infection creates scar tissue in the subarachnoid space and results in a communication problem. However, intraventricular infection may cause scarring in the aqueduct, foramen of Monro, and exit foramina of the fourth ventricle resulting in a noncommunicating-type hydrocephalus. Similar to posthemorrhagic hydrocephalus, the treatment depends on the imaging characteristics. Success rates remain low in cases of infants with postinfectious hydrocephalus treated with ETV.[14,15] Failure of ETV in these instances is thought to be due to thickening of the leptomeninges and third ventricular floor from scarring.[16,17,18]

11.3.9 Idiopathic Normal Pressure Hydrocephalus

In cases of idiopathic normal pressure hydrocephalus, impaired CSF flow is due to abnormalities in ventricular compliance as opposed to mechanical obstruction. In light of this, VPS remains the traditional treatment option. However, studies have shown good efficacy from ETV in some instances. Gangemi et al

reported improvement of 69.1% of patients, with no change in 21.8% and continued deterioration in 9.1%.[19] It should be noted that this study may give a false assurance of the efficacy of ETV as the authors did not make the distinction between those patients with true normal pressure hydrocephalus and LOVA (long-standing overt ventriculomegaly of adulthood).

11.3.10 Age

Studies have found age to be the best predictor of success for ETV. Patients younger than 1 year have a higher chance of failure, and those younger than 1 month have an even higher rate of failure.[10,20] These age ranges impart the lowest scores in calculation of the ETVSS.

11.3.11 Contraindications to ETV

Relative contraindications include age less than 6 months, a prohibitively small third ventricle, presumed communicating hydrocephalus, previous history of infection, thickened third ventricular floor, and abnormal third ventricular anatomy on imaging. However, these are relative contraindications. Patients with these conditions are increasingly presented in the literature with positive outcomes from ETV. Alternative options should be considered in patients with a large massa intermedia, such as those with spina bifida (▶ Fig. 11.7), those with an

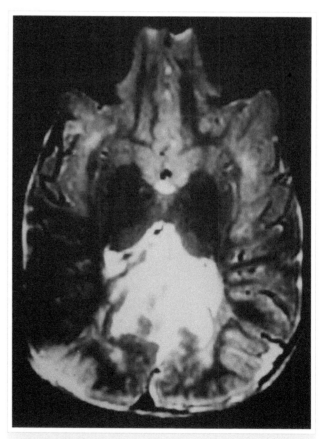

Fig. 11.7 Axial T2 MRI demonstrating hydrocephalus pattern in a patient with spina bifida.

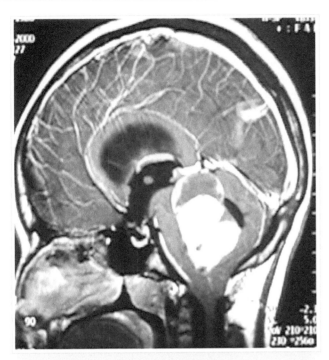

Fig. 11.8 Sagittal T1 gadolinium-enhanced MRI demonstrating a large posterior fossa tumor with resultant effaced interpeduncular cisterns.

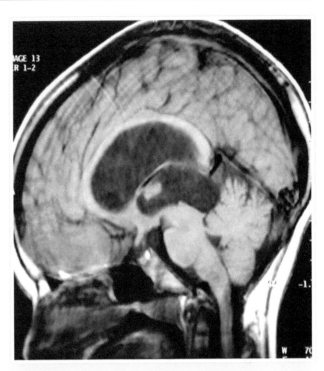

Fig. 11.9 Sagittal T1 unenhanced MRI demonstrating a thickened third ventricular floor.

effaced interpeduncular cistern (▶ Fig. 11.8), and those with a thickened floor (▶ Fig. 11.9). Also, care should be taken in patients with obstruction above the third ventricle, distal to the interpeduncular cistern, or no clear obstruction on preoperative imaging, as the utility of ETV is limited. In the authors' experience, negative prognosticators include patients who are post-meningitis, tumor with meningeal involvement, post-IVH of prematurity, and any history of infection.

11.4 Complication Avoidance

ETV carries with it a morbidity rate in the range of 6 to 21%, and an abort rate between 0.4 and 26%.[21] Mortality from complications is rare, but is most often associated with subarachnoid hemorrhage from damage to the basilar complex or late failure.[22]

It is important to recognize that bradycardia and rarely asystole may occur secondary to manipulation of the third ventricle. This can happen with unchecked irrigation into the third ventricle as a result of the scope itself blocking egress of fluid from both foramina of Monro. It may also occur from pressure on an unforgiving third ventricular floor. Care must be taken to consistently check cardiac monitoring, use warmed lactated ringers solution to irrigate, ensure that irrigation channels are clear to allow the egress of fluid, and avoid excessive traction on the floor and subsequently the walls of the hypothalamus. The best way to manage this problem is to have the anesthesiologist turn up the volume of the electrocardiogram (ECG) machine with commencement of the operation.

Excessive traction on the hypothalamus can lead to other serious complications, including diabetes insipidus, hyperphagia, loss of thirst, amenorrhea, hyperkalemia, hyponatremia, and even death.[23,24,25,26,27] Often times, complications are temporary. The normal third ventricular floor consists of a thin median raphe, void of neural pathways, and the hypothalamus. Hence, theoretically, the thinned-out floor observed with hydrocephalus consists of stretched functional neural tissue and therefore it becomes imperative to try to avoid placement of the stoma anywhere but in the midline. With this in mind, a common problem with ETV is when the surgeon places the stoma through the thinnest part of the floor. Although this is tempting, the thinnest part may be behind the basilar bifurcation/tip and therefore unsafe. The safest zone for the placement of the hole is anterior to the underlying vascular complex, posterior to the infundibular recess, posterior to the dorsum sella, and in the midline. When the floor is opaque and the underlying structures are invisible, the best way to estimate the safe zone is by dividing the floor between the infundibular recess anteriorly and the mammillary bodies posteriorly, into thirds. The safest zone is between the anterior and middle third. Care should also be taken in consideration of instruments for floor fenestration (see Technique section below).

Damage to the fornices is one of the most common complications encountered.[28,29] This most often occurs with movement of the endoscope from the lateral to the third ventricle, within the third ventricle, or its removal from the third ventricle. Damage to the fornices can result in memory impairment, with bilateral damage resulting in greater impairment. It can also occur when the lateral ventricle is initially cannulated or when the contralateral ventricle is erroneously entered instead of the third ventricle. Techniques to avoid forniceal injury include accurate burr hole placement, using a standard brain needle to enter into the ventricle versus directly with an endoscope, choosing an endoscope with a smaller diameter if encountering a small foramen of Monro, and taking care when using a flexible endoscope to return to the neutral position before removal.

Perhaps, vascular injury is the most feared complication. This occurs when the basilar artery or its branches are violated. Though rare, it can have devastating consequences. There is an increased risk of injury if the floor of the third ventricle is opaque or is entered too posteriorly, or if there is imprecise enlargement of the stoma. However, the most common error that results in vascular injury is the technique by which the surgeon penetrates the floor. This is arguably the most controversial aspect of ETV. Almost every "sharp" technique has resulted in basilar artery injury. "Sharp" techniques to penetrate the floor include the use of closed grabbing forceps, monopolar and bipolar coagulation devices, stylets, a Fogarty balloon catheter with the stylet within its lumen, laser probes, and other instruments that may be passed down the working channel of the endoscope. Given the devastating consequences of a basilar artery injury and the very uncommon permanent complications of traction on the floor of the third ventricle, the senior author strongly recommends a blunter technique (see Technique section below). Using an endoscopic sheath with smooth, rather than sharp, walls may also prevent damage to surrounding vessels. Another safe tactic includes placing the sloping face of the angled scope posteriorly when entering the floor so that the branches of the basilar artery can be pushed safely away in the event the bifurcation is encountered. In general, minor hemorrhage can be controlled by gentle irrigation, but can rarely result in procedure abortion. This is most often due to damage of ependymal vessels upon entry into the third ventricle. It is important that in the case of visual obstruction the surgical instruments are minimally moved, as surrounding structures are easily injured. Using a small brain needle to tap the ventricles before insertion of the sheath is advisable to avoid injury from passing a large endoscope sheath into surrounding eloquent brain. If hemorrhage occurs, as mentioned, irrigate gently and generously. If this fails, consider tamponading the source of bleeding with the endoscope or directly coagulating the bleeding vessel. As a last resort, the CSF can be briefly removed from the ventricles and replaced with air to allow for easier visualization and coagulation. Major vascular damage includes direct trauma to the basilar artery or its branches, subarachnoid, intraventricular, or intracerebral hemorrhage, pseudoaneurysm formation at the basilar tip, and arterial or venous infarcts, all of which may require immediate cessation of the procedure.[30,31]

CSF leaks can be due to raised ICP, but also due to failure of the ETV.[23] This can be avoided by wound closure in a layered fashion, and the use of Gelfoam to plug the cortical opening.[22,28] Care must be taken not to allow the Gelfoam to enter into the ventricular system.

Subdural hygromas are a rarely reported complication of ETV, and are likely to occur more commonly than they are reported.[32,33] They are observed more frequently when a large diameter endoscope is used. Proposed mechanisms include the rapid loss of CSF causing collapse of the cortical mantle and subsequent widening of the subdural space into which CSF can collect.[30] Blood in the subdural space can also occur due to loss of CSF and brain collapse. Subdural hematomas are usually small in size, but occasionally are large and symptomatic.[34] These complications can be avoided by expanding the ventricles before removing the sheath from the lateral ventricle, placing Gelfoam into the cortical opening, avoiding lumbar and ventricular drainage postoperatively, and ensuring hemostasis before closure.

Cranial neuropathies due to ETV are also a rare complication. When encountered, usually the oculomotor and abducens nerves are affected.[30] These nerves can be compressed when the floor is pushed downward, but they mostly occur when the instrumentation deviates off the midline. Care must be taken to not excessively stretch the floor upon entering and to not enter too deeply past the floor. It is the authors' recommendation to make an impression on the floor of the third ventricle before perforating to be able to visualize where the stoma will be placed.

Other complications include perioperative fever (commonly due to blood in the ventricles), ventriculitis, seizures, infection, and intracerebral hemorrhage.

11.5 Technical Nuances/Clinical Pearls

11.5.1 Preoperative Planning

Planning should be based on the study of MRI imaging with cine sequences to identify the location of obstruction and the basilar artery with respect to the third ventricle.[22]

The surgical equipment required is composed of several components, including an endoscope within a sheath with light source, the endoscope tower, and an irrigation source with warmed Ringer's solution, as well as endoscopic-specific instrumentation, including an instrument for fenestration of the floor of the third ventricle if necessary and a balloon catheter for enlarging the stoma. Three types of endoscopes are available to choose from, based on operator preference (▶ Table 11.2). The video/control tower consists of a high-definition camera unit, a low-heat-generating light source (usually xenon), a digital recording device, and an irrigation unit (although the senior author prefers manual irrigation). The surgeon and staff should be familiarized with the equipment, and make sure it is in working order before starting the procedure. If one is to use a balloon catheter to expand the stoma, it is good practice to check that the balloon inflates before inserting the scope into the patient. The placement of equipment is important to ensure an unobstructed view for the surgeon. The monitor should be placed directly in front of the surgeon and operating staff to allow clear visualization. The patient is placed supine with their head placed on a horseshoe headrest in a neutral position and elevated 30 degrees to the horizontal plane. A Mayfield clamp may be used for neuronavigation purposes, but is not preferred by the authors.

Table 11.2 Advantages and disadvantages of the three different endoscopes currently in use

Rigid endoscope	Semi-flexible	Flexible
Wide angle view	Less wide angled than rigid scope	Small diameter
Best quality of vision Image can be magnified without losing resolution Instruments can be passed through	Intermediate resolution between rigid and flexible scopes	Lower quality of image May be difficult to pass instruments through Resolution decreases with higher magnifications
Can only be used for targets in a straight trajectory from the site of insertion		Operator can look around corners

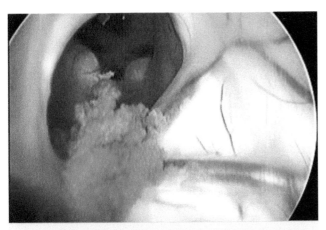

Fig. 11.10 Endoscopic view demonstrating major anatomical landmarks of the lateral ventricle, including the fornix, the foramen of Monro, and the thalamostriate and septal veins.

11.5.2 Irrigation

Close monitoring and maintenance of irrigation is essential for successful ETV. Irrigation not only maintains the ventricle size, but also is required to control minor bleeding and maintain visibility. Ringer's solution warmed to 36 °C should be used. A channel for egress of fluid should be clear and constantly monitored to avoid increased ICP. This is particularly important when the scope is within the third ventricle, where the scope can obstruct the foramen of Monro and raised ICP can lead to bradycardia and asystole.[35] If continuous irrigation is used, the flow rate should be less than 15 mL/minute.

11.5.3 Technique

The location of the burr hole is generally placed on the nondominant side, just anterior to the coronal suture and 3 cm from the midline. The dura is sharply opened in a cruciate fashion and the edges coagulated; then the pia is opened and bleeding is controlled. A brain needle is placed into the ventricle, followed by the scope within a sheath along the same tract. At this point, major landmarks should be identified including the fornix, the

foramen of Monro, and the thalamostriate and septal veins (▸ Fig. 11.10). The choroid plexus will be found projecting forward to the foramen and then passing posteriorly to lie under the roof of the third ventricle (▸ Fig. 11.10). Once the third ventricle is entered, the lateral walls of the anterior thalamus and hypothalamus will be visualized. They are joined by the massa intermedia. Posteriorly will be the pineal body, the habenular commissure, the posterior commissure, and the cerebral aqueduct (▸ Fig. 11.11), although with the anteriorly pointing trajectory, one should not be able to visualize these structures. Gentle irrigation should be used to clear hemorrhages if they occur, with the use of bipolar cautery if necessary. In an anterior-to-posterior direction, the following structures are identified: lamina terminalis, optic chiasm, infundibular recess, tuber cinereum, thinned-out floor, mammillary bodies, and the posterior perforated substance. On average, in an adult the foramen of Monro is approximately 6 cm from the dura mater via this approach. The safe zone in the third ventricle for perforation is identified, anterior to the mammillary bodies, and the underlying basilar tip is visible through the transparent floor and just posterior to the infundibular recess. Care is taken to identify and avoid the basilar artery, located just anterior and inferior to the mammillary bodies (▸ Fig. 11.12). Targeting perforation just posterior to the infundibular recess helps avoid the basilar complex below the floor. Perforation of the floor is completed using the scope itself. The authors use a 30-degree scope which has a pointed end and a sloping face. The pointed end is anterior, with the sloping face looking posteriorly. If the floor is thick and unforgiving and traction results in bradycardia or if the interpeduncular space is limited and does not allow the passage of a 4-mm scope, then the authors recommend a "sharper" technique such as initial perforation with a blunt instrument such as grabbing forceps, followed by balloon dilatation of the stoma with 0.2 mL of fluid. An example of such a balloon is a no. 3 French Fogarty balloon catheter. The stoma is widened to greater than 4 mm, as small holes do close over time (▸ Fig. 11.13). The authors prefer not to advance the balloon below the floor or to pull back while the balloon is inflated. Advancement into the interpeduncular cistern should be limited to avoid damage to the basilar complex, its branches, and the oculomotor nerve. An endoscope is passed into the cistern for better visualization. Arachnoid bands or an imperforated

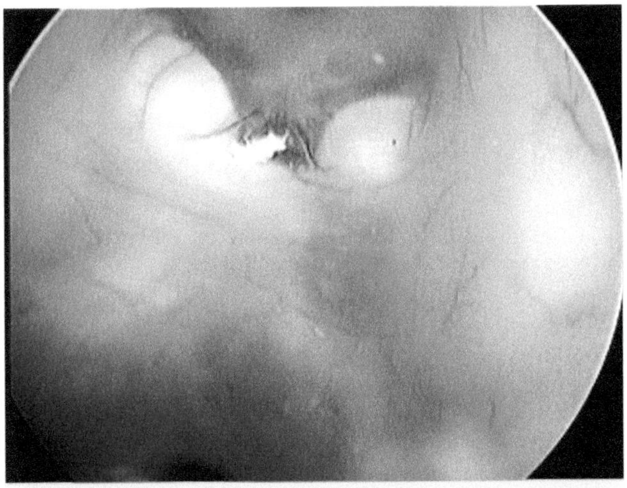

Fig. 11.11 A posterior endoscopic view demonstrating the pineal body, the habenular commissure, the posterior commissure, and the cerebral aqueduct.

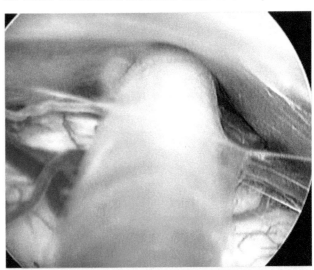

Fig. 11.12 Endoscopic view demonstrating the basilar artery, located just anterior and inferior to the mammillary bodies.

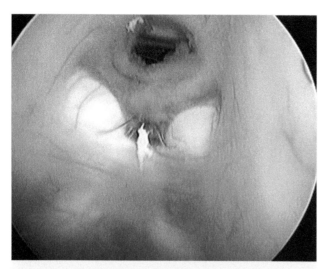

Fig. 11.13 Endoscopic view demonstrating the ventriculostomy enlarged using a number 3 French Fogarty balloon.

Table 11.3 Rate of endoscopic third ventriculostomy patency as related to age

Age	n	Patency rates
<1 mo	13	0%
1–6 mo	19	41%
6 mo to 2 y	22	58%
2–15 y	50	78%
15–30 y	38	79%
>30 y	42	71%

membrane of Liliequist can be bluntly dissected. Examine for pulsatile flow indicative of good CSF egress. Ensure clear hemostasis. The parenchymal hole is plugged with a piece of Gelfoam as is the burr hole opening. The incision is closed in a layered fashion. In the event of intraoperative bleeding or previous shunt, some surgeons prefer the use of an extraventricular drain. Drainage is also utilized in cases of bleeding to prevent clot formation. When used in a patient with a previous shunt, it is recommended to gradually increase the pressure setting and monitor ICP and clinical status. The authors do not prefer the routine placement of an extraventricular drain postoperatively.

11.5.4 Postoperative Monitoring

Observation in an intensive care setting for 24 hours is recommended. Postoperative CT scans can be taken, but often continued ventriculomegaly can be detected in the early postoperative period as CSF pathways may take several weeks to reestablish.[28] Postoperative MRI should be obtained within 2 months of the procedure to observe for resolution of hydrocephalus or transependymal flow, and patients should be monitored for signs of failure to ensure symptomatic improvement.[22,23] A flow void in the third ventricle can often be seen. An MRI with cine sequences can help better visualize CSF flow, but in the authors' experience MRI imaging is not a reliable tool, as it depends on many variables, including the placement of region of interest, end-tidal CO_2 and continuous positive airway pressure, and techniques of acquisition. As mentioned, long-term follow-up is mandatory, as ETV is more prone to fail than VPS in the first 3 months, but then has been shown to have a clear advantage over VPS.[36]

11.6 Authors' Institutional Experience

In a study from the authors' home institution, 205 consecutive patients were included who had an ETV as long as 22.6 years earlier.[8] There were 21 intraoperative failures (10%).

The ETV was presumed to have failed if it was revised, a shunt was inserted, or the patient died from hydrocephalus. The etiology of the hydrocephalus included 80 patients with primary aqueductal stenosis, 35 patients with secondary aqueductal stenosis, 30 patients with myelomeningocele, 26 patients with infection or IVH, and 7 with other causes. A total of 68 patients were previously shunted. ▸ Table 11.3 shows 5-year patency as a function of age. ▸ Fig. 11.14 plots the reliability of the 184 surgically successful ETV procedures stratified according to age group. After adjustment for age, the following factors did not significantly affect long-term patency: a prior history of shunt insertion ($n = 68$), previous shunt infection ($n = 12$), surgeon, surgical method, or pathogenesis of hydrocephalus. Complications were noted in 11.2%. Serious complications were noted in five patients (2.4%).

11.7 Final Thoughts/Expert Recommendations

Third ventriculostomy is increasingly becoming accepted as an effective option for noncommunicating hydrocephalus. In our experience, even patients with complex shunt histories may become shunt-free following ETV. It is of utmost importance to impart careful patient selection, but all patients with

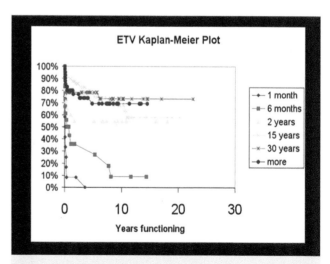

Fig. 11.14 Plot of the reliability of the 184 surgically successful ETV procedures stratified according to age group.

noncommunicating hydrocephalus should initially be considered. Important points include the following:

- Preoperative imaging should show noncommunicating hydrocephalus.
- Surgical technique should avoid thermal or sharp perforation of the floor.
- Floor perforation should maintain midline approach, and ensure adequate size of the stoma (greater than 4 mm).
- Adequate postoperative time should be given for the CSF pathways to open.
- Clinical, and not necessarily radiological, improvement is the goal of treatment.
- Success from selected patients should be > 70%.
- Long-term follow-up is essential as late failures are well documented.

References

[1] Dandy WE. Extirpation of the choroid plexus of the lateral ventricles in communicating hydrocephalus. Ann Surg. 1918; 68(6):569–579

[2] Dandy W. An operative procedure for hydrocephalus. Bull Johns Hopkins Hosp. 1922; 33:189–190

[3] Dandy W. Surgery of the Brain. Hagerstown, MD: W.F. Prior Co.; 1945

[4] Scarff JE. Endoscopic treatment of hydrocephalus: Description of a ventriculoscope and preliminary report of cases. Arch Neurol Psychiatry. 1936; 35 (4):853–861

[5] Nulsen FE, Spitz EB. Treatment of hydrocephalus by direct shunt from ventricle to jugular vein. Surg Forum. 1951; •••:399–403

[6] Vries JK. An endoscopic technique for third ventriculostomy. Surg Neurol. 1978; 9(3):165–168

[7] Jones RF, Stening WA, Brydon M. Endoscopic third ventriculostomy. Neurosurgery. 1990; 26(1):86–91, discussion 91–92

[8] Kadrian D, van Gelder J, Florida D, et al. Long-term reliability of endoscopic third ventriculostomy. Neurosurgery. 2005; 56(6):1271–1278, discussion 1278

[9] Vulcu S, Tschabitscher M, Mueller-Forell W, Oertel J. Transventricular fenestration of the lamina terminalis: the value of a flexible endoscope: technical note. J Neurol Surg A Cent Eur Neurosurg. 2014; 75(3):207–216

[10] Durnford AJ, Kirkham FJ, Mathad N, Sparrow OC. Endoscopic third ventriculostomy in the treatment of childhood hydrocephalus: validation of a success score that predicts long-term outcome. J Neurosurg Pediatr. 2011; 8(5): 489–493

[11] Massimi L, Pravatà E, Tamburrini G, et al. Endoscopic third ventriculostomy for the management of Chiari I and related hydrocephalus: outcome and pathogenetic implications. Neurosurgery. 2011; 68(4):950–956

[12] Hayhurst C, Osman-Farah J, Das K, Mallucci C. Initial management of hydrocephalus associated with Chiari malformation Type I–syringomyelia complex via endoscopic third ventriculostomy: an outcome analysis. J Neurosurg. 2008; 108(6):1211–1214

[13] McLone DG. Care of the neonate with a myelomeningocele. Neurosurg Clin N Am. 1998; 9(1):111–120

[14] Baldauf J, Fritsch MJ, Oertel J, Gaab MR, Schröder H. Value of endoscopic third ventriculostomy instead of shunt revision. Minim Invasive Neurosurg. 2010; 53(4):159–163

[15] Baldauf J, Oertel J, Gaab MR, Schroeder HW. Endoscopic third ventriculostomy in children younger than 2 years of age. Childs Nerv Syst. 2007; 23 (6):623–626

[16] Constantini S, Siomin V. Re: Death after late failure of endoscopic third ventriculostomy: a potential solution. Neurosurgery. 2005; 56(3):E629

[17] Siomin V, Cinalli G, Grotenhuis A, et al. Endoscopic third ventriculostomy in patients with cerebrospinal fluid infection and/or hemorrhage. J Neurosurg. 2002; 97(3):519–524

[18] Siomin V, Constantini S. Endoscopic third ventriculostomy in tuberculous meningitis. Childs Nerv Syst. 2003; 19(5)(–)(6):269

[19] Gangemi M, Maiuri F, Naddeo M, et al. Endoscopic third ventriculostomy in idiopathic normal pressure hydrocephalus: an Italian multicenter study. Neurosurgery. 2008; 63(1):62–67, discussion 67–69

[20] Kulkarni AV, Drake JM, Kestle JR, Mallucci CL, Sgouros S, Constantini S, Canadian Pediatric Neurosurgery Study Group. Predicting who will benefit from endoscopic third ventriculostomy compared with shunt insertion in childhood hydrocephalus using the ETV Success Score. J Neurosurg Pediatr. 2010; 6(4):310–315

[21] Iantosca MR, Hader WJ, Drake JM. Results of endoscopic third ventriculostomy. Neurosurg Clin N Am. 2004; 15(1):67–75

[22] Recinos PFJG, Recinos VR. Endoscopic third ventriculostomy. In: Quinones-Hinojosa, ed. Schmidek and Sweet: Operative Neurosurgical Techniques. 6 ed. Philadelphia, PA: Elsevier Health Sciences; 2012:1143–1150

[23] Hader WJ, Walker RL, Myles ST, Hamilton M. Complications of endoscopic third ventriculostomy in previously shunted patients. Neurosurgery. 2008; 63(1) Suppl 1:ONS168–ONS174, discussion ONS174–ONS175

[24] Teo C. Third ventriculostomy in the treatment of hydrocephalus: experience with more than 120 cases. In: Hellwig D, Bauer BL, eds. Minimally Invasive Techniques for Neurosurgery: Current Status and Future Perspectives. Berlin: Springer; 1998:73–76

[25] Pierre-Kahn A, Renier D, Bombois B, Askienay S, Moreau R, Hirsch JF. Role of the ventriculocisternostomy in the treatment of non-communicating hydrocephalus [in French]. Neurochirurgie. 1975; 21(7):557–569

[26] Vaicys C, Fried A. Transient hyponatriemia complicated by seizures after endoscopic third ventriculostomy. Minim Invasive Neurosurg. 2000; 43(4):190–191

[27] Anandh B, Madhusudan Reddy KR, Mohanty A, Umamaheswara Rao GS, Chandramouli BA. Intraoperative bradycardia and postoperative hyperkalemia in patients undergoing endoscopic third ventriculostomy. Minim Invasive Neurosurg. 2002; 45(3):154–157

[28] Teo C. Complications of endoscopic third ventriculostomy. In: Cinalli G, Sainte-Rose C, Maixner WJ, eds. Pediatric Hydrocephalus. Milano: Springer Milan; 2005:411–420

[29] Schroeder HW, Gaab MR. Intracranial endoscopy. Neurosurg Focus. 1999; 6(4):e1

[30] Schroeder HW, Niendorf WR, Gaab MR. Complications of endoscopic third ventriculostomy. J Neurosurg. 2002; 96(6):1032–1040

[31] McLaughlin MR, Wahlig JB, Kaufmann AM, Albright AL. Traumatic basilar aneurysm after endoscopic third ventriculostomy: case report. Neurosurgery. 1997; 41(6):1400–1403, discussion 1403–1404

[32] Freudenstein D, Wagner A, Ernemann U, Duffner F. Subdural hygroma as a complication of endoscopic neurosurgery–two case reports. Neurol Med Chir (Tokyo). 2002; 42(12):554–559

[33] Wiewrodt D, Schumacher R, Wagner W. Hygromas after endoscopic third ventriculostomy in the first year of life: incidence, management and outcome in a series of 34 patients. Childs Nerv Syst. 2008; 24(1):57–63

[34] Mohanty A, Anandh B, Reddy MS, Sastry KV. Contralateral massive acute subdural collection after endoscopic third ventriculostomy - a case report. Minim Invasive Neurosurg. 1997; 40(2):59–61

[35] Cinalli G. Endoscopic third ventriculostomy. In: Cinalli G, Sainte-Rose C, Maixner WJ, eds. Pediatric Hydrocephalus. Milano: Springer Milan; 2005:361–388

[36] Kulkarni AV, Drake JM, Mallucci CL, Sgouros S, Roth J, Constantini S, Canadian Pediatric Neurosurgery Study Group. Endoscopic third ventriculostomy in the treatment of childhood hydrocephalus. J Pediatr. 2009; 155(2):254–9.e1

12 Management of Colloid Cysts: Moderator

Tatsuhiro Fujii and Gabriel Zada

Summary

Colloid cysts are nonneoplastic epithelial masses that may cause obstruction of the cerebrospinal fluid flow pathways, thereby resulting in obstructive (noncommunicating) hydrocephalus. When treatment is indicated, surgical intervention remains the mainstay as there are no viable medical or radiosurgery-based options. Historically, surgical treatment of colloid cysts involves a wide variety of approaches and techniques, ranging from simple cyst fenestration or aspiration to full cyst excision, and from minimally invasive stereotactic or endoscopic approaches to traditional open microsurgical craniotomy for cyst excision. In this chapter, we discuss the advantages and pitfalls of endoscopic versus microsurgical approaches in the treatment of colloid cysts.

Keywords: colloid cyst, third ventricle, transcortical, interhemispheric, transcallosal, intraventricular, neuroendoscopy, stereotactic

12.1 Introduction

Colloid cysts are nonneoplastic epithelial masses that typically arise from the roof of the third ventricle near the foramen of Monro.[1] Although often asymptomatic and discovered incidentally, colloid cysts may cause obstruction of the cerebrospinal fluid flow pathways, thereby resulting in obstructive (noncommunicating) hydrocephalus.[1,2] Additional signs and symptoms may result from mass effect on surrounding structures and may include memory loss, gait instability, and vision loss.[3,4] Sudden loss of consciousness and death have also been rarely reported as outcomes in patients with colloid cysts.[5,6,7]

Clinical decision making in patients with colloid cysts must include a thorough evaluation of patient history, neurological exam findings, and imaging characteristics. Key patient characteristics such as patient age and medical comorbidities must guide the goals of any recommended treatment. Imaging features (such as cyst size) and the presence of hydrocephalus are also key clinical features that should guide decision making.[8,9] In many patients with small, incidental colloid cysts discovered incidentally and without imaging evidence of hydrocephalus, serial monitoring may be employed as a useful strategy.[10,11] When treatment is indicated, surgical intervention remains the mainstay as there are no viable medical or radiosurgery-based options. Historically, surgical treatment of colloid cysts involves a wide variety of approaches and techniques, ranging from simple cyst fenestration or aspiration to full cyst excision, and from minimally invasive stereotactic or endoscopic approaches (▶ Fig. 12.1) to traditional open microsurgical craniotomy for cyst excision. It is important to remember that the tool utilized for visualization is independent of the actual surgical approach, and a spectrum of overlapping approaches and tools for visualization (e.g., microscope, endoscope, exoscope) may be appropriately paired to provide a tailored and individualized plan for optimal surgical success and safety. Nevertheless, because

surgical approaches to the third ventricle have traditionally been defined by their complex anatomy and depth, there has been considerable interest in the development of minimally invasive surgical options for pathology of this region, so as to avoid

complications associated with transcortical approaches or brain retraction that are inherent to open microsurgical approaches.[12] Generally speaking, the limitations of these approaches that neurosurgeons have had to overcome include a lack of adequate visualization or an ability to perform two-handed microdissection and coagulation.

12.2 Evolution and Spectrum of Surgical Options for Colloid Cysts

12.2.1 Traditional (Open) Microsurgical Craniotomy for Colloid Cysts

The traditional neurosurgical mainstay for treatment of symptomatic colloid cysts includes one of a variety of approaches to the third ventricle. The two most commonly employed open surgical approaches to the lateral/third ventricles and foramen of Monro are the interhemispheric/transcallosal and frontal transcortical approaches.[12] Other open microsurgical approaches to the third ventricle that are used less commonly for colloid cysts include a subfrontal translamina terminalis approach and a posterior approach such as a supracerebellar/

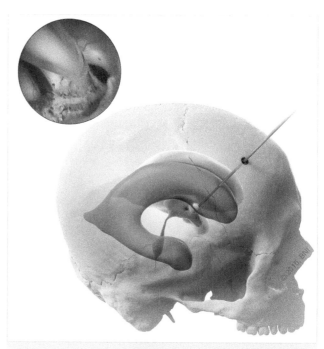

Fig. 12.1 Illustration showing trajectory for endoscopic resection of colloid cysts at the foramen of Monro. (Used with permission from Barrow Neurological Institute, Phoenix, AZ.)

infratentorial approach.[13,14,15] Generally speaking, although open craniotomy offers major benefits including wider surgical access, ability to operate within an air medium, and use of traditional neurosurgical instruments for bimanual microdissection, several key limitations include requirement for a larger incision and craniotomy, increased need for brain retraction, limitations in optics and illumination, and potentially increased risk of postoperative cerebral edema or seizures.[12]

The transcortical approach to the lateral ventricle and foramen of Monro is a standard approach that provides excellent access to colloid cyst pathology. Once access of the lateral ventricle is achieved, the operation proceeds within an air medium, and the cyst can be fenestrated, drained, and carefully dissected from the roof of the third ventricle and internal cerebral veins. The major drawbacks of this approach are the need to traverse normal cortical and subcortical brain tissue and retract this tissue for the duration of the cyst excision.[16] Access of the ventricle may be facilitated with the use of neuronavigation. At this depth, illumination and surgical access/instrumentation may be partially limiting features of the operation, but the ability to utilize standard neurosurgical instruments (e.g., bipolar forceps and microinstruments) provides an additional level of comfort and assurance to the surgeon. The ability to perform standard microdissection of the cyst capsule and appropriately address any bleeding vessels following cyst removal has historically translated into high rates of complete cyst excision rather than partial excision or fenestration, thereby likely translating into more long-term, definitive outcomes for patients with colloid cysts.[17]

Similarly, the interhemispheric transcallosal approach to the lateral ventricle augmented by a transchoroidal approach to the roof of the third ventricle is a nuanced and refined approach to treating colloid cysts. Similar to the transcortical approach, the interhemispheric transcallosal approach offers ability for fine microdissection in an air medium, and affords the surgeon an opportunity to directly address any sources of bleeding using standard neurosurgical electrocautery devices. The drawbacks of the interhemispheric transcallosal approach include a major requirement for brain retraction, occasional sacrifice or risk of injury to major veins or venous sinuses, and risk of injury to other key anatomical structures including distal anterior cerebral artery vessels, the fornices, and the internal cerebral veins.[11,12] As with the transcortical approach, safety and efficiency may be improved using neuronavigation.

In an effort to simplify surgical access to colloid cysts of the third ventricle and partially ameliorate some of the challenges and risks discussed above, an evolution of stereotactic and endoscopic techniques has been underway for the better part of a century in neurosurgery. Over the past few decades, a confluence in the development of optical and surgical technology has allowed neurosurgeons to safely and definitively treat colloid cysts and other intraventricular pathology without the need for open craniotomy and with minimization of brain retraction and surgical access.[18]

Early attempts for minimally invasive treatment of colloid cysts involved needle aspiration procedures guided by stereotactic systems.[19] Although feasibility was demonstrated and patient symptoms often improved, this methodology was inherently limited by a lack of direct surgical observation and a high risk of cyst reaccumulation and symptom recurrence. Nevertheless, the principles developed by pioneering surgeons using developing stereotactic and endoscopic systems paved the way for more recent techniques facilitated by their experience and the addition of improved instrumentation and optical technology, as well as more streamlined stereotactic guidance.

12.2.2 Intraventricular Neuroendoscopy for Colloid Cysts

Intraventricular neuroendoscopy has undergone a punctuated development for over a century, often in conjunction with refinements and the availability of surgical technology at any given time.[20] In recent years, unparalleled visualization and illumination subserved by refinements in miniaturization of optical technology, charge-coupled devices, and fiberoptics have lent themselves to neuroendoscopic access of intraventricular pathology. The major benefits of neuroendoscopic approaches to colloid cysts include smaller incisions, burr hole access, no need for brain retraction, and unparalleled illumination.[21,22] This minimal access approach provides additional downstream benefits to patients, including faster recovery, shorter hospital stays, reduced pain, and reduced risk of infections. Although visualization may be pristine when using the endoscope, it is easily threatened on account of the fluid medium the operation is performed in and the risk of any blood products obscuring necessary visualization. Additional limitations to purely neuroendoscopic colloid cyst excision include a steep learning curve, lack of stereotactic visualization, requirement for highly specialized instrumentation and optical equipment, obscuration of visualization with bleeding when working within a fluid medium, current inability to perform two-handed dissection and bipolar electrocautery, and a need for a surgical assistant to drive the endoscope.[23] When uncomplicated, a neuroendoscopic colloid cyst excision is a graceful and rewarding operation. However, even small complications or challenges associated with intraoperative bleeding or visualization may be highly frustrating and potentially risky, and overcoming the learning curve required to prevent or address these issues may be a formidable challenge for some surgeons.

Despite these inherent challenges, with sufficient experience and a refined technique, overcoming the learning curve associated with neuroendoscopic techniques and successful excision of colloid cysts using neuroendoscopic approaches can be successfully realized. This technique may rely on deliberate single-instrument cautery and dissection of the cyst from the roof of the third ventricle and venous anatomy, prior to delivering the cyst capsule in its entirety. Following cyst excision, venous bleeding is often controlled with sustained irrigation and leaving an external ventricular catheter in place, rather than targeted bipolar cautery that can be performed with open approaches. For these reasons, full colloid cyst excision may not be safely achievable using neuroendoscopic approaches, thereby resulting in subtotal cyst excision in some cases, which portend a higher risk of symptomatic colloid cyst recurrence/progression.[24,25] In other cases, conversion from neuroendoscopic to open interhemispheric or transcortical approaches has been successfully reported.[26,27]

Despite these limitations, numerous successful surgical case series of neuroendoscopic management of colloid cysts have been reported,[28,29] and future developments in optical technology and surgical instrumentation for intraventricular neuroendoscopic procedures will likely shape the ability to safely and effectively resect colloid cysts with less requirement for open approaches. These may include reliance on multiport approaches to facilitate improved instrument mobility, and optimized electrocautery devices.

12.2.3 Channel-Based Approaches to the Lateral Ventricles and Colloid Cysts: A Happy Medium?

In more recent years, stereotactic channel-based exoscopic approaches to the ventricular system have allowed surgeons to take advantage of the benefits of both open and endoscopic approaches when addressing colloid cysts.[30] More specifically, navigable surgical channel-based ports have allowed surgeons to target the lateral ventricle transcortically using minicraniotomies, transsulcal access, improved circumferential brain retraction, and exoscopic illumination/optics, while also allowing two-handed dissection within an air medium.[30] Channel-based excision of colloid cysts has evolved rapidly over the past one to two decades, and remains another viable and evolving option in the catalogue of surgical techniques that may be employed for colloid cysts.

12.3 Surgical Decision Making in Patients with Colloid Cysts

Among the options discussed above (including nonsurgical treatment/observation), many patient and imaging characteristics need to be considered prior to providing a recommendation to a patient and family.[2,9] This in part depends on the surgical goals that must be individualized for each patient. As an example, in an older, symptomatic patient the goal of surgery may be alleviation of mass effect and symptoms, and partial cyst excision with aspiration and drainage may be a successful and safer option where a less invasive approach is preferred. In contrast, for younger patients, full excision may be a priority given the risk of recurrence and desire for a sustained, definitive intervention.

Factors that lend themselves to nonsurgical management in patients with colloid cysts include incidental discovery, lack of signs/symptoms, advanced patient age or presence of comorbidities, small size (often < 1 cm), and lack of hydrocephalus. Factors that lend themselves to neuroendoscopic approaches include presence of hydrocephalus or ventriculomegaly, small cyst size, location near the foramen of Monro, and first-time operation. Conversely, transcortical (exoscopic or microscopic) or interhemispheric approaches should be considered for any complicating features such as recurrent cyst, small ventricle

size, large or calcified cysts, or those located more posteriorly when endoscopic access is limiting.[31]

12.4 Final Thoughts and Recommendations

Ideally, neurosurgeons treating patients with colloid cysts will be prepared to tailor a neurosurgical approach to any given patient's pathology, priorities, and preferences using numerous available permutations of optical equipment and surgical access. Consistent reliance on a single approach (open or endoscopic) may not be in any single patient's best interest. Consideration of all the key factors discussed in this section, along with the required breadth and versatility in a given surgeon or team's comprehensive approach to treating patients with colloid cysts, will allow for customized treatments based on an individual's presenting features. Surgeons ideally suited for treating patients with complex third ventricular pathology will ideally be versatile in endoscopic and open surgical approaches, and can make appropriate recommendations for patients based on these factors without bias or restrictions based on experience or learning curve limitations. As optical and minimally invasive surgical technology continues to improve, we will likely see continued refinement and implementation of these approaches. Nevertheless, traditional open craniotomy for colloid cysts will always remain a safe, effective, and often definitive approach for colloid cysts when treated in experienced centers, and will especially remain viable options for larger, more complex, or multiple recurrent cysts.

References

[1] Beaumont TL, Limbrick DD, Jr, Rich KM, Wippold FJ, II, Dacey RG, Jr. Natural history of colloid cysts of the third ventricle. J Neurosurg. 2016; 125 (6):1420–1430

[2] Doron O, Feldman Z, Zauberman J. MRI features have a role in pre-surgical planning of colloid cyst removal. Acta Neurochir (Wien). 2016; 158(4):671–676

[3] de Witt Hamer PC, Verstegen MJ, De Haan RJ, et al. High risk of acute deterioration in patients harboring symptomatic colloid cysts of the third ventricle. J Neurosurg. 2002; 96(6):1041–1045

[4] Camacho A, Abernathey CD, Kelly PJ, Laws ER, Jr. Colloid cysts: experience with the management of 84 cases since the introduction of computed tomography. Neurosurgery. 1989; 24(5):693–700

[5] Byard RW. Variable presentations of lethal colloid cysts. J Forensic Sci. 2016; 61(6):1538–1540

[6] Godano U, Ferrai R, Meleddu V, Bellinzona M. Hemorrhagic colloid cyst with sudden coma. Minim Invasive Neurosurg. 2010; 53(5–6):273–274

[7] Büttner A, Winkler PA, Eisenmenger W, Weis S. Colloid cysts of the third ventricle with fatal outcome: a report of two cases and review of the literature. Int J Legal Med. 1997; 110(5):260–266

[8] Weaver KJ, McCord M, Neal D, et al. Do tumor and ventricular volume predict the need for postresection shunting in colloid cyst patients? J Neurosurg. 2016; 125(3):585–590

[9] Rangel-Castilla L, Chen F, Choi L, Clark JC, Nakaji P. Endoscopic approach to colloid cyst: what is the optimal entry point and trajectory? J Neurosurg. 2014; 121(4):790–796

[10] Pollock BE, Huston J, III. Natural history of asymptomatic colloid cysts of the third ventricle. J Neurosurg. 1999; 91(3):364–369

[11] Kondziolka D, Lunsford LD. Microsurgical resection of colloid cysts using a stereotactic transventricular approach. Surg Neurol. 1996; 46(5):485–490, discussion 490–492

[12] Milligan BD, Meyer FB. Morbidity of transcallosal and transcortical approaches to lesions in and around the lateral and third ventricles: a single-

institution experience. Neurosurgery. 2010; 67(6):1483–1496, discussion 1496

[13] Konovalov AN, Pitskhelauri DI. Infratentorial supracerebellar approach to the colloid cysts of the third ventricle. Neurosurgery. 2001; 49(5):1116–1122, discussion 1122–1123

[14] Desai KI, Nadkarni TD, Muzumdar DP, Goel AH. Surgical management of colloid cyst of the third ventricle–a study of 105 cases. Surg Neurol. 2002; 57 (5):295–302, discussion 302–304

[15] Konovalov AN, Gorelyshev SK. Surgical treatment of anterior third ventricle tumours. Acta Neurochir (Wien). 1992; 118(1–2):33–39

[16] Szmuda T, Słoniewski P, Szmuda M, Waszak PM, Starzyńska A. Quantification of white matter fibre pathways disruption in frontal transcortical approach to the lateral ventricle or the interventricular foramen in diffusion tensor tractography. Folia Morphol (Warsz). 2014; 73(2):129–138

[17] Sampath R, Vannemreddy P, Nanda A. Microsurgical excision of colloid cyst with favorable cognitive outcomes and short operative time and hospital stay: operative techniques and analyses of outcomes with review of previous studies. Neurosurgery. 2010; 66(2):368–374, discussion 374–375

[18] Couldwell WT, Apuzzo ML. Initial experience related to the use of the Cosman-Roberts-Wells stereotactic instrument. Technical note. J Neurosurg. 1990; 72(1):145–148

[19] Apuzzo ML, Chandrasoma PT, Zelman V, Giannotta SL, Weiss MH. Computed tomographic guidance stereotaxis in the management of lesions of the third ventricular region. Neurosurgery. 1984; 15(4):502–508

[20] Zada G, Liu C, Apuzzo ML. "Through the looking glass": optical physics, issues, and the evolution of neuroendoscopy. World Neurosurg. 2013; 79(2) Suppl: S3–S13

[21] Boogaarts H, El-Kheshin S, Grotenhuis J. Endoscopic colloid cyst resection: technical note. Minim Invasive Neurosurg. 2011; 54(2):95–97

[22] Boogaarts HD, Decq P, Grotenhuis JA, et al. Long-term results of the neuroendoscopic management of colloid cysts of the third ventricle: a series of 90 cases. Neurosurgery. 2011; 68(1):179–187

[23] Qiao L, Souweidane MM. Purely endoscopic removal of intraventricular brain tumors: a consensus opinion and update. Minim Invasive Neurosurg. 2011; 54(4):149–154

[24] Grondin RT, Hader W, MacRae ME, Hamilton MG. Endoscopic versus microsurgical resection of third ventricle colloid cysts. Can J Neurol Sci. 2007; 34 (2):197–207

[25] Sheikh AB, Mendelson ZS, Liu JK. Endoscopic versus microsurgical resection of colloid cysts: a systematic review and meta-analysis of 1,278 patients. World Neurosurg. 2014; 82(6):1187–1197

[26] Osorio JA, Clark AJ, Safaee M, et al. Intraoperative conversion from endoscopic to open transcortical-transventricular removal of colloid cysts as a salvage procedure. Cureus. 2015; 7(2):e247

[27] Greenlee JD, Teo C, Ghahreman A, Kwok B. Purely endoscopic resection of colloid cysts. Neurosurgery. 2008; 62(3) Suppl 1:51–55, discussion 55–56

[28] Margetis K, Souweidane MM. Endoscopic treatment of intraventricular cystic tumors. World Neurosurg. 2013; 79(2) Suppl:19.e1–19.e11

[29] Nduom EK, Sribnick EA, Ormond DR, Hadjipanayis CG. Neuroendoscopic resection of intraventricular tumors and cysts through a working channel with a variable aspiration tissue resector: a feasibility and safety study. Minim Invasive Surg. 2013; 2013:471805

[30] Eliyas JK, Glynn R, Kulwin CG, et al. Minimally invasive transsulcal resection of intraventricular and periventricular lesions through a tubular retractor system: multicentric experience and results. World Neurosurg. 2016; 90:556–564

[31] Two A, Christian E, Mathew A, Giannotta S, Zada G. Giant, calcified colloid cyst of the lateral ventricle. J Clin Neurosci. 2016; 24:6–9

13 Management of Colloid Cysts: Microscope

Joseph A. Osorio and Michael W. McDermott

Summary

Open microsurgical approaches have been the gold standard in treatment of colloid cysts of the third ventricle. Bimodal dexterity and sharp microsurgical dissection afforded via a microsurgical approach allow for potential complete resection of these cysts. In this chapter, we describe technical nuances and complication avoidance techniques in the treatment of this complex disease.

Keywords: colloid cysts, microsurgical, resection, interhemispheric, transcortical

13.1 Open Microsurgical Perspective

13.1.1 Introduction

Operative techniques for the removal of third ventricular colloid cysts have evolved over time, and currently there are a variety of surgical approaches that are utilized, and the optimal approach is debated. Recommendations for definitive surgical removal can range from endoscopy through a burr-hole opening to open craniotomy approaches that include either an interhemispheric transcallosal approach or a transcortical-transventricular approach.[1,2,3] Open craniotomy results have shown an acceptable incidence of complications along with complete removal of cyst capsule and cyst contents, which has resulted in a low recurrence rate. In this chapter, we will describe a case example where the open surgical technique using a microsurgical transcortical-transventricular approach was utilized for a successful gross total resection of cyst and cyst capsule. We will focus on the arguments that favor an open craniotomy, specifically the transcortical-transventricular technique, the nuances involved in achieving a successful operative resection, and a review of the literature that currently favors the open microscopic approach.

13.1.2 Case Example

A 28-year-old man while traveling had new onset of headaches, nausea, and vomiting. A subsequent workup revealed a large third ventricular cyst consistent with a colloid cyst. He subsequently had the cyst removed endoscopically at a different facility; the operative report description detailed complete cyst aspiration, but a small amount of cyst capsule adherent to bilateral fornices was not able to be resected. A 12-month follow-up after an initial endoscopic removal showed a large recurrence of the third ventricular cyst measuring > 1 cm. The patient now presented to our facility, and we recommended to have the cyst removed using an open microsurgical approach, using purely a transcortical-transventricular approach. The patient was neurologically intact.

An intraoperative transcortical-transventricular approach was used to obtain access to this colloid cyst, which primarily resided within zone 2 and zone 3 (a classification that we will describe later in this text). The choroid plexus and the foramen of Monro were identified (▶ Fig. 13.1). The corridor of the dissection was expanded by coagulation and cutting of choroid plexus and extension past septal vein. Our dissection is extended to anterior margin of the medial atrial vein (leaving this vein patent). This allowed for a careful isolation and dissection of the blood supply of the colloid cyst with a successful gross total resection. ▶ Fig. 13.1 provides intraoperative images of this dissection within the lateral and third ventricle.

Intraoperative placement of an external ventricular drain (EVD) was secured, and was left in place until the cerebral spinal fluid (CSF) had cleared. The EVD was removed on postoperative day (POD) 3, and the patient was discharged on POD 4.

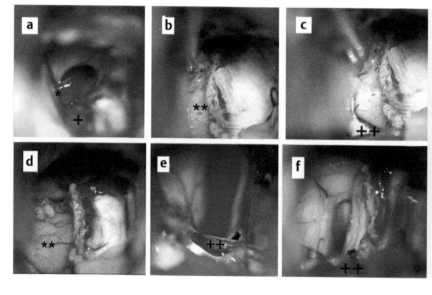

Fig. 13.1 Intraoperative images from transcortical-transventricular approach for zone 2 cyst. **(a)** Initial exposure into ventricle showing foramen of Monro, choroid plexus (+), and septal vein (*) on left. **(b)** After coagulation and cutting of choroid plexus and extension past septal vein, therefore foramen of Monro appearing wider, with colloid cyst (**) adjacent to thalamostriate vein. **(c)** Zone 2 dissection is extended to anterior margin of the lateral atrial vein (++) that is left intact; colloid cyst (**) is noted encompassing all of zone 2. **(d)** Colloid cyst (**) is carefully isolated from its adjacent blood supply. **(e)** Lateral atrial vein (++) is preserved, and **(f)** wide exposure obtained after careful resection.

There were no complications and the patient returned home neurologically intact. He has remained without recurrence.

13.1.3 Advantages of the Open Microsurgical Traditional Approach

The open transcortical-transventricular microsurgical approach provides a traditional corridor with a microscope and the surgeon working bimanually down a narrow opening directly upon the colloid cyst within the third ventricle. The most favorable advantage of this approach is the ability for a single surgeon to utilize both hands for the most delicate portion of the resection, without the use of cameras or assistants, which are required for the endoscopic approach. The ability to perform bimanual microdissection allows for an improved ability to manipulate or work near critical structures; it provides better control of bleeding and also the ability to widen the operative corridor if needed. In addition, the capsule of the cyst can be grasped with one instrument and dissected from attachments in the roof of the third ventricle with a separate instrument; an endoscope would only allow for a single instrument to be used at one time.

Large colloid cysts are often not accessible entirely through the foramen of Monro, and require a larger operative corridor for microdissection and resection of the colloid cyst capsule. A larger operative corridor can be achieved by opening along the roof of the third ventricle by microdissection of the tinea fornix via a transchoroidal approach. This approach is best performed under direct microscopic visualization using bimanual microdissection. The expansion of the foramen of Monro posteriorly using this approach is a delicate operation around critical structures and vessels. Expanding the operative corridor is an advantage and an added capacity of the open microsurgical approach.

The definitive operation for a colloid cyst involves complete resection of contents and most importantly the cyst capsule to avoid recurrence. This should be performed without damage to the surrounding structures that include critical venous structures and the fornix. The open microsurgical approach provides the best amount of operative freedom together with direct control, which in our experience allows the most success in complete access and removal of the cyst capsule, ultimately resulting in the fewest recurrences.

Many of the advantages that are in favor of an open microsurgical approach when comparing open to an endoscopic approach can be made for both the transcortical-transventricular approach and the midline transcallosal approach. We favor the transcortical-transventricular approach because the time for the approach is shorter, the difficulty of the anatomic dissection is lower, the risk to the parasagittal veins is lower, and the overall neurological complication rate is lower (▶ Table 13.1).

Table 13.1 Comparison between open microsurgical approaches: transcortical versus transcallosal

	Transcortical	Transcallosal
Surgical time for approach	Shorter	Longer
Difficulty of anatomic dissection	Lower	Higher
Risk to parasagittal veins	Lower	Higher
Neurologic complication rate	Lower	Higher

13.1.4 Disadvantages of the Endoscope

The endoscopic approach is favored because of the small operative corridor and speedier recovery, but the major drawback to this approach is the inability to completely excise the cyst capsule, with resultant higher recurrence rates and need for repeat surgery. The increase in cyst recurrence using this method is a result of operating through a narrow corridor and utilizing techniques to attempt to obliterate the cyst capsule, such as coagulation of the capsule, for segments of the capsule that are too difficult to remove through an endoscopic approach.

The endoscopic approach is usually a two-surgeon technique, operator and navigator. The limiting factors for endoscopy are the single working channel and a trajectory for the instruments that is parallel to the line of sight of the endoscope. Opening of the tinea choroidea in the roof of the third ventricle cannot be done safely with the endoscope technique. When using this technique for larger cysts, the surgeon often plans for coagulation of the cyst capsule and aspiration of cyst contents, which makes recurrence a very realistic possibility. Capsule excision is quite different than capsule coagulation, and although the latter has the ability to reduce the chance of recurrence, the rate varies and is not zero. It has been shown that, in the hands of very experienced endoscopic neurosurgeons, the rate of capsule excision may approach that of open cranial operations.[4,5] Although associated with high rates of complete cyst removal, some have noted that it may be difficult with larger cysts[6] or cysts that are further posterior in the third ventricle.

The fornix is a critical structure that often is abutting the superior and anterior aspects of cyst, either because of direct adhesion or because of the size and extent of the cyst. For the endoscopic approach, forniceal adhesion is a particular challenge because separating the cyst from the fornix is often done by coagulation, and direct coagulation could injure the fornix. Also, when using the endoscopic approach for larger cysts within the third ventricle, the fornix is also at risk because of simple manipulation of the instruments at the foramen of Monro compressing and injuring this surrounding structure. The direct compression is often a result of restricting the operative corridor to the foramen of Monro, without expanding this opening.

13.1.5 Patient Selection

Age at the time of an operative intervention plays an important role in choosing an approach because the potential for recurrence is higher for younger patients because of longer life expectancy. For this reason, we would recommend offering the most definitive approach that would result in a gross total resection of cyst contents and cyst capsule for patients with longer life expectancies. In our experience, gross total resection is best achieved using an open transcortical-transventricular microsurgical excision.

Cyst size is also an important factor to consider when selecting the operative approach. Careful planning using the preoperative magnetic resonance imaging (MRI) can demonstrate the extent of the cyst within the third ventricle. We have previously created an anatomical zone classification that was created for surgeons to understand the operative boundaries when enlarging the operative corridor along the roof of the third ventricle by microdissection of the tinea fornicea via a transchoroidal approach. ▶ Fig. 13.2 is an illustration showing the zone classification, and we will later describe in detail the anatomical boundaries of the three zones. For colloid cysts

that are larger in size, we have noted that they often extend posteriorly into zone 2 and zone 3. For these in particular, we would recommend an open transcortical-transventricular microsurgical approach.

Recurrent colloid cysts are often operations that are more challenging and would benefit from a bimanual microdissection. In particular, it commonly involves a detailed microdissection of the roof of the third ventricle behind the foramen to free the adhesions that frequently will involve the most vital structures including the venous drainage and the fornix. An open transcortical-transventricular microsurgical approach would allow for careful resection and manipulation under direct visualization.

In summary, we believe that an open transcortical-transventricular microsurgical excision is a superior approach for younger patients, for patients with large cysts that fill the third ventricle, or for those with recurrence after prior treatment. The open microsurgical technique, coupled with modern image-guided systems, provides a safe, effective, and direct approach with the best chances for a gross total resection. Our approach to patients with colloid cysts based on our experience is summarized in ▶ Table 13.2.

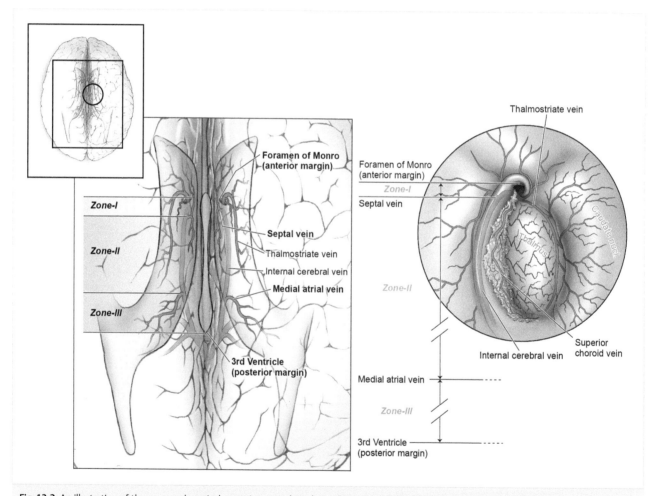

Fig. 13.2 An illustration of the proposed surgical operative zones based on relationships defined by the anterior column of the fornix, the septal vein, and the lateral atrial vein. Zone 1 extends from the anterior column of the fornix back to the anterior margin of the septal vein.

Table 13.2 Recommendations for surgical treatment based on colloid cysts size and patient age

Age	Surgical zone (size)	Treatment option(s)
Younger	1	Endo/TC-TV
	2,3	TC-TV
Older	1	Endo
	2,3	Endo/TC-TV

Note: Size: zone 1 = smaller; zone 2,3 = larger. Options: Endo = endoscopic removal; TC-TV = transcortical-transventricular.

13.1.6 Complication Avoidance

Preoperative planning is critical in avoiding complications when approaching a third ventricular colloid cyst using the open craniotomy transcortical-transventricular microsurgical approach. It is important to minimize the subcortical dissection to the ventricle, and choosing an optimal tract and entry point is essential in achieving this goal. Using modern image-guided systems, a well-prepared entry point and trajectory are chosen on the middle frontal gyrus.

Cyst decompression is often performed first so that the cyst capsule can be easily identified and excised safely. Collapse of the cyst creates a plane around the capsule that allows for small vessels attached to the capsule of the colloid cyst to be coagulated with the bipolar and divided with straight microscissors. For larger cysts in zone 2, further dissection is required to divide small vessels from the roof of the third ventricle supplying the capsule.

Following successful resection of the colloid cyst, a small septostomy is created to facilitate CSF flow across the lateral ventricles. Finally, the ventricular cavity is inspected for any bleeding, and our practice is to always place an EVD into the frontal horn of the lateral ventricle in order to evacuate any surgical bleeding that may exist within the ventricle in the postoperative period.

It is also possible to suture closed the surface corticectomy where the pia arachnoid has been coagulated. In our experience, since introducing this additional step, we have not had a single case of symptomatic subdural hygroma requiring additional treatment.

13.1.7 Technical Nuances

The desired trajectory is an important initial selection by the surgeon, and this should encompass an understanding of the planned extent of resection and opening into the third ventricle. An orthogonal trajectory aimed at the foramen of Monro should be placed upon the middle frontal gyrus.

In order to carry out the dissection along the selected path after choosing the entry cortical point, a rubber catheter is introduced using an image-guided stylet and trajectory into the ventricle, and subsequently left in place as an identifier for the proper dissection tract. This allows for not only an image-guided trajectory, but also a place-holder for that path that is used during the subcortical dissection. The subcortical dissection is carried along the rubber catheter. Overall, this technique facilitates achieving the smallest cortical opening desired. The operative microscope is subsequently used for the subcortical dissection, and blunt dissection is favored over electrocautery or suction, so that a pronounced tract is not created.

Extending the opening posteriorly at the foramen of Monro, and gaining access into the third ventricle, will allow for the resection of larger colloid cysts. Based on past experience with these cysts in the roof of the third ventricle, we designed a classification of surgical operative zones based on relationships defined by the anterior column of the fornix, the septal vein, and the medial atrial vein.

- Zone 1: Zone 1 extends from the anterior column of the fornix back to the anterior margin of the septal vein (▶ Fig. 13.2). Small colloid cysts can be completely removed in this zone by opening the tinea choroidea between the fornix medially and the choroid plexus laterally. Without division of the septal vein, a few additional millimeters of exposure of the roof of the third ventricle can be achieved in this way (▶ Fig. 13.2).
- Zone 2: Zone 2 extends from the anterior margin of the septal vein to the anterior margin of the medial atrial vein. Access to this zone requires isolation, coagulation, and division of the septal vein, preserving the patency of the thalamostriate and internal cerebral veins. Once the septal vein is coagulated, the tinea fornicea can be opened along the roof of the third ventricle, lateral to the body of the fornix and medial to the choroid plexus and internal cerebral veins. Large cysts in this zone can be carefully isolated from their blood supply from the posterior medial choroidal arteries, and the cyst wall can be excised completely (▶ Fig. 13.2).
- Zone 3: Zone 3 extends from the medial atrial vein back to the posterior third ventricle. The medial atrial vein is the posterior limit of the dissection in the roof of the third ventricle but the aqueduct and posterior third ventricle can be easily seen.

13.1.8 Literature Review/Evidence in Favor of Microscopic Approach

Open microscopic removal of colloid cysts, by either transcortical or transcallosal approach, is associated with a very high rate of complete removal including the cyst capsule that approaches 100%.[1,3,7,8] When deciding between the microscopic approach via the transcortical and transcallosal corridor, the surgeon must decide which approach is less morbid. Traditionally, there has been a concern that the transcortical approach is associated with a higher rate of seizures than with the transcallosal approach. Milligan and Meyer et al reviewed the Mayo Clinic experience with surgical approaches to lesions around the third ventricle.[9] The transcallosal approach carried a 4.4-fold increased risk of seizures in the postoperative period compared to the transcortical approach. Hassaneen et al, in reporting the morbidity of transcallosal approaches to tumors of the third ventricle, found that 34% of patients had a neurologic complication, and that sacrifice of parasagittal veins was the likely influencing factor associated with the risk of complications.[10] The transcortical approach fortunately does not involve sacrifice of cortical veins, and this likely is the reason for the difference in complications.

In contrast to the open microsurgical approach, endoscopic removal is associated with a lower rate of complete removal of cyst, ranging from 10 to 53%.[1,2,7,11,12,13] Grondin et al compared their endoscopic and microsurgical experience for colloid cysts. Complete resection of the cyst capsule was achieved in 12% of the endoscopic group and 100% of the microsurgical group

($p < 0.001$). The complication rate was higher in the microsurgical group (32.2 vs. 8.3%; $p < 0.001$) but the recurrence rate was lower (0.6 vs. 3.3%; $p < 0.003$). Horn et al compared the endoscopic to the transcallosal microsurgical approach and found that there was no residual on postoperative scans in 53% of endoscopic and 94% of transcallosal cases. In a publication of the Italian cooperative study of endoscopic colloid cyst removal in 11 centers reporting on 61 patients, the planned technique was coagulation of capsule and cyst aspiration. Capsule excision was achieved in 9.8% and the recurrence rate was 11.4%. Recently, Hoffman et al reported on the significance of cyst remnants after endoscopic colloid cyst resection, reporting their experience and summarizing the literature.[14] Across all studies of endoscopic treatment, the recurrence rate was 6.3% with a mean time to recurrence of 51 months and a morbidity rate of 13.9%. In the hands of very experienced endoscopic neurosurgeons, the rate of capsule excision may approach that of open cranial operations.[4,5] A supraorbital endoscopic modification has been proposed to improve visualization of the likely area of cyst adhesion to the third ventricular wall; however, this was not associated with improved rates of complete removal.[15] Others have used frame-based or frameless stereotaxy to place a tubular retractor transfrontally for microscopic removal of colloid cysts.[6,16,17] Although associated with high rates of complete cyst removal, some have noted that it may be difficult with larger cysts.[6]

While Horn et al noted a low rate of complete cyst removal with endoscopy compared to transcallosal approaches,[7] they also demonstrate significantly lower operating room time and hospital stay and, therefore, propose that endoscopic removal is appropriate to attempt as the first approach to remove a colloid cyst. If the cyst recurs, then open surgery should be attempted. In the large series by Greenlee et al, 6 out of 35 attempted endoscopic colloid cyst operations were converted into open minicraniotomy.[4] One was due to equipment malfunction, but the others were due to forniceal adhesion and the need for improved visualization. All cases were associated with complete removal, suggesting that transfrontal open cranial approaches are efficacious as intraoperative salvage procedures. The effects of conversion to open surgery on the procedure and outcome were not directly compared.

The goal of complete cyst removal including the capsule is to prevent recurrence. However, this has not been conclusively proven as many operations described in case series with subtotal removal do not result in recurrence. Nevertheless, Grondin et al performed a systematic review of the literature comparing open cranial and endoscopic approaches and reported a statistically significant increase in recurrence with endoscopic approaches (3 vs. 0.6%).[1] This suggests that complete removal may be optimal treatment for these lesions.

13.1.9 Clinical Pearls

- An open transcortical microsurgical approach can be an effective technique for achieving a gross total resection of a colloid cyst within the third ventricle.
- The transcortical-transventricular approach should always be coupled with the use of an image-guided catheter insertion into the ventricle as a guide to subcortical dissection.

- The open microsurgical approach allows the surgeon the benefit of utilizing bimanual operative dissection, which increases the chances of a safe resection of cysts of all sizes, including those that are large and adherent to critical surrounding structures.
- The benefit in offering a definitive therapy upfront for younger patients and patients with large cysts that fill the third ventricle is avoiding a recurrence as well as need for further surgery.
- In the setting of a failed endoscopic resection, an open transcortical excision should be considered as a safe and effective technique for recurrent colloid cysts.

References

[1] Grondin RT, Hader W, MacRae ME, Hamilton MG. Endoscopic versus microsurgical resection of third ventricle colloid cysts. Can J Neurol Sci. 2007; 34 (2):197–207

[2] Longatti P, Godano U, Gangemi M, et al. Italian neuroendoscopy group. Cooperative study by the Italian neuroendoscopy group on the treatment of 61 colloid cysts. Childs Nerv Syst. 2006; 22(10):1263–1267

[3] Sampath R, Vannemreddy P, Nanda A. Microsurgical excision of colloid cyst with favorable cognitive outcomes and short operative time and hospital stay: operative techniques and analyses of outcomes with review of previous studies. Neurosurgery. 2010; 66(2):368–374, discussion 374–375

[4] Greenlee JD, Teo C, Ghahreman A, Kwok B. Purely endoscopic resection of colloid cysts. Neurosurgery. 2008; 62(3) Suppl 1:51–55, discussion 55–56

[5] Engh JA, Lunsford LD, Amin DV, et al. Stereotactically guided endoscopic port surgery for intraventricular tumor and colloid cyst resection. Neurosurgery. 2010; 67(3) Suppl Operative:ons198–ons204, discussion ons204–ons205

[6] Barlas O, Karadereler S. Stereotactically guided microsurgical removal of colloid cysts. Acta Neurochir (Wien). 2004; 146(11):1199–1204

[7] Horn EM, Feiz-Erfan I, Bristol RE, et al. Treatment options for third ventricular colloid cysts: comparison of open microsurgical versus endoscopic resection. Neurosurgery. 2007; 60(4):613–618, discussion 618–620

[8] Desai KI, Nadkarni TD, Muzumdar DP, Goel AH. Surgical management of colloid cyst of the third ventricle–a study of 105 cases. Surg Neurol. 2002; 57 (5):295–302, discussion 302–304

[9] Milligan BD, Meyer FB. Morbidity of transcallosal and transcortical approaches to lesions in and around the lateral and third ventricles: a single-institution experience. Neurosurgery. 2010; 67(6):1483–1496, discussion 1496

[10] Hassaneen W, Suki D, Salaskar AL, et al. Immediate morbidity and mortality associated with transcallosal resection of tumors of the third ventricle. J Clin Neurosci. 2010; 17(7):830–836

[11] Boogaarts HD, Decq P, Grotenhuis JA, et al. Long-term results of the neuroendoscopic management of colloid cysts of the third ventricle: a series of 90 cases. Neurosurgery. 2011; 68(1):179–187

[12] Kehler U, Brunori A, Gliemroth J, et al. Twenty colloid cysts–comparison of endoscopic and microsurgical management. Minim Invasive Neurosurg. 2001; 44(3):121–127

[13] Hellwig D, Bauer BL, Schulte M, Gatscher S, Riegel T, Bertalanffy H. Neuroendoscopic treatment for colloid cysts of the third ventricle: the experience of a decade. Neurosurgery. 2003; 52(3):525–533, discussion 532–533

[14] Hoffman CE, Savage NJ, Souweidane MM. The significance of cyst remnants after endoscopic colloid cyst resection: a retrospective clinical case series. Neurosurgery. 2013; 73(2):233–237, discussion 237–239

[15] Delitala A, Brunori A, Russo N. Supraorbital endoscopic approach to colloid cysts. Neurosurgery. 2011; 69(2) Suppl Operative:ons176–ons182, discussion ons182–ons183

[16] Cohen-Gadol AA. Minitubular transcortical microsurgical approach for gross total resection of third ventricular colloid cysts: technique and assessment. World Neurosurg. 2013; 79(1):207.e7–207.e10

[17] Kondziolka D, Lunsford LD. Microsurgical resection of colloid cysts using a stereotactic transventricular approach. Surg Neurol. 1996; 46(5):485–490, discussion 490–492

14 Management of Colloid Cysts: Endoscope

Sheri K. Palejwala and Peter Nakaji

Summary

The endoscopic approach is the preferred default technique for the resection of third ventricular colloid cysts, with the open microsurgical technique reserved for a certain subset of lesions. We advocate the use of a bimanual, dual-instrument endoscopic technique, which allows for adequate surgical maneuverability to achieve both cyst resection and management of any potential complications. Furthermore, the minimally invasive technique decreases retraction of critical structures such as the fornices, internal cerebral veins, cingulate gyrus, and normal frontal cortex, thereby significantly lessening the main sources of morbidity associated with microsurgical colloid cyst management. Finally, with advancements in neuroendoscope technology, improvements in endoscopic instruments, and greater surgical training in endoscopy, complete cyst wall resection rates of 80 to 100% are feasible, such that previous arguments against the endoscopic technique due to incompleteness of resection are not applicable in the modern era. Given the lower surgical impact and the associated morbidity to surrounding structures and steadily increasing rates of complete resection, endoscopic colloid cyst management should remain the first-line treatment, with microsurgery reserved for a subset of cases.

Keywords: colloid cyst, endoscopic, fornix, interhemispheric, minimally invasive surgery, neuroendoscope, third ventricle, transcallosal; transcortical; transventricular

14.1 Endoscopic Perspective

14.1.1 Introduction

Colloid cysts comprise 0.5 to 2% of all brain tumors and are typically located within the third ventricle.[1,2] Due to their location, they can block the flow of cerebrospinal fluid (CSF) at one or both foramina of Monro, and thereby present with obstructive hydrocephalus, producing headache, nausea, and emesis.[3] Described frequently in the literature, sudden coma and death is the most feared complication, presumably occurring due to acute obstructive hydrocephalus, at a rate of 3.1 to 10%.[3,4,5,6,7] As a result, the preferred treatment is often surgical management, especially with large lesions and in the presence of ventriculomegaly.[3,8] Third ventricular colloid cysts are typically treated definitively with transcallosal or transcortical resection, or more conservatively with stereotactic cyst fenestration and aspiration, or ventriculoperitoneal shunting.[8] With the increasingly widespread use of intracranial neuroendoscopy, endoscopic colloid cyst resection has gained popularity over the past three decades, with comparable results to the open transcranial approaches and decreased surgical impact and resultant morbidity.[8,9]

14.1.2 Open Microsurgical Approaches

The two most commonly utilized surgical approaches to third ventricular colloid cysts include the interhemispheric transcallosal and transcortical-transventricular approaches, which are often held as the gold standard.[4] Open microsurgical approaches have a significantly greater likelihood of complete cyst wall resection, but come at the cost of greater associated morbidity.[4,7,9] The controversy in the use of open microsurgical colloid cyst resection lies in whether the more completeness of resection justifies the added morbidity of the more extensive approach. Ultimately, the decision is subjective and depends on the experience and expertise of the surgeon and the preferences of the patient.

Transcallosal Approach

The transcallosal approach provides an excellent view into the superior aspects of the third ventricle, where most colloid cysts occur.[9] Understandably, high rates of gross total resection can be achieved from this wide exposure and use of a standard bimanual microsurgical technique. A large meta-analysis of 1,278 patients reported a complete resection rate (without intraoperative evidence of any cyst wall remnants) of 96.8%, significantly higher than that of the endoscopic group (58.2%, $p < 0.0001$). However, the access afforded by the transcallosal approach is time-consuming and can lead to additional morbidity. This primarily stems from prolonged retraction of critical structures such as the fornices, which can cause short-term memory impairment, deep cerebral veins leading to venous infarction, or the cingulate gyri, which can cause mutism.

Horn et al described 55 patients who underwent either a transcallosal or endoscopic colloid cyst resection and found the transcallosal approach was associated with a significantly higher operative time (174 vs. 267 minutes, $p < 0.05$) and longer hospital length of stay (5.4 vs. 6.3 days, $p < 0.05$).[7] More importantly, the transcallosal approach is associated with greater morbidity than the endoscopic approach, including postoperative seizures, short-term memory deficits from forniceal injury, internal cerebral vein damage causing venous infarction, transient hemiparesis, disconnection syndrome, or mutism from bilateral cingulate gyrus retraction injury, and infection.[4,7,9]

Transcortical Approach

The transcortical-transventricular approach for the resection of a colloid cyst was first described by Dandy in 1921.[10] Since the advent of microsurgical technique, mortality has decreased drastically, from 19% to less than 1% in the modern era.[4,9] However, the morbidity of this approach is not insignificant. Firstly, when pursuing a deep surgical target, the field of view and light penetrance offered by a standard surgical microscope are limited, such that often a large frontal corticectomy is required, with extensive removal of otherwise normal, nonpathologic brain tissue.[11] This is likely the cause for the relatively high rates of postoperative seizures at 10.4%, compared to 0.3% with endoscopy.[9] Overall, the large meta-analysis showed significantly higher rates of complications, including seizures, infection, memory deficits, venous infarct, and hemiparesis, with the microsurgical transcortical approach at 24.5% relative to the transcallosal (14.4%) and endoscopic (10.5%) approaches.[9] Across comparisons of open microsurgical (transcallosal and transcortical) and endoscopic approaches for the resection of colloid cysts, the complication rates are relatively low and somewhat variable across studies; however, they all consistently reported greater morbidity in the cohort undergoing open approaches over those patients who had an endoscopic resection.[3,4,7,9,12]

14.1.3 Endoscopic Approach

In 1983, Powell et al first described the endoscopic aspiration of a colloid cyst.[13] Since then there have been over three decades of improvement in the technology, techniques, and training, such that neuroendoscopic resection is now safer and more efficacious.[4] Numerous comparative series have noted that the endoscopic approach is associated with a shorter operative time, faster recovery, and decreased complication rate owing to a smaller cortical incision, with a decreased rate of postoperative seizures, hydrocephalus, meningitis, and memory loss.[4,7]

Historically, the largest drawback of the endoscopic approach is the significantly decreased rate of complete resection (53–64.9%) in comparison to open transcranial approaches (94–100%).[4,7,9] Expectedly, the recurrence and reoperation rates were also higher in endoscopy groups (3.9 and 3.0%, respectively) compared to the microsurgical cohort (1.5 and 0.4%, respectively, $p < 0.0003$ and $p < 0.0006$, respectively). However, many of these larger analyses include studies that are several decades old, evaluating surgeries performed even earlier, where the goals of neuroendoscopy were often simply for cyst aspiration and decompression of the ventricular system.[9,14]

Given the burgeoning field of neuroendoscopy and drive toward minimally invasive neurosurgery over the past several decades, these high recurrence rates might not be representative of more modern techniques. This is especially true of the drastically improved visualization and maneuverability of modern neuroendoscopes and the wide variety of endoscopic instruments now available. Furthermore, the surgical learning curve is being more quickly overcome with early exposure to endoscopic technique and its widespread application throughout neurosurgical subspecialties and institutions.[4] Expectedly, newer endoscopic studies demonstrated 80 to 100% rates of complete cyst resection, and several groups demonstrated increasing rates of complete surgical resection as experience with the endoscopic approach grew within their respective series.[4,15,16,17]

Modern studies also incorporate the use of stereotactic neuronavigation, which has become ubiquitous throughout neurosurgery.[7,8,14,17] This allows for greater specificity in the placement of the burr hole craniotomy and trajectory planning, so as to lessen the surgical impact on the nascent brain parenchyma, minimize manipulation of critical structures, and improve access to the surgical target.[8] More importantly, stereotaxis allows the craniotomy to be tailored to the patient's individual pathoanatomy and substantially increases the likelihood of complete surgical resection.[8,14,17]

In a minority of cases in which endoscopic resection is subtotal, remnants are left along critical structures to lessen the potential morbidity of further dissection.[17] These remnants can be observed with serial imaging or the patient can undergo subsequent resection(s) for management. Cyst wall remnants can be difficult to detect on neuroimaging, such that many have proposed that the degree of resection should be determined by direct intraoperative intraventricular visualization.[9] However, colloid cyst recurrence has also been reported in instances where the surgeons felt they achieved gross total resection based on intraoperative intraventricular inspection.[4,9] Colloid cyst recurrence typically occurs in the setting of known, larger residual often intentionally left behind on the fornices, internal cerebral veins, third ventricular walls, or other critical structures. Cyst recurrence typically presents within 2 years of initial resection, although more distant recurrences have been described. Most recurrences are symptomatic with headache, memory loss, or other symptoms of obstructive hydrocephalus. Therefore, all patients should be followed regularly, clinically and radiographically, to assess for cyst recurrence, irrespective of the surgical approach and even if gross total resection was felt to be achieved. It is also important to note here that reoperation for recurrence can be performed via an endoscopic or microsurgical approach, and repeat endoscopy has been reported to be safe and efficacious, and often led to complete resection.[4]

14.1.4 Endoscopic Technique

Surgical technique, especially in the setting of emerging technology, should be continuously developing. Our strategy for the management of colloid cysts has evolved to an anterolateral approach using a bimanual, dual-instrument endoscopic technique focusing on complete cyst wall resection.[17] Several technical presuppositions underlie our advocacy of the endoscopic technique: dual instruments, surgeon facility with endoscopic sharp dissection techniques, and image guidance. The approach should be as far lateral and anterior as allowed by the head of the caudate to facilitate a direct view of the underside of the roof of the third ventricle.[8,17] A review of the technique that we use will help inform the reader of the method that we are advocating against the open approach. This description also reveals the reasoning behind the limitations that can sometimes make the endoscopic approach less favorable for a complete resection.

Stereotactic neuronavigation is used to customize the starting point, which on average is 4.2 cm lateral to midline and 4.6 cm anterior to the coronal suture.[8] The most anterolateral trajectory afforded by the head of the caudate is then taken to provide access to the roof of the third ventricle and to come under the arch of the fornix as much as possible. We most frequently perform our approach on the nondominant, right side, unless the pathology asymmetrically favors the left.[17] However, a very left approach carries some risk to language due the endangerment of Broca's area; in some cases, this may lead to a shift back to a right approach or an open one. In our hands, a rigid 6-mm 30-degree endoscope is used with two 1.4-mm working channels, a single 2.2-mm channel, and a 2.4-mm optic channel (MINOP TM System; Aesculap, Tuttlingen, Germany).[3] Naturally, there are other endoscope options that will also serve. With the help of image guidance, the endoscope is directed into the frontal horn of the lateral ventricle. Once the cyst is encountered, bipolar electrocautery is used for coagulation; the cyst is then punctured and gently aspirated. The cyst wall is resected using pediatric flexible graspers for gentle traction along with endoscopic microscissors for sharp dissection or bipolar electrocautery. While the assistant holds the endoscope as a dynamic "scope holder," a standard bimanual technique is employed through the working channels of the neuroendoscope.[3,17] Septum pellucidotomy should certainly be considered with the endoscopic technique to prevent the rare case of foraminal obstruction turning into unilateral trapped ventricle. Using this technique, we have achieved complete resection in 82% of cases, with near-total, radiographically complete resection in 95% of colloid cysts.[17]

In addition to historically lesser rates of complete cyst wall resection, another criticism of the endoscopic technique has been the dependence on fuller dilated ventricles. However, a study showed that 16 patients with normal-sized ventricles underwent endoscopic colloid cyst resection with comparable safety and efficacy to their hydrocephalic counterparts.[3] Neuroendoscopy, however, still presents a steep learning curve, and endoscopic colloid cyst resection in the setting of normal-sized ventricles lies on the more difficult end of the spectrum. We recommend not advancing the endoscope through smaller foramina of Monro and not tackling more challenging cases until the surgeon has acquired sufficient experience with more straightforward lesions.[3] Lesions in the classic location, at the foramen of Monro itself, are most favorable, whereas those more posteriorly located in the third ventricle or in an interforniceal or interseptal position should be considered for a microsurgical approach or drainage only.

14.1.5 Indications and Limitations

The endoscopic approach allows for rapid decompression of the cyst and the often dilated ventricular system. It can allow 80 to 100% rates of complete cyst wall resection, and long-term studies are needed to reflect the likely lower rates of recurrence and reoperation resulting from these improved resection rates.[4,15,16,17] Despite this, there are some limitations of the endoscopic approach in achieving a complete resection, including a larger cyst size (> 1.5 cm), flattened fornices indicating greater cyst–forniceal adherence, less common cyst locations including the posterior third ventricle and interseptal locations, and finally left-sided cysts (▶ Table 14.1).[18] These are not strict contraindications of the endoscopic technique per se; rather, they are preoperative factors that might indicate a decreased likelihood of complete resection via the endoscopic approach. As such, the surgeon may be inclined to pursue a microsurgical transcallosal technique instead or to counsel the patient more thoroughly on the likelihood of residual, recurrence, and reoperations.

Table 14.1 Indications for selecting either an endoscopic or microsurgical technique for colloid cyst resection

	Endoscopic	Microsurgical
Cyst diameter	< 1.5 cm	> 1.5 cm
Fornices	Rounded	Thinned/flattened
Side of best access	Right or central	Left
Location	Anterior/foramen of Monro	Interseptal or posterior third ventricle

On the other hand, we advocate the endoscopic technique be used as first-line treatment, with a goal of maximal safe resection. If the endoscopic access is felt to be insufficient for cyst wall resection or complication management, the surgeon can always convert to an open approach. A study evaluating four cases of colloid cyst resection that were converted from an endoscopic to a microsurgical transcortical approach cited tougher cyst wall consistency and technical issues with the endoscope as the primary causes for conversion.[19] As the technology improves and both surgeons and surgical teams become more facile with the use of endoscopy, these issues are expected to be less prevalent. We believe that conversion to a microsurgical technique, though seldom necessary, remains a viable option, especially for challenging cases or for surgeons just starting to incorporate neuroendoscopy into their armamentarium for the management of colloid cysts or other intraventricular lesions. Furthermore, in the event of subtotal resection, any residual cyst wall can be monitored with serial magnetic resonance imaging (MRI) or resected using a repeat endoscopic approach or a microsurgical interhemispheric transcallosal approach.[3,4,7,17]

Essentially, the objective is not for the surgeon to commit to a single surgical approach and cling to it dogmatically throughout his or her career. Rather, it is important to understand the nuanced technicalities of all the surgical management strategies available along with the indications for nonsurgical management, such that the surgeons can decide alongside their patients which strategy is most applicable to the specific pathoanatomy at hand.

14.1.6 Case Examples

Two illustrative cases are provided. The first shows a "classic" good candidate for an endoscopic approach, in that the colloid cyst is moderate in size, presents with associated hydrocephalus, is subforniceal in location, and is located at the foramen of Monro.

The second is an intraseptal interforniceal cyst, which is unfavorable for definitive endoscopic resection (and perhaps for any approach except drainage and fenestration).

Case 1

A 56-year-old man presented with progressive headache and imbalance, and began vomiting on the day of admission. Computed tomography (CT) (not shown) and then MRI disclosed a colloid cyst of the third ventricle (▶ Fig. 14.1a,b). An external ventricular drain was placed, which provided immediate relief of the patient's symptoms. He was taken for a right-sided endoscopic resection the next day. Note that on imaging the cyst is moderate in size (about 12 mm in greatest dimension), below the fornices (and hence more easily separable), and at the foramen of Monro (and hence accessible to the endoscope without choroidal fissure dissection). The presence of enlarged ventricles makes a more anterolateral angle of approach possible, which allows the surgeon better access to the underside of the fornices, where the point of attachment is. The patient underwent uncomplicated and total removal with no impact on his memory (▶ Fig. 14.1c).

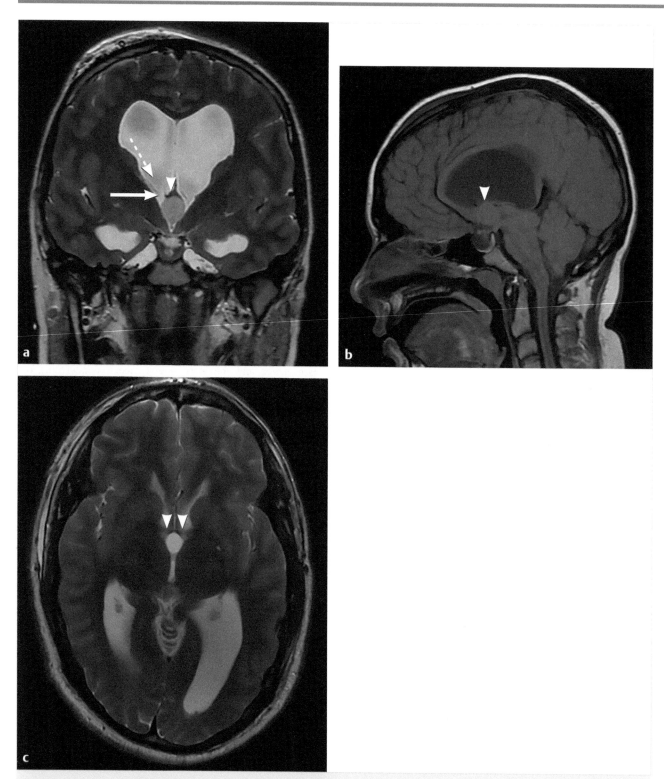

Fig. 14.1 **(a)** Coronal T2-weighted MRI at the level of the foramen of Monro shows the ventricles are large, allowing a shallower approach over the head of the caudate (*dashed line arrow*), the foramen of Monro is large and open on the right (*solid arrow*), and the cyst is below the fornices (*arrowhead*) within the third ventricle. **(b)** Sagittal T1-weighted MRI without gadolinium through the midline shows there is a small separation between the arch of the fornix and the cyst (*arrowhead*), further supporting the idea that it will be separable. **(c)** Postoperative MRI shows complete removal of the cyst with a space where the cyst used to be with excellent preservation of the fornices (*arrowheads*). (Used with permission from Barrow Neurological Institute, Phoenix, AZ.)

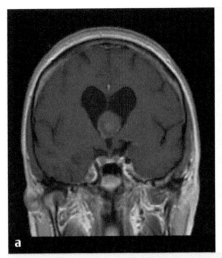
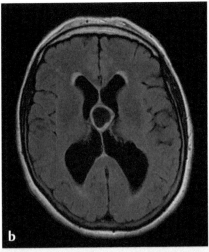
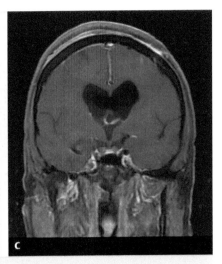

Fig. 14.2 **(a)** Coronal T1-weighted with gadolinium MRI of the brain shows a large colloid cyst, which is up between the fornices rather than down in the third ventricle. **(b)** Axial FLAIR MRI confirms the colloid cyst is between the fornices and up between the leaflets of the septum. **(c)** Postoperative coronal T1-weighted with gadolinium MRI shows collapse of the cyst and preservation of the fornices. Persistent ventriculomegaly is seen that partially resolved on subsequent imaging. (Used with permission from Barrow Neurological Institute, Phoenix, AZ.)

Case 2

A 66-year-old woman presented with increasing memory difficulty and a known history of colloid cyst, which was seen to have expanded on serial imaging. She also had progressive headaches. MRI shows that the cyst is large and between the leaflets of the septum pellucidum and the fornices (▶ Fig. 14.2**a**, **b**). After some discussion, an interhemispheric transcallosal craniotomy was recommended, which the patient underwent without complication. The cyst was drained, and the wall was fenestrated but not resected in toto because it was adherent over a long stretch of the fornix bilaterally (▶ Fig. 14.2**c**). Initially, the patient had short-term memory problems, which subsequently cleared to better than her preoperative baseline by 2 weeks postoperatively. She is being monitored with serial imaging with the expectation that the cyst has a higher than usual possibility of recurring in the future.

14.1.7 Conclusion

Colloid cysts are a pathology that is as likely to excite controversy as any in neurosurgery. This stems largely from the fact that there are two good options for management, microsurgical and endoscopic, and the high stakes involved. The potential risks between acute coma and death from CSF obstruction must be weighed against damage to the fornices with attendant impairment of short-term memory. There are virtues to each approach and risks that differ slightly with either. However, in sum we believe that the endoscopic approach is the preferred default technique, with the open microsurgical technique reserved for a certain subset of colloid cysts. A high degree of facility with both techniques is essential. Arguably, this is harder to achieve for the endoscopic technique because the general techniques of microsurgery are more easily practiced and transferable to open surgery than the less commonly used skills of complex intraventricular neuroendoscopy. With advancements in the technology of neuroendoscopes and instruments, and the increasing numbers of neurosurgeons specializing in neuroendoscopy and minimally invasive techniques, the surgical morbidity of endoscopic approaches remains low, while the efficacy is ever-improving.

References

[1] Batnitzky S, Sarwar M, Leeds NE, Schechter MM, Azar-Kia B. Colloid cysts of the third ventricle. Radiology. 1974; 112(2):327–341

[2] Little JR, MacCarty CS. Colloid cysts of the third ventricle. J Neurosurg. 1974; 40(2):230–235

[3] Wait SD, Gazzeri R, Wilson DA, Abla AA, Nakaji P, Teo C. Endoscopic colloid cyst resection in the absence of ventriculomegaly. Neurosurgery. 2013; 73(1) Suppl Operative:ons39–ons46, ons46–ons47

[4] Boogaarts HD, Decq P, Grotenhuis JA, et al. Long-term results of the neuroendoscopic management of colloid cysts of the third ventricle: a series of 90 cases. Neurosurgery. 2011; 68(1):179–187

[5] Beaumont TL, Limbrick DD, Jr, Rich KM, Wippold FJ, II, Dacey RG, Jr. Natural history of colloid cysts of the third ventricle. J Neurosurg. 2016; 125 (6):1420–1430

[6] Byard RW. Variable presentations of lethal colloid cysts. J Forensic Sci. 2016; 61(6):1538–1540

[7] Horn EM, Feiz-Erfan I, Bristol RE, et al. Treatment options for third ventricular colloid cysts: comparison of open microsurgical versus endoscopic resection. Neurosurgery. 2007; 60(4):613–618, discussion 618–620

[8] Rangel-Castilla L, Chen F, Choi L, Clark JC, Nakaji P. Endoscopic approach to colloid cyst: what is the optimal entry point and trajectory? J Neurosurg. 2014; 121(4):790–796

[9] Sheikh AB, Mendelson ZS, Liu JK. Endoscopic versus microsurgical resection of colloid cysts: a systematic review and meta-analysis of 1,278 patients. World Neurosurg. 2014; 82(6):1187–1197

[10] Dandy W. Benign Tumors in the Third Ventricle of the Brain: Diagnosis and Treatment. Springfield, IL: Williams and Wilkins; 1933

[11] Teo C, Nakaji P. Neuro-oncologic applications of endoscopy. Neurosurg Clin N Am. 2004; 15(1):89–103

[12] Grondin RT, Hader W, MacRae ME, Hamilton MG. Endoscopic versus microsurgical resection of third ventricle colloid cysts. Can J Neurol Sci. 2007; 34 (2):197–207

[13] Powell MP, Torrens MJ, Thomson JLG, Horgan JG. Isodense colloid cysts of the third ventricle: a diagnostic and therapeutic problem resolved by ventriculoscopy. Neurosurgery. 1983; 13(3):234–237

[14] Gaab MR. Colloid cysts: endoscopic or microsurgical resection? World Neurosurg. 2014; 82(6):1017–1019

[15] Birski M, Birska J, Paczkowski D, et al. Combination of neuroendoscopic and stereotactic procedures for total resection of colloid cysts with favorable neurological and cognitive outcomes. World Neurosurg. 2016; 85:205–214

[16] Bergsneider M. Complete microsurgical resection of colloid cysts with a dual-port endoscopic technique. Neurosurgery. 2007; 60(2) Suppl 1:ONS33–ONS42, discussion ONS42–ONS43

[17] Wilson DA, Fusco DJ, Wait SD, Nakaji P. Endoscopic resection of colloid cysts: use of a dual-instrument technique and an anterolateral approach. World Neurosurg. 2013; 80(5):576–583

[18] Azab WA, Salaheddin W, Alsheikh TM, Nasim K, Nasr MM. Colloid cysts posterior and anterior to the foramen of Monro: Anatomical features and implications for endoscopic excision. Surg Neurol Int. 2014; 5:124

[19] da C F Pinto PH, Nigri F, Gobbi GN, Caparelli-Daquer EM, Caparelli-Daquer E. Conversion technique from neuroendoscopy to microsurgery in ventricular tumors: Technical note. Surg Neurol Int. 2016; 7(32) Suppl 31: S785–S789

15 Intracranial Arachnoid Cyst Fenestration versus Shunting

Brian L. Anderson, Mark Iantosca, and Brad E. Zacharia

Summary

Intraventricular arachnoid cysts are congenital lesions, which can grow over time and result in obstructive hydrocephalus. When symptomatic, treatment paradigms involve cyst fenestration versus shunting. Due to their variable locations, no single approach can address the totality of arachnoid cyst treatment. With continued advancement in techniques and technology, neuroendoscopy now offers an alternative to open microsurgical approaches for a variety of cranial pathologies with minimal disruption of normal tissue and an excellent morbidity profile. In this chapter, we describe the various treatment paradigms and their associated advantages and pitfalls.

Keywords: arachnoid cyst, endoscopic, shunt, fenestration

15.1 Introduction

Arachnoid cysts represent the most commonly identified intracranial cysts and are responsible for about 1% of all intracranial lesions. The etiology of arachnoid cysts remains a topic of debate, and a wide range of explanations have been offered ranging from infectious to traumatic, with most experts now generally accepting that the origin is likely congenital. These abnormalities arise from mesenchyme and appear as duplication of the otherwise normal arachnoid membrane. Their function as a mass lesion is hypothesized from various physiologic pathways including a ball-valve mechanism, osmotic gradient distribution, and fluid hypersecretion, to name a few. They are often seen in association with underlying hydrocephalus, perhaps explaining treatment failure despite successful fenestration.

Since their discovery in the early 1800s, most have considered them an incidental and generally benign finding. Their identification in the setting of various neurologic symptoms has continued to raise questions regarding their clinical significance. Advancements in neuroradiology and the increasing numbers of radiologic studies performed have led to an increase in identification as well. Traditional management strategies have included observation with and without radiographic follow-up as well as surgical intervention in select cases. A conservative strategy of observation is further bolstered by the fact that natural history studies demonstrate a low rate of cyst growth, which approaches zero in patients older than 4 years of age.[1,2]

Due to their variable locations, no single approach can address the totality of arachnoid cyst treatment. In part, due to continued advancement in techniques and technology, neuroendoscopy now offers an alternative to open microsurgical approaches for a variety of cranial pathologies with minimal disruption of normal tissue and an excellent morbidity profile. In particular, the treatment of intraventricular and cystic pathology has been revolutionized by the advent of neuroendoscopy. Excellent visualization is achieved within the ventricular system and cystic structures and adequate working area is typically encountered. The coupling of neuronavigation has further advanced these techniques and increased their safety profile and is now considered routine and preferred for an array of benign and malignant neurologic conditions.

In this chapter, we will discuss our strategy for the evaluation and treatment of arachnoid cysts, including considerations and recommendations for surgical intervention. We will emphasize the role that neuroendoscopy now plays and address the advantages and disadvantages of this technique while providing technical nuances and clinical pearls.

15.2 Epidemiology

Historical estimates of the prevalence of arachnoid cysts range from 0.5 to 4%.[3,4] With increased availability of advanced radiographic imaging, a number of prevalence studies have now been reported in both the pediatric and adult populations. In 2010, Al-Holou et al evaluated nearly 12,000 pediatric magnetic resonance imaging (MRI) studies and found an overall incidence of 2.6%, with a greater incidence in males compared to females (3.8 and 1.8%, respectively). The most common locations were the middle and posterior fossa accounting for the majority of lesions. Much less common were cysts along the convexity, intraventricular, and suprasellar, accounting for 4% each. A predilection for the left hemisphere was also noted with 47% compared to 27% on the right, and the remainder were found in the midline.[2]

In 2013, Al-Holou et al reported findings of a similar study performed in adults. Over 48,000 adults underwent MRI and were evaluated for arachnoid cysts. Similar to the pediatric population, an increased prevalence was noted in males compared with females (1.8 vs. 1.1%). Variations by location included a dominance of posterior fossa cysts, with 38% affecting the cerebellum and another 7% located in the cerebellopontine angle. Middle fossa cysts accounted for 34% and were responsible for the strong left-sided predominance.[1] The natural history was evaluated in 203 patients with an average follow-up of 3.3 years, finding symptom development in only 1% of patients. This is consistent with other natural history studies that indicate a low risk of progression in incidentally found arachnoid cysts, with the highest risk found in patients younger than 5 years.[4,5,6]

15.3 Pathogenesis

The prevailing theory points to a congenital origin for arachnoid cysts, with multiple studies reporting their discovery as early as the first trimester of development.[7,8,9,10] Histologic studies have reported the presence of a duplication of the normal arachnoid at the limit of the cyst, giving rise to the cyst wall.[9,11,12] This potential space is filled with fluid to create the cyst cavity. A congenital origin is further supported by the presence of other developmental defects that can be present concurrently. The diversity of cyst locations raises doubt that any one theory can explain the formation of all arachnoid cysts. Theories for the formation of intraventricular cysts note the presence of scattered rests of arachnoid cells within the ventricular system, while others suggest the membrane of Liliequist as the origin of the cysts in the suprasellar location.[13]

Theories to explain the growth and pressure elevations found in some patients have been reported. Some authors suggest a one-way valve-type fluid system to explain this finding, while others suggest hypersecretion of entrapped fluid.[14,15,16,17] Increased protein concentration found within cysts have suggested that an osmotic component may play a role.[18] A full explanation is still lacking and why a small fraction progress to clinical relevance remains a mystery.

15.4 Clinical Presentation

The majority of arachnoid cysts are found incidentally on cranial imaging obtained for presumably unrelated reasons. A multitude of studies agree on a symptomatic rate of approximately 5% of radiographically identified arachnoid cysts.[1,2,3,4] Symptoms attributed to the presence of an arachnoid cyst are usually secondary to mass compression of local structures or elevated intracranial pressure. Infants most often present with signs and symptoms of hydrocephalus. In older children and adults, headache is the most common presenting symptom, with nausea and vomiting, lethargy, and sixth cranial nerve palsies found less often.[19,20,21,22,23,24] Other symptoms specific to location include visual disturbances and pituitary dysfunction for suprasellar cysts, nystagmus and other cranial nerve findings for cerebellopontine angle cysts, and obstructive hydrocephalus for intraventricular or quadrigeminal plate cysts. Multiple other neurologic complaints associated with arachnoid cysts have been reported, but the sensitivity and specificity of any one individual finding are often difficult to pin on the arachnoid cyst.[20,25,26,27]

The most concerning complication reported to have association with arachnoid cysts is intracranial hemorrhage. When this occurs, intracystic hemorrhage may be seen with symptoms associated with sudden mass effect. Most commonly, the presentation is chronic and subdural hygromas are typically identified.[28,29,30] Hemorrhage presentation in this population is often more benign and protracted than even chronic subdural hematoma. The risk of hemorrhage in nontemporal arachnoid cysts is remote, with overall hemorrhage rates of the order of 0.1%. Thus, there remains little evidence to justify prophylactic surgery. Trauma has been suggested to increase the risk of hemorrhage but reports of a true association are mixed.[31,32] We feel that hemorrhage is a risk with or without clear antecedent trauma, and it remains unclear that limiting activity mitigates that risk. We consider continued participation in athletics safe but a frank discussion of the data with the patient and family is suggested.[33]

Estimates of seizure rates in patients with arachnoid cyst are reported as high as 10 to 30%.[2,20,34] Causation is difficult to determine, as seizure is a common indication for many of the imaging studies that resulted in identification of the cyst. Temporal lobe epilepsy was naturally felt to result from middle fossa arachnoid cysts but the correlations have been limited. One notable finding has been the increased rate of cortical dysplasia in one-quarter of patients found to have cyst formation.[35,36,37] This may confound the association between arachnoid cysts and seizure disorders. Arai et al reported the findings of 77 patients treated for middle fossa arachnoid cysts. Thirty-four percent of patients had a preoperative diagnosis of epilepsy, and 54% had abnormal findings on electroencephalogram (EEG). The patients underwent cyst-peritoneal shunt placement without significant complication. Only one patient has resolution of seizures, while four had increased medication needs. Seventy-one percent had unchanged or worsened findings on EEG.[20] Moreover, the authors also demonstrated no improvement in behavioral issues or developmental delay with surgical intervention, speaking to the limited efficacy of treatment to reverse developmental deficits.[34] While there may be an association between the presence of an arachnoid cyst and epilepsy, causality appears to be lacking and treatment perhaps dubious.

15.5 Imaging Findings

The increasing frequency of radiographic evaluation is largely responsible for the heightened awareness of the presence of arachnoid cysts. Computed tomography (CT) and MRI evaluation provide relevant information in the workup of symptomatic and asymptomatic patients. CT imaging is particularly helpful when concern for cystic hemorrhage or associated calcification is present. Incidental, nonhemorrhagic arachnoid cysts should mirror cerebrospinal fluid (CSF) in density and appearance. If the finding is in a location of concern, an MRI study should be completed to rule out other potential pathology including dermoid or epidermoid cysts, neurenteric cysts, porencephalic cysts, and other cystic-appearing lesions. MRI findings are consistent with CSF in all sequences including FLAIR (fluid-attenuated inversion recovery) and diffusion-weighted imaging, which is helpful in the differentiation of the other cystic etiologies mentioned (▶ Fig. 15.1, ▶ Fig. 15.2, ▶ Fig. 15.3, ▶ Fig. 15.4). To better evaluate arachnoid cysts for communicative flow, phase-contrast cine flow imaging studies have been reported with some success.[38,39] Cisternography may also be used to demonstrate communication with adjacent structures, but this practice is no longer routinely utilized and has been supplanted in large part by novel MRI techniques.[39,40] Careful evaluation of adjacent structures for edema and compression is required. The presence of ventriculomegaly or other findings

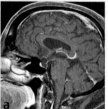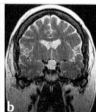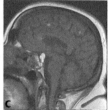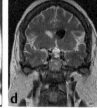

Fig. 15.1 Sellar/suprasellar arachnoid cyst presenting with progressive visual disturbance. **(a)** Preoperative sagittal T1-weighted MRI with contrast; note the gland pushed anteriorly and inferiorly. **(b)** Preoperative coronal T2-weighted MRI; note mild superior displacement of the optic chiasm. **(c,d)** Postoperative MRI with fat noted within the arachnoid cyst.

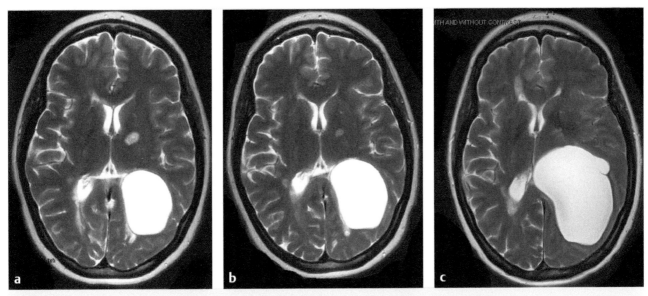

Fig. 15.2 (a-c) Serial preoperative axial T2-weighted MRI of a left parietal periventricular cyst demonstrating steady interval growth with resultant local mass effect. Note the thin membrane between the cyst and the left atrium of the lateral ventricle.

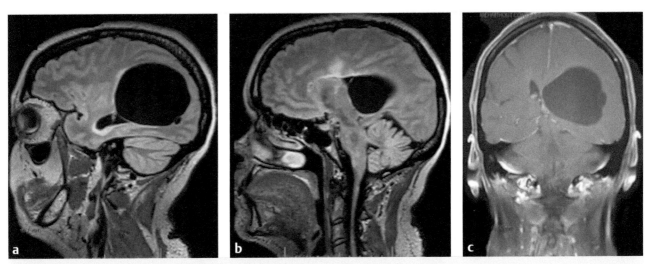

Fig. 15.3 Preoperative sagittal **(a,b)** and coronal **(c)** MRI demonstrating the periventricular cyst. Note the thin membrane separating the cyst from both the atrium and the temporal horn of the lateral ventricle.

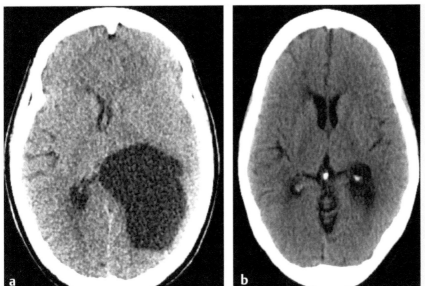

Fig. 15.4 Pre- **(a)** and postoperative **(b)** operative noncontrast CT scan demonstrating significant cyst decompression and reduction in regional mass effect following fenestration.

that could indicate hydrocephalus must be reconciled. Correlation of imaging findings to clinical presentation will improve the likelihood of treatment success.

15.6 To Treat or Not to Treat

The question of whether to surgically treat an arachnoid cyst requires careful consideration of the goals of intervention and the likelihood that this can be achieved with an acceptable risk of complication. It has now been well established that most arachnoid cysts are discovered incidentally with little concern for frank neurologic involvement.[1,2,3,4,19] With a prevalence as high as 1 to 3% in patients undergoing cranial imaging, many are likely to present with any number of complaints common to the general population and their association must be considered on a case-by-case basis.

Key findings that should not be readily dismissed include evidence of hydrocephalus, cranial neuropathy, significant local mass effect or edema, new-onset seizure, and significant cranial remodeling. Rarely, we have had to intervene on a young child with progressive skull deformity from a large temporal cyst based primarily on potential disfigurement and social stigma. This group represents a relatively small portion of those found to have an arachnoid cyst but should not be overlooked. The most difficult patients to manage are those who present with less convincing symptoms, which are not readily attributed to the presence of the arachnoid cyst. Chronic headache, intermittent cognitive symptoms, dizziness, and gait disturbances and developmental delays may be found coincidentally, but their association is often questionable. There are a variety of opinions on the role that surgical intervention plays in this group. Findings in the pediatric population are more likely to be treated with surgery than their similar adult comparison given the increased difficulty in accurately following subtle symptoms and the concern regarding long-term sequelae, even despite the lack of compelling data supporting intervention.

Mørkve et al recently reported their findings of a prospective evaluation of 90 patients undergoing surgical treatment of symptomatic arachnoid cysts. Outcome measures focused on the symptoms of headache and dizziness, with pre- and postoperative assessments performed. They found a significant reduction in both dizziness and headache complaints in treated patients. Intervention was predominantly open surgical fenestration. Twenty percent of patients were lost to follow-up and were therefore not accounted for introducing significant bias, but their findings may support intervention to reduce the symptoms of headache and dizziness.[41]

While a small minority within pediatric neurosurgery have advocated for prophylactic intervention in an effort to reduce the risk of subsequent hemorrhage, we feel it is safe to say that surgery is rarely, if ever, indicated prophylactically for reduction of hemorrhage risk. There are mixed studies regarding the true risk of hemorrhage and some suggest the risk of hemorrhage is not reduced by preemptive intervention.[42,43] While there is near-complete agreement to conservatively manage asymptomatic arachnoid cysts, symptom presentation and radiographic correlation should be carefully evaluated and a determination for treatment rendered on a case-by-case basis.

15.7 Evolution of Surgical Treatment

Several options exist for patients who present with appropriate indications for surgical intervention. Conceptually, all procedures aim to reduce the pressure of the fluid content within the arachnoid cyst. Initial efforts, limited by technology, were centered on an open approach with craniotomy and fenestration of the cyst wall to provide communication of the cyst contents with the other subarachnoid and/or ventricular spaces.[19,34,44] Rarely are aggressive attempts made to strip the entirety of the cyst wall, although a small piece can be sent for histologic analysis should one be suspicious of a sinister pathology. Shunting procedures offer a relatively simple means to divert fluid accumulation within the cyst by means of a technique that is common to nearly all neurosurgeons and presents a low risk of upfront complication, although there remains an ever-present risk of hardware malfunction and/or infection.[20,45,46]

More recently, endoscopic approaches with cyst wall fenestration have emerged as an option capable of the benefits provided by open surgery and with a minimally invasive approach similar to shunt placement.[26,43,47,48] The trend toward endoscopic treatment of intracranial pathology is consistent with the efforts of neurosurgeons from the origin of the specialty and follows a typical pattern seen throughout our history and all neurosurgical subspecialties.[49,50,51,52] Historical approaches were limited by the technology of the times, but we have incorporated new technologies to minimize soft-tissue and brain disruption, facilitate safe surgical approaches, and improve patient outcomes. In particular, advances in endoscopy including improved optics, advanced light sources, and the creation of bimanual endoscopic instrumentation have combined with the pioneering spirit of neurosurgeons to rapidly grow the field of neuroendoscopy. We feel the endoscopic approach to arachnoid cysts is a natural evolution in the management of these lesions and warrants consideration as the first-line surgical treatment modality.

15.8 Modern Decision-Making Algorithm

While the breadth of anatomic locations and clinical presentations of arachnoid cysts precludes a formulaic management strategy, we feel that organizing treatment approaches based on anatomic location provides a framework for the neurosurgeon to approach these lesions. This is by no means comprehensive and we are cautious to not be draconian regarding the use of a single strategy.

15.8.1 Sellar/Parasellar

Sellar and parasellar arachnoid cysts comprise a relatively rare category of arachnoid cysts, making up approximately 3% of this group. These patients frequently present with visual dysfunction and/or constitutional symptoms. MRI typically demonstrates a cystic lesion in the sella with CSF density, without abnormal enhancement, upward bowing of the diaphragm sella, and thinning of the pituitary gland (▶ Fig. 15.1).

These have been traditionally managed via a supratentorial craniotomy and wide fenestration into the basal cisterns. When a lesion is predominately suprasellar and does not have an easily accessible boundary with a ventricular cavity, we find microsurgical fenestration via a supraorbital eyebrow craniotomy most appropriate. We have, however, adopted the technique of McLaughlin et al for addressing predominately sellar arachnoid cysts.[53] Early attempts at wide endonasal fenestration of sellar arachnoid cysts were associated with a relatively high rate of serious complications.[54,55,56] The current technique provides a simplified endoscopic endonasal approach to eliminate CSF flow into the arachnoid cyst without creating or expanding the arachnoid opening into the basal cisterns. This goal is accomplished by opening into and obliterating the arachnoid cyst with abdominal fat to reinforce a defective diaphragma sella or arachnoid diverticulum (▶ Fig. 15.1**b**). While this technique is contrary to the traditional method, we have obtained good early results consistent with those of McLaughlin and colleagues.[53] We believe this to be a rational alternative to management of predominately sellar arachnoid cysts with a favorable morbidity profile and high degree of efficacy.

15.8.2 Intraventricular/Periventricular

This is a heterogeneous group of patients as arachnoid cysts can form anywhere within the ventricular system itself and extraventricular cysts frequently have a border with the ventricular system. These lesions often come to attention due to symptoms of increased intracranial pressure secondary to hydrocephalus. With very rare exception, we find that the endoscopic approach is ideal for these cysts. When working within the cystic or ventricular cavity, one is provided with ample working room to visualize regional anatomy. With the use of modern intraventricular endoscopic instruments, one is able to complete a wide fenestration between the cystic structure and normal ventricular passageways or resect the cyst in its entirety (although this is often not required). If there is suspicion of a neoplasm, a piece of the cyst wall can easily be sampled and sent for pathologic analysis. Moreover, the endoscopic approach allows one to address concomitant hydrocephalus via septal fenestration or endoscopic third ventriculostomy when needed.

15.8.3 Temporal/Posterior Fossa

Although the most common locations for arachnoid cysts, these are less often associated with concordant symptomatic presentation. As such, these cyst types only infrequently require surgical intervention. As discussed above, there are some data that support treatment of temporal arachnoid cysts to improve quality of life, but this study has significant methodological flaws and the jury is still out in this regard.[41] When these do require surgical intervention, we favor cyst fenestration over cystoperitoneal shunting. As noted earlier, we make every effort to avoid permanent hardware implantation given the risks of hardware failure and infection. While cyst fenestration can be accomplished with endoscopic guidance, we often find that a minicraniotomy and use of the operating microscope provide excellent exposure, visualization, and simpler manipulation of tissue than a purely endoscopic approach. We always have the endoscope setup, however, as endoscopic assistance can be

quite helpful, especially to see around corners with a limited calvarial opening.

15.9 Endoscopic Surgical Management

Given the wide variation in cyst presentation and location, we cannot touch on every nuance in the management of all lesions; however, we will present a case of an arachnoid cyst that is illustrative of a few of the key factors to consider with an endoscopic arachnoid cyst fenestration. Prior to pursuing any neuroendoscopic procedure, one must familiarize himself/herself with the wide array of equipment necessary to safely perform this surgery. We primarily utilize the MINOP Modular Neuroendoscopy System from Aesculap, but have also utilized the LOTTA System from Storz. Both provide excellent optics and a wide range of endoscopic instruments, allow for bimanual instrumentation, and provide both straight and 30-degree optics. For all but the most complex of cases, we prefer to utilize a two-surgeon approach, with the surgeon utilizing the instruments and an assistant driving the endoscope. For longer or more complex cases, an endoscope holder can be utilized, and there are a wide range of these on the market. Unfortunately, a full discussion of the various neuroendoscopic systems is beyond the scope of this chapter.

15.10 Case Example

Our patient is a 50-year-old woman with a longstanding history of multiple sclerosis, which has been recently controlled with medication. In routine follow-up with her neurologist, she noted mild cognitive dysfunction and progressive imbalance. She undergoes at least twice yearly MRI for follow-up of her disease and a slowly enlarging left parietal cyst was noted, prompting referral to neurosurgery (▶ Fig. 15.1).

On neurological examination, the patient was largely intact. One could not tease out significant cognitive deficits, although the patient noted she was not as sharp as she was a few months ago. We did, however, identify a new partial right homonymous hemianopsia. Her MRI demonstrated a 7.2 × 5.2 cm parieto-occipital cyst (▶ Fig. 15.1, ▶ Fig. 15.2). The cyst abutted the wall of the atrium of the lateral ventricle and exerted significant regional mass effect. This resulted in early uncal herniation and trapping of the left temporal horn (▶ Fig. 15.2). In 2013, this cyst had measured 3.5 × 4.7 cm (▶ Fig. 15.2**a**) and was thus clearly enlarging.

While the etiology of this cyst was not entirely clear, one might speculate that this developed from a previous multiple sclerosis plaque. Regardless, given her clear neurological deficit and subjective decline, we agreed that directly addressing the cyst was the most prudent course of action. We discussed the three prevailing options: (1) open surgical cyst fenestration, (2) endoscopic cyst fenestration, and (3) cyst-peritoneal shunting. We personally reserve cyst shunting for patients who have failed at least one attempt at cyst fenestration. The hardware complications and the nonphysiologic shunting are undesirable and we feel this renders shunting a second-line treatment. Open surgical resection can offer more robust working angles and the ability to use traditional bimanual surgical techniques. One is often able to achieve a more robust fenestration with an open procedure, although the relative merits of this are not clear. In cases with a multiplicity of complex cysts, an open approach may be favored. Similarly, in cases with a large burden of hemorrhage or infectious material, an open approach may facilitate visualization. The above notwithstanding, our preference is to proceed with endoscopic cyst fenestration whenever we feel it is technically feasible and this is clearly the preferred approach for cysts within or adjacent to dilated portions of the ventricular system.

We ultimately decided to pursue a left parietal endoscopic cyst fenestration. The patient was positioned supine with a right-sided shoulder bump to allow her head to rotate to the right and expose the left parietal boss. We registered the Stealth AxiEM frameless, pinless neuronavigation system based on a preoperatively obtained stereotactic CT scan. Given the large size of this cyst and the minimal overlying cortex, we chose an entry point that would allow for traversing minimal cortex and facilitate easy cyst entry. We then chose a target where the cyst wall abutted the atrium of the lateral ventricle. This trajectory was reviewed on the Stealth system and the target distance was noted.

The entry point was then identified on the scalp and a 3-cm linear incision was marked. After instillation of local anesthetic, the incision was made down to the skull. A standard perforator was used to make a single burr hole. We then placed the Stealth AxiEM stylet in a ventricular catheter. A minimal dural opening was performed and the catheter was advanced via Stealth navigation to the target depth. We then passed the MINOP ventriculoscope adjacent to the catheter and followed it under direct visualization. We could see that the catheter had penetrated the deep cyst wall. We utilized the endoscope and obturator to further pierce the cyst membrane. Choroid plexus was seen confirming entry into the lateral ventricle. The fenestration was further enlarged with the endoscope. Immaculate hemostasis was noted and the endoscope was withdrawn. A single piece of Gelfoam was placed in the burr hole and the scalp was closed in the usual fashion.

The patient did very well postoperatively with improvement in her subjective neurologic symptoms. At about 3 months postoperatively, she has improvement in her visual field deficit. CT demonstrated significant decrease in the size of the cyst, now measuring $4.3 \times 3 \times 1.5$ cm with reduced mass effect (▶ Fig. 15.4).

15.11 Technical Nuances

There are a multitude of factors that one must take into consideration when addressing intracranial cysts via an endoscopic approach. The minimally invasive nature of endoscopic fenestration can be viewed in both a positive and a negative light. Given its inherent limitations, one must take additional steps in preparation.

As with all of neurosurgery, preoperative evaluation of the imaging is crucial. In particular, the cyst location, size, relationship to ventricular or cisternal spaces, and presence of hemorrhage should be noted. The regional compression of brain and/or ventricular spaces should also be identified. In general, we prefer an approach from the ventricular system into the cyst,

rather than vice versa, as it is easier to fenestrate into a bulging cyst. It is also important to note the location of choroid plexus and vascular structures in relationship to one's proposed trajectory.

While we have come to rely heavily on neuronavigation and find it crucial in these cases, there are several caveats. We most commonly utilize the frameless AxiEM system, but any navigation system can be adapted for neuroendoscopic use. The advantage of the AxiEM system is that it obviates the need for a direct line of site, which can often pose an issue with odd trajectories. Moreover, the system is navigated from the tip of the probe and as such is not subject to issue regarding bending and misalignment of the probe. Although solid metal can interfere with the AxiEM system, we have found that it works well through the working channel of the MINOP endoscope and thus one can directly track the camera in real time. Neuronavigation is particularly useful when fenestrating from a smaller into a larger structure to provide a perpendicular approach to the cyst wall facilitating safe fenestration.

Most importantly, one must consider how the brain will shift once the cyst is fenestrated. This can render neuronavigation inaccurate and unreliable. Therefore, in cases in which a small target is identified, we will oftentimes pass a ventricular catheter along the trajectory under neuronavigation to serve as a guide for endoscope insertion as we feel this is when our navigation is most accurate. We will also try and minimize the dural opening essentially creating a seal around the endoscope. This avoids additional egress of CSF and deflation of the cyst during surgery.

15.12 Clinical Pearls

- Test *all* equipment and verify navigation/registration thoroughly prior to incision/insertion.
- Complex cases require advanced and subspecialized neuroendoscopic equipment. The key features include superb optics, continuous ingress and egress of irrigation/CSF, and a wide array of endoscopic instruments including bipolar and monopolar cautery.
- Closely evaluate preoperative imaging for cyst characteristics, location, and regional anatomy.
- Maintain an orthogonal head position (i.e., 0 or 90 degrees) when possible during surgery as this facilitates an understanding of ventricular/cyst anatomy.
- Minimize the dural opening to avoid significant egress of CSF.
- When possible, fenestrate from a smaller into a larger structure.
- Perform the most anatomically critical portion of the operation first, when navigation is likely to be most accurate.
- Prioritize operative goals in the event of ventricular collapse or bleeding that obscures anatomy. For instance, fenestration for the relief of hydrocephalus may take precedence over a biopsy, which may produce bleeding and hinder effective fenestration.
- Attempt bleeding control by direct pressure with the scope head and irrigation prior to utilizing cautery that can potentially worsen bleeding or cause thermal damage to adjacent structures.

15.13 Pitfalls

- Preparation is critical. Have bipolar endoscopic cautery available in the event of bleeding that cannot be controlled with irrigation.
- It is quite easy to become disoriented especially once the cyst decompresses.

References

[1] Al-Holou WN, Terman S, Kilburg C, Garton HJ, Muraszko KM, Maher CO. Prevalence and natural history of arachnoid cysts in adults. J Neurosurg. 2013; 118(2):222–231

[2] Al-Holou WN, Yew AY, Boomsaad ZE, Garton HJ, Muraszko KM, Maher CO. Prevalence and natural history of arachnoid cysts in children. J Neurosurg Pediatr. 2010; 5(6):578–585

[3] Katzman GL, Dagher AP, Patronas NJ. Incidental findings on brain magnetic resonance imaging from 1000 asymptomatic volunteers. JAMA. 1999; 282 (1):36–39

[4] Weber F, Knopf H. Incidental findings in magnetic resonance imaging of the brains of healthy young men. J Neurol Sci. 2006; 240(1–2):81–84

[5] Candela S, Puerta P, Alamar M, et al. Epidemiology and classification of arachnoid cysts in children [in Spanish]. Neurocirugia (Astur). 2015; 26 (5):234–240

[6] Huang JH, Mei WZ, Chen Y, Chen JW, Lin ZX. Analysis on clinical characteristics of intracranial arachnoid cysts in 488 pediatric cases. Int J Clin Exp Med. 2015; 8(10):18343–18350

[7] De Keersmaecker B, Ramaekers P, Claus F, et al. Outcome of 12 antenatally diagnosed fetal arachnoid cysts: case series and review of the literature. Eur J Paediatr Neurol. 2015; 19(2):114–121

[8] Goksu E, Kazan S. Spontaneous shrinkage of a suprasellar arachnoid cyst diagnosed with prenatal sonography and fetal magnetic resonance imaging: case report and review of the literature. Turk Neurosurg. 2015; 25(4):670–673

[9] Youssef A, D'Antonio F, Khalil A, et al. Outcome of fetuses with supratentorial extra-axial intracranial cysts: a systematic review. Fetal Diagn Ther. 2016; 40 (1):1–12

[10] Bretelle F, Senat MV, Bernard JP, Hillion Y, Ville Y. First-trimester diagnosis of fetal arachnoid cyst: prenatal implication. Ultrasound Obstet Gynecol. 2002; 20(4):400–402

[11] Cotes C, Bonfante E, Lazor J, et al. Congenital basis of posterior fossa anomalies. Neuroradiol J. 2015; 28(3):238–253

[12] Rengachary SS, Watanabe I. Ultrastructure and pathogenesis of intracranial arachnoid cysts. J Neuropathol Exp Neurol. 1981; 40(1):61–83

[13] Fox JL, Al-Mefty O. Suprasellar arachnoid cysts: an extension of the membrane of Liliequist. Neurosurgery. 1980; 7(6):615–618

[14] Helland CA, Aarhus M, Knappskog P, et al. Increased NKCC1 expression in arachnoid cysts supports secretory basis for cyst formation. Exp Neurol. 2010; 224(2):424–428

[15] Dagain A, Lepeintre JF, Scarone P, Costache C, Dupuy M, Gaillard S. Endoscopic removal of a suprasellar arachnoid cyst: an anatomical study with special reference to skull base. Surg Radiol Anat. 2010; 32(4):389–392

[16] Berle M, Wester KG, Ulvik RJ, et al. Arachnoid cysts do not contain cerebrospinal fluid: A comparative chemical analysis of arachnoid cyst fluid and cerebrospinal fluid in adults. Cerebrospinal Fluid Res. 2010; 7:8

[17] Santamarta D, Aguas J, Ferrer E. The natural history of arachnoid cysts: endoscopic and cine-mode MRI evidence of a slit-valve mechanism. Minim Invasive Neurosurg. 1995; 38(4):133–137

[18] Sandberg DI, McComb JG, Krieger MD. Chemical analysis of fluid obtained from intracranial arachnoid cysts in pediatric patients. J Neurosurg. 2005; 103(5) Suppl:427–432

[19] Helland CA, Wester K. A population-based study of intracranial arachnoid cysts: clinical and neuroimaging outcomes following surgical cyst decompression in children. J Neurosurg. 2006; 105(5) Suppl:385–390

[20] Arai H, Sato K, Wachi A, Okuda O, Takeda N. Arachnoid cysts of the middle cranial fossa: experience with 77 patients who were treated with cystoperitoneal shunting. Neurosurgery. 1996; 39(6):1108–1112, discussion 1112–1113

[21] Rajesh S, Bhatnagar S, Chauhan U, Gupta S, Agarwal N, Kasana V. Arachnoid cyst of the cavum velum interpositum in a septuagenarian: radiological features and differential diagnosis. Neuroradiol J. 2014; 27(2):154–157

[22] Pradilla G, Jallo G. Arachnoid cysts: case series and review of the literature. Neurosurg Focus. 2007; 22(2):E7

[23] Hershey AD, Powers SW, Bentti AL, LeCates S, deGrauw TJ. Characterization of chronic daily headaches in children in a multidisciplinary headache center. Neurology. 2001; 56(8):1032–1037

[24] Cherian J, Viswanathan A, Evans RW. Headache and arachnoid cysts. Headache. 2014; 54(7):1224–1228

[25] Rico-Cotelo M, Diaz-Cabanas L, Allut AG, Gelabert-Gonzalez M. Intraventricular arachnoid cyst [in Spanish]. Rev Neurol. 2013; 57(1):25–28

[26] Hinojosa J, Esparza J, Muñoz MJ, Valencia J. Endoscopic treatment of suprasellar arachnoid cysts [in Spanish]. Neurocirugia (Astur). 2001; 12(6):482–488, discussion 489

[27] Alexiou GA, Sfakianos G, Prodromou N. Giant suprasellar arachnoid cyst with head bobbing. Mov Disord. 2013; 28(9):1216

[28] Kertmen H, Gürer B, Yilmaz ER, Sekerci Z. Chronic subdural hematoma associated with an arachnoid cyst in a juvenile taekwondo athlete: a case report and review of the literature. Pediatr Neurosurg. 2012; 48(1):55–58

[29] Kawanishi A, Nakayama M, Kadota K. Heading injury precipitating subdural hematoma associated with arachnoid cysts–two case reports. Neurol Med Chir (Tokyo). 1999; 39(3):231–233

[30] Demetriades AK, McEvoy AW, Kitchen ND. Subdural haematoma associated with an arachnoid cyst after repetitive minor heading injury in ball games. Br J Sports Med. 2004; 38(4):E8

[31] Zuckerman SL, Prather CT, Yengo-Kahn AM, Solomon GS, Sills AK, Bonfield CM. Sport-related structural brain injury associated with arachnoid cysts: a systematic review and quantitative analysis. Neurosurg Focus. 2016; 40(4):E9

[32] Strahle J, Selzer BJ, Geh N, et al. Sports participation with arachnoid cysts. J Neurosurg Pediatr. 2016; 17(4):410–417

[33] Liu Z, Xu P, Li Q, Liu H, Chen N, Xu J. Arachnoid cysts with subdural hematoma or intracystic hemorrhage in children. Pediatr Emerg Care. 2014; 30(5): 345–351

[34] Ciricillo SF, Cogen PH, Harsh GR, Edwards MS. Intracranial arachnoid cysts in children. A comparison of the effects of fenestration and shunting. J Neurosurg. 1991; 74(2):230–235

[35] Sener RN. Coexistence of schizencephaly and middle cranial fossa arachnoid cyst: a report of two patients. Eur Radiol. 1997; 7(3):409–411

[36] Vaquerizo-Madrid J. Sylvian arachnoid cysts, temporal lobe hypoplasia and epileptic encephalopathy [in Spanish]. Rev Neurol. 1999; 29(12):1188–1189

[37] Arroyo S, Santamaria J. What is the relationship between arachnoid cysts and seizure foci? Epilepsia. 1997; 38(10):1098–1102

[38] Battal B, Kocaoglu M, Bulakbasi N, Husmen G, Tuba Sanal H, Tayfun C. Cerebrospinal fluid flow imaging by using phase-contrast MR technique. Br J Radiol. 2011; 84(1004):758–765

[39] Yildiz H, Erdogan C, Yalcin R, et al. evaluation of communication between intracranial arachnoid cysts and cisterns with phase-contrast cine MR imaging. AJNR Am J Neuroradiol. 2005; 26(1):145–151

[40] Galassi E, Tognetti F, Gaist G, Fagioli L, Frank F, Frank G. CT scan and metrizamide CT cisternography in arachnoid cysts of the middle cranial fossa: classification and pathophysiological aspects. Surg Neurol. 1982; 17(5):363–369

[41] Mørkve SH, Helland CA, Amus J, Lund-Johansen M, Wester KG. Surgical decompression of arachnoid cysts leads to improved quality of life: a prospective study. Neurosurgery. 2016; 78(5):613–625

[42] Levy ML, Wang M, Aryan HE, Yoo K, Meltzer H. Microsurgical keyhole approach for middle fossa arachnoid cyst fenestration. Neurosurgery. 2003; 53(5):1138–1144, discussion 1144–1145

[43] Spacca B, Kandasamy J, Mallucci CL, Genitori L. Endoscopic treatment of middle fossa arachnoid cysts: a series of 40 patients treated endoscopically in two centres. Childs Nerv Syst. 2010; 26(2):163–172

[44] Ozgur BM, Aryan HE, Levy ML. Microsurgical keyhole middle fossa arachnoid cyst fenestration. J Clin Neurosci. 2005; 12(7):804–806

[45] Gangemi M, Colella G, Magro F, Maiuri F. Suprasellar arachnoid cysts: endoscopy versus microsurgical cyst excision and shunting. Br J Neurosurg. 2007; 21(3):276–280

[46] Gangemi M, Seneca V, Colella G, Cioffi V, Imperato A, Maiuri F. Endoscopy versus microsurgical cyst excision and shunting for treating intracranial arachnoid cysts. J Neurosurg Pediatr. 2011; 8(2):158–164

[47] Tamburrini G, D'Angelo L, Paternoster G, Massimi L, Caldarelli M, Di Rocco C. Endoscopic management of intra and paraventricular CSF cysts. Childs Nerv Syst. 2007; 23(6):645–651

[48] Enchev Y, Oi S. Historical trends of neuroendoscopic surgical techniques in the treatment of hydrocephalus. Neurosurg Rev. 2008; 31(3):249–262

[49] Rowland NC, Sammartino F, Lozano AM. Advances in surgery for movement disorders. Mov Disord. 2017; 32(1):5–10

[50] Hardesty DA, Ponce FA, Little AS, Nakaji P. A quantitative analysis of published skull base endoscopy literature. J Neurol Surg B Skull Base. 2016; 77(1):24–31

[51] Beyer-Berjot L, Aggarwal R. Toward technology-supported surgical training: the potential of virtual simulators in laparoscopic surgery. Scand J Surg. 2013; 102(4):221–226

[52] Suri A, Patra DP, Meena RK. Simulation in neurosurgery: past, present, and future. Neurol India. 2016; 64(3):387–395

[53] McLaughlin N, Vandergrift A, Ditzel Filho LF, et al. Endonasal management of sellar arachnoid cysts: simple cyst obliteration technique. J Neurosurg. 2012; 116(4):728–740

[54] Cavallo LM, Prevedello D, Esposito F, et al. The role of the endoscope in the transsphenoidal management of cystic lesions of the sellar region. Neurosurg Rev. 2008; 31(1):55–64, discussion 64

[55] Dubuisson AS, Stevenaert A, Martin DH, Flandroy PP. Intrasellar arachnoid cysts. Neurosurgery. 2007; 61(3):505–513, discussion 513

[56] Saeki N, Tokunaga H, Hoshi S, et al. Delayed postoperative CSF rhinorrhea of intrasellar arachnoid cyst. Acta Neurochir (Wien). 1999; 141(2):165–169

16 Endoscopic Aqueductal Stenting

Steffen K. Fleck and Henry W. S. Schroeder

Summary

Cerebral aqueductal stenosis from a variety of congenital or acquired diseases can result in obstructive hydrocephalus. The 1920s saw the first attempts at treating supratentorial hydrocephalus due to aqueductal stenosis. Modern approaches have relied heavily on cerebrospinal fluid diversion procedures but carry the risk of shunt failure and revision. Alternatives include reopening the natural fluid resorption pathways using cerebral aqueductal stenting. In this chapter, we discuss the surgical indications, nuances, complication avoidance, and alternatives to cerebral aqueductal stenting.

Keywords: aqueductoplasty, aqueductal stenosis, hydrocephalus, isolated fourth ventricle, neuroendoscopy

16.1 Introduction

16.1.1 General Overview

Although Magendie was the first to describe an occlusion of the aqueduct of Sylvius (iter) (1842), Touche appears to be the first author to draw the connection between hydrocephalus and obliteration of the aqueduct.[1] Spiller and later Guthrie speculated that inflammation was the cause of aqueductal occlusion and hydrocephalus.[2,3,4]

The 1920s saw the first attempts at treating supratentorial hydrocephalus due to aqueductal stenosis (AS). As Dandy explained it, "The treatment of the hydrocephalus must be directed toward an attack on the cause of the disease." He performed the first aqueduct reconstructions in two infants. He exposed the fourth ventricle by separating the divided surfaces of the cerebellum, and after piercing the aqueduct with a steel catheter, he inserted a rubber catheter from the fourth ventricle through the aqueduct, and then left it in place for 2 to 3 weeks.[4]

Various other authors reported their experiences as well (Greenwood, 1944; Norlén, 1949; Elvidge, 1966; Turnball and Drake, 1966; Crosby, 1973).[5,6,7,8,9,10,11,12] Leksell, for example, reported a large series of 62 patients with AS who were surgically treated. In his early cases, the aqueduct was catheterized from a suboccipital approach. The rubber catheter was then left in place for several days, and guided out through the neck muscles. Later, he developed a method of catheterizing the aqueduct with a soft rubber catheter and then permanently placing a tantalum spiral tube within the aqueduct.[12] Subsequently, Lapras et al reported a large series of 74 patients who were treated between 1964 and 1983 by way of direct suboccipital surgery in a sitting position. They used a specially designed catheter which diminished the risk of catheter dislocation. The authors concluded that, using this technique, between 50 and 60% of patients could remain shunt-independent.[13] For microsurgical procedures, such as aqueduct canalization and fenestration of the fourth ventricle outlets, transcerebellar, transtentorial, and transhiatus approaches have all been shown as viable options. Additionally, readjustment of supratentorial overdrainage as a possible cause of aqueductal obstruction has been discussed.[14,15,16,17,18,19]

16.1.2 Etiology of Aqueductal Stenosis Including Isolated (or "Trapped") Fourth Ventricle

Hydrocephalus is caused by AS in 10 to 40% in adults and in 15 to 60% in children.[20,21,22,23,24] Intraventricular hemorrhages, infections or inflammation, and local or disseminating tumor diseases (e.g., carcinomatous meningitis) are the main causes of AS and/or isolated (or "trapped") fourth ventricle (IFV).[25,26] The aqueduct may also passively collapse under pressure from distended lateral ventricles—a secondary cause of aqueductal obstruction rather than a primary stenosis.[27] Overdrainage of an existing shunt system can also cause occlusion of the aqueduct. This complication can occur following supratentorial shunting procedures (which produce initial improvement) and is likely due to the development of adhesions and the narrowing of the aqueductal walls in the presence of ependymal inflammation.[16,28,29]

IFV may also develop after initially sufficient supratentorial shunting procedures.[30] Fourth ventricle outlet obstruction (FVOO) can be associated with congenital foramen of Magendie obstructions, Chiari I malformations, or Dandy–Walker malformations. Ongoing cerebrospinal fluid (CSF) production from the choroid plexus and ependyma within the fourth ventricle or a valvelike mechanism in the aqueduct, combined with proximal obstruction of the aqueduct and distal obstruction of the foramina of Magendie and Luschka, leads to a progressive dilation of the fourth ventricle.[15,31] When this occurs, the brainstem becomes compressed against the clivus and the cerebellum against the tentorium.[15,30,32,33,34,35]

16.1.3 Classification of Aqueductal Stenosis (According to Therapy Options)

In 1949, Russel classified congenital AS into four categories based on the pathology: (1) forking, (2) simple primary stenosis (true narrowing), (3) septum formation, and (4) gliotic stenosis.[36,37] AS can also be differentiated as follows to reflect the most appropriate neuroendoscopic strategy:
- *Membranous occlusion*: This involves a proximal ampullary dilatation of the prestenotic aqueduct.
- *Tumor or cyst related*: Here, the obstruction evolves either directly from tectal gliomas or secondarily from pineal region processes such as cysts, pinealomas, or germinomas.
- *IFV*: This is caused by an occlusion of both the aqueduct and foramina of Luschka and Magendie.

16.1.4 Signs and Symptoms

Generally, the signs and symptoms of intracranial hypertension caused by a hydrocephalus include headache, nausea, vomiting, seizures, ataxia, and decrease of consciousness. The symptoms can occur acutely but also chronically in longstanding hydrocephalus. Late-onset idiopathic AS usually presents with ataxia, dementia, or urinary incontinence, as is observed in patients with normal pressure hydrocephalus. Pediatric patients with hydrocephalus may present with splaying sutures and bulged fontanels, increasing head circumferences, lethargy, spasticity, opisthotonus, bradycardia, apneic episodes, and sucking weakness. Palsies of certain nerves (oculomotor, trochlear, abducens, facial, bulbar) or Parinaud's syndrome might also occur, especially in cases of IFV.[15,37] Tonsillar herniation, which is consistent with an acquired Chiari malformation and hydromyelia formation, can occur too; this is due to longstanding enlargement of CSF spaces within the posterior fossa.[38]

16.2 Evolution of Neuroendoscopic Treatment Options

16.2.1 Treatment Options: Overview

Various procedures have been developed for the specific treatment of IFV.[14,15,39,40,41] CSF diversionary procedures involve placement of intracranial shunt system catheters. Possible approaches include midline transvermian, lateral cerebellar, transaqueductal (anterograde or retrograde), transforaminal (Magendie), and transcortical (tentorial hiatus). Microsurgical techniques (fourth ventriculocisternostomy) for treating IFV include fenestration via the posterior fossa, with or without stent placement in the spinal subarachnoid space, as well as placement of a transcerebellar catheter that is connected to a supratentorial shunt system.[14,15,40,42,43] Endoscopic interventions aim to achieve a more physiological flow of CSF than is possible with extracranial shunting. They also seek to equalize pressure between the CSF compartments and to avoid the introduction of foreign material like shunts, which are well known for their long-term complications.[37,44,45,46] As endoscopic equipment has improved during the last 25 years, neuroendoscopic techniques have evolved in parallel, leading to improved outcomes and resulting in a number of new treatment options for a variety of cranial diseases. Endoscopic third ventriculostomy (ETV) is now the most widely employed endoscopic procedure for treating obstructive hydrocephalus due to AS in both adults and children.[47,48] The limitations of this procedure, however, must be noted,[48,49] and the value of endoscopic aqueduct restoration is still being debated.

16.2.2 Endoscopic Aqueductoplasty

Endoscopic aqueductoplasty (EAP) with stenting is a treatment alternative for both triventricular obstructive hydrocephalus due to AS and for IFV. This procedure has also been established during the last decades and, in the hands of an experienced neurosurgeon, has been proven to be both safe and effective.[34,50,51,52,53] Recent long-term evaluations of aqueductoplasty without stent implantation, however, have shown disappointingly low success rates in the treatment of triventricular hydrocephalus due to AS.[50,54,55]

The main endoscopic options are:
• Aqueductoplasty with stenting (anterograde or retrograde).

• Interventriculostomy (lateral or third ventricle to fourth ventricle) with stenting.
• ETV (for triventricular obstructive hydrocephalus).

Endoscopically, an internal CSF diversion channel can be created with cannulation or aqueductoplasty (with or without stent) or by performing a fenestration of the superior medullary velum. Depending on the size of the supratentorial ventricles, either a supra- or infratentorial (antegrade or retrograde) approach can be taken.[10,33,35,46,56,57,58,59,60,61,62,63] In cases of an IFV, aqueductal stenting can be performed to establish a connection with an existing shunt to the lateral ventricles. This treatment approach offers a stable clinical course.[32] The stent can be placed using a rigid endoscope. Due to the curved course of the aqueduct, steerable endoscopes bear certain advantages and may be safer.[46,64]

16.3 Endoscopic Techniques

16.3.1 Antegrade Transventricular Approach

Aqueductoplasty with Stenting

When the individual anatomy allows, we favor a supratentorial approach. The patient lies supine under general anesthesia, and the head is generally positioned in a horseshoe-shaped headrest. When neuronavigation is employed, sharp fixation with a Mayfield clamp may be necessary. With young children, we secure the head with tape. Additionally, the head is slightly elevated and anteflected to avoid excessive CSF loss.

In most cases (baring contraindications), we administer a perioperative single-shot antibiotic prophylaxis (cefuroxime) 30 minutes before skin incision. We perform our endoscopic procedures with a rod-lens ventriculoscopic system (LOTTA system; Karl Storz, Tuttlingen, Germany), which includes a larger (Standard LOTTA) and a smaller (Little LOTTA) ventriculoscope.[65] The smaller scope (diameter: 3.6 mm) is usually used for aqueductoplasty and ETV. Flexible scopes are useful for inspecting distal segments of the aqueduct but are not frequently used in our clinic. We prefer to utilize holding devices (e.g., pneumatic arm: Pointsetter; Mitaka, Co., Tokyo, Japan) rather than relying on "freehand" guidance.

The position of the individual burr hole is determined on the basis of information obtained from high-resolution (sagittal) magnetic resonance imaging (MRI). Neuronavigation (in our department: BrainLAB, Heimstetten, Germany) can also be used to help determine the optimal trajectory. Here, a line considering the foramen of Monro and the entry point of the aqueduct should be envisioned. In the majority of cases, the burr hole is located 3 to 5 cm anterior to the coronal suture. In adults, the burr hole is approximately 1 to 2 cm off-midline, with an age-dependent deviation in children. The size of the foramen of Monro, the bottleneck of this procedure, determines which side is used for the approach. A preexisting catheter can serve as a further helpful intraventricular landmark.

After stepwise incision and opening of the dura, we confirm the trajectory using a Cushing needle. The sheath with trocar is inserted into the frontal horn of the lateral ventricle, which is reached after 4 to 5 cm in adults. The trocar is then removed, and the endoscope is introduced. Tiny hemorrhages disappear within minutes under continuous irrigation. The choroid plexus, the thalamostriate vein, and the foramen of Monro are then identified, and the endoscope is carefully advanced, under visual control, through the foramen into the third ventricle. The edges of the endoscopic sheath must always remain visible (with the endoscope retracted into the trocar) during navigation through the ventricle, especially when passing through the foramen of Monro. If the foramen is narrow, the endoscope is guided along the top of the plexus, which is gently pressed downward. For further anatomical orientation within the third ventricle, 30- and 45-degree inspection optics are sometimes useful. Finally, the diagnostic scope is replaced with the operating scope.

A noninflated balloon catheter (no. 3 French Fogarty) is used to widen the aqueduct. Here, the balloon must be inflated very carefully (with much less inflation than in ETV). Additionally, the catheter should be filled with fluid (not air) to avoid a possible pop-up enlargement of the balloon. Bending the tip of the catheter can also help accommodate the slightly curved shape of the aqueduct and variations in individual anatomy.

We always inspect the aqueduct using rigid optics (2-mm diameter; 0, 30, and 45 degrees) or use a flexible scope for visualizing the choroid plexus of the fourth ventricle. Additionally, a steerable endoscope can be used to perforate distal membranous occlusions. When the endoscope is positioned within the aqueduct (and occluding it), care must be taken to avoid forced irrigation, as this can lead to a devastating overload of the fourth ventricle.

After opening the aqueduct, a stent such as an 8 French ventricular catheter (Cordis Corp., Miami, FL, or Bactiseal, Codman Corp, Raynham, MA) should be placed. We prefer to advance the catheter without a stylet in order to minimize the risk of midbrain injury. The optimal length must be estimated based on preoperative MRI, future head growth in young children, and expected impact of CSF compartment changes. Additional perforations along the stent will ensure adequate communication between CSF cavities. Additional holes in the aqueduct, however, are not recommended as ependymal or glial scarring can occur.

The stent can be placed under direct visual control via the working channel, using the standard LOTTA system. Grasping forceps can be used to keep the stent in place while removing the ventriculoscope and endoscopic sheath. Otherwise, the stent can be placed in the fourth ventricle by way of gentle manipulation: after removing the working channel, the catheter is guided alongside a 0-degree inspection endoscope. Reevaluation with a 0-degree inspection optic or a flexible scope can confirm correct placement of the stent. We connect the catheter with a **burr hole reservoir** (e.g., Integra Neurosciences Implants, France) or with a preexisting shunt system, making it possible to take pressure measurements and CSF specimens if needed. Recently, we have begun using Tachosil to promote periosteal and galeal closure as a means of preventing CSF fistulas.

Interventriculostomy

Interventriculostomy is an endoscopic option in cases where an IFV is bulging through the quadrigeminal cistern into the tentorial hiatus. Here, it is necessary to pass through the posterior part of the third or lateral ventricle and the roof of the fourth ventricle. The basal and internal veins and tectal plate, which are usually significantly displaced superiorly and laterally, are particularly vulnerable.[15,33,38,40] Therefore, fenestration should only be attempted if a translucent membrane is present.[59] A stent is recommended to help avoid reocclusion.

Endoscopic Transventricular Transaqueductal Magendie and Luschka Foraminoplasty

Neuroendoscopy with a flexible scope is an alternative to microsurgical suboccipital craniotomy and rigid endoscopy in the management of primary or secondary FVOO. Longatti et al used a flexible endoscope for successful transventricular transaqueductal fenestration of the foramen of Magendie.[66] Torres-Corzo et al also reported on a large series of Magendie foraminoplasties. Additionally, they were the first to describe foraminoplasties of foramen of Luschka in patients in whom an ETV was not feasible due to nonpatent basal subarachnoid spaces or to the occurrence of primary FVOO. This method is both safe and feasible, with 65.3% of patients improving clinically and having significantly better outcomes.[67]

16.3.2 Retrograde Aqueductoplasty via an Infratentorial Approach (Endoscopic Trans-Fourth Ventricle Aqueductoplasty)

Indication

The indication for an *anterior* transventricular approach may be limited in cases of (1) slit ventricles, (2) certain anatomical restrictions that preclude ETV (very thick floor of the third ventricle, narrow space between mammillary bodies and dorsum sellae, herniation of the floor into the sella, proximity of basilar artery and floor, small foramen of Monro), or (3) distal AS.[68] In these cases, *retrograde* cannulation of the aqueduct with an infratentorial approach can be an option.

Several authors have described their techniques, which include developing specially designed catheters (Lapras) for cannulation of the aqueduct.[11,13,69] A suboccipital approach using rigid or steerable scopes, when performed in an experienced neuroendoscopic clinic, is both safe and effective. It is also particularly suited for treating IFV.[37,56,59,60,68,70] Cinalli et al, however, noted that the suboccipital (paramedian) approach also has its limits, due to the lack of orientation and often distorted anatomy.[35] Furthermore, patients with Chiari malformation type II are not candidates for the trans-fourth approach.[71] The potential benefit of the posterior fossa approach (opening of the fourth ventricle outlet in IFV, for example) must be balanced against its greater invasiveness. Even combined procedures (ETV and infratentorial approach for EAP and stenting) have been reported to reverse the flow of CSF from the fourth into the third ventricle and ultimately into the interpeduncular cistern.[72]

Technique

A small suboccipital craniectomy is performed with the patient in a prone or sitting position. Some authors prefer to use an additional median straight skin incision, marking a trajectory from the foramen of Magendie to the aqueduct, far from the craniectomy site where the endoscope is inserted.[60] The bilateral tonsils are elevated with retractors, and space for the rigid neuroendoscope is prepared. A rigid 0-degree endoscope is inserted into the fourth ventricle. After careful exploration of the choroid plexus and the caudal end of the aqueduct, a 3 French Fogarty catheter can be passed through the aqueduct. A stent can then be placed under endoscopic control and attached to the dura or connected with an existing shunt system. In this way, a connection via Y-connector to the same valve system ensures equilibration of pressure levels between the supra- and infratentorial CSF spaces. When a trapped fourth ventricle is very large and the cerebellar cortex is thin, we prefer to insert the endoscope via a paramedian burr hole directly into the enlarged fourth ventricle. This procedure is straightforward and avoids microsurgical splitting of the tonsils.

16.4 Surgical Outcomes of Endoscopic Techniques

16.4.1 Obstructive Triventricular Hydrocephalus

ETV and EAP (with or without stenting), even simultaneously, are increasingly being used to treat obstructive triventricular hydrocephalus due to AS.[47,50,53,73,74,75,76] Compared to ETV, aqueductoplasty has the advantage of restoring a more physiological CSF pathway. Additionally, the arachnoid membranes, which sometimes cause ETV failure when they interfere with CSF circulation below the floor of the third ventricle, are not usually encountered around the aqueduct. The anatomy of the basilar artery and its branches, as well as injury to the hypothalamus in cases of a thickened third ventricle floor, may increase the risks or even hinder an ETV. Manipulation within the aqueduct meanwhile carries the potential risk of midbrain damage and possibly certain neurological deficits. Obviously, the risk will substantially increase with the length of the occlusion.

The success rate for ETV in terms of long-term reclosure rate is satisfactory. ETV studies that include pediatric patients with obstructive hydrocephalus report success rates between 33 and 82.2%. A variety of factors influence the chances of success: AS, no history of hemorrhage or infection, and no previous shunt history are in general positive predictors of a good outcome, whereas a younger age is a predictor of a poorer outcome.[77,78,79,80,81] The age-dependency of success has already been shown for ETV/choroid plexus coagulation in patients with AS-related hydrocephalus.[82]

Initially, the success rates of EAP in carefully selected patients were reported at between 69 and 100% without mortality.[34,50,52,53,76] In the long term, however, EAP has been shown to fail frequently, even long after the operation, due to reclosure of the aqueduct. Reclosure has even occurred in cases with ideal anatomy and thin membranous occlusions.[50,55,76,83] To date, we have observed a clinically significant reclosure rate after EAP without stenting of 55% in our patients, which is in accordance with the literature. Stent placement is now generally recommended as a means of substantially improving the chances of

sufficient drainage in the long term and preventing an occlusion of the lumen.

16.4.2 Isolated Fourth Ventricle

Due to the rare occurrence of IFV, the existing publications are largely based on small retrospective cohort studies.[35,37,38,57,59,60,84] EAP alone (without stenting) for therapy of an IFV has been reported to fail frequently. Success, defined as clinical improvement without the need for reoperation, was found in only up to one-third of patients, with failure owing to restenosis of the aqueduct.[33,35] When subsequent stenting was performed, however, the failure rate was much lower (around 15%).[32] Other authors reported success rates of more than 70% after stent placement.[38] When a trans-fourth ventricular aqueductoplasty with stenting was performed, all patients demonstrated stable clinical improvement over the mean follow-up period of 90.8 months.[60]

A radiologically evident decrease in fourth ventricle size has been reported to occur in 10 to 50%,[33,57] 76%,[60] and in 100% of the patients, although none of the IFV returned to their normal size.[59] Recently, Fallah et al[85] performed an individual participant data meta-analysis to determine the efficacy and safety of EAP (without concomitant ETV or CSF shunt) with respect to patient age, pathogenesis, surgical approach, and stent usage. The authors found 14 eligible articles reporting on 137 patients. Seventy-five percent of patients did not require a second CSF diversion procedure. According to the multivariate analysis, older age at surgery, congenital pathogenesis, and stent usage were independent predictors of a good outcome.

Overall, with careful individualized preoperative planning, EAP with stenting (from supratentorial or infratentorial) and interventriculostomy with stenting have become safe, feasible, and accepted treatment methods when performed by experienced neurosurgeons. Longer AS or tumor-related obstructions should be treated with ETV.[32]

16.4.3 Possible Reasons for Aqueductal Reclosure after EAP

EAP can normalize CSF flow within the aqueduct at least in the short term. MRI studies have demonstrated that patients who have undergone EAP have the same CSF flow within the aqueduct as healthy volunteers. Furthermore, flow rate through the restored aqueduct has been shown to be significantly lower than through the stoma of an ETV; simultaneous ETV does not appear to influence the flow rate within the aqueduct after EAP.[86]

We suggest that a higher flow through the aqueduct reduces the risk of reclosure. This point is supported by the observation that the post-ETV reclosure rate seems to be higher when the membrane of Liliequist has not been adequately opened. After wider fenestration during repeated ETV, we observed a long-lasting patency of the stoma.[54] Interestingly, flow through the ventriculostoma after ETV is only minimally reduced due to a simultaneous EAP. Although we might expect a stronger reduction of flow through the ETV, the flow is nearly the same.

The diameter of the aqueduct is obviously much smaller than the opening after ETV. Additionally, the aqueduct is longer and tube-shaped. Thus, the risk of developing relevant obstructions seems to be much greater for aqueductoplasty than for ETV. This is in accordance with the law of Hagen–Poiseuille, which states that flow through a tube is mainly determined by its diameter and is inversely related to its length. This translates into lower outflow resistance after ETV and higher outflow resistance through the restored aqueduct. Other studies show comparable results.[87,88] The stroke volume was found to be significantly greater in ventriculostomas, compared to in the aqueducts of a healthy control group.[89] However, even some patients with high flow rates through the restored aqueduct develop post-EAP reclosures, making flow observations a poor predictor of success. More than 90 years ago, Dandy stated that "strictures of the aqueduct of Sylvius recur after any attempt to restore the lumen,"[90] and this observation seems to still hold true today. Ultimately, we conclude that ETV is the therapy of choice for the treatment of hydrocephalus due to AS. In cases of IFV, this endoscopic procedure in combination with stent placement is also clearly indicated.[54,55]

16.5 Endoscopic Surgical Management

16.5.1 Indication and Choice of Treatment Options: Patient Selection

In general, worsening clinical symptoms (as described above) or progressive enlargement of the CSF compartments will ultimately necessitate an operation. For obstructive triventricular hydrocephalus caused by AS, a widening of the lateral and third ventricle, caudal bulging of the floor of the third ventricle, bowing of the lamina terminalis, periventricular intensity changes showing transependymal CSF accumulation, widening of the prestenotic aqueduct, and a diminished cortical sulcus profile are typical radiological signs of ongoing hydrocephalus. In these cases, a clear indication to operate evolves as the typical hydrocephalus symptoms develop.

Surgical treatment of IFV is indicated due to increasing pressure to the brainstem and cerebellum.[15,30,91,92] Symptomatic patients suffer from intracranial hypertension and brainstem or cerebellar signs. However, even with a marked dilatation of the fourth ventricle a longstanding stable clinical and radiological course is also possible ("compensated trapped fourth ventricle").[16,61,93] The individual anatomy, patient history (including cause of the pathology), estimated risk of complications, and personal experience with certain techniques will influence the individualized treatment choice.

16.5.2 Preoperative Planning and Considerations: Anatomic Eligibility for EAP/Stenting

The modality of choice for visualizing the CSF compartments is MRI. Particularly helpful are high-resolution T2-weighted techniques that allow for qualitative assessment of flow through the aqueduct (e.g., CISS [constructive interference in steady state] or FIESTA [fast imaging employing steady-state acquisition]). Additionally, cardiac-gated cine phase-contrast MRI allows for quantitative evaluation of CSF flow and can thus be used to determine the patency of the aqueduct or ventriculostoma.[54,94] Even high-resolution MRI, however, may fail to reveal the underlying cause of a tetraventricular hydrocephalus (intraventricular vs. extraventricular or absorptive). Under these circumstances, MRI ventriculography following intraventricular gadolinium administration might provide additional diagnostic information.[95] Other details with respect to preoperative planning and determining anatomic eligibility for EAP/stenting are described below (avoidance of complications.).

16.6 Postoperative Care and Follow-up

Careful postoperative observation for one night on an intensive care unit or intermediate care unit is essential. In addition to early postoperative failure, late failure with rapid neurological deterioration is also possible. For these reasons, long-term follow-up is recommended, similar to patients undergoing an ETV. Our routine protocol includes:
- MRI with flow studies 1 day postoperatively (to confirm correct position of the stent and determine the size of the ventricular compartments).
- Clinical examination 10 to 14 days after discharge.
- Follow-up examination including MRI with flow studies after 3 months.
- Annual clinical and radiological follow-ups.

16.7 Case Examples

16.7.1 Case 1

History and Treatment

A normally developed child presented with lethargy, opisthotonus, and sucking weakness 5 days after birth without signs or symptoms of sepsis. The initial transcranial ultrasound showed enlarged lateral and third ventricles. The first emergency operation performed was an endoscopic lavage through a frontal burr hole. This revealed ventriculitis caused by *Streptococcus agalactiae*, and intravenous antibiotic therapy was initiated. Endoscopic lavage was repeated over the course of the following weeks. A Rickham reservoir was then implanted, followed by a subgaleal shunt. Here, the intent was to avoid frequent punctures and also to decrease protein levels in preparation for subsequent ventriculoperitoneal (VP) shunting.

At the age of 6 weeks, the (initially normal) fourth ventricle enlarged into a space- occupying compartment, leading to brainstem irregularities, including apneic episodes (▶ Fig. 16.1). We decided to perform aqueductal stenting combined with VP shunt implantation (and connected both). Intraoperatively, an obstruction of the aqueduct was noted. It was possible to properly place the stent in the fourth ventricle via the aqueduct under visual control using a rigid 2-mm 0-degree inspection optic. Postoperatively, a transient disconjugate eye movement disorder resolved completely. At last follow-up of 18 months, the sizes of all ventricles remained stable despite the upward movement of the tip of the stent due to the age-dependent head enlargement. A typical multiloculated cystic intracranial

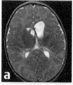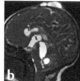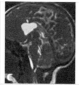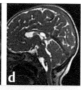

Fig. 16.1 Preoperative **(a)** axial and **(b)** sagittal T2 MRI demonstrating an enlarged isolated fourth ventricle, associated with AS; intermittent subgaleal CSF accumulation (shunt), with supratentorial CSF spaces remaining stable over the course of 3 weeks. **(c)** A properly placed aqueductal stent; decrease in size of the fourth ventricle. **(d)** Prepontine enlarged cyst; the tip of the aqueductal stent has migrated upward due to the physiological head enlargement.

disease also evolved, and enlargement of a prepontine cyst necessitated two microsurgical fenestrations from a retrosigmoid approach. At present, the girl shows nearly normal psychomotoric development.

Discussion

We believe that there was no sufficient microsurgical means of treating an IFV. Neuroendoscopy allowed for a much less invasive operation at the age of 6 weeks. In this case, the only possible microsurgical strategies would have involved an infratentorial approach to the fourth ventricle with the aim of opening its outlet and leaving a separate shunt in situ. Here, however, the widened supratentorial ventricles offered the best means of treating the AS. In such situations, neuronavigation can provide great assistance with orientation, especially when the anatomy is distorted. This is usually the case in postinfectious multiloculated hydrocephalic patients. Furthermore, this case illustrates the need for careful follow-up and, as is often the case, the need for a combination of various surgical techniques.

16.7.2 Case 2

History and Treatment

A 2-year-old boy suffered from a progressive and space-occupying IFV (► Fig. 16.2). At the age of 4 weeks, he was shunted due to posthemorrhagic triventricular hydrocephalus with AS. The clinical follow-up demonstrated a stable course despite a retarded clinical status. Because of the increasing size of a developing trapped fourth ventricle, motoric function was impaired, with increasing ataxia, worsening of seizures, and

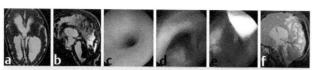

Fig. 16.2 Preoperative **(a)** axial and **(b)** sagittal T2 MRI demonstrating revealing enlarged supratentorial ventricles, and a space-occupying trapped fourth ventricle, as well as occlusion of the aqueduct. **(c)** An endoscopic view (rigid 2-mm 0-degree optic): membranous occlusion of the aqueduct, prestenotic dilatation of the aqueduct. **(d)** An endoscopic view into the fourth ventricle (rigid 30° diagnostic optic, 2 mm); **(e)** properly placed stent within the fourth ventricle. **(f)** Postoperative MR imaging showing a properly placed stent in the fourth ventricle; size of fourth ventricle decreased.

new apneic episodes. We decided to perform an antegrade aqueductoplasty with stenting. A thin membranous occlusion was opened, a stent was placed, and the procedure was uneventful. The frequency of seizures and ataxia decreased, and apneic episodes stopped. As is typical, the size of fourth ventricle decreased but did not reach a normal size.

Discussion

With a constellation of a thin membranous aqueductal occlusion, in combination with enlarged ventricles, antegrade stenting was a safe and feasible treatment option. A direct infratentorial microsurgical approach to the fourth ventricle, in contrast, would have been more invasive. Furthermore, postoperative infratentorial scarring can reduce the chances of success of this procedure. An additional infratentorial catheter can also increase the risk of dysfunction/obstruction of the shunt system, as it can lead to decreased flow within the fourth ventricle if not used as a stent connecting supra- and infratentorial CSF spaces.

16.7.3 Case 3

History and Treatment

A 35-year-old male patient presented 7 years status post resection of a giant right-sided temporal oligoastrocytoma (WHO II°) (► Fig. 16.3). After treatment of postoperative postinfectious hydrocephalus with a VP shunt, he had been clinically stable, free of complaints, and had returned to his job as a car driver. After this long stable course, he developed a rapidly progressive deterioration of consciousness. MRI revealed a contrast-enhancing progressive tumor, suggestive of a high-grade glioma with carcinomatous gliosis. As a result of mass effect by the tumor, the fourth ventricle had become isolated and space-occupying. We decided to immediately operate on the IFV via a supratentorial approach. We performed aqueductal stenting and connected the stent with the preexisting VP shunt. The procedure was straightforward. Neuronavigation and the existing proximal shunt catheter were useful for intraoperative orientation, as the intraventricular gliotic scarring and distorted anatomy and obscured the usual anatomical orientation landmarks. Initially, the patient showed postoperative improvement but then died 4 weeks later from the rapidly progressive glioma.

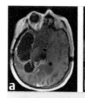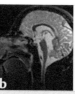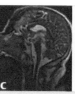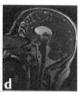

Fig. 16.3 **(a)** T1 MRI demonstrating a left temporal cyst after tumor resection, and ubiquitous contrast enhancement. **(b)** T2 MRI (CISS) showing a profound upward bulging of the fourth ventricle with distorted anatomy around the aqueduct, difficult trajectory for reaching the aqueduct via an infratentorial approach. Postoperative **(c)** sagittal T2 MRI (CISS) revealing the position of the aqueductal stent within the fourth ventricle, and **(d)** size reduction of the fourth ventricle.

Discussion

After balancing the pros and cons of an infratentorial procedure, we ultimately decided on an endoscopic supratentorial transforaminal approach. The aim was to connect the new stent with the preexisting VP shunt in order to achieve equilibration between the CSF compartments. In view of the initial MRI, it was unclear how aqueductal stenting could be performed. The anatomy was severely distorted due to gliotic scarring, but the preexisting proximal catheter helped with orientation, and neuronavigation provided additional information. A microsurgical (possibly endoscope-assisted) opening of the fourth ventricle outlet might have been an option. The trajectory to the caudal orifice of the aqueduct, however, was very cranially orientated (nearly 90 degrees to the axial level of the foramen magnum) due to the profound upward bulging of the fourth ventricle. We also wanted to avoid double proximal catheters. Finally, the anatomy at the distal end of the aqueduct did not provide sufficient orientation for safely introducing an aqueductal stent. Unfortunately, none of the possible procedures were able to change the final outcome of the patient.

16.8 Avoiding Complications

Several potential complications must be mentioned. General complications of endoscopic procedures with implants include CSF space infection, subdural effusion, and dysfunction of implanted material (such as migration, occlusion, and disconnection). Additionally, complications directly associated with the anatomical conditions near the aqueduct are midbrain injuries, disconjugate eye movement, Parinaud's syndrome, and oculomotor and trochlear palsy.[37,96] The risks involved in placing of a fourth ventricle catheter are significant and may occur directly in association with the operation or at a later time due to postoperative expansion of the brain.

Recently, a descending transtentorial herniation (herniation of supratentorial structures through the tentorial hiatus into the posterior fossa) was described as a result of the presence of a two shunt system (supra- and infratentorial) with the same pressure level after treatment of trapped fourth ventricle.[61] This phenomenon is already well known to occur after lumbar punctures in the presence of elevated supratentorial pressure.[97,98] Postoperative complication rates (namely disconjugate eye movements, more transient than permanent) have been reported at between 11.4 and 25%.[38,59,60] In their recent meta-analysis, Fallah et al found a morbidity of 22% (mainly ophthalmoparesis and hemorrhage), and no mortality after EAP. The incidence of newly developed ophthalmoparesis was nearly identical in procedures with and without stenting (5.19 vs. 5.17%).[85] ▶ Table 16.1 summarizes several points, and technical nuances, to be considered for avoiding procedural complications.

16.9 Technical Nuances

It is of utmost importance to consider the individual anatomy when planning EAP/stenting. First, the ventricular size must allow for handling of the endoscope without an increased risk to the surrounding structures. Furthermore, the size of the foramen of Monro must permit the passage of the endoscope. These points will essentially determine the choice of endoscope used in the procedure. Smaller rigid or steerable endoscopes are recommended, particularly for newborns and young children. The foramina of Monro should also be examined on coronal and sagittal MR images to determine the optimal approach.[99] Furthermore, it is of utmost importance to clarify the individual anatomy of the aqueduct: on average, the cerebral aqueduct is 15 mm in length with a diameter that varies between 0.5 and 2.8 mm along its course in adults. For children, the measured data are age-dependent. In general, the aqueduct is ventrally concave, which is important to consider when advancing the catheter or endoscope. Sometimes it is advisable to bend the tip of the balloon catheter to follow the shape of the aqueduct and avoid a via falsa. In hydrocephalic patients, however, the individual anatomy is always variable, and a careful, individualized study of the preoperative imaging as described above is indispensable.

Table 16.1 Summary of technical nuances to be considered for avoiding procedural complications

Preoperative planning		
Anatomical eligibility	Size of ventricles (left/right)	Decision making for endoscopic antegrade or retrograde approach
	Size of foramen of Monro (left/right)	
	Extent/entity of aqueductal stenosis	
Imaging	Use neuronavigation based on high-resolution MRI	
Burr hole location	Individual position with respect to foramen of Monro and spatial orientation of aqueduct	
Intraoperative clues		
Irrigation	Avoid while endoscope within the aqueduct	
Fogarty balloon catheter	Bending the tip according to aqueductal anatomy	
Stent	Appropriate length	
	Additional perforations/not at level of aqueduct	
	Connect with burr hole reservoir existing shunt	

Navigation systems help plan the trajectory in patients where the ventricles are not significantly enlarged. Moreover, navigation is helpful when anatomic intraventricular landmarks are distorted—where orientation would otherwise be difficult or even impossible. In patients with shunt-related slit ventricles, an externalization of the shunt 48 to 72 hours before the operation under strict intracranial pressure monitoring can help enlarge the ventricles;[59,100] we do not, however, advocate this technique. Additionally, a change of the valve of an existing shunt may be needed.[57]

16.10 General Advantages/ Disadvantages of Neuroendoscopic versus Microsurgical Procedures

In general, endoscopic techniques, compared to microsurgical techniques, are a much less invasive option of treating a variety of pathologies. The HD visualization that is now available allows for greatly improved image quality. Operations on deeper structures can be more tailored, permitting an intervention with a smaller craniotomy or even just a burr hole. As the main point to be mentioned, rigid scopes with different angles (e.g., 6, 30, 45, and 70 degrees) and steerable scopes allow for better visualization of surrounding anatomical structures. With microsurgery, the field of visualization is restricted, offering only a straight view of deeper structures. Endoscopically, even hidden areas can be safely explored.

With endoscopy, the estimated CSF loss is usually less severe and more controlled than with open microsurgery, as continuous fluid irrigation is possible. On the other hand, endoscopy has limitations in maneuvering the instruments within the working channel. Furthermore, bleeding can greatly impair endoscopic visualization. Tiny bleeds, however, are usually self-limiting and will stop under continuous irrigation. For more severe hemorrhages, we use the small chamber irrigation technique.[101]

16.11 Clinical Pearls and Conclusion

According to our experience, neuroendoscopic techniques should be seriously considered when treating any type of obstructive hydrocephalus. Any microsurgical approach has an increased risk, and shunts harbor more long-term complications. ETV is the gold standard for treating hydrocephalus caused by AS. Simple aqueductoplasty has a disappointingly high rate of reclosure and cannot be recommended. Aqueductal stenting is the therapy of choice for a trapped fourth ventricle. Ideally, the stent is simultaneously used with shunt catheter, which is often necessary. However, in non–shunt-dependent patients, simple aqueductal stenting is sufficient for treating an IFV. It is of utmost importance that the stent be fixed to a burr hole reservoir to prevent stent migration. Retrograde aqueductoplasty and stent placement is required in cases of supratentorial slit ventricles. Aqueductal stenting usually offers a stable long-term clinical course, and although the long-term success rates are promising, life-long surveillance is still mandatory.

16.12 Acknowledgments

We thank Marc Matthes, MSc, for careful preparations of the figures, and Samantha Taber for editing the English text. We thank Soenke Langner, MD, PhD, for providing MR images.

References

[1] Touche M. Hydrocéphale Interne (Présentartion de Piéces). Bull Mem Soc Med Hop Paris. 1902(19):141–144

[2] Spiller WG. Two cases of partial internal hydrocephalus from closure of the interventricular passages: with remarks on bilateral contractures caused by a unilateral cerebral lesion. Am J Med Sci. 1902; 124:144–155

[3] Guthrie LG. Hydrocephalus. Practitioner. 1910; 32:47

[4] Dandy W. The diagnosis and treatment of hydrocephalus resulting from strictures of the aqueduct of sylvius. Surg Gynecol Obstet. 1920; 31:340–358

[5] Greenwood J, Jr.. Cicatricial occlusion of aqueduct. Dis. Nerv. System. 1944; 5:139–141

[6] Norlen G. Contribution to the surgical treatment of inoperable tumours causing obstruction of the Sylvian aqueduct. Acta Psychiatr Neurol. 1949; 24 (3-4):629–637

[7] Elvidge A. Interventriculostomy in stenosis of the aqueduct. As presented at meeting of the Canadian Neurological Society, Edmonton, Canada, June, 1964. J Neurosurg. 1966; 24:11–23

[8] Turnbull IM, Drake CG. Membranous Occlusion of the Aqueduct of Sylvius. J Neurosurg. 1966; 24(1):24–34

[9] Crosby RMN, Henderson CM, Paul RL. Catheterization of the cerebral aqueduct for obstructive hydrocephalus in infants. Journal of Neurosurg. 1973; 38(5):596–601

[10] Mottolese C, Szathmari A, Ginguene C, Simon E, Ricci-Franchi AC. Endoscopic aqueductoplasty. J Neurosurg. 2007; 106(5) Suppl:414–416, author reply 416–418

[11] Lapras C, Poirier N, Deruty R, Bret P, Jyeux O. Catheterization of the sylvian aqueduct. Its present role in the surgical treatment of sylvian aqueduct stenosis of PCF tumors, and of syringomyelia [French]. Neurochirurgie. 1975; 21(2):101–109

[12] Leksell L. A surgical procedure for atresia of the aqueduct of Sylvius. Acta Psychiatr Neurol. 1949; 24(3)(–)(4):559–568

[13] Lapras C, Bret P, Patet JD, Huppert J, Honorato D. Hydrocephalus and aqueduct stenosis. Direct surgical treatment by interventriculostomy (aqueduct canulation). J Neurosurg Sci. 1986; 30(1)(–)(2):47–53

[14] Dollo C, Kanner A, Siomin V, Ben-Sira L, Sivan J, Constantini S. Outlet fenestration for isolated fourth ventricle with and without an internal shunt. Childs Nerv Syst. 2001; 17(8):483–486

[15] Harter DH. Management strategies for treatment of the trapped fourth ventricle. Childs Nerv Syst. 2004; 20(10):710–716

[16] James HE. Spectrum of the syndrome of the isolated fourth ventricle in posthemorrhagic hydrocephalus of the premature infant. Pediatr Neurosurg. 1990 – 1991; 16(6):305–308

[17] Oi S, Matsumoto S. Isolated fourth ventricle. J Pediatr Neurosci. 1986; 2:125–133

[18] Scotti G, Musgrave MA, Fitz CR, Harwood-Nash DC. The isolated fourth ventricle in children: CT and clinical review of 16 cases. AJR Am J Roentgenol. 1980; 135(6):1233–1238

[19] Longatti P, Marton E, Magrini S. The marionette technique for treatment of isolated fourth ventricle: technical note. J Neurosurg Pediatr. 2013; 12 (4):339–343

[20] Tisell M. How should primary aqueductal stenosis in adults be treated? A review. Acta Neurol Scand. 2005; 111(3):145–153

[21] Hirsch JF, Hirsch E, Sainte Rose C, Renier D, Pierre-Khan A. Stenosis of the aqueduct of Sylvius. Etiology and treatment. J Neurosurg Sci. 1986; 30(1)(–) (2):29–39

[22] Jellinger G. Anatomopathology of non-tumoral aqueductal stenosis. J Neurosurg Sci. 1986; 30(1)(–)(2):1–16

[23] Robertson IJ, Leggate JR, Miller JD, Steers AJ. Aqueduct stenosis–presentation and prognosis. Br J Neurosurg. 1990; 4(2):101–106

[24] Tisell M, Edsbagge M, Stephensen H, Czosnyka M, Wikkelsø C. Elastance correlates with outcome after endoscopic third ventriculostomy in adults with hydrocephalus caused by primary aqueductal stenosis. Neurosurgery. 2002; 50(1):70–77

[25] Ang BT, Steinbok P, Cochrane DD. Etiological differences between the isolated lateral ventricle and the isolated fourth ventricle. Childs Nerv Syst. 2006; 22(9):1080–1085

[26] Oi S, Matsumoto S. Pathophysiology of aqueductal obstruction in isolated IV ventricle after shunting. Childs Nerv Syst. 1986; 2(6):282–286

[27] Williams B. Is aqueduct stenosis a result of hydrocephalus? Brain. 1973; 96 (2):399–412

[28] Foltz EL, Shurtleff DB. Conversion of communicating hydrocephalus to stenosis or occlusion of the aqueduct during ventricular shunt. J Neurosurg. 1966; 24(2):520–529

[29] Spennato P, Cinalli G, Carannante G. Multiloculated hydrocephalus. In: Cinall G, Maixner WJ, Saint-Rose C, eds. Pediatric Hydrocephalus. Milan: Springer; 2004:219–244

[30] Hawkins JC, III, Hoffman HJ, Humphreys RP. Isolated fourth ventricle as a complication of ventricular shunting. Report of three cases. J Neurosurg. 1978; 49(6):910–913

[31] Rekate HL. Hydrocephalus classification and pathophysiology. In: McLone DG, ed. Pediatric Neurosurgery: Surgery of the Developing Nervous System. Philadelphia, PA: Saunders; 2001:457–474

[32] Fritsch MJ, Schroeder HW. Endoscopic aqueductoplasty and stenting. World Neurosurg. 2013; 79(2) Suppl:20.e15–20.e18

[33] Fritsch MJ, Kienke S, Manwaring KH, Mehdorn HM. Endoscopic aqueductoplasty and interventriculostomy for the treatment of isolated fourth ventricle in children. Neurosurgery. 2004; 55(2):372–377, discussion 377–379

[34] Fritsch MJ, Kienke S, Mehdorn HM. Endoscopic aqueductoplasty: stent or not to stent? Childs Nerv Syst. 2004; 20(3):137–142

[35] Cinalli G, Spennato P, Savarese L, et al. Endoscopic aqueductoplasty and placement of a stent in the cerebral aqueduct in the management of isolated fourth ventricle in children. J Neurosurg. 2006; 104(1) Suppl:21–27

[36] Russel DS. Observations on the Pathology of Hydrocephalus. Special Report Series No. 265, Medical Research Council. London: HM Stationery Office; 1949

[37] da Silva LR, Cavalheiro S, Zymberg ST. Endoscopic aqueductoplasty in the treatment of aqueductal stenosis. Childs Nerv Syst. 2007; 23(11):1263–1268

[38] Ogiwara H, Morota N. Endoscopic transaqueductal or interventricular stent placement for the treatment of isolated fourth ventricle and pre-isolated fourth ventricle. Childs Nerv Syst. 2013; 29(8):1299–1303

[39] Chai WX. Long-term results of fourth ventriculo-cisternostomy in complex versus simplex atresias of the fourth ventricle outlets. Acta Neurochir (Wien). 1995; 134(1–2):27–34

[40] Montes JL, Clarke DB, Farmer JP. Stereotactic transtentorial hiatus ventriculoperitoneal shunting for the sequestered fourth ventricle. Technical note. J Neurosurg. 1994; 80(4):759–761

[41] Sharma RR, Pawar SJ, Devadas RV, Dev EJ. CT stereotaxy guided lateral transcerebellar programmable fourth ventriculo-peritoneal shunting for symptomatic trapped fourth ventricle. Clin Neurol Neurosurg. 2001; 103(3):143–146

[42] Udayakumaran S, Biyani N, Rosenbaum DP, Ben-Sira L, Constantini S, Beni-Adani L. Posterior fossa craniotomy for trapped fourth ventricle in shunt-treated hydrocephalic children: long-term outcome. J Neurosurg Pediatr. 2011; 7(1):52–63

[43] Villavicencio AT, Wellons JC, III, George TM. Avoiding complicated shunt systems by open fenestration of symptomatic fourth ventricular cysts associated with hydrocephalus. Pediatr Neurosurg. 1998; 29(6):314–319

[44] Guertin SR. Cerebrospinal fluid shunts. Evaluation, complications, and crisis management. Pediatr Clin North Am. 1987; 34(1):203–217

[45] Benzel EC, Reeves JD, Kesterson L, Hadden TA. Slit ventricle syndrome in children: clinical presentation and treatment. Acta Neurochir (Wien). 1992; 117(1–2):7–14

[46] Sansone JM, Iskandar BJ. Endoscopic cerebral aqueductoplasty: a transfourth ventricle approach. J Neurosurg. 2005; 103(5) Suppl:388–392

[47] Jones RF, Kwok BC, Stening WA, Vonau M. The current status of endoscopic third ventriculostomy in the management of non-communicating hydrocephalus. Minim Invasive Neurosurg. 1994; 37(1):28–36

[48] Jones RF, Stening WA, Brydon M. Endoscopic third ventriculostomy. Neurosurgery. 1990; 26(1):86–91, discussion 91–92

[49] Schroeder HW, Warzok RW, Assaf JA, Gaab MR. Fatal subarachnoid hemorrhage after endoscopic third ventriculostomy. Case report. Neurosurg Focus. 1999; 6(4):e4

[50] Erşahin Y. Endoscopic aqueductoplasty. Childs Nerv Syst. 2007; 23(2):143–150

[51] Miki T, Nakajima N, Wada J, Haraoka J. Indications for neuroendoscopic aqueductoplasty without stenting for obstructive hydrocephalus due to aqueductal stenosis. Minim Invasive Neurosurg. 2005; 48(3):136–141

[52] Schroeder HW, Gaab MR. Endoscopic aqueductoplasty: technique and results. Neurosurgery. 1999; 45(3):508–515, discussion 515–518

[53] Schroeder HW, Oertel J, Gaab MR. Endoscopic aqueductoplasty in the treatment of aqueductal stenosis. Childs Nerv Syst. 2004; 20(11–12):821–827

[54] Schroeder C, Fleck S, Gaab MR, Schweim KH, Schroeder HW. Why does endoscopic aqueductoplasty fail so frequently? Analysis of cerebrospinal fluid flow after endoscopic third ventriculostomy and aqueductoplasty using cine phase-contrast magnetic resonance imaging. J Neurosurg. 2012; 117 (1):141–149

[55] Schroeder HW, Oertel J, Gaab MR. Endoscopic treatment of cerebrospinal fluid pathway obstructions. Neurosurgery. 2007; 60(2) Suppl 1:ONS44–ONS51, discussion ONS51–ONS52

[56] Matula C, Reinprecht A, Roessler K, Tschabitscher M, Koos WT. Endoscopic exploration of the IVth ventricle. Minim Invasive Neurosurg. 1996; 39 (3):86–92

[57] Schulz M, Goelz L, Spors B, Haberl H, Thomale UW. Endoscopic treatment of isolated fourth ventricle: clinical and radiological outcome. Neurosurgery. 2012; 70(4):847–858, discussion 858–859

[58] Shin M, Morita A, Asano S, Ueki K, Kirino T. Neuroendoscopic aqueductal stent placement procedure for isolated fourth ventricle after ventricular shunt placement. Case report. J Neurosurg. 2000; 92(6):1036–1039

[59] Teo C, Burson T, Misra S. Endoscopic treatment of the trapped fourth ventricle. Neurosurgery. 1999; 44(6):1257–1261, discussion 1261–1262

[60] Gallo P, Szathmari A, Simon E, et al. The endoscopic trans-fourth ventricle aqueductoplasty and stent placement for the treatment of trapped fourth ventricle: long-term results in a series of 18 consecutive patients. Neurol India. 2012; 60(3):271–277

[61] Frassanito P, Markogiannakis G, Di Bonaventura R, Massimi L, Tamburrini G, Caldarelli M. Descending transtentorial herniation, a rare complication of the treatment of trapped fourth ventricle: case report. J Neurosurg Pediatr. 2015; 16(5):540–544

[62] Torres-Corzo J, Rodriguez-Della Vecchia R, Rangel-Castilla L. Trapped fourth ventricle treated with shunt placement in the fourth ventricle by direct visualization with flexible neuroendoscope. Minim Invasive Neurosurg. 2004; 47(2):86–89

[63] Geng J, Wu D, Chen X, Zhang M, Xu B, Yu X. Aqueduct stent placement: indications, technique, and clinical experience. World Neurosurg. 2015; 84 (5):1347–1353

[64] Little AS, Zabramski JM, Nakaji P. Simplified aqueductal stenting for isolated fourth ventricle using a small-caliber flexible endoscope in a patient with neurococcidiomycosis: technical case report. Neurosurgery. 2010; 66(6) Suppl Operative:373–374, discussion 374

[65] Schroeder HW. A new multipurpose ventriculoscope. Neurosurgery. 2008; 62(2):489–491, discussion 491–492

[66] Longatti P, Fiorindi A, Feletti A, Baratto V. Endoscopic opening of the foramen of magendie using transaqueductal navigation for membrane obstruction of the fourth ventricle outlets. Technical note. J Neurosurg. 2006; 105 (6):924–927

[67] Torres-Corzo J, Sánchez-Rodríguez J, Cervantes D, et al. Endoscopic transventricular transaqueductal Magendie and Luschka foraminoplasty for hydrocephalus. Neurosurgery. 2014; 74(4):426–435, discussion 436

[68] Gawish I, Reisch R, Perneczky A. Endoscopic aqueductoplasty through a tailored craniocervical approach. J Neurosurg. 2005; 103(5):778–782

[69] Goel A, Pandya SK. A shunting procedure for cerebrospinal fluid fistula, employing cannulation of the third and fourth ventricles. Br J Neurosurg. 1993; 7(3):299–302

[70] Toyota S, Taki T, Oshino S, et al. A neuroendoscopic approach to the aqueduct via the fourth ventricle combined with suboccipital craniectomy. Minim Invasive Neurosurg. 2004; 47(5):312–315

[71] Rekate HL. Endoscopic fourth ventricular aqueductoplasty. J Neurosurg. 2005; 103(5):773–774, discussion 774–775

[72] Ferrer E, de Notaris M. Third ventriculostomy and fourth ventricle outlets obstruction. World Neurosurg. 2013; 79(2) Suppl:20.e9–20.e13

[73] Baldauf J, Oertel J, Gaab MR, Schroeder HW. Endoscopic third ventriculostomy in children younger than 2 years of age. Childs Nerv Syst. 2007; 23 (6):623–626

[74] Gangemi M, Donati P, Maiuri F, Longatti P, Godano U, Mascari C. Endoscopic third ventriculostomy for hydrocephalus. Minim Invasive Neurosurg. 1999; 42(3):128–132

[75] Hopf NJ, Grunert P, Fries G, Resch KD, Perneczky A. Endoscopic third ventriculostomy: outcome analysis of 100 consecutive procedures. Neurosurgery. 1999; 44(4):795–804, discussion 804–806

[76] Oka K, Yamamoto M, Ikeda K, Tomonaga M. Flexible endoneurosurgical therapy for aqueductal stenosis. Neurosurgery. 1993; 33(2):236–242, discussion 242–243

[77] Cinalli G, Sainte-Rose C, Chumas P, et al. Failure of third ventriculostomy in the treatment of aqueductal stenosis in children. Neurosurg Focus. 1999; 6 (4):e3

[78] Warf BC, Tracy S, Mugamba J. Long-term outcome for endoscopic third ventriculostomy alone or in combination with choroid plexus cauterization for congenital aqueductal stenosis in African infants. J Neurosurg Pediatr. 2012; 10(2):108–111

[79] Bisht A, Suri A, Bansal S, et al. Factors affecting surgical outcome of endoscopic third ventriculostomy in congenital hydrocephalus. J Clin Neurosci. 2014; 21(9):1483–1489

[80] Sufianov AA, Sufianova GZ, Iakimov IA. Endoscopic third ventriculostomy in patients younger than 2 years: outcome analysis of 41 hydrocephalus cases. J Neurosurg Pediatr. 2010; 5(4):392–401

[81] Javadpour M, Mallucci C, Brodbelt A, Golash A, May P. The impact of endoscopic third ventriculostomy on the management of newly diagnosed hydrocephalus in infants. Pediatr Neurosurg. 2001; 35(3):131–135

[82] Kulkarni AV, Drake JM, Mallucci CL, Sgouros S, Roth J, Constantini S, Canadian Pediatric Neurosurgery Study Group. Endoscopic third ventriculostomy in the treatment of childhood hydrocephalus. J Pediatr. 2009; 155(2):254–9.e1

[83] Schroeder HW, Oertel J, Gaab MR. Incidence of complications in neuroendoscopic surgery. Childs Nerv Syst. 2004; 20(11–12):878–883

[84] Sagan LM, Kojder I, Poncyljusz W. Endoscopic aqueductal stent placement for the treatment of a trapped fourth ventricle. J Neurosurg. 2006; 105(4) Suppl:275–280

[85] Fallah A, Wang AC, Weil AG, Ibrahim GM, Mansouri A, Bhatia S. Predictors of outcome following cerebral aqueductoplasty: an individual participant data meta-analysis. Neurosurgery. 2016; 78(2):285–296

[86] Schroeder HW, Schweim C, Schweim KH, Gaab MR. Analysis of aqueductal cerebrospinal fluid flow after endoscopic aqueductoplasty by using cine phase-contrast magnetic resonance imaging. J Neurosurg. 2000; 93(2): 237–244

[87] Stoquart-El Sankari S, Lehmann P, Gondry-Jouet C, et al. Phase-contrast MR imaging support for the diagnosis of aqueductal stenosis. AJNR Am J Neuroradiol. 2009; 30(1):209–214

[88] Dinçer A, Yildiz E, Kohan S, Memet Özek M. Analysis of endoscopic third ventriculostomy patency by MRI: value of different pulse sequences, the sequence parameters, and the imaging planes for investigation of flow void. Childs Nerv Syst. 2011; 27(1):127–135

[89] Bargalló N, Olondo L, Garcia AI, Capurro S, Caral L, Rumia J. Functional analysis of third ventriculostomy patency by quantification of CSF stroke volume by using cine phase-contrast MR imaging. AJNR Am J Neuroradiol. 2005; 26 (10):2514–2521

[90] Dandy W. An operative procedure for hydrocephalus. Bull Johns Hopkins Hosp. 1922; 33:189–190

[91] Oi S, Abbott R. Loculated ventricles and isolated compartments in hydrocephalus: their pathophysiology and the efficacy of neuroendoscopic surgery. Neurosurg Clin N Am. 2004; 15(1):77–87

[92] Rademaker KJ, Govaert P, Vandertop WP, Gooskens R, Meiners LC, de Vries LS. Rapidly progressive enlargement of the fourth ventricle in the preterm infant with post-haemorrhagic ventricular dilatation. Acta Paediatr. 1995; 84(10):1193–1196

[93] Udayakumaran S, Panikar D. Postulating the concept of compensated trapped fourth ventricle: a case-based demonstration with long-term clinicoradiological follow-up. Childs Nerv Syst. 2012; 28(5):661–664

[94] Kulkarni AV, Drake JM, Armstrong DC, Dirks PB. Imaging correlates of successful endoscopic third ventriculostomy. J Neurosurg. 2000; 92(6): 915–919

[95] Joseph VB, Raghuram L, Korah IP, Chacko AG. MR ventriculography for the study of CSF flow. AJNR Am J Neuroradiol. 2003; 24(3):373–381

[96] Spennato P, O'Brien DF, Fraher JP, Mallucci CL. Bilateral abducent and facial nerve palsies following fourth ventricle shunting: two case reports. Childs Nerv Syst. 2005; 21(4):309–316

[97] Oyelese AA, Steinberg GK, Huhn SL, Wijman CA. Paradoxical cerebral herniation secondary to lumbar puncture after decompressive craniectomy for a large space-occupying hemispheric stroke: case report. Neurosurgery. 2005; 57(3):E594–, discussion E594

[98] Samadani U, Huang JH, Baranov D, Zager EL, Grady MS. Intracranial hypotension after intraoperative lumbar cerebrospinal fluid drainage. Neurosurgery. 2003; 52(1):148–151, discussion 151–152

[99] O'Brien DF, Javadpour M, Collins DR, Spennato P, Mallucci CL. Endoscopic third ventriculostomy: an outcome analysis of primary cases and procedures performed after ventriculoperitoneal shunt malfunction. J Neurosurg. 2005; 103(5) Suppl:393–400

[100] Boschert JM, Krauss JK. Endoscopic third ventriculostomy in the treatment of shunt-related over-drainage: Preliminary experience with a new approach how to render ventricles navigable. Clin Neurol Neurosurg. 2006; 108(2):143–149

[101] Manwaring JC, El Damaty A, Baldauf J, Schroeder HW. The small-chamber irrigation technique (SCIT): a simple maneuver for managing intraoperative hemorrhage during endoscopic intraventricular surgery. Neurosurgery. 2014; 10 Suppl 3:375–379, discussion 379

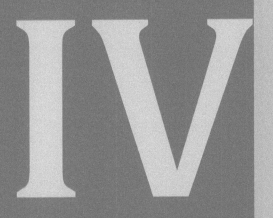

IV

17 Decompression of Cranial Nerves: Microscope

Nayan Lamba, Hasan A. Zaidi, and Robert F. Spetzler

Summary

Microvascular decompression is an effective method to relieve symptoms of cranial nerve compression or brainstem compression as a result of pulsatile vascular compression. Microsurgical visualization techniques have been the mainstay of treatment for nearly 50 years. In comparison with endoscopic approaches, the microscope allows for maximal surgical freedom and comparable craniotomy size, and it provides familiarity for surgeons adept at microsurgical dissection. In this chapter, we discuss the history and indications of microvascular decompression and its advantages over endoscopic approaches for decompression of cranial nerves.

Keywords: brainstem, cranial nerves, decompression, endoscope, microscope, microvascular

17.1 Microsurgical Perspective

17.1.1 Introduction

Vascular compression syndromes arise when pulsatile blood vessels directly compress cranial nerves (CNs), and this compression results in mechanical irritation and injury to the myelin of the nerves.[1,2] Trigeminal neuralgia (TN), hemifacial spasm (HFS), vestibulocochlear neuralgia, and glossopharyngeal neuralgia are the most common neurovascular compression syndromes.[1] Other examples include Meniere disease, vertigo, tinnitus, spasmodic torticollis, and brainstem vascular compression.[2] Each is caused by compression of a different set of vessels and leads to a unique set of symptoms. The most common syndromes are described below.

The trigeminal nerve (CN V) is a mixed sensory motor CN responsible for sensory innervation of the face and motor functions of the masticatory and tensor veli palatine muscles.[3] TN most often occurs when the superior cerebellar artery (SCA), anterior inferior cerebellar artery (AICA), or venous structures compress the trigeminal nerve.[1] This compression syndrome is characterized by paroxysmal, shocklike facial pain that is abrupt in onset and termination.[1,4] Pain occurs in the unilateral V2 or V3 dermatomal distribution of the trigeminal nerve and is triggered by otherwise harmless sensory stimuli.[1,4]

The facial nerve (CN VII) is also a mixed nerve. It controls the muscles of facial expression, conveys the sensation of taste from the anterior two-thirds of the tongue, and supplies parasympathetic fibers to the nasal mucosa and to the submandibular, sublingual, and lacrimal glands.[3] HFS occurs when the facial nerve is compressed by the AICA, posterior inferior cerebellar artery (PICA), vertebral artery, or less often by venous structures.[1] This compression syndrome results in involuntary synchronous spasms of one side of the face. Spasms usually begin around the eye and involve muscles supplied by the facial nerve.[1]

The vestibulocochlear nerve (CN VIII) is a pure sensory nerve that is responsible for the sensation of hearing via its cochlear component and balance via its vestibular component.[3] Vestibular paroxysmia occurs when the AICA or venous structures compress the CN VIII.[1] Compression results in episodic attacks of acute vertigo and disequilibrium that may be accompanied by tinnitus.

Finally, the glossopharyngeal nerve (CN IX) is a mixed sensory, motor, and parasympathetic nerve that carries sensory information from the posterior tongue, oropharyngeal, and ear regions; chemoreceptor and baroreceptor information from the carotid body and sinuses; and motor information to fibers of the ipsilateral parotid gland.[3] Glossopharyngeal neuralgia occurs because of compression of the glossopharyngeal nerve by the PICA, vertebral artery, or venous structures.[1] This compression causes intense, unilateral, paroxysmal pain in the sensory distribution of the glossopharyngeal nerve.

17.1.2 History and Evolution of Microvascular Decompression of Cranial Nerves

In the 1920s, the accepted approach for treating TN was the Spiller–Frazier approach, in which nerves were approached in the middle fossa and divided at the foramen ovale and foramen rotundum all the way to the gasserian ganglion.[5] However, despite sparing of the upper ganglion and first branch of the trigeminal nerve, this approach was associated with high rates of facial paralysis and keratitis. Nevertheless, it remained the mainstay of treatment for the next 50 years.[5]

Around the same time, neurosurgeon Walter Dandy developed a new approach that would become the first example of microvascular decompression (MVD) for TN.[5] His suboccipital cerebellar surgical approach involved complete or partial sectioning of the trigeminal nerve within the posterior fossa instead of the middle fossa.[5] Notably, this approach allowed for the preservation of touch sensation and had a much lower rate of facial paralysis than the Spiller–Frazier approach.[5] When Dandy published the report of his technique, he merely commented on the "random arterial loops" that seemed to block his view of the sensory root of the trigeminal ganglion, not realizing that these loops might be the source of the neuralgia.[6] It was only after he had performed about 250 trigeminal neurectomies via the cerebellar approach that he realized that the mass effect from these vascular loops was likely the cause of the pathology.[5] In an analysis of 215 cases, Dandy found that some mass effect had an impact on the root entry zone of the trigeminal nerve in 60% of cases; in 66 cases, compression was caused by the SCA, and in 30 cases, compression was caused by the petrosal vein.[7] Despite his intensive work toward gaining an understanding of the pathophysiology of TN, Dandy did not publish again on these hypotheses after 1934.[5]

In the 1950s, a neurosurgeon in Copenhagen, Palle Taarnhoj, revisited Dandy's approaches.[5] He utilized a temporal approach involving exposure of the middle fossa via a temporal craniectomy, followed by division of the dura over the posterior portion of the ganglion and root.[5] This decompressive approach, like Dandy's, allowed for resolution of TN without facial paralysis or sensory loss, and Taarnhoj's ideas soon made their way to the United States.[5] In 1959, James Gardner of the Cleveland Clinic quickly adapted the decompressive approach and published a case series of 100 patients in which he demonstrated that 67 patients had complete resolution of their tic douloureux after recovery from anesthesia.[5,8] Like Dandy, Gardner also advocated for the vascular compression hypothesis, stating that the source of damage to the trigeminal root might be anomalous arteries, aneurysms, basilar impressions, or posterior neoplasms.[5]

With the advent of the technology needed to visualize these structures, this hypothesis finally gained widespread acknowledgment in the 1960s.[2,5] In the late 1960s, Peter Jannetta introduced the operating microscope to the decompressive procedure for TN, enabling direct visualization of the arteries and veins that were compressing the trigeminal nerve.[5] In a report of five patients with TN, he described exposure of the nerve through the tentorium and the use of a binocular dissecting microscope for visualization.[9] He found that the trigeminal nerve was compressed by small arteries, most likely the branches of the SCA, and in four of five cases, he was able to free this artery from the arachnoid membrane and move it away from the trigeminal nerve.[5,9] Jannetta applied a similar microscopic approach to relieving HFS in a 41-year-old man via coagulation and division of a small pontomedullary vein that was compressing the facial nerve.[10] Jannetta's targeted approach against the compressing vein provided the patient with permanent relief from HFS. In 1977, Jannetta reported on his use of microsurgical decompression in patients with CN neuralgias, which demonstrated the continued success of his approach.[10] Of 61 patients treated for TN via the microscopic approach, 57 experienced complete resolution of pain following surgery. Moreover, of the 45 patients with classical HFS, 38 had an excellent response, reporting no spasm or weakness. Jannetta's microsurgical decompression approach has since become the gold standard for the treatment of cerebellopontine angle neuralgias, including TN, HFS, acoustic nerve dysfunction, and glossopharyngeal neuralgia.[5,10,11,12]

17.1.3 Cranial Nerve Vascular Compression Syndromes

Trigeminal Neuralgia

CN vascular compression syndromes occur when blood vessels directly contact and irritate the CN at its root exit or entry zone from the brainstem.[3,5,13,14] This mechanical conflict occurs in the cerebellopontine angle between the root entry zone of the nerve at the brainstem and its exit out of the posterior fossa.[15]

The most common compressive vessels in patients with TN are the SCA, followed by the AICA, and less frequently loops of the basilar artery, the vertebral artery, or the PICA.[16] Although it occurs less frequently than arterial compression, venous compression can also occur, most notably caused by the superior petrosal vein.[16]

In addition to mechanical stimulation, demyelination at the site of compression is thought to play a role in TN pathogenesis.[17] Numerous animal studies and biopsy analyses have demonstrated demyelination at the site of nerve compression.[18] Jannetta hypothesized that the perception of pain in these patients arises because of compression-induced demyelination and the subsequent spread of impulses at these sites of demyelination.[19] Additional studies have demonstrated that patients with TN may also have plaques within the trigeminal nerve.[20] A final piece of evidence relating demyelination to the pathogenesis of TN is that the incidence of TN is higher in patients with multiple sclerosis.[20] Although most patients benefit from MVD, a subgroup of patients do not achieve symptomatic relief after decompression (even when a vessel is clearly involved).[17] Thus, it is likely that both microvascular compression and demyelination play a role in the pathogenesis of TN.[17]

First-line treatments for TN are pharmacologic, consisting of sodium channel blockers such as carbamazepine and oxcarbazepine.[1,4,21] Sodium channel blockers are effective in most TN patients but may be associated with numerous adverse effects, such as drowsiness, dizziness, rash, and tremor.[4] In patients often requiring high doses to achieve pain relief, these adverse effects worsen and ultimately lead to treatment failure as patients reduce their doses.[4] Other medications that have demonstrated efficacy for TN, albeit to a lesser degree, include baclofen, lamotrigine, and pimozide.[21]

For medically refractory patients, surgery can be considered.[4,21] Surgical techniques include percutaneous procedures on the gasserian ganglion (i.e., percutaneous rhizotomy), Gamma Knife surgery (GKS), and MVD. Percutaneous rhizotomy involves the penetration of the foramen ovale with a cannula followed by the controlled creation of a lesion in the trigeminal ganglion or root via radiofrequency thermocoagulation, chemical injection, or mechanical compression using a balloon. Most (90%) patients experience pain relief from rhizotomy, with 68 to 85% of patients remaining pain-free at 1-year follow-up, 54 to 64% pain-free at 3-year follow-up, and 50% pain-free at the 5-year mark.[21]

GKS is a noninvasive option that involves focusing a beam of radiation at the trigeminal root in the posterior fossa.[21] Because it has a relatively low adverse effects profile and does not require open surgery, GKS has gained popularity as a primary treatment for TN.[5] Various studies demonstrate that GKS can achieve pain relief at 1 year after operation in 69 to 89% of patients.[21,22] Several studies have also reported high rates of initial pain relief, with as many as 71 to 90% of patients reporting immediate relief after surgery.[5,22] However, the weakness of GKS lies in its poor long-term and adverse effects profile. Facial numbness has been reported in 20 to 32% of patients after GKS.[5] Moreover, in a review of 10 GKS studies, the pain-free period that patients experienced lasted 8 to 50 months, and 5-year recurrence rates were 11 to 53%.[22]

The last option for TN treatment is MVD. MVD is a neurosurgical procedure in which a craniotomy is performed to reach the vessels in the posterior fossa that are compressing the trigeminal nerve.[4,21] Immediate pain relief after surgery is tremendous, with relief rates of 80 to 98%.[4,21,22] Most notable is the long period of pain relief after MVD. In a review of 13 MVD studies, the overall pain-free duration lasted more than 5 years.[22] Moreover, recurrence rates were lower with MVD than with GKS, falling to 8 to 38%.[22] Of the major procedural interventions available for TN, MVD offers the longest period of pain relief and the greatest patient satisfaction rate.[4,5,22]

Although craniotomy and MVD have emerged as the gold standards for medically refractory TN, it should be noted that many patients with TN are poor craniotomy candidates due to older age and medical comorbidities.[23] In such patients, stereotactic radiosurgery, despite being less efficacious than MVD, should be considered.

Hemifacial Spasm

Treatments for HFS include both pharmacologic and surgical options. Oral medications, such as carbamazepine and benzodiazepines, have poor efficacy in treating HFS. Botulinum toxin injections have demonstrated success in 76 to 100% of patients, with a major drawback being the relatively brief period of relief (only 10–31 weeks). Therefore, over time, patients require multiple, lifelong injections for sustained disease control. Other limitations include higher doses needed over time, as well as an adverse effects profile consisting of orbicularis oris paralysis, ptosis, and lagophthalmos.[24]

If botulinum toxin injections are not tolerated by patients with HFS, MVD may be considered. This neurosurgical approach involves placement of Teflon sponges between the compressed nerve and culprit blood vessels, which allows the nerve to be released from any ectopic excitation or irritation due to compression by a vessel (▶ Fig. 17.1).[24] A 2012 systematic review of the safety and efficacy of MVD pooled results from 22 studies on 5,685 patients and found that 91.1% of patients experienced complete HFS symptom resolution following surgery; moreover, for the studies reporting a 5-year mean follow-up, 87.6% of patients reported symptom resolution.[24] Although complications were relatively rare, transient facial palsy occurred in 9.5% of patients, transient hearing deficits in 3.2% of patients, and cerebrospinal fluid leak in 1.4% of patients. Permanent complications were even rarer, with a 2.3% rate of hearing deficit and 0.9% rate of facial palsy.

Glossopharyngeal Neuralgia

Like TN and HFS, glossopharyngeal neuralgia can also be treated by pharmacologic or surgical means. Because common analgesic therapy is ineffective, the mainstay of pharmacologic treatment consists of anticonvulsants such as phenytoin and carbamazepine. For patients with a poor response to these medications, surgical treatment is indicated. Neurosurgical treatments available for glossopharyngeal neuralgia include open craniotomy with vagus nerve (CN X) and glossopharyngeal nerve (CN IX) rhizotomy or neurotomy and a percutaneous approach with radiofrequency rhizotomy, trigeminal tractotomy, or nucleotomy. MVD is also an option.[25,26]

A 2002 study followed outcomes in 20 patients treated with MVD for glossopharyngeal neuralgia and demonstrated immediate and long-term success rates of greater than 90%.[27] A study conducted in 2004 demonstrated a 98% pain-relief rate after MVD.[28] Long-term follow-up (median, 12.7 years) was available for 29 patients, 28 (97%) of whom still had pain relief. Finally, a 2010 review article that described outcomes in 21 patients with glossopharyngeal neuralgia found that 90% of MVD patients experienced complete symptom relief at a median follow-up of 4 years.[26]

In comparison to MVD, rhizotomy and GKS treatments for glossopharyngeal neuralgia are not as robust.[26,29] Rhizotomy is

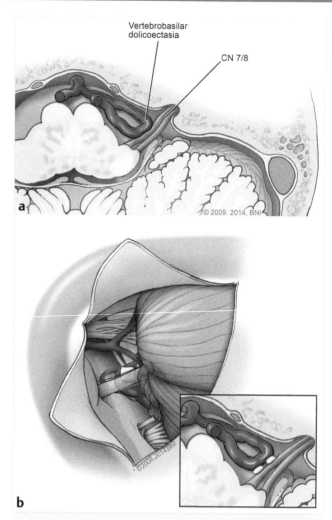

Fig. 17.1 Illustration demonstrating **(a)** axial view: a large dolichoectatic vertebral artery compressing the cranial nerve VII–VIII complex resulting in hemifacial spasm. **(b)** Posterolateral view: Teflon pledgets are used to relieve pulsatile vascular compression of the artery against the facial nerve (inset: axial view). (Used with permission from Barrow Neurological Institute, Phoenix, AZ.)

associated with high rates of postoperative hoarseness and dysphagia.[29,30] A 2013 review compared postoperative complications and long-term pain control in patients undergoing MVD or rhizotomy and found that, while rhizotomy offered improved long-term pain control compared to MVD (87 vs. 85%, respectively, at mean follow-up times of about 4.5 years), rhizotomy was associated with higher rates of vagus nerve dysfunction (25 vs. 13.2%).[30] A 2016 study that tracked outcomes in 22 patients who received GKS for glossopharyngeal neuralgia demonstrated a 63% rate of pain relief 1 year after the procedure, dropping to 49% by 2 years and 38% at 3 to 5 years.[29] Together, these studies indicate the overall superiority of MVD over rhizotomy and radiosurgery in terms of long-term pain relief.

17.1.4 Operative Findings

In light of the pathophysiology of CN compression syndromes, the intraoperative identification of an offending vessel during MVD is essential. In a series of patients for whom no vascular compression was found intraoperatively, the rate of not identifying an offending vessel during MVD varied substantially, from 3 to 90%.[31] When an offending vessel was not found, various approaches were undertaken by the operating surgeons, with partial sensory root resection being the most common.[31] Other options included MVD, neurolysis, or whole nerve division.[31] The authors advocated for MVD over ablative procedures in such scenarios because ablation carries the risk of causing significant sensory deficits.[31] In their study, two of five patients for whom no vessel was identified still reported complete pain resolution after 1 operation; the remaining three patients underwent reoperation, after which they, too, reported resolution of pain.[31] Their pain relief was thought to be caused by the potential effect of simply manipulating the nerve during the operation and relieving any abnormal brainstem activity, despite the absence of a vessel causing compression.[31]

Despite symptom improvement in the short term, some studies have demonstrated higher rates of pain recurrence in patients with no identifiable compression during their initial operation.[31,32] In one study, pain recurrence was 11.8% at 12 months and 43.2% at 48 months in such patients; these rates are higher than the rates for patients with identifiable compressing vessels.[32]

17.1.5 Case Presentation

A 55-year-old man presented to Barrow Neurological Institute with a multiple-year history of left facial spasms that were recalcitrant to conservative management. He began having botulinum toxin injections 2 years before presentation and reported that his symptoms initially improved for up to 5 months at a time after injections. As the duration of symptom relief after injections shortened, he required nearly monthly injections but each injection had reduced efficacy. Imaging was notable for a vascular loop adjacent to the fascial–vestibulocochlear (CN VII-VIII) complex (▶ Fig. 17.2a). After extensive discussions on the risks and benefits of surgery, the patient decided to proceed with surgical intervention. After sedation and intubation, leads monitoring somatosensory evoked potentials and auditory evoked potentials for the trigeminal and facial nerves and the brainstem were placed, and baseline monitoring was recorded. The patient's head was then placed in a Mayfield head clamp and rotated to the right to reveal the left periauricular region. A computer neuronavigation system was then registered using the contours of the scalp, and accuracy was confirmed with known anatomical landmarks. The transverse sigmoid junction was marked, and an incision was planned in this region. Neuronavigation guidance permitted a small incision and craniotomy, similar to that used for endoscopic procedures. The craniotomy was performed using a high-speed pneumatic drill, with exposure of the inferior aspects of both the transverse and sigmoid sinuses (▶ Fig. 17.2b). A T-shaped dural opening was made using a No. 15 blade, and the dura was tacked to the bone to mobilize the lip of the sigmoid sinus, which can often obstruct visualization during access to the basal cisterns. The operating microscope was moved into position, and the remainder of the procedure was performed using microscopic visualization. Sharp microdissection was used to open the posterior fossa arachnoid membrane, with special attention focused on performance of early release of cerebrospinal fluid to permit brain relaxation. No fixed retraction was used during the procedure. Sharp microdissection was used to release any adhesions to neurovascular structures, and the CN VII–VIII complex was identified exiting the porus acusticus. Blunt dissectors were used to explore the proximal segment of the facial nerve. A loop of the AICA was identified as impinging on the facial nerve as it exited the brainstem. A Teflon interpositional graft was placed between the vessel and the nerve. The cisternal segment of the facial nerve was then explored to confirm that no additional vessels were compressing the nerves (▶ Fig. 17.2c–f). Microscopic visualization allowed for an excellent view of the proximal segment of the nerve, but visualization of the cisternal segment of the facial nerve required manipulation of CN VIII. The dura and skin were closed in a watertight fashion. Postoperatively, the patient experienced minimal postoperative pain and had complete resolution of his HFS spasms. At the 6-month follow-up, his symptom relief was stable, and he was weaned off anticonvulsant medications.

17.1.6 Advantages of the Microscopic Approach

Comparison of Postoperative Success: Maintenance of Pain Relief

The endoscopic approach to MVD is rarely employed, and the microscopic approach is considered the standard of care.[5,11,33] Thus, few large-scale studies have examined outcomes in patients undergoing fully endoscopic nerve decompression. Outcomes reported in those studies are comparable to outcomes reported for the microscopic approach. Kabil et al[34] demonstrated a 93% complete relief rate in 118 patients with long-term follow-up of 3 years after endoscopic trigeminal decompression. Yadav et al[35] reported a 94% partial and 90% complete pain relief rate in 51 endoscopically treated patients undergoing trigeminal nerve decompression. Setty et al[36] reported a 98% complete pain relief rate ($n = 56$) at a mean 32-month follow-up in 57 patients who were treated with endovascular decompression for TN.

When microscopic surgery and endoscopic surgery success rates are compared, they are similar for HFS.[37] However, perhaps more meaningful are rates from studies using the microscopic approach, given the larger numbers of patients and longer follow-up times documented in these studies. Barker et al[37] reported an 86% excellent HFS relief rate at 1-month follow-up in 612 patients who were treated for HFS; the response rate remained high at 86% at 10-year follow-up. In a study evaluating long-term outcomes in 1,032 patients who underwent microscopic surgery for TN or HFS between 1976 and 1991, immediate postoperative cure rates were 92.9 to 98.3%, and at follow-up times of 5 years or more, success rates were 80.3 to 89%.[38] Finally, in the Barker et al[13] study of 1,185 patients treated via microscope for TN, 82% of patients had complete relief and 16% had partial relief immediately following the operation; at 1-year follow-up, 75% still had complete relief and 9% had partial relief; at 10-year follow-up, 64% had complete relief and 4% had partial relief. The microscopic approach to CN decompression has thus proven effective in large cohorts of patients, providing both immediate and maintenance relief.[13,37,38]

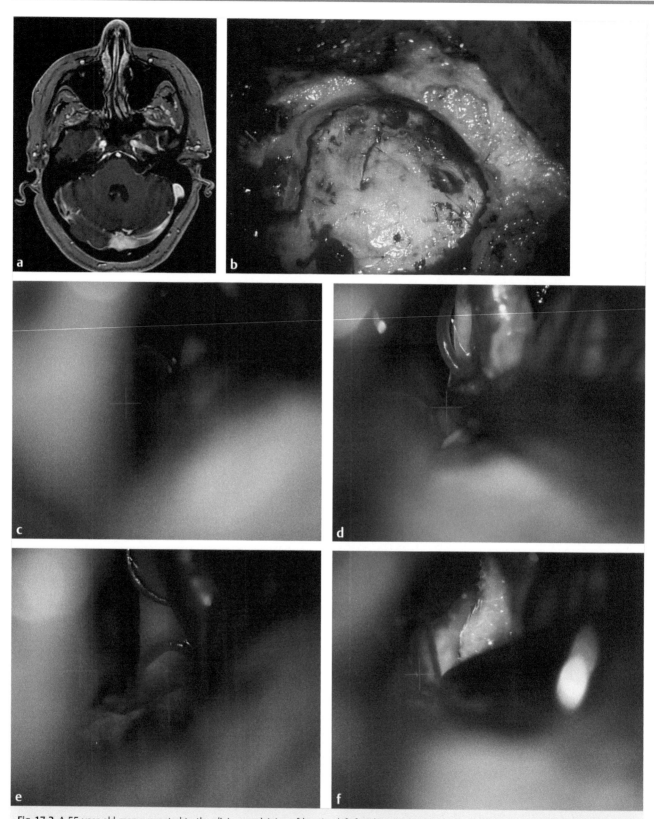

Fig. 17.2 A 55-year-old man presented to the clinic complaining of burning left facial pain in the V2 and V3 dermatomal distributions that conservative management failed to alleviate. **(a)** A preoperative magnetic resonance image demonstrates a vascular loop adjacent to the left trigeminal nerve (cranial nerve [CN] V). **(b)** The intraoperative photograph demonstrates a small craniotomy centered at the transverse–sigmoid junction. **(c)** The arachnoid membrane was widely opened, and the CN identified. **(d)** Microsurgical dissection past Dandy's vein allows identification of CN V, which was followed proximally to the brainstem. **(e)** A small vessel loop was identified ventral to the brainstem exit zone of CN V, and **(f)** an interpositional Teflon pledget was placed between the vascular loop and the nerve. Postoperatively, the patient experienced no perioperative complications and had complete resolution of his burning facial pain. (Used with permission from Barrow Neurological Institute, Phoenix, AZ.)

In a comparison of patient outcomes after microscopic versus endoscopic surgery, Lee et al[33] found that the endoscope offered better visualization of the offending vessels than the operating microscope. The vessels compressing the CNs could not be identified in 7% of the endoscopy cases compared to 11% of the microscopy cases. However, the increased visualization seemed to have no effect on postoperative outcomes, as both groups of patients reported 70 to 80% rates of improvement in pain intensity and 85% in activities of daily living, with 80% pain control at 3-year follow-up.

Although data providing a direct comparison of the two techniques are sparse, these studies collectively demonstrate that despite potential visualization enhancements offered by the endoscopic approach, both techniques provide patients with excellent relief rates postoperatively and at long-term follow-up.[13,33,34,35,36,37,38]

Technical Advantages of the Microscopic Approach

Despite the superiority of visualization that is largely cited as the primary advantage of the endoscopic approach over the microscopic approach for brainstem decompression, the microscopic approach remains the standard.[11] Studies suggest that the microscope may allow for operative maneuverability superior to that of the endoscope. In addition, visualization is limited even with the endoscopic approach; for example, because the endoscope is usually deep within the surgical field and only captures images anterior to its tip, visualization behind the surgical field of view is poor. This anterior surgical view makes the insertion and removal of instruments from the operative field more dangerous and increases the likelihood of vessel and neural tissue injury.[11] Moreover, the microscope offers binocular depth perception superior to that afforded by the endoscope.

17.1.7 Disadvantages of the Endoscopic Approach

Technical Limitations

The endoscopic approach has numerous technical limitations. Notably, the endoscopic approach has visual restraints, including poor depth perception of the surgical field and blind spots, and space constraints due to the endoscope itself taking up space in an already small surgical field.[11,14,33] In addition, the heat generated at the tip of the endoscope may result in damage to adjacent structures.[33]

The endoscope is also difficult to use when trying to stop intraoperative bleeding, with the added complication of blood staining the telescope and fogging the lens.[11,14,39] Preventing or overcoming this limitation when it arises involves additional procedural steps, such as intermittent irrigation of the lens and involvement of an assistant.[39] These steps inevitably increase the time required for the procedure. Moreover, proper positioning and maneuvering by the assistant require significant practice and have a steep learning curve.

Technical Expertise

Overall, one significant limitation of the endoscopic approach is the technical expertise required. Endoscopic decompression requires bimanual dexterity, and thus significant practice on cadavers or models is likely to be required before a surgeon can perform endoscopic decompressions effectively.[36,39] Moreover, as in the example of a bleeding complication, the surgeon holding the endoscope would not have the bimanual dexterity needed for the procedure—the approach is therefore limited by the need for an assistant.[36,39]

Patient Selection

As described above, surgical treatment of CN compression syndromes is warranted for individuals who are refractory to medical therapy, and it provides success rates of 75 to 98%.[31,32] For patients undergoing MVD, those with severe vascular compression at the root entry zone have better results after MVD than those with milder compression; moreover, patients with arterial as opposed to venous compression have better outcomes.[31,32]

Complication Avoidance

Postoperative complications after MVD include cochlear, vestibular, facial, and abducens nerve dysfunction, as well as hearing loss, hyperpathia, and hyperesthesia.[13,40,41] Minor complications, including aching pain, sensory loss, and mild or transient CN dysfunction, have been reported at rates of 2 to 7%.[4] Hearing is affected at rates of 0.8 to 16.2%.[4,10,12,13,14] Facial palsies and numbness occur in 1 to 9.1% of patients.[12,13,14] Overall, more serious complications are even less common, with stroke rates of 0.3 to 1.7%, a cerebellar hematoma rate of 1.7%, and an edema rate of 0.5%.[4,10,13] Moreover, mortality rates are low, ranging from 0.1 to 1.7%.[4,10,12,13]

Numerous methods have been proposed to avoid MVD complications. One method involves close brainstem response monitoring throughout the operation. For example, it is recommended that auditory brainstem responses be monitored for signs of nerve damage, such as > 1-ms delay of the latency of the fifth wave or a 40% reduction of amplitude.[40] Since the introduction of intraoperative monitoring of brainstem evoked responses at the end of the 20th century, complications have become less frequent.[13,42] The rate of ipsilateral hearing loss, for example, decreased from 3% before 1980 to 1% after 1980.[13]

Other considerations to avoid complications involve technical precision and meticulous attention to detail. Damage to the cochlear and vestibular nerves can be prevented by performing traction perpendicular to the axis of the acoustic nerve.[40] Extreme care should be exercised when near an offending artery to prevent damage to the facial nerve, the abducens nerve, and the lower CNs.[40] The AICA should be handled with care to protect the facial nerve. Additionally, the vertebrobasilar artery must be meticulously handled to avoid hypofunction of the abducens nerve. Therefore, a limited prosthesis should be used when replacing the vertebrobasilar artery to avoid stressing the abducens nerve.[40] Finally, lower CN dysfunction most often occurs when the nerves are manipulated or damaged by heat from a bipolar coagulator. Damage to the nerves can be minimized by covering them with a wet Cottonoid before using the coagulator.[40] Another strategy is to use a narrow suction tube, which may allow the surgeon a greater degree of space and mobility within which to work, allowing for more careful manipulation and avoidance of injury.[12]

One of the most troublesome postoperative sequelae after MVD is postoperative cerebellar edema, which may occur because of inappropriate retraction of the cerebellum or because of intraoperative trauma to the superior petrosal veins.[40] Damage from cerebellar retraction may be prevented by fully opening the cerebellar cisterns and removing as much cerebrospinal fluid as possible.[40] Moreover, the cerebellar retraction time should be less than 5 minutes. Retraction of the cerebellum should be extremely gentle and, if possible, a suction tube should be used in place of a retractor.[40] Venous trauma can be prevented by carefully cutting the arachnoid membrane covering the veins to allow vessel movement.[40] Fibrin glue should be used to ensure proper drainage of the veins into their major sinus.[40] If cerebellar edema occurs, it must be dealt with immediately via ventricular drainage or posterior fossa decompression surgery.[40] Overall, it is imperative to limit the duration and extent of retraction to prevent cerebellar injury by performing the entire operation through a small incision in less than 2 hours.[42]

Although it is essential to prevent such complications and to address them immediately should they arise, we underscore that serious complications during and after MVD are rare. MVD remains the gold standard for treatment of microvascular CN compression because of its excellent success rate.[12]

References

[1] Donahue JH, Ornan DA, Mukherjee S. Imaging of vascular compression syndromes. Radiol Clin North Am. 2017; 55(1):123–138

[2] Jannetta PJ. The history of microvascular decompression surgery. In: Li ST, Zhong Jun, Selukha R, eds. Microvascular Decompression Surgery: New York, NY: Springer; 2016:1–7

[3] Haller S, Etienne L, Kövari E, Varoquaux AD, Urbach H, Becker M. Imaging of neurovascular compression syndromes: trigeminal neuralgia, hemifacial spasm, vestibular paroxysmia, and glossopharyngeal neuralgia. AJNR Am J Neuroradiol. 2016; 37(8):1384–1392

[4] Maarbjerg S, Di Stefano G, Bendtsen L, Cruccu G. Trigeminal neuralgia - diagnosis and treatment. Cephalalgia. 2017; 37(7):648–657

[5] Patel SK, Liu JK. Overview and history of trigeminal neuralgia. Neurosurg Clin N Am. 2016; 27(3):265–276

[6] Dandy WE. The treatment of trigeminal neuralgia by the cerebellar route. Ann Surg. 1932; 96(4):787–795

[7] Dandy WE. Concerning the cause of trigeminal neuralgia. Am J Surg. 1934; 24:447–455

[8] Gardner WJ, Miklos MV. Response of trigeminal neuralgia to decompression of sensory root; discussion of cause of trigeminal neuralgia. J Am Med Assoc. 1959; 170(15):1773–1776

[9] Jannetta PJ. Arterial compression of the trigeminal nerve at the pons in patients with trigeminal neuralgia. J Neurosurg. 1967; 26(1):159–162

[10] Jannetta PJ. Observations on the etiology of trigeminal neuralgia, hemifacial spasm, acoustic nerve dysfunction and glossopharyngeal neuralgia. Definitive microsurgical treatment and results in 117 patients. Neurochirurgia (Stuttg). 1977; 20(5):145–154

[11] Piazza M, Lee JY. Endoscopic and microscopic microvascular decompression. Neurosurg Clin N Am. 2016; 27(3):305–313

[12] Xia L, Zhong J, Zhu J, et al. Effectiveness and safety of microvascular decompression surgery for treatment of trigeminal neuralgia: a systematic review. J Craniofac Surg. 2014; 25(4):1413–1417

[13] Barker FG, II, Jannetta PJ, Bissonette DJ, Larkins MV, Jho HD. The long-term outcome of microvascular decompression for trigeminal neuralgia. N Engl J Med. 1996; 334(17):1077–1083

[14] Cui ZL. Zhipei. Advances in microvascular decompression for hemifacial spasm. J Otol. 2015; 10(1):1–6

[15] Broggi M, Acerbi F, Ferroli P, Tringali G, Schiariti M, Broggi G. Microvascular decompression for neurovascular conflicts in the cerebello-pontine angle: which role for endoscopy? Acta Neurochir (Wien). 2013; 155(9):1709–1716

[16] Matsushima KJ, Xiaochun R, Albert L. Microsurgical anatomy for microvascular decompression. In: Li ST, Zhong J; Sekula RF, eds. Microvascular Decompression Surgery. New York, NY: Springer; 2016

[17] Frederickson AMG, Michael S, Sekula RF. Pathogenesis of trigeminal neuralgia. In: Li ST, Zhong J; Sekula RF, eds. Microvascular Decompression Surgery. New York, NY: Springer; 2016

[18] Grasso G, Landi A, Alafaci C. A novel pathophysiological mechanism contributing to trigeminal neuralgia. Mol Med. 2016; 22:452–454

[19] Jannetta PJ, McLaughlin MR, Casey KF. Technique of microvascular decompression. Technical note. Neurosurg Focus. 2005; 18(5):E5

[20] Love S, Coakham HB. Trigeminal neuralgia: pathology and pathogenesis. Brain. 2001; 124(Pt 12):2347–2360

[21] Cruccu G, Gronseth G, Alksne J, et al. American Academy of Neurology Society, European Federation of Neurological Society. AAN-EFNS guidelines on trigeminal neuralgia management. Eur J Neurol. 2008; 15(10):1013–1028

[22] Parmar M, Sharma N, Modgill V, Naidu P. Comparative evaluation of surgical procedures for trigeminal neuralgia. J Maxillofac Oral Surg. 2013; 12(4): 400–409

[23] Kondziolka D, Zorro O, Lobato-Polo J, et al. Gamma Knife stereotactic radiosurgery for idiopathic trigeminal neuralgia. J Neurosurg. 2010; 112(4): 758–765

[24] Miller LE, Miller VM. Safety and effectiveness of microvascular decompression for treatment of hemifacial spasm: a systematic review. Br J Neurosurg. 2012; 26(4):438–444

[25] Teixeira MJ, de Siqueira SR, Bor-Seng-Shu E. Glossopharyngeal neuralgia: neurosurgical treatment and differential diagnosis. Acta Neurochir (Wien). 2008; 150(5):471–475, discussion 475

[26] Kandan SR, Khan S, Jeyaretna DS, Lhatoo S, Patel NK, Coakham HB. Neuralgia of the glossopharyngeal and vagal nerves: long-term outcome following surgical treatment and literature review. Br J Neurosurg. 2010; 24(4): 441–446

[27] Patel A, Kassam A, Horowitz M, Chang YF. Microvascular decompression in the management of glossopharyngeal neuralgia: analysis of 217 cases. Neurosurgery. 2002; 50(4):705–710, discussion 710–711

[28] Sampson JH, Grossi PM, Asaoka K, Fukushima T. Microvascular decompression for glossopharyngeal neuralgia: long-term effectiveness and complication avoidance. Neurosurgery. 2004; 54(4):884–889, discussion 889–890

[29] Kano H, Urgosik D, Liscak R, et al. Stereotactic radiosurgery for idiopathic glossopharyngeal neuralgia: an international multicenter study. J Neurosurg. 2016; 125 Suppl 1:147–153

[30] Rey-Dios R, Cohen-Gadol AA. Current neurosurgical management of glossopharyngeal neuralgia and technical nuances for microvascular decompression surgery. Neurosurg Focus. 2013; 34(3):E8

[31] Baechli H, Gratzl O. Microvascular decompression in trigeminal neuralgia with no vascular compression. Eur Surg Res. 2007; 39(1):51–57

[32] Revuelta-Gutiérrez R, López-González MA, Soto-Hernández JL. Surgical treatment of trigeminal neuralgia without vascular compression: 20 years of experience. Surg Neurol. 2006; 66(1):32–36, discussion 36

[33] Lee JY, Pierce JT, Sandhu SK, Petrov D, Yang AI. Endoscopic versus microscopic microvascular decompression for trigeminal neuralgia: equivalent pain outcomes with possibly decreased postoperative headache after endoscopic surgery. J Neurosurg. 20 17; 126(5):1676–1684

[34] Kabil MS, Eby JB, Shahinian HK. Endoscopic vascular decompression versus microvascular decompression of the trigeminal nerve. Minim Invasive Neurosurg. 2005; 48(4):207–212

[35] Yadav YR, Parihar V, Agarwal M, Sherekar S, Bhatele P. Endoscopic vascular decompression of the trigeminal nerve. Minim Invasive Neurosurg. 2011; 54 (3):110–114

[36] Setty P, Volkov AA, D'Andrea KP, Pieper DR. Endoscopic vascular decompression for the treatment of trigeminal neuralgia: clinical outcomes and technical note. World Neurosurg. 2014; 81(3)(–)(4):603–608

[37] Barker FG, II, Jannetta PJ, Bissonette DJ, Shields PT, Larkins MV, Jho HD. Microvascular decompression for hemifacial spasm. J Neurosurg. 1995; 82(2): 201–210

[38] Kondo A. Follow-up results of microvascular decompression in trigeminal neuralgia and hemifacial spasm. Neurosurgery. 1997; 40(1):46–51, discussion 51–52

[39] Kher Y, Yadav N, Yadav YR, Parihar V, Ratre S, Bajaj J. Endoscopic vascular decompression in trigeminal neuralgia. Turk Neurosurg. 20 17; 27(6):998–1006

[40] Kondo A. Outcome evaluation and postoperative management. In: Li STZ, Raymond SF, eds. Microvascular Decompression Surgery. New York, NY:: Springer; 2016:171–176

[41] Oesman C, Mooij JJ. Long-term follow-up of microvascular decompression for trigeminal neuralgia. Skull Base. 2011; 21(5):313–322

[42] McLaughlin MR, Jannetta PJ, Clyde BL, Subach BR, Comey CH, Resnick DK. Microvascular decompression of cranial nerves: lessons learned after 4400 operations. J Neurosurg. 1999; 90(1):1–8

18 Decompression of Cranial Nerves: Endoscope

Andrew I. Yang and John Y. K. Lee

Summary

Experience in endoscopic microvascular decompression (MVD) of cranial nerves (CN) has been primarily in the management of trigeminal neuralgia. The panoramic view offered by endoscopy has been associated with enhanced identification of neurovascular conflict (NVC) when compared to the microscope. Endoscopy may have most utility in cases of NVC along the medial/inferior aspects of the proximal nerve, or the medial aspect of the distal nerve; in cases of compression by a diminutive vein; and in cases of a low/prominent petrous ridge. Endoscopy can allow the surgeon to more confidently rule out NVC, which would inform subsequent surgical interventions such as internal neurolysis. Endoscopic MVD is a safe alternative to the traditional MVD with a microscope, and is at least as equally effective in terms of pain outcomes.

Keywords: cranial nerves, vascular compression, endoscope

18.1 Endoscopic Perspective

18.1.1 History and Physical Examination

Case 1

The patient is a 27-year-old female with a history of right-sided trigeminal neuralgia (TN) for 1 year. She reported episodes of sharp, shooting pain in the right V2 and V3 distributions, and denied any facial numbness. Triggers included touch, talking, chewing, and cold temperature. The pain episodes had been refractory to medical management with carbamazepine and gabapentin. The patient was deemed to be a good candidate for endoscopic microvascular decompression (MVD).

Case 2

The patient is a 32-year-old female with a history of right-sided TN for 18 years. She reported episodes of sharp, shooting pain in the right V2 distribution that felt like shards of glass. Triggers included eating, talking, and brushing teeth. She denied any facial numbness. The patient had been started on carbamazepine, but was weaned off the drug due to its side effects, and had not resumed due to pregnancy and nursing. The patient was deemed to be a good candidate for endoscopic MVD.

18.1.2 Intraoperative Management

Case 1

The patient was placed in the lateral decubitus position, with the head placed in three-pin fixation. The head was flexed two fingerbreadths from the sternum and rotated 70 to 80 degrees away from the right side in order to maintain the angle of the vertex parallel to the floor.

A linear incision was made inferior to the junction of the transverse and sigmoid sinuses, and soft-tissue dissection was done in the subperiosteal plane to the digastric groove. A burr hole was placed posterior to the superior aspect of the insertion of the digastric muscle with a cutting drill bit, and extended toward the junction of the sinuses with a Kerrison rongeur and matchstick cutting burr. Any mastoid air cells entered during drilling were filled with bone wax.

The dura was opened in a **C**-shaped manner, and flapped towards the sigmoid sinus. A 2.7-mm outer-diameter scope (Storz, Culver City, CA) was used for visualization, secured at the head of the bed with a pneumatic holding arm (Mitaka Kohki Co., Tokyo, Japan). The endoscope was advanced in the anteroinferior direction with dynamic retraction on the cerebellum, using a sterile glove and patty combination to protect the cerebellar pial surface. The suction and microdissection instruments (Storz) were advanced parallel to the endoscope.

The arachnoid sheath around cranial nerves (CNs) XI, X, and XI was sharply dissected, allowing adequate time for cerebrospinal fluid (CSF) egress. The petrosal vein was identified, followed by CNs VIII and V. The superior cerebellar artery (SCA) was identified compressing CN V on its cephalad aspect (▶ Fig. 18.1**a**). The endoscope was advanced to offer a panoramic view of the cerebellopontine angle (CPA) (▶ Fig. 18.1**b**). The SCA was mobilized (▶ Fig. 18.1**c**), once again with sharp arachnoid dissection, and two pieces of Teflon were used to decompress CN V (▶ Fig. 18.1**d**). The SCA was also noted to be compressing the distal/caudal aspect of CN V (▶ Fig. 18.1**d**), which was not originally visualized due to a prominent suprameatal petrous tubercle. In fact, due to the confines of the working space, this branch of the SCA was dissected away from CN V with one hand holding the endoscope and the other the round knife (▶ Fig. 18.1**e**), and then decompressed using an additional piece of Teflon (▶ Fig. 18.1**f**). After hemostasis was achieved, the dura was primarily repaired and supplemented with a collagen allograft. Cranioplasty was done with bone cement contoured to the defect (< 5 cm).

The patient was transferred to the neurological intensive care unit for close observation overnight, and discharged on postoperative day 4. She reported relief in facial pain on postoperative day 0.

Case 2

In this case, the petrosal vein was cauterized and cut to allow for adequate visualization and decompression. Whenever possible, the senior author (J.Y.K.L.) prefers not to sacrifice the petrosal vein. Although this maneuver is generally considered safe, some instances of postoperative hemorrhage may be the result of venous engorgement or venous infarction, and as such every effort is made to avoid its sacrifice. In this case, however, the corridor to the CPA was very tight due to a broad-based petrous tubercle, which obscured view of CN V (▶ Fig. 18.2**a**). The SCA on the cephalad side (▶ Fig. 18.2**b,c**) and a small distal traversing petrosal vein were noted to compress CN V. The vein was only seen after the endoscope was advanced past the petrous tubercle (▶ Fig. 18.2**d**). The distal vein was once again dissected away from CN V with one hand holding the endoscope and the other the round knife (▶ Fig. 18.2**e**). The endoscope allowed the surgeon to address all instances of neurovascular conflict (NVC) (▶ Fig. 18.2**f**).

The patient was discharged on postoperative day 3.

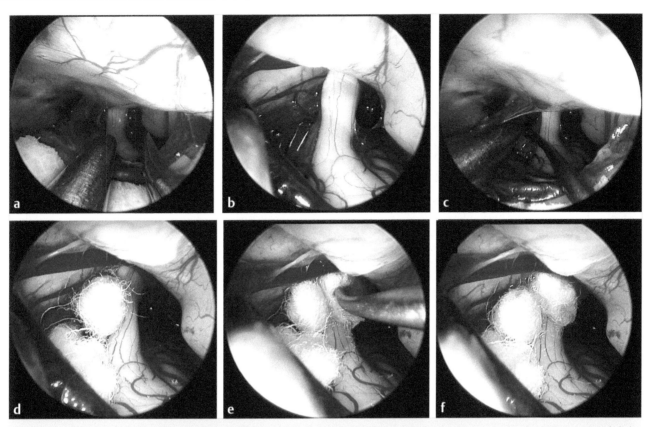

Fig. 18.1 (a–f) Intraoperative endoscopic images from case 1. **(a)** Superior cerebellar artery (SCA) compresses cranial nerve (CN) V at its cephalad aspect. **(b)** Endoscope advanced. **(c)** SCA mobilized with sharp arachnoid dissection. **(d)** CN V decompressed with two pieces of Teflon. **(e)** SCA also compressed CN V at its distal/caudal aspect, which was treated with additional piece of Teflon. **(f)** Endoscope shows decompression of CN V.

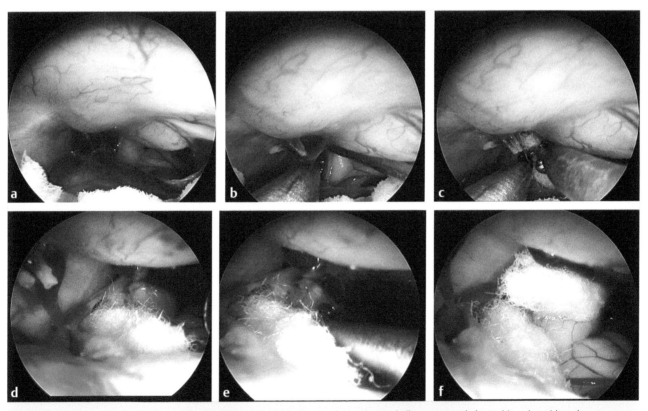

Fig. 18.2 (a–f) Intraoperative endoscopic images from case 2. **(a)** The corridor to the cerebellopontine angle limited by a broad-based petrous tubercle. **(b)** Superior cerebellar artery (SCA) compresses cranial nerve (CN) V at its cephalad aspect. **(c)** CN V decompressed with Teflon. **(d)** Endoscope advanced past the petrous tubercle, revealing a small distal traversing petrosal vein compressing CN V. **(e)** Distal vein dissected away from CN V with round knife. **(f)** Endoscope shows decompression of CN V.

18.1.3 Surgical Outcomes

At the 1-month postoperative follow-up, both patients reported no episodes of TN pain. They also reported no facial numbness or hearing loss, and were gradually returning to full activity.

18.1.4 Advantages of Endoscopic Approach and Disadvantages of Microscopic Approach for the Case Illustrations

The endoscopic approach requires a smaller craniectomy (~1.5 cm) and dural opening (< 1.0 cm), and hence a smaller skin incision and less muscle dissection. As the bone work does not need to extend as anterolateral as in the microscopic approach (~5 cm),[1] there is less mastoid air cell disruption with the endoscopic approach. Even with the copious application of bone wax, disruption of the mastoid air cells can increase the risk of postoperative CSF leaks, which in a large series had an incidence of 2.17%.[2]

The CPA is a small space, often requiring significant retraction in addition to arachnoid dissection to visualize CN V. Hence, with the panoramic view afforded by the endoscope, retraction on the cerebellum, brainstem, and acousticofacial bundle can be eliminated or at least minimized, reducing the risk of injury to these structures from focal ischemia or mechanical tension.

With the traditional microscopic approach, retraction on the cerebellum can lead to hemorrhage and contusions in 0.68% of cases in a large series for decompression of CNs V, VII, and XI/X.[2] Concomitant tension on the acousticofacial bundle led to hearing loss in 1.4% of cases in the same series. In particular, hearing loss was noted in 0.97% of CN V cases. The degree of retraction can be reduced by adequate bony exposure, often requiring partial removal of the mastoid bone. However, this incurs the additional risk of a postoperative CSF leak.

Successful decompression of CN V requires identification of all NVC along the root entry zone, which is variable in length and can extend to the distal nerve as it enters Meckel's cave. With the traditional microscopic approach, NVC can be particularly hard to visualize on the medial and inferior aspects of the proximal nerve, and the medial aspect of the distal nerve. Indeed, higher rates of NVC visualization with the endoscope have been reported in the literature.[3,4,5,6]

Recurrence of TN is a known risk of MVD, although annual rates of recurrence are less than 2% at 5 years and less than 1% at 10 years.[7] Veins or small arteries are the most commonly found compressive vessels in reoperations. These findings may represent new vascular loops that form as part of the progressive vessel changes that take place with normal aging,[8] vascular loops that were neglected due to their diminutive size or absence of nerve distortion (i.e., arteries or veins that are only in contact with or close to the nerve),[9] or perhaps occult vascular compressions that were difficult to visualize with only the microscope.

In addition to identification of all NVC, the adequacy of the decompression itself with Teflon can be more exhaustively assessed with the endoscope. Furthermore, in cases where NVC is definitively ruled out, the surgeon can appropriately employ alternate techniques, e.g., internal neurolysis, to achieve the best outcome possible.[10]

18.1.5 Patient Selection (Authors' Experience)

Initially, endoscopic MVD was performed in patients with a relatively wider corridor to the CPA. These include the elderly, i.e., patients with a degree of cerebellar atrophy, and those with a small petrous tubercle. The first 14 cases at our institution were endoscope-assisted operations, in which the microscope was the primary visualization tool, with the endoscope utilized as an adjunct. Currently, however, all TN cases are done with a fully endoscopic approach, demonstrating the steep learning curve for the surgeon. In fact, as the provided cases are meant to illustrate, the endoscopic approach is particularly relevant in patients whose anatomy presents a narrow working space. These include young patients and patients with Chiari malformations, who have a tight posterior fossa.

Reoperations for vascular compression can also be performed safely and effectively using a purely endoscopic approach. Although scar dissection can take additional time, careful attention to hemostasis allows for effective visualization and decompression without additional risk.

18.1.6 Complication Avoidance, Technical Nuances, and Clinical Pearls

The dural opening for the endoscopic approach needs to be only 1 cm in diameter (▶ Fig. 18.3b). Hence, external anatomical landmarks should be utilized to minimize the size of the skin incision, muscle dissection, and bony exposure. The superior aspect of the insertion of the digastric muscle is a consistent landmark, whereas the mastoid emissary vein is inconsistent. Placement of the burr hole just posterior to the digastric notch allows the dural incision at the junction of the transverse and sigmoid sinuses. In this way, the craniectomy (▶ Fig. 18.3a) defect in the majority of our endoscopic MVD cases can be covered with a burr hole cap.

A pneumatic holding arm (Mitaka Kohki Co.) for the endoscope, with a figure "4" arrangement of the joints,[11] allows the surgeon to perform bimanual microsurgery (▶ Fig. 18.3c). A triangle with the endoscope parked at the apex (12 o'clock position), the suction in the left hand (7 o'clock position), and the microinstrument in the right (5 o'clock position) is maintained both proximally at the dura and distally at the petrous temporal bone to avoid clashing of instruments (▶ Fig. 18.3d). In cases with a very prominent petrous tubercle, it can be impossible to fit the endoscope and both instruments in the CPA. In such cases, bimanual surgery must be compromised to accommodate the endoscope.

Introduction of instruments proximal to the endoscope is blind. Hence, care must be taken to introduce instruments parallel to the scope, maintaining a triangle both proximally and distally. By visualizing where instruments should appear prior to their arrival on the screen, and confirming that they emerge at the appropriate positions, injury to adjacent structures and instrument clashing can be minimized. In particular, a portion of CNs VII/VIII is always kept in view when introducing the left- and right-hand instruments distally to work on CN V.

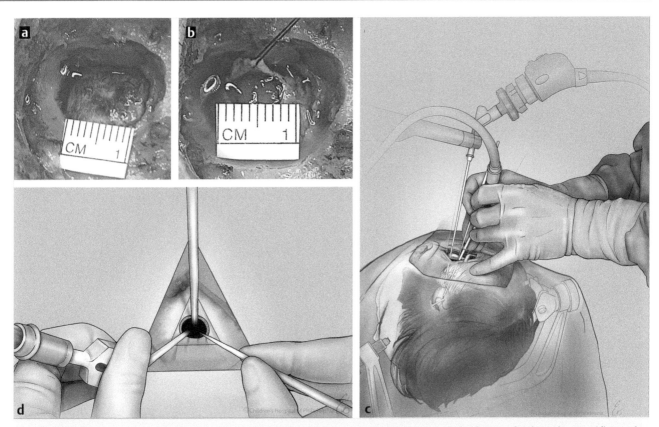

Fig. 18.3 (a) Size of craniectomy. **(b)** Size of dural opening. **(c)** Bimanual microsurgery with a pneumatic holding arm for the endoscope. **(d)** Triangle method. (Reproduced with permission from artist Eo Trueblood. Copyright Stream Studios/The Children's Hospital of Philadelphia.)

Gentle, dynamic elevation of the cerebellum is done with a sterile glove plus cottonoid patty to allow for CSF egress, specifically by releasing the arachnoid in the medial CPA and cerebellomedullary cisterns. Alternatively, CSF can be drained through a lumbar puncture in the operating room prior to incision, although we have not found this additional procedure necessary for the endoscopic approach.

A 2.7-mm 0-degree endoscope (Storz) is utilized, as opposed to the standard 4-mm sinus endoscope, to maximize working space. Debris accumulating at the distal portion of the endoscope can obscure visualization. This can be mitigated with an irrigation sheath (Medtronic Zomed, Jacksonville, FL). We have opted to omit the irrigating sheath, however, to further maximize maneuverability in the tight confines of the CPA. Intensity of the endoscope light source is kept at 25 to 50% to minimize the risk of thermal injury to the surrounding structures.

Both straight and angled endoscopes allow visualization of occult NVC in the medial/inferior aspects of the proximal nerve and the medial aspect of the distal nerve toward Meckel's cave, particularly in cases of CN V positioned medial to a low/prominent petrous ridge. These areas are particularly difficult to explore with the microscope. Hence, the endoscopic approach allows the surgeon to better identify NVC or to more confidently rule out NVC. This is particularly important when techniques such as internal neurolysis can be employed in the absence of NVC, or when compression is primarily venous without deformation of the nerve. Thirty-degree angled endoscopes have offered the optimal balance between improved visualization and maneuverability.

In addition, angled endoscopes are useful in identifying anatomy between CNs VII and IX, in particular for decompression of CN VII (hemifacial spasm), nervus intermedius (geniculate neuralgia), CN VIII (tinnitus, positional vertigo; particularly within the internal auditory canal), and CN IX (glossopharyngeal neuralgia) (▶ Fig. 18.4). For instance, a 30-degree medially directed (downward on screen) endoscope provides visualization of the root entry zone of CNs VII/VIII without retraction on the flocculus of the cerebellum, which can result in traction on CN VIII.

Venous compression is often identified distally.[12] It is important to remember that the root entry zone can extend to the distal CN V, near its entrance into Meckel's cave. Curved instruments can aid dissection in this area. Instruments with gentle curvature (Sephernia microscissors; Storz) are most useful as instruments are generally introduced into the CPA parallel to the shaft of the endoscope, whereas instruments with an aggressive curvature may be unwieldy.

18.1.7 Literature Review/Evidence in Favor of Endoscopic Approach

The literature for endoscopic MVD is largely limited to case reports and case series. In one of the larger series of 255 patients, pain outcomes and complication rates for endoscopic MVD were shown in addition to pooled data from several large microscopic MVD series.[13] At the 3-year follow-up, 95% of patients experienced "complete" pain relief, defined as 98% pain relief without the need for medications. Although no

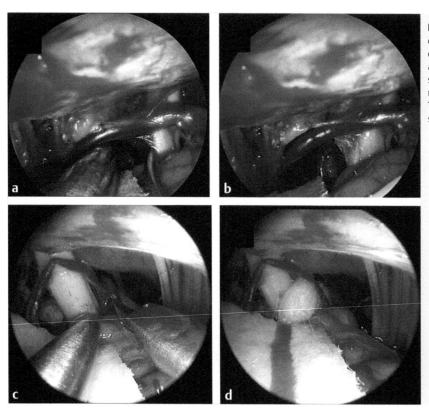

Fig. 18.4 **(a)** In a case of hemifacial spasm, cranial nerve (CN) VII is compressed at its root entry zone by the anterior inferior cerebellar artery (AICA). **(b)** Endoscope shows decompression of CN VII. **(c)** In a patient with geniculate neuralgia, nervus intermedius is sectioned. **(d)** The same patient also presented with hemifacial spasm. CN VII is decompressed from AICA.

statistical comparisons were made, this compared favorably to the 80% of patients who experienced "complete" relief with microscopic MVD. Complications including facial nerve injury, facial numbness from CN V manipulation, hearing loss, and CSF leak also compared favorably for the endoscopic approach, although once again no statistical testing was conducted.

Two centers have retrospectively compared the two cohorts in a retrospective, nonrandomized, noncontemporaneous fashion. In both studies, surgery was performed by a single surgeon at the same hospital, and the time period separating the two cohorts was relatively short. In the first report, only length of stay was statistically compared, and was found to be shorter for the endoscopic cohort (2.4 vs. 4.4 days).[14]

The second report statistically compared pain outcomes and complications between the two cohorts.[15] Pain outcomes were measured with the quantitative, validated pain outcome tool, the Penn Facial Pain Scale (PFPS, previously Brief Pain Inventory —Facial).[16] The PFPS measures three domains of pain: pain intensity, interference with activities of daily life, and interference with facial function. Prior to intervention, the two groups were equally balanced in all three domains with severe intensity and severe interference. At a mean follow-up of 2.4 and 1.3 years for the microscopic and endoscopic groups, respectively, there were no significant differences in pain outcomes as measured by the PFPS. Improvements in both cohorts surpassed patient-reported minimum clinically important differences in all three domains of the PFPS.[17]

On Cox regression analysis, there was no significant difference between the two groups in terms of actuarial freedom from facial pain recurrence, with 80% pain control at 3 years. Complication rates were very low, with the only significant difference between the two cohorts being the lower incidence

of headaches at 1-month follow-up in the endoscopic cohort (7 vs. 21%). In this series, there was no difference in length of stay. These data conclude that endoscopic MVD is a safe alternative to microscopic MVD, and is at least equivalent in pain outcomes.

As the first principle of CN decompression is to find all compressive vessels, endoscopy can be expected to lead to improved pain outcomes. Indeed, the use of endoscopy has been reported to reveal NVC that was not visualized using the microscope in 8 to 27% of cases in several other reports.[3,4,5,6] The association between superior identification of NVC and improved pain outcomes, however, has yet to be shown conclusively.

Recently, it has been proposed that NVC is neither necessary nor sufficient for TN. Preoperative magnetic resonance imaging/ angiography (MRI/MRA) has been shown to reveal no NVC in 29 and 18% of patients with TN type 1 and type 2, respectively.[18] Identification of all points of potential NVC is paramount because there are several therapeutic alternatives for TN once NVC has been definitively ruled out.

Interventions for TN in the absence of NVC include percutaneous ablative therapies delivered to the gasserian ganglion (e.g., radiofrequency gangliolysis, chemoablation using glycerol, physical ablation using balloon microcompression), and stereotactic radiosurgery. In addition, a partial sensory rhizotomy, in which the lateral one-half to two-thirds of the sensory root is transected, can also be performed upon a negative exploration. Finally, another option is internal neurolysis (aka "brushing" or "combing"), in which all or portions of the TN are divided longitudinally along its fibers.

Given the availability of several therapeutic options for TN in the absence of NVC, it is paramount to assess NVC with a high degree of sensitivity and specificity. Preoperative MRI has been noted to have a sensitivity and specificity of 96% for TN1, and 90 and 66%, respectively, for TN2.[18] This study utilized surgical exploration with a microscope as the gold standard, and thus repetition of this study with endoscopic surgical exploration as the gold standard is warranted. Ultimately, however, preoperative MRI may not be sensitive or specific enough to base surgical decision-making, and employment of these alternate surgical techniques should follow upon a negative surgical exploration with the endoscope.

References

[1] Cohen-Gadol AA. Microvascular decompression surgery for trigeminal neuralgia and hemifacial spasm: naunces of the technique based on experiences with 100 patients and review of the literature. Clin Neurol Neurosurg. 2011; 113(10):844–853

[2] McLaughlin MR, Jannetta PJ, Clyde BL, Subach BR, Comey CH, Resnick DK. Microvascular decompression of cranial nerves: lessons learned after 4400 operations. J Neurosurg. 1999; 90(1):1–8

[3] Jarrahy R, Berci G, Shahinian HK. Endoscope-assisted microvascular decompression of the trigeminal nerve. Otolaryngol Head Neck Surg. 2000; 123 (3):218–223

[4] Teo C, Nakaji P, Mobbs RJ. Endoscope-assisted microvascular decompression for trigeminal neuralgia: technical case report. Neurosurgery. 2006; 59(4) Suppl 2:E489–E490, discussion E490

[5] Yadav YR, Parihar V, Agarwal M, Sherekar S, Bhatele P. Endoscopic vascular decompression of the trigeminal nerve. Minim Invasive Neurosurg. 2011; 54 (3):110–114

[6] Chen MJ, Zhang WJ, Yang C, Wu YQ, Zhang ZY, Wang Y. Endoscopic neurovascular perspective in microvascular decompression of trigeminal neuralgia. J Craniomaxillofac Surg. 2008; 36(8):456–461

[7] Barker FG, II, Jannetta PJ, Bissonette DJ, Larkins MV, Jho HD. The long-term outcome of microvascular decompression for trigeminal neuralgia. N Engl J Med. 1996; 334(17):1077–1083

[8] Ugwuanyi UCPC, Kitchen ND. The operative findings in re-do microvascular decompression for recurrent trigeminal neuralgia. Br J Neurosurg. 2010; 24 (1):26–30

[9] Cho DY, Chang CG, Wang YC, Wang FH, Shen CC, Yang DY. Repeat operations in failed microvascular decompression for trigeminal neuralgia. Neurosurgery. 1994; 35(4):665–669, discussion 669–670

[10] Ko AL, Ozpinar A, Lee A, Raslan AM, McCartney S, Burchiel KJ. Long-term efficacy and safety of internal neurolysis for trigeminal neuralgia without neurovascular compression. J Neurosurg. 2015; 122(5): 1048–1057

[11] Lang S-S, Chen HI, Lee JYK. Endoscopic microvascular decompression: a stepwise operative technique. ORL J Otorhinolaryngol Relat Spec. 2012; 74 (6):293–298

[12] El-Garem HF, Badr-El-Dine M, Talaat AM, Magnan J. Endoscopy as a tool in minimally invasive trigeminal neuralgia surgery. Otol Neurotol. 2002; 23 (2):132–135

[13] Kabil MS, Eby JB, Shahinian HK. Endoscopic vascular decompression versus microvascular decompression of the trigeminal nerve. Minim Invasive Neurosurg. 2005; 48(4):207–212

[14] Artz GJ, Hux FJ, Larouere MJ, Bojrab DI, Babu S, Pieper DR. Endoscopic vascular decompression. Otol Neurotol. 2008; 29(7):995–1000

[15] Lee JYK, Pierce JT, Sandhu SK, Petrov D, Yang AI. Endoscopic versus microscopic microvascular decompression for trigeminal neuralgia: equivalent pain outcomes with possibly decreased postoperative headache after endoscopic surgery. J Neurosurg. 2016(July):1–9

[16] Lee JYK, Chen HI, Urban C, et al. Development of and psychometric testing for the Brief Pain Inventory-Facial in patients with facial pain syndromes. J Neurosurg. 2010; 113(3):516–523

[17] Sandhu SK, Halpern CH, Vakhshori V, Mirsaeedi-Farahani K, Farrar JT, Lee JYK. Brief pain inventory–facial minimum clinically important difference. J Neurosurg. 2015; 122(1):180–190

[18] Lee A, McCartney S, Burbidge C, Raslan AM, Burchiel KJ. Trigeminal neuralgia occurs and recurs in the absence of neurovascular compression. J Neurosurg. 2014; 120(5):1048–1054

19 Clipping of Cerebral Aneurysms: Moderator

Hasan A. Zaidi and Robert F. Spetzler

Summary

Microsurgical clipping has long been considered the gold standard approach for the treatment of cerebral aneurysms. It provides durable obliteration of flow into the aneurysm. Over the past two decades, endovascular coiling has evolved as a minimally invasive approach for the treatment of these lesions. In this chapter, we describe the evolution and history of the management of cerebral aneurysms, as well as our institutional experience in the treatment of this pathology.

Keywords: endoscopic, pineal region, posterior fossa, supracerebellar infratentorial

19.1 Moderator

19.1.1 Introduction

The history of intracranial aneurysm surgery is brief, spanning less than a century. Within such a short time, surgery for intracranial aneurysms has evolved rapidly, due in large part to technological advances that transformed neurosurgical practice in the 20th century. The surgical microscope provides greater illumination and magnification of the surgical bed, and improved metal alloy designs allow better clip reconstruction techniques and durable rates of aneurysm obliteration. The advent of endovascular therapy in the 1990s gave rise to alternative treatment paradigms for various intracranial aneurysms, and treatment options improved with each new generation of embolysates. Today, the frontiers of intracranial aneurysm surgery are marked by techniques that combine traditional clip occlusion with novel surgical approaches. Endonasal surgery, in particular, has evolved from simple approaches to sellar lesions to extended endonasal approaches that allow access to a wide range of complex ventral skull base tumors. As extended endonasal approaches and skull base repair techniques have improved, and as neurosurgeons have become more experienced with them, the opportunity has emerged to approach vascular lesions using a minimally invasive corridor and previously well-established microsurgical clipping techniques.

19.1.2 Epidemiology and Natural History of Intracranial Aneurysms

Autopsy and imaging series suggest that the overall incidence of intracranial aneurysms in the general population is 2 to 3.6%[1] and that the incidence does not vary dramatically by country of origin or ethnicity. Although these lesions are relatively rare in young persons, their prevalence increases dramatically in persons older than 30 years, with important predisposing traits being smoking, hypertension, and sex.[1] Women and persons with a family history of either ruptured or unruptured cerebral aneurysms have an increased incidence of unruptured intracranial aneurysms, which suggests a genetic predisposition to development of these lesions. The contribution of genetic factors is thought to be multifactorial, with experts suggesting that approximately 10% of all ruptured aneurysms are associated with inherited factors.[2] The risk of hemorrhage among patients with known incidental intracranial aneurysms is difficult to determine because of the lack of rigorous prospective follow-up studies. A pooled analysis of 4,705 patients with 6,556 unruptured aneurysms (length of follow-up, 26,122 patient-years) determined that the overall annual risk of rupture is 1.2% over 5-year follow-up.[3] The authors also found a statistically significant increased risk for aneurysmal rupture in this cohort for female sex, age older than 60 years, aneurysm location in the posterior circulation, Japanese or Finnish descent, and aneurysm size > 5 mm.

The incidence of subarachnoid hemorrhage in patients with a ruptured aneurysm is reported to be 6 to 10 cases per 100,000 person-years,[4] with a higher incidence among Finnish, northern Swedish, and Japanese populations (approximately 16–20 cases per 100,000 person-years).[5] The initial hemorrhage is often devastating, with nearly 50% of patients dying either before reaching the hospital or during the immediate perioperative period. Approximately one-half of those who do survive will suffer from irreversible brain damage,[6] often as a result of the initial hemorrhage or from delayed cerebral vasospasm. The most common location for ruptured aneurysms is the anterior communicating artery (31%), followed by the middle cerebral artery bifurcation (26%), the proximal internal carotid artery or the posterior communicating artery (13%), and the basilar bifurcation (4%). In general, ruptured aneurysms are larger than unruptured aneurysms (8 vs. 4 mm).[7]

After the hemorrhage of an intracranial aneurysm, its highest risk for rerupture is over the next 24 hours, at a rate of approximately 4 to 7%. In the following 2 weeks, the cumulative daily risk is 1 to 2% per day, for a total risk of rerupture of 30 to 35% in the first month without surgical or endovascular obliteration of the aneurysm.[8] Rerupture carries a mortality rate of 35%. Between 50 and 75% of patients with an aneurysmal subarachnoid hemorrhage have clinical or radiographic evidence of cerebral vasospasm, which occurs in a delayed fashion approximately 3 to 5 days after the initial hemorrhage. Without treatment, nearly one-half of these patients will develop ischemic neurologic complications from delayed vasospasm.

19.1.3 Modern Treatment Paradigms for Intracranial Aneurysms

In modern practice, two well-accepted methods for treating intracranial aneurysms are used: open craniotomy for microsurgical clip occlusion and endovascular embolization. For patients with unruptured aneurysms, the goal of surgical intervention is threefold: (1) to preserve the parent vessel, (2) to obliterate flow to the aneurysm documented by angiographic confirmation, and (3) to reduce complication rates such that the risk of intervention is maintained well below the risks associated with the natural history of the disease. Reducing the likelihood of complications is critical, especially because the risk of rupture for aneurysms is exceedingly low. In determining the treatment for an unruptured aneurysm, one must carefully consider the risk of the intervention, as the risks vary by treatment modality.

Transcranial Microsurgical Clipping

Over the past 40 years, advances in microsurgical anatomy, surgical technology, and skull base surgery have transformed open microsurgical clipping from a high-risk procedure into a time-tested treatment for intracranial aneurysms (▶ Fig. 19.1).[6] This transformation has occurred in large part because clip occlusion yields durable aneurysm obliteration rates, with several groups[9,10] reporting low rates (0.18–0.4%) of subarachnoid hemorrhage after clip occlusion. However, the risks of perioperative morbidity and mortality vary dramatically from study to study because of differences in surgeon experience and types of aneurysms treated. In a meta-analysis of 2,568 unruptured aneurysms of all types treated between 1966 and 1996, Raaymakers et al[11] reported a mortality rate of 2.6% (95% confidence interval [CI], 2–3.3) and a permanent morbidity rate of 10.9% (95% CI, 9.6–12.2). In addition to surgeon experience and hospital case volume, several predictors of surgical outcomes have been identified. Solomon et al[12] reported that larger aneurysms were associated with a greater risk of morbidity and mortality: 0% for aneurysms ≤ 10 mm in diameter, 6% for aneurysms 10 to 25 mm, and 20% for aneurysms > 25 mm. In addition, they reported higher rates of complications for posterior circulation aneurysms than for anterior circulation aneurysms (50 vs. 13%). Takahashi[13] also reported that patients with unruptured aneurysms who were older than 80 years had higher rates of perioperative morbidity and mortality. Nevertheless, open microsurgical clipping offers durable rates of aneurysm obliteration and acceptable rates of perioperative morbidity and mortality for select patients, and it remains the gold standard to which other treatment modalities are compared.

Endovascular Treatment

In the early 1990s, the advent of Guglielmi detachable coils brought about a new age in the treatment of vascular diseases.[14,15] Endovascular coil embolization has steadily gained in popularity within the neurosurgical community largely because of its ability to provide rapid access to vascular pathology via a minimally invasive approach without requiring a craniotomy and its associated risks. Endovascular coil embolization is ideal for older patients and for patients with comorbid conditions that place them at higher risk of perioperative medical complications. Despite these advantages, early studies demonstrated relatively dismal obliteration rates for aneurysms. Koivisto et al[16] and Vanninen et al[17] performed a prospective randomized controlled trial and found that only 50% of aneurysms demonstrated angiographic obliteration after the first procedure, with permanent complications of 4.0%. As interventionalists have gained experience with stent-assisted and balloon-assisted coiling, and as coil designs have improved, coil embolization has evolved into a viable treatment alternative for a range of vascular lesions using a minimally invasive approach. However, despite these advances, certain anatomical features can make endovascular therapy less suitable. The presence of tortuous vessels or distal lesions may make microcatheter access impossible. Aneurysms that incorporate the parent vessel into the dome,

aneurysms that have wide necks, and blisterlike aneurysms can make endovascular coiling challenging or impossible in certain circumstances, even with balloon or stent assistance. Partially thrombosed aneurysms increase the risk of recurrent disease as a result of coil impaction and shift. Coil embolization may also be less suitable in patients whose symptoms are related to mass effect and in patients who have cranial neuropathy due to giant, partially thrombosed aneurysms.

19.1.4 Frontiers of Vascular Neurosurgery: Endoscopic Endonasal Approaches for Cerebral Aneurysms

As endoscopic skull base surgeons have become more adept at minimally invasive ventral approaches, the opportunity has emerged for combining these skills with previously well-established open cranial microsurgical clipping techniques for the treatment of vascular lesions. The minimally invasive ventral approaches provide an attractive alternative to open traditional cranial approaches: direct ventral access to pathology that does not require an incision, retractors, or direct exposure of the brain. As endoscopic surgical techniques have steadily improved over time, so have open microsurgical approaches. "Mini" open approaches that minimize approach-related morbidity can provide microvascular surgeons with the delicate bimodal control necessary for exposing and dissecting vascular pathology without impeding surgical dexterity (▶ Fig. 19.1).[18] This ability is in direct contrast to that of endonasal approaches, whereby surgical fidelity and maneuverability are inherently limited in a confined surgical corridor, with a high risk for instrument conflict and inadvertent vascular injury. Open microsurgical approaches do not compromise proximal vascular control, which is essential for vascular neurosurgery, and such control may be limited in certain endoscopic endonasal approaches. Furthermore, retractorless microsurgical approaches for vascular lesions have reduced approach-related morbidity in the treatment of deep-seated vascular lesions,[19] further closing the gap and reducing the potential advantages afforded by the endonasal approaches. Endoscopic endonasal approaches for vascular lesions also require large exposures and skull base reconstruction techniques that are not yet perfected. Since the development of vascularized nasoseptal flaps, the rate of cerebrospinal fluid leaks after extended endonasal approaches has improved dramatically. However, even in the best hands, the rates of cerebrospinal fluid leaks and meningitis can be prohibitively high, approaching 30 and 20%, respectively.[20] These complications are nearly nonexistent in open cranial approaches. Lastly, developing a combined, coordinated team effort that focuses on endonasal vascular pathology can provide logistical challenges, particularly in the case of ruptured aneurysms, which necessitate surgical obliteration within 24 hours. Despite these disadvantages, endoscopic endonasal surgery may be a viable treatment alternative in the future for select patients with lesions that are not ideally suited for traditional microsurgical or endovascular approaches. As experience with endonasal vascular approaches grows, these indications may expand to other vascular lesions, but large-scale clinical studies are necessary to assess their true efficacy over time-tested treatment modalities.

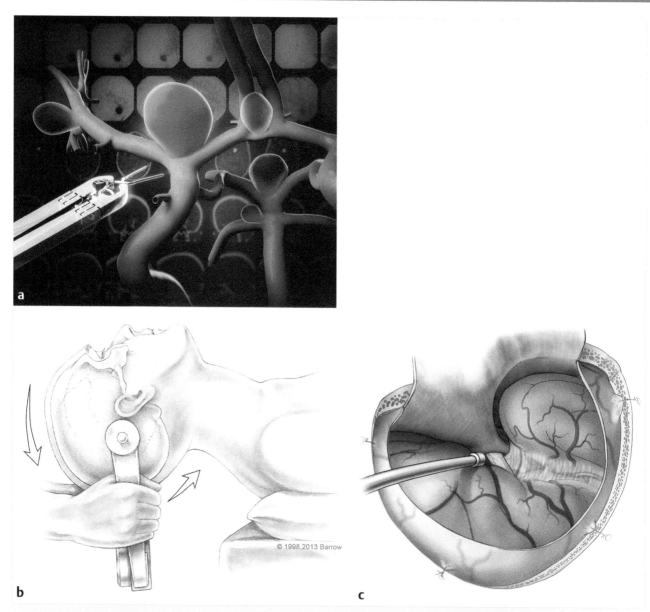

Fig. 19.1 (a) Artist's illustration depicts a stylized image of aneurysms and how an aneurysm is approached for clipping. Background design shows magnetic resonance images that guide the neurosurgeon. (b) Artist's illustration demonstrating patient positioning for microneurosurgical clipping of intracranial aneurysms. Visualization can be improved using gravity retraction by elevating the patient's shoulder, extending the neck, and rotating the head approximately 10–15 degrees to the contralateral side. (c) Artist's illustration demonstrating the intracranial view after a modified orbitozygomatic craniotomy. The frontotemporal lobes are exposed, and the sylvian fissure is widely dissected. The patient positioning allows the frontal lobe to "fall away" from the temporal lobe without the use of fixed retractors. Open microsurgical techniques conducted in this manner obviate retraction-related injury to the brain while maximizing visualization, operative maneuverability, and surgeon comfort during the duration of the case. (Used with permission from Barrow Neurological Institute, Phoenix, AZ.)

19.1.5 Final Thoughts/Expert Recommendations

Although endoscopic endonasal vascular surgery dramatically minimizes approach-related morbidity and provides direct access to vascular pathology, large-scale studies have not yet been conducted to compare the efficacy and safety of these approaches to those of well-established traditional open cranial or endovascular routes. In most cases, the added morbidity of large endonasal exposures to access these lesions, with their concomitant risk of cerebrospinal fluid leak, may not warrant these approaches because the potential complications exceed the risks associated with untreated unruptured aneurysms. Finally, limited surgical dexterity in a confined endonasal corridor with the higher risk of instrument conflict and the impracticality of rapidly deploying an endonasal vascular surgery or skull base team, even at high-volume centers, limit its large-scale applicability in the broader neurosurgical community. However, as endonasal techniques and technology improve, these novel approaches may become a reasonable option for a select group of patients who would otherwise not be ideal candidates for traditional treatment paradigms.

References

[1] Vlak MH, Algra A, Brandenburg R, Rinkel GJ. Prevalence of unruptured intracranial aneurysms, with emphasis on sex, age, comorbidity, country, and time period: a systematic review and meta-analysis. Lancet Neurol. 2011; 10 (7):626–636

[2] Feigin VL, Rinkel GJ, Lawes CM, et al. Risk factors for subarachnoid hemorrhage: an updated systematic review of epidemiological studies. Stroke. 2005; 36(12):2773–2780

[3] Wermer MJ, van der Schaaf IC, Algra A, Rinkel GJ. Risk of rupture of unruptured intracranial aneurysms in relation to patient and aneurysm characteristics: an updated meta-analysis. Stroke. 2007; 38(4):1404–1410

[4] Linn FH, Rinkel GJ, Algra A, van Gijn J. Incidence of subarachnoid hemorrhage: role of region, year, and rate of computed tomography: a meta-analysis. Stroke. 1996; 27(4):625–629

[5] Fogelholm R, Hernesniemi J, Vapalahti M. Impact of early surgery on outcome after aneurysmal subarachnoid hemorrhage. A population-based study. Stroke. 1993; 24(11):1649–1654

[6] Chen PR, Frerichs K, Spetzler R. Natural history and general management of unruptured intracranial aneurysms. Neurosurg Focus. 2004; 17(5):E1

[7] Lehecka M, Frosen J, Korja M, et al. Intracranial aneurysms. In: Kalani MYS, Nakaji P, Spetzler RF, eds. Neurovascular Surgery. 2nd ed. New York, NY: Thieme; 2015:457–467

[8] Pakarinen S. Incidence, aetiology, and prognosis of primary subarachnoid haemorrhage. A study based on 589 cases diagnosed in a defined urban population during a defined period. Acta Neurol Scand. 1967; 43 Suppl 29:29–, 1–28

[9] Asgari S, Wanke I, Schoch B, Stolke D. Recurrent hemorrhage after initially complete occlusion of intracranial aneurysms. Neurosurg Rev. 2003; 26 (4):269–274

[10] Lozier AP, Kim GH, Sciacca RR, Connolly ES, Jr, Solomon RA. Microsurgical treatment of basilar apex aneurysms: perioperative and long-term clinical outcome. Neurosurgery. 2004; 54(2):286–296, discussion 296–299

[11] Raaymakers TW, Rinkel GJ, Limburg M, Algra A. Mortality and morbidity of surgery for unruptured intracranial aneurysms: a meta-analysis. Stroke. 1998; 29(8):1531–1538

[12] Solomon RA, Fink ME, Pile-Spellman J. Surgical management of unruptured intracranial aneurysms. J Neurosurg. 1994; 80(3):440–446

[13] Takahashi T. The treatment of symptomatic unruptured aneurysms. Acta Neurochir Suppl (Wien). 2002; 82:17–19

[14] Guglielmi G, Viñuela F, Dion J, Duckwiler G. Electrothrombosis of saccular aneurysms via endovascular approach. Part 2: Preliminary clinical experience. J Neurosurg. 1991; 75(1):8–14

[15] Guglielmi G, Viñuela F, Sepetka I, Macellari V. Electrothrombosis of saccular aneurysms via endovascular approach. Part 1: Electrochemical basis, technique, and experimental results. J Neurosurg. 1991; 75(1):1–7

[16] Koivisto T, Vanninen R, Hurskainen H, Saari T, Hernesniemi J, Vapalahti M. Outcomes of early endovascular versus surgical treatment of ruptured cerebral aneurysms. A prospective randomized study. Stroke. 2000; 31 (10):2369–2377

[17] Vanninen R, Koivisto T, Saari T, Hernesniemi J, Vapalahti M. Ruptured intracranial aneurysms: acute endovascular treatment with electrolytically detachable coils–a prospective randomized study. Radiology. 1999; 211 (2):325–336

[18] Yagmurlu K, Safavi-Abbasi S, Belykh E, et al. Quantitative anatomical analysis and clinical experience with mini-pterional and mini-orbitozygomatic approaches for intracranial aneurysm surgery. J Neurosurg. 201 7; 127(3):646–659

[19] Sun H, Safavi-Abbasi S, Spetzler RF. Retractorless surgery for intracranial aneurysms. J Neurosurg Sci. 2016; 60(1):54–69

[20] Gardner PA, Vaz-Guimaraes F, Jankowitz B, et al. Endoscopic endonasal clipping of intracranial aneurysms: surgical technique and results. World Neurosurg. 2015; 84(5):1380–1393

20 Clipping of Cerebral Aneurysms: Microscope and Endoscope

Francisco Vaz-Guimaraes, Paul A. Gardner, Juan C. Fernandez-Miranda, Eric W. Wang, and Carl H. Snyderman

Summary

The endoscopic endonasal approach has been widely accepted for many skull base pathologies but has been used only very sparingly for treating cerebral aneurysms. Select, medially projecting paraclinoidal internal carotid aneurysms may be best suited for this approach but require an experienced team with significant experience with both open aneurysm clipping and endonasal surgery.

Keywords: endoscopic endonasal, aneurysm, clipping, paraclinoid carotid

20.1 Endoscopic and Microscopic Perspective

20.1.1 Illustrative Case

History and Physical

A 45-year-old female smoker, with a positive family history for intracranial aneurysm rupture, presented to the emergency department with a history of sudden-onset headache 1 day before admission. She had no comorbidities and also denied drug allergies. On neurological examination, she displayed signs of meningeal irritation and no focal neurological deficits. A computed tomography (CT) scan revealed a Fisher II spontaneous subarachnoid hemorrhage (SAH) (▸ Fig. 20.1a). A four-vessel cerebral angiogram revealed a 7-mm left paraclinoid aneurysm projecting superomedially (▸ Fig. 20.1b–d). The patient underwent microsurgical clipping via an endoscopic endonasal approach (EEA).

Intraoperative Management

Initially, a frontal external ventricular drain was placed following standard technique. Sequentially, the patient was placed supine with her head fixed in a three-pin radiolucent head holder, rotated approximately 25 degrees toward the right side and in slight extension. Image-guided CT angiography was registered and a right femoral sheath was placed and prepared for intraoperative angiography. The midface and abdomen were prepped and draped and antibiotic prophylaxis was administered with a third-generation cephalosporin.

An endoscopic endonasal transsellar-transcavernous-transplanum approach with continuous neurophysiologic monitoring (i.e., somatosensory evoked potentials) was performed. A right-sided, vascularized nasoseptal flap was harvested. Then, a wide sphenoidotomy and a posterior septectomy were performed to allow bimanual, binostril access to the sphenoid sinus. At this point, proximal vascular control was achieved by performing the transsellar-transcavernous portion of the operation. The bone over the sella turcica, distal portion of the left paraclival segment of the internal carotid artery (ICA), and parasellar (paraclinoid) segments of the ICA was removed. This maneuver exposed the most anterior aspect of the medial wall of the cavernous sinus. The sellar dural opening was carefully extended into the cavernous sinus, which was partially thrombosed following injection of flowable hemostatic agents. Thus, the intracavernous segment of the ICA was exposed and proximal vascular control achieved (▸ Fig. 20.2a).

Next, the transplanum portion of the operation was performed. Bone over the tuberculum sellae and planum sphenoidale was removed. Doppler was used for accurate localization of the aneurysm before the dura covering the sella and planum sphenoidale were opened. The aneurysm neck was dissected free from the ophthalmic and superior hypophyseal arteries after opening of the distal dural ring at the level of the diaphragm sellae (▸ Fig. 20.2b–e). One straight clip was applied across the neck of the aneurysm using a single-shaft clip applier introduced through the ipsilateral nostril (▸ Fig. 20.2f).

The Doppler demonstrated the presence of blood flow at the level of the aneurysmal dome (▸ Fig. 20.3a). Two additional

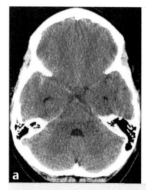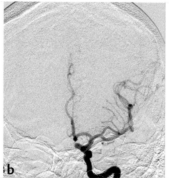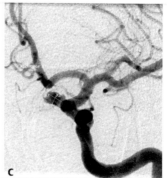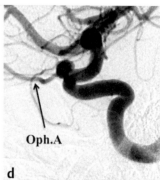

Fig. 20.1 Preoperative radiological studies. **(a)** CT scan without contrast revealing subarachnoid hemorrhage; **(b,c)** cerebral angiography, anteroposterior view, revealing a paraclinoidal aneurysm projecting superomedially; **(d)** cerebral angiography, lateral view, showing the aneurysm arising immediately distal to the ophthalmic artery (Oph.A).

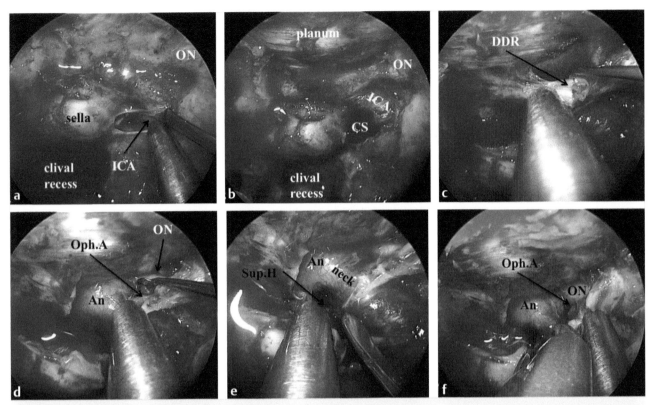

Fig. 20.2 Endoscopic endonasal aneurysm clipping. Intraoperative pictures with a 0-degree endoscope. **(a)** Proximal vascular control is gained via the medial cavernous sinus (ON: optic nerve). **(b)** Transnasal craniotomy. Bone from the planum sphenoidale all the way down to sella was removed (CS: cavernous sinus). **(c)** Opening of the dura of the planum and distal dural ring (DDR). **(d)** This maneuver gives access to the ophthalmic artery and the distal neck of the aneurysm (An), which has been dissected. Note the position of the optic nerve. **(e)** Dissection of the proximal neck of the aneurysm with clear visualization of the superior hypophyseal artery (Sup.H). **(f)** Placement of the first clip under endoscopic control. The clip is precisely placed across the neck of the aneurysm while preserving the ophthalmic and superior hypophyseal arteries.

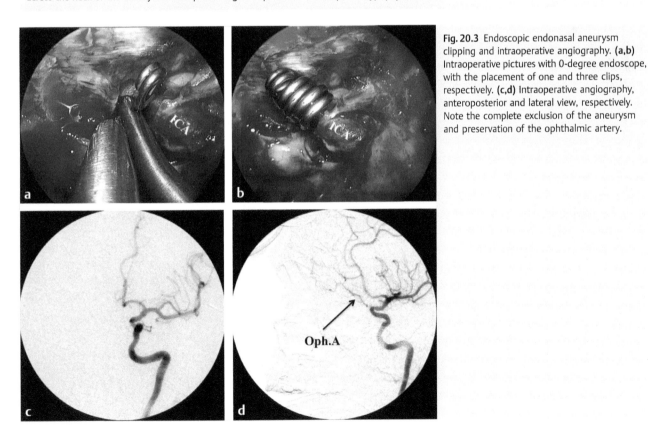

Fig. 20.3 Endoscopic endonasal aneurysm clipping and intraoperative angiography. **(a,b)** Intraoperative pictures with 0-degree endoscope, with the placement of one and three clips, respectively. **(c,d)** Intraoperative angiography, anteroposterior and lateral view, respectively. Note the complete exclusion of the aneurysm and preservation of the ophthalmic artery.

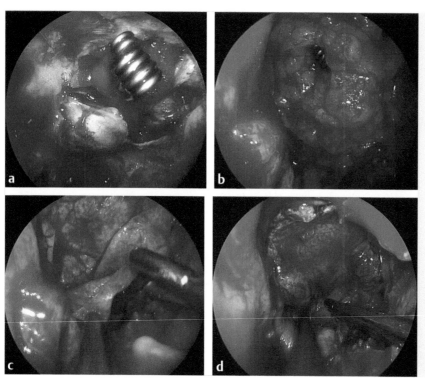

Fig. 20.4 (a–d) Endoscopic skull base reconstruction.

straight clips were placed with no change in the Doppler signal (▶ Fig. 20.3**b**). After dissecting the dome of the aneurysm, it was realized that the anterior cerebral arteries were in contact with the aneurysm wall and thereby sonating through it. At this point, an intraoperative angiography was done, which showed the complete exclusion of the aneurysm (▶ Fig. 20.3**c, d**).

Skull base reconstruction was done in a multilayer fashion using a combination of an inlay Duragen graft (▶ Fig. 20.4**a**), an autologous fat graft placed around the clips, which was then covered by a piece of collagen porcine intestinal biomatrix (▶ Fig. 20.4**b, c**). Finally, the vascularized nasoseptal flap was placed over the entire reconstruction (▶ Fig. 20.4**d**) and secured with Duraseal tissue glue and packing.

Surgical Outcome

The patient had an uneventful recovery and the postoperative course was uncomplicated. The ventricular drain was removed following usual SAH protocol (weaning during intensive care unit observation for vasospasm). The patient was discharged after vasospasm observation on postoperative day 11 with no complaints or neurological deficits. At 3-month follow-up after consultation, she remained neurologically intact.

20.1.2 Endoscopic Endonasal Approach for Paraclinoid Aneurysms

Advantages

Due to its anterior midline trajectory and wide, magnified view provided by the endoscope, the EEA provides a superior view of and corridor for paraclinoid aneurysms that project medially while obviating manipulation of the optic apparatus.[1,2] Clip placement across the neck of the aneurysm, variably through the ipsilateral (usually) or contralateral nostril, is simplified because its blades are perpendicular to the neck and generally precisely parallel to the paraclinoid ICA, which is the preferred clip positioning for aneurysms arising at curves in the outer wall of the parent vessel.[3] A simple straight clip may be sufficient for most aneurysms.

Given the superior control of the superior hypophyseal artery and perforator branches to the optic nerve and chiasm, the risk of inadvertent clip occlusion is greatly minimized, thus decreasing the likelihood of postoperative hypopituitarism and vision loss. Vision is further protected by the complete lack of optic nerve manipulation. Direct proximal vascular control of the cavernous ICA can be relatively easily obtained by performing a transcavernous approach without the necessity of removal of the anterior clinoid process or a separate incision for dissection of the cervical ICA.[1] Opening of the medial compartment of the cavernous sinus via EEAs is associated with a very low risk of new postoperative cranial neuropathies (i.e., oculomotor palsy)[4] as opposed to the opening of the roof of the cavernous sinus during microscopic approaches.[5] Additional advantages of the EEA for surgical clipping of paraclinoid aneurysms are the absence of brain retraction and, potentially, a more comfortable postoperative recovery with excellent cosmetic results.

Disadvantages

There is a long learning curve associated with endoscopic endonasal skull base surgery.[6] The lack of a skull base team with significant anatomic and clinical experience with these operations is a main contraindication for endonasal aneurysm clipping.

The two-dimensional visualization of the operative field provided by the endoscope may cause spatial disorientation in less experienced surgeons. Working through the relatively deep and narrow endonasal corridor may be an additional challenge because of hindrance of instruments. Furthermore, adequate visualization of the operative field may be very difficult in cases of intraoperative aneurysm rupture. In fact, the ability to manage a major vascular injury may be compromised due to limited surgical maneuverability and poor visualization.[7]

The lack of surgical instruments specifically designed for endonasal cerebrovascular surgery is also a disadvantage. Current clip appliers have limitations on angles of application or removal. If a clip slips into a different angle over the dome of the aneurysm, reengaging such a clip is technically challenging. The use of multiple clips may also greatly reduce working space. Moreover, clips often protrude into the sphenoid sinus and make skull base reconstruction more difficult, thus increasing the risks of postoperative cerebrospinal fluid (CSF) leakage and meningitis.[1]

Finally, distal vascular control may be difficult to establish in cases of large aneurysms and, therefore, a craniotomy may be necessary to provide such control.[1,2,8] Cerebral revascularization and vessel anastomosis cannot be performed via an endoscopic endonasal route and vascular repair options are limited. Finally, paraclinoid aneurysms projecting laterally under the anterior clinoid process are not amenable to endoscopic endonasal clipping.

20.1.3 Microscopic Approach for Paraclinoid Aneurysms

Advantages

The microscopic, craniotomic approach for clipping of paraclinoid aneurysms is safe, effective, and reliable, and is associated with relatively low morbidity and mortality rates. Surgical series have been reported by many medical centers worldwide, thus attesting its prominent role in the treatment of paraclinoid aneurysms.[9,10,11,12,13,14,15,16,17,18,19,20,21,22,23,24,25,26] The pterional approach and its variants are among the most versatile and widely used surgical approaches in neurosurgical practice. Therefore, most neurosurgeons have familiarity with this type of exposure, as opposed to the EEA to the skull base. The 3D microscopic visualization of the operative field provided by the surgical microscope also minimizes the risk of spatial disorientation within the operative field.

Surgical maneuverability is superior compared to the EEA and may be further enhanced by performing extensive dissection of the subarachnoid cisterns for CSF release and supplementing the pterional approach with orbital and zygomatic osteotomies.[27] Due to this larger exposure and increased working space, the aneurysm may be approached by a variety of different surgical angles and trajectories, which facilitates aneurysm mobilization and dissection as well as clip placement and removal. Furthermore, cases requiring cerebral revascularization or vascular anastomosis can be only performed via microscopic approaches.

In terms of paraclinoid aneurysms, all types of aneurysm, regardless of size (i.e., small vs. giant) and dome projection (i.e., superior, inferior, medial, or lateral), are amenable for surgical clipping via microscopic approaches.

Disadvantages

Proximal vascular control requires a separate cervical incision or exposure of the ICA along the floor of the middle fossa at the Glascock's triangle, which is technically challenging. Moreover, adequate exposure of the proximal neck of the aneurysm often requires removal of the anterior clinoid process (▶ Fig. 20.5). The anterior clinoidectomy may elicit cavernous sinus bleeding through its roof along the carotid-oculomotor membrane. Given its proximity with the oculomotor nerve, postoperative diplopia may occur.

Mobilization of the optic nerve may be necessary for adequate aneurysm exposure, especially for those projecting medially. This maneuver is associated with increased risk of postoperative vision loss. Inadvertent clip occlusion of the superior hypophyseal artery and perforator branches to the optic

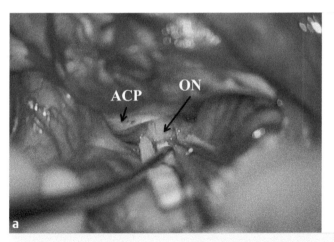
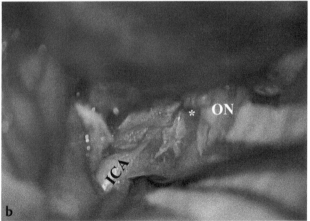

Fig. 20.5 (a,b) Left pterional approach for paraclinoid aneurysm projecting medially. Intraoperative microscopic view. Note that following removal of the anterior clinoid process (ACP), the paraclinoid segment of the ICA may be exposed and the distal neck of the aneurysm may easily be dissected. However, its proximal neck (*) is not fully visualized.

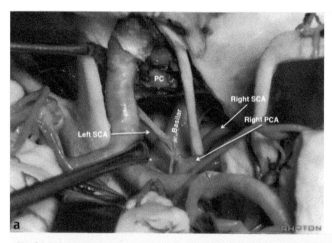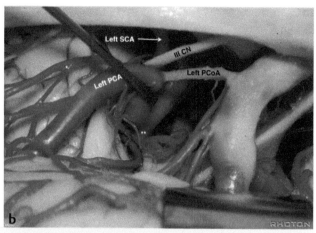

Fig. 20.6 Anterior transcavernous and subtemporal approaches (*The Rhoton Collection*). (a) Right anterior transcavernous approach. Proximal vascular control is achieved after removal of the posterior clinoid (PC) process. Note that the exposure of the left superior cerebellar artery (SCA) and left posterior cerebral artery (asterisk) is slightly limited. (b) Left subtemporal approach. Exposure of the ipsilateral posterior cerebral artery (PCA) and SCA is easily obtained, while exposure of the contralateral arteries is limited. In this specimen, only the origin of the PCA (double asterisk) is exposed (*The Rhoton Collection*).

chiasm is more likely to occur via microscopic approaches compared to EEAs due to poor visualization of these midline structures. Brain retraction and dissection, although can often be performed atraumatically, is an inherent disadvantage of microscopic approaches and may be more difficult in the setting of SAH. Due to the necessity of a more extensive tissue dissection, patients are more likely to complain of pain and discomfort during their postoperative recovery. Finally, microscopic approaches may be associated with poor cosmetic results in the case of palsy of the frontal branch of the facial nerve, atrophy of the temporalis muscle, and orbital asymmetry.[28]

20.1.4 Patient Selection: Our Experience

Clipping of intracranial aneurysms via EEAs is only indicated in a few, well-selected cases.[1,2] In our experience, other than medially projecting, paraclinoid aneurysms, two types of aneurysms may be considered for endoscopic endonasal clipping.

Low-Lying Basilar Apex Aneurysms

Proximal vascular control in low-lying basilar apex aneurysms may be problematic when approached transcranially. A transcavernous approach with removal of the posterior clinoid process, which is often associated with oculomotor nerve palsy, is required in order to achieve adequate exposure of the basilar trunk for vascular control (▶ Fig. 20.6a).[4] Moreover, distal control of the contralateral posterior cerebral and superior cerebellar arteries may be difficult if clipping is performed via a lateral subtemporal approach (▶ Fig. 20.6b).[29] Given the direct anterior midline trajectory of the endonasal route, wide access to the prepontine cistern and therefore adequate exposure of the basilar trunk and its major branches are readily achieved. If necessary, a posterior clinoidectomy may be performed endonasally to increase surgical maneuverability and access to the interpeduncular cistern.[30,31]

Proximal Posterior Circulation Aneurysms Situated Ventral to the Brainstem

Adequate microsurgical exposure of posterior circulation (i.e., vertebrobasilar) aneurysms situated ventral to the brainstem may be also troublesome. Although proximal vascular control may be easily obtained via a posterolateral approach (i.e., far-lateral approach), distal vascular control and exposure of the aneurysm neck may be very limited (▶ Fig. 20.7).[32] As previously mentioned, the endonasal route provides adequate proximal and distal vascular control and complete exposure of the aneurysm.

Regardless of the approach (endoscopic or microscopic), surgical clipping is often easier in small and unruptured aneurysms. Nevertheless, the presence of ruptured or large/giant aneurysm is not considered a contraindication for endoscopic endonasal clipping, although the risk of intraoperative rupture and unsuccessful clipping may be significantly higher. Therefore, careful preoperative analysis of clinical, anatomical, and radiological findings is of utmost importance before electing to proceed with endoscopic endonasal clipping of intracranial aneurysms.

20.1.5 Complication Avoidance

The avoidance of complication in aneurysm surgery begins with the development of a contingency plan. Intraoperative angiography and the ability to convert to a microscopic approach have to be available at all times. For some cases, this means even clipping and preparing for craniotomy. Moreover, the basic principles of cerebrovascular surgery (i.e., vascular control, sharp microdissection, aneurysm mobilization and dissection, minimal iatrogenic ischemia) must be strictly followed throughout the entire endoscopic procedure.[33]

Following careful patient selection, a surgical team with significant combined experience with endoscopic, skull base, and cerebrovascular surgery is needed to safely conduct the operation. Endoscopic endonasal cerebrovascular surgery is

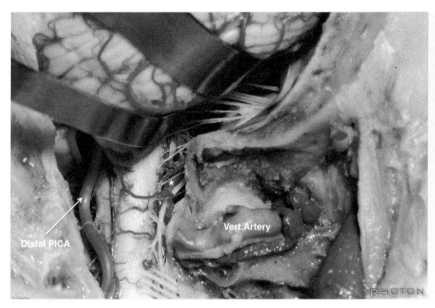

Fig. 20.7 Far-lateral approach (*The Rhoton Collection*). Right far-lateral approach. Note that control of the vertebral artery is more difficult distally (*) as the artery enters into the premedullary cistern just anterior to the ventral surface of the medulla (*The Rhoton Collection*).

considered a "level V" procedure,[34] which is among the most complex endoscopic endonasal operations and therefore more often associated with complications and adverse outcomes.

Proximal vascular control must be obtained as soon as possible, especially for ruptured aneurysms. This consists of exposing the cavernous segment of the ICA for paraclinoid aneurysms, and the vertebral arteries and basilar trunk for posterior circulation aneurysms. These require transcavernous and wide transclival approaches, respectively. Once vascular control is achieved and surgical approach completed, binostril bimanual dissection of the aneurysm, including its neck, perforator branches, and the parent vessel, must be performed following traditional microsurgical techniques. These include cutting and spreading with microscissors with blunt tips, and probing with a slightly curved or angled extended microdissector. Once such dissection is completed, clip blades are properly positioned and gently released across the aneurysm neck.

Proper incorporation of the clip into the skull base reconstruction is key to minimize the risk of postoperative CSF leakage, the most common complication. The recommended multilayer reconstruction must include complete clip coverage with an autologous fat graft. This interposed fat graft tends to nullify the risk of erosion of the vascularized flap by the clip, especially for those protruding into the sphenoid sinus. Moreover, the flap must be large enough to cover not only the dural opening but also the entire sphenoid, including planum sphenoidale and sella, and the entire clival recess for paraclinoid and posterior circulation aneurysms, respectively.[1] Temporary CSF diversion (i.e., lumbar drain) is often recommended for 3 days.

20.1.6 Technical Nuances

The technical tenets of endoscopic endonasal cerebrovascular surgery include adequate exposure, bimanual microsurgical dissection, and proper skull base reconstruction. It requires profound anatomical knowledge, significant training, and experience with endoscopic endonasal surgery and the development

of "team skills." These procedures are usually performed in close collaboration between neurosurgeons and otolaryngologists/head and neck surgeons working together simultaneously throughout the entire operation (i.e., exposure, dissection, clipping, reconstruction).

Nevertheless, working through the relatively deep and narrow endonasal surgical corridor may be problematic. Limited surgical maneuverability and poor visualization are the potential consequences of increased hindrance of instruments. To overcome this "sword fight," the use of both nares (binostril approach), wide exposure, and close and continued communication between the surgeons are imperative. Among different surgical techniques for endoscopic endonasal surgery, bimanual-binarial dissection with dynamic endoscopy, in which one surgeon is fully dedicated to a two-handed dissection using both nostrils, and the other surgeon is fully dedicated to endoscope guidance, provides the best option for replicating microsurgery. In a laboratory investigation, we have demonstrated that this technique has the potential to improve surgical performance while emphasizing endoscope guidance and microsurgical dissection.[34]

To improve access and working space, a posterior septectomy and right middle turbinectomy are routinely performed. This maneuver facilitates general endonasal exposure and bimanual-binarial dissection by minimizing visual obscuration of the endoscope by the intervening nasal septum and enlarges the nasal cavity, thus allowing more room for the endoscope.

Surgery starts with harvesting of a large vascularized nasoseptal flap.[35] The tendency is to create a flap based on the size of the dural defect required to clip the aneurysm, which is often small, especially for a paraclinoidal aneurysm. However, the need to first cover the clips with other auto- or allograft leaves the flap to cover the entire sinus and it should be made as large as possible to allow this. In cases of posterior circulation aneurysm, a medial maxillectomy may be also performed in order to displace the flap laterally into the maxilla and allow full endonasal exposure of the inferior clivus.

As with the sinus exposure, the bony exposure should be as wide as possible. Bone over critical structures is drilled or "eggshelled" with frequent irrigation. It is then carefully peeled away with dissectors or the footplate of a rongeur, rather than biting it away. This is especially important over the ICA or aneurysm. Bone should be removed well beyond (several millimeters) the structure of interest to ensure proper access. For instance, exposure of the dura covering Meckel's cave allows lateral displacement of the paraclival segment of the ICA, thus increasing working space and surgical maneuverability; exposure of the most anterior dura of the planum sphenoidale allows its retraction, which also increases working space to the suprasellar region; a posterior clinoidectomy increases surgical access to the interpeduncular cistern and the basilar bifurcation. This technique allows safe exposure of the cavernous sinus wall and skeletonization of the paraclival and paraclinoid segments of the ICA. Cavernous sinus and basilar plexus bleeding may be efficiently controlled with flowable hemostatic agents.[7]

Before dural opening, Doppler may be used to identify the exact location of the aneurysm and avoid inadvertent injury. For paraclinoid aneurysms, the distal dural ring must by bluntly and carefully opened in order to provide adequate exposure of the ophthalmic artery and distal neck of the aneurysm (▶ Fig. 20.2c). In cases of large aneurysms, limited exposure of the distal neck and impossibility of distal vascular control must be anticipated and a combined pterional approach planned if necessary. Aneurysm dissection must follow traditional microsurgical techniques. During this delicate dissection, the position of the endoscope is of great importance. Placing the endoscope in a fixed holder greatly limits the view, which is best achieved through slow, careful dynamic endoscopy, moving in concert with the dissection. Slow and gentle movements, coordinated with the dissection, are necessary to allow for a clear view of the aneurysm, parent vessel, perforator branches, and dissecting instruments. A 6-Fr Fukushima-style tapered teardrop suction (usually with a slight upward bend at the tip), hold by the nondominant hand of the neurosurgeon, enables blunt dissection while keeping the operative field clear from blood and CSF.

Once aneurysm dissection is completed, clip placement must be planned. The use of straight clips is recommended given the anterior midline trajectory of the endonasal approach and limited maneuverability. Curved clips may be useful for paraclinoid aneurysms whose neck displays an anteroposterior trajectory.[1] For basilar apex aneurysms, a bayonet clip may facilitate visualization by shifting the clip applier away from the line of sight. Temporary clipping and trapping under burst suppression may be necessary for large aneurysms.

The skull base reconstruction must be performed as previously described. Two details must be further emphasized: an autologous fat graft must be interposed between the clip and the nasoseptal flap to avoid flap erosion and perforation; and the flap should be large enough to cover the entire sphenoid.

20.1.7 Clinical Pearls

To minimize hindrance of instruments and increase working space, the endonasal corridor must be expanded as much as possible. In paraclinoid aneurysms, the parasellar bone removal can be extended all the way to the Meckel's cave and should include an optic canal decompression to the optic strut. For basilar apex aneurysms, removal of the dorsum sellae and posterior clinoids via an extra- or interdural pituitary transposition is key (intradural transposition must be avoided to minimize the risk of hypopituitarism). For vertebral artery aneurysms, a lateral inferior extension (i.e., endoscopic endonasal transclival "far-medial" approach) is necessary.[36,37] By doing these "expanded" approaches, the exposed dura and associated structures can be gently retracted to increase working space, thereby allowing a safer and more comfortable bimanual microdissection. Moreover, these expansions of exposure also allow for the use of 0-degree endoscopes for almost all cases. The straight view provided by these endoscopes facilitates microdissection by minimizing the risk of spatial disorientation, which may occur when working with angled endoscopes. Occasionally, an angled endoscope will allow extra room for instrumentation when working on the basilar apex or aneurysms with a paramedian projection.

Hindrance of instruments may be also minimized by dynamic endoscopy. In a laboratory investigation, we have demonstrated that microsurgical dissection is significantly improved when endoscope guidance/positioning is performed by a co-surgeon rather than using an endoscope holder. By continuously adjusting endoscope position, the co-surgeon may increase working space by moving the endoscope sideways while still keeping appropriate distance from the region of interest, optimizing field of view, and minimizing the risk of spatial disorientation by enhancing depth perception.[34]

For paraclinoid aneurysms, opening of the distal dural ring is necessary to allow unimpeded access to the ophthalmic artery and distal neck of the aneurysm. Removing the bone that covers the paraclinoid segment of the ICA also allows gentle lateralization of the vessel, increases working space, and facilitates distal vascular control. Dissection of the proximal neck of the aneurysm must be performed with extreme caution, especially for more proximal aneurysms closely related with the diaphragma sellae. This situation may increase the risk of inadvertent aneurysm neck injury.[1] Because the perforator branches are projecting medially, their preservation is facilitated.

Wide exposure of the suprasellar-infrachiasmatic region can be easily obtained endonasally. On the other hand, exposure of the suprachiasmatic region (i.e., chiasmatic cistern) and aneurysms of the anterior communicating artery (AComA) complex may be limited by frontal lobe sagging (▶ Fig. 20.8). Furthermore, the anterior cerebral artery may be located superior and lateral to the optic nerve, thus making proximal vascular control more difficult and increasing the risk of optic nerve injury. Although we do not have personal experience with endonasal clipping of AComA aneurysms, we believe that the indications for endonasal clipping are restricted to small midline aneurysms projecting superiorly, as described by Froelich et al[38] and Yildirim et al,[45] or inferiorly. Clipping of aneurysms projecting anteriorly and posteriorly may be challenging given the interposed aneurysm dome between the surgeons and the neck of the aneurysm, and

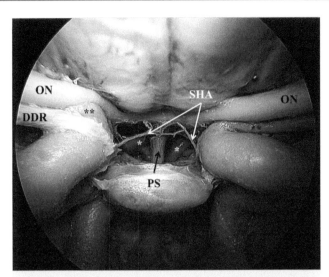

Fig. 20.8 Endoscopic endonasal exposure of the infrachiasmatic and suprachiasmatic regions. Note the basal surface of the frontal lobe limiting exposure of the suprachiasmatic region and AComA complex. On the other hand, a wide exposure of the infrachiasmatic region and its contents (PS, pituitary stalk; SHA, superior hypophyseal artery) is obtained endonasally. Note that removal of the distal dural ring (DDR) exposes the ophthalmic artery (**). *Posterior cerebral arteries within the interpeduncular cistern (further exposure may be obtained by performing an *inter*dural pituitary transposition).

limited control of perforator branches, respectively. Posterior displacement of the optic chiasm by tumors arising in the sella-suprasellar region may facilitate endonasal exposure of the AcomA complex.[45]

High-lying basilar apex aneurysms are not a good indication for endoscopic endonasal clipping. Exposure of the aneurysm within the interpeduncular cistern is restricted and distal vascular control is limited. The use of angled endoscopes may be required throughout the operation with its inherent disadvantages. A more direct visualization may be obtained by performing a full *intra*dural pituitary transposition, but at the expense of an increased likelihood of postoperative hypopituitarism (▶ Fig. 20.8). On the other hand, EEA for clipping of low-lying basilar apex is a valid option compared with traditional microscopic approaches given the advantages previously described in the section "Patient Selection: Our Experience."

20.1.8 Literature Review/Evidence in Favor of Endoscopic Approach

EEAs for aneurysm clipping are very rarely reported. To date, only 24 aneurysms in 22 patients reported in 10 manuscripts have been treated by these means.[1,8,38,39,40,41,42,43,44,45] These include 12 paraclinoid, 3 basilar apex, 3 AComA, 2 basilar trunk, 2 posterior cerebral artery (PCA), 1 posterior inferior cerebellar artery (PICA), and 1 vertebral artery aneurysm. Two patients presented with two aneurysms. Eleven patients

had their aneurysms incidentally discovered, while seven presented with spontaneous SAH and four with focal neurological deficits. Twenty-two aneurysms were successfully clipped, while two required further treatment (repeated surgery for clipping and endovascular coiling for residual neck). Postoperative CSF leak was the most common postoperative complication (5 patients, 22.7%), followed by meningitis (3 patients) and lacunar stroke (2 patients with basilar apex and 1 patient with PCA aneurysms). A major stroke was reported in one patient with a basilar apex aneurysm. Proximal and distal vascular control could be obtained in all cases. A giant paraclinoid aneurysm required a combined pterional approach for distal vascular control.

Among the 15 anterior circulation aneurysms (13 patients), all of them were successfully clipped endonasally. Two patients experienced postoperative CSF leak (15.4%), and a new endoscopic approach was necessary for repair. There were no cases of new postoperative vision loss, hypopituitarism, or ICA occlusion (i.e., stroke). On the other hand, of the nine posterior circulation aneurysms (nine patients), three developed postoperative CSF leak (33.3%), two required additional treatment for residual neck (22.2%), and four patients suffered a postoperative stroke (44.4%) due to injury of perforating branches. ▶ Table 20.1 summarizes these surgical reports/series.

Comparatively, patients with posterior circulation aneurysms have a significant increased risk of neurological disability due to injury of perforator branches ($p = 0.0172$, Fisher's exact test) compared to patients with anterior circulation aneurysms. The risk of postoperative CSF leak ($p = 0.609$, Fisher's exact test) and incomplete treatment requiring additional endovascular treatment ($p = 0.375$, Fisher's exact test) was similar between both groups. Posterior circulation aneurysms were larger than anterior circulation aneurysms (median: 9 ± 5.07 mm vs. 5.5 ± 5.87 mm, respectively) although this difference was not statistically significant ($p = 0.7381$, 95% confidence interval, -5.95 to 4.29).

These findings suggest that paraclinoid aneurysms projecting medially are the most suitable cases for endoscopic endonasal clipping. Posterior circulation aneurysms, especially basilar apex and PCA aneurysms whose neck is located above the level of the dorsum sellae and posterior clinoids, are often associated with postoperative neurological complications (i.e., perforator injuries) and the decision to operate them through an endonasal route must be critically analyzed. On the other hand, basilar trunk, proximal anterior inferior cerebellar artery (AICA), vertebrobasilar junction, and vertebral artery aneurysms are also potentially better options for endoscopic clipping because the endonasal route inherently provides a superior surgical exposure of midline structures compared to microscopic approaches. Additionally, the microscopic exposure of these aneurysms and surrounding structures, which is often poor, usually requires extensive tissue dissection and larger craniotomies (e.g., combined transpetrosal–middle fossa approach) and is associated with a higher risk of inadvertent cranial nerve injuries.

Table 20.1 Endoscopic endonasal clipping of intracranial aneurysms

Author	Patient	Clinical picture	Local/size (mm)	Growth direction	Previous treatment	Neurologic Complication	Outcome
Kassam et al 2006	51,F	Focal deficits	Verteb/11	Ventral BS surf.	Endovasc	None	Complete recovery
Kassam et al 2007	56,F	Incidental finding	Sup Hyp/5	Medial	None	None	Complete recovery
Kitano and Taneda 2007	58,F	Incidental finding	ACom/n.a	n.a.	None	None	Complete recovery
Enseñat et al 2011	74,F	SAH	PICA/ 1.2	Ventral BS surf.	None	CSF leak	Complete recovery
Froelich et al 2011	55,M	Incidental finding	ACom/7	Superior	None	None	Complete recovery
Germanwala and Zanation 2011	42,F	SAH	Ophth/ 5 Paracl/10	S.medial P.medial	None	None	Complete recovery
Drazin et al 2012	59,F	SAH	Bas. Tr/ 4	VentralBS surf.	Endovasc	None	Repeat surgery for reclipping
Somanna et al 2015	42,F	SAH	Bas. Ap/10	Posterosuperior	None	None	Endovascular coiling for residual neck
	70,F	SAH	Bas. Ap/5	Superior	None	Lacunar stroke	Neurological disability
	35,M	Focal deficits	PCA/9.4	Superior	None	Stroke CSF leak Meningitis	Neurological disability
	50,M	SAH	Bas. Tr/9	Ventral BS surf.	None	None	Complete recovery
Gardner et al 2015	42,F	Incidental findings	Ophth/3.5	I.medial	None	None	Complete recovery
	74,M	CN palsy	PCA/19	Ventral BS surf.	None	CSF leak Meningitis Lacunar stroke	Mild disability
	43,F	Incidental finding	Sup Hyp/5	Medial	None	CSF leak	Complete recovery
	47,F	Incidental finding	Bas.Ap/9	Posterosuperior	None	Lacunar stroke	Complete recovery
	45,M	Vision loss Hypopituitarism	Ophth/giant Ophth/5	Superomedial	None	None	Complete recovery
	73,F	Incidental finding	Ophth/6	Medial	None	CSF leak Meningitis	Complete recovery
	45,F	SAH	Ophth/7	Superomedial	None	None	Complete recovery
	34,F	Incidental finding	Ophth/4	Medial	None	None	Complete recovery
	55,F	Incidental finding	Sup.Hyp/11	Medial	None	None	Complete recovery
	42,F	Incidental finding	Sup.Hyp	Inferomedial	None	None	Complete recovery
Yildirim et al 2015	72,F	Incidental finding	ACom	Anterosuperior	None	None	Complete recovery

Abbreviations: Bas. Ap, basilar apex; Bas. Tr, basilar trunk; BS, brainstem; CN, cranial nerve; Endovasc, endovascular; F, female; I.medial, inferomedial; M, male; n.a., not available; Ophth, ophthalmic artery; Paracl, paraclinoid segment; P.medial, posteromedial; S.medial, superomedial; Sup Hyp, superior hypophyseal artery; Verteb, vertebral artery.

20.1.9 Literature Review/Evidence in Favor of Microscopic Approach

Microscopic approaches for aneurysm clipping remain as a safe and effective treatment option despite continued advancement of endovascular techniques. Several large recent surgical series, including more than 4,000 patients, have reported successful clipping of paraclinoid and posterior circulation aneurysms[10,11, 12,13,14,15,16,17,18,19,20,21,22,23,24,25,26,46,47,48,49,50,51,52,53,54,55,56,57,58,59,60, 61,62,63,64] (▶ Table 20.2 and ▶ Table 20.3). Moreover, if direct aneurysm clipping is precluded for anatomic reasons, aneurysm wrapping and/or vascular bypass followed by parent vessel occlusion may be safely performed.

Paraclinoid aneurysms tend to harbor wide necks and often emanate from the parent vessel in close relationship with the superior hypophyseal and ophthalmic arteries. Furthermore, these aneurysms may project superiorly toward the optic nerves (ophthalmic aneurysms), inferiorly toward the roof of the cavernous sinus (ventral aneurysms), medially toward the diaphragma sellae (superior hypophyseal and carotid cave aneurysms), and laterally (subclinoid aneurysms) underneath the anterior clinoid process. All types of aneurysms, including those giant aneurysms projecting in multiple directions, are amenable for successful clipping through microscopic approaches. Drilling of the anterior clinoid process, unroofing of the optic canal, and opening of the falciform ligament and distal dural ring allows significant mobilization of the ICA or optic nerve, thus facilitating aneurysm neck dissection and clipping. For medially projecting aneurysm, a contralateral approach may be considered. Laterally projecting aneurysms are usually the most difficult to properly clip and superiorly projecting ones are the most commonly associated with intraoperative rupture.

Table 20.2 Microsurgical series of patients with paraclinoid aneurysms

Series	No. of patients	Total occlusion	Mortality
Hoh et al 2001	179	94.1%	2.8%
Barami et al 2003	61	n.a.	1.6%
Iihara et al 2003	35	73.5%	n.a.
Silveira et al 2004	51	90.2%	0%
Khan et al 2005	75	96.1%	0%
Liu et al 2008	38	92.1%	5.3%
Raco et al 2008	104	93.2%	0%
Xu et al 2008	36	90.9%	5.6%
Fulkerson et al 2009	126	79.4%	0.8%
Eliava et al 2010	83	90.4%	3.6%
Sharma et al 2010	78	n.a.	0%
Son et al 2010	24	n.a.	0%
Xu et al 2010	51	90.9%	3.9%
Nanda and Javalkar 2011	80	92.6%	8.7%
Colli et al 2013	95	96.1%	7.4%
Lai and Morgan 2013	169	95.1%	0.6%
Matano et al 2016	127	93.7%	0%

Table 20.3 Microsurgical series of patients with posterior circulation aneurysms

Series	No. of patients	Total occlusion	Mortality
Sundt 1990	157	n.a.	13.4%
Peerless et al 1996	1,476	n.a.	5.7%
Morcos and Heros 1997	145	n.a.	3.4%
Samson et al 1999	302	95%	8.9%
Kitazawa et al 2001	11	100%	0%
Seifert et al 2001	24	100%	8.3%
D'Ambrosio et al 2004	20	100%	0%
Gonzalez et al 2004	32	90.6%	6.3%
Honda et al 2004	10	100%	0%
Lozier et al 2004	98	92%	6.1%
Al-khayat et al 2005	52	100%	1.9%
Krisht et al 2007	50	100%	2%
Sanai et al 2008	217	95.4%	7.2%
Lai and Morgan 2012	256	n.a.	9.2%
Singh et al 2012	20	100%	15%
Shi et al 2013	41	100%	2.4%
McLaughlin and Martin 2014	18	100%	0%
Nanda et al 2014	62	91.9%	
Lehto et al 2015	190	n.a.	n.a.
Nair et al 2015	13	100%	7.7%

Posterior circulation aneurysms are among the most difficult ones to treat surgically given their rarity, intricate relationship with critical neurovascular structures, and relative deep and narrow operative field. Nonetheless, the role of microscopic approaches for clipping of posterior circulation aneurysms is well established. Among major surgical series, microscopic approaches play a major role for the successful treatment of basilar apex, proximal PCA (i.e., P1 segment), superior cerebellar artery, distal AICA, and PICA aneurysms. The wide surgical access and increased maneuverability provided by modern cranial base microscopic approaches enable the neurosurgeon to safely tackle the aneurysm while preserving perforating branches under clear visualization and proper vascular control.

The rates of complete aneurysm occlusion and surgery-related mortality of paraclinoid aneurysms varied from 73.5 to 96.1% (mean, 90.6%; median, 92.1%) and from 0 to 8.7% (mean, 2.5%; median, 1.6%), respectively, according to major recent microsurgical series encompassing more than 1,400 patients (▶ Table 20.2). Among posterior circulation aneurysms, including more than 2,700 aneurysms from different sites along the vertebrobasilar system, rates of complete aneurysm occlusion and mortality varied from 90.6 to 100% (mean, 97.5%; median, 100%) and from 0 to 13.4% (mean, 4.7%; median, 4.5%) (▶ Table 20.3).

It is also important to mention that the surgical endoscope may be used during microscopic approaches to enhance visualization of the operative field. The endoscope is mainly used before and after clip placement to check for completeness of aneurysm clipping and preservation of perforating branches, especially for large and anatomically complex lesions. Eventually, aneurysm dissection and clipping may be performed solely under endoscopic visualization.[65]

Compared with endovascular treatment, microsurgical clipping of intracranial aneurysms still remains as a competitive option for several reasons. Patients presenting with compressive symptom are generally more likely to benefit from surgical clipping rather than coiling due to immediate cessation of mass effect following clipping. Moreover, although the use of advanced endovascular techniques, such as balloon remodeling, stent assistance, and, more recently, flow diversion (i.e., pipeline embolization devices), has increased total occlusion rates, rates of immediate aneurysm occlusion, residual aneurysm, recanalization/recurrence, and retreatment compare largely unfavorably to microsurgical series. The use of antiplatelet agents to decrease the risk of thromboembolic complications and symptomatic ischemia following the use of stents and flow diversion devices is associated with an increased risk of symptomatic intracranial hemorrhage. Finally, the procedural and long-term risks of these modern techniques remain high or unknown and longer International Subarachnoid Aneurysm Trial (ISAT) follow-up has shown potential loss of benefit of coiling compared to clipping.

20.1.10 Conclusion

Careful case selection is of paramount importance in choosing an EEA for aneurysm clipping. The principles of cerebrovascular surgery must be maintained and surgical exposure must be wide enough to allow for bimanual dissection with proximal and distal vascular control obtained as soon as possible. Overall, paraclinoid aneurysms projecting medially, low-lying basilar apex aneurysms (below the level of the posterior clinoids), and vertebrobasilar aneurysms whose neck lies ventral to the brainstem are the most suitable for this type of approach. Given the very limited number of patients treated this way, there is no definitive evidence in the medical literature to recommend this kind of surgical treatment. Endoscopic endonasal aneurysm clipping must be performed only by experienced surgical teams in very rare, well-selected cases. Despite its limited role, this treatment modality must be considered part of the armamentarium of the cerebrovascular neurosurgeons in dealing with these challenging aneurysms.

References

[1] Gardner PA, Vaz-Guimaraes F, Jankowitz B, et al. Endoscopic endonasal clipping of intracranial aneurysms: Surgical technique and results. World Neurosurg. 2015; 84(5):1380–1393

[2] Vaz-Guimaraes F, Gardner PA, Fernandez-Miranda JC, Wang E, Snyderman CH. Endoscopic endonasal skull base surgery for vascular lesions: a systematic review of the literature. J Neurosurg Sci. 2016; 60(4):503–513

[3] Rhoton AL Jr. Aneurysms. Neurosurgery. 2002; 51:S121–S158

[4] Koutourousiou M, Vaz Guimaraes Filho F, Fernandez-Miranda JC, Wang EW, Snyderman CH, Gardner PA. Endoscopic endonasal surgery for tumors of the cavernous sinus: Experience of 234 cases. J Am Coll Surg. 2014; 219(3) Suppl:S68

[5] Seoane E, Tedeschi H, de Oliveira E, Wen HT, Rhoton AL, Jr. The pretemporal transcavernous approach to the interpeduncular and prepontine cisterns: microsurgical anatomy and technique application. Neurosurgery. 2000; 46(4):891–898, discussion 898–899

[6] Snyderman C, Kassam A, Carrau R, Mintz A, Gardner P, Prevedello DM. Acquisition of surgical skills for endonasal skull base surgery: a training program. Laryngoscope. 2007; 117(4):699–705

[7] Vaz-Guimaraes F, Su SY, Fernandez-Miranda JC, Wang EW, Snyderman CH, Gardner PA. Hemostasis in endoscopic endonasal skull base surgery. J Neurol Surg B Skull Base. 2015; 76(4):296–302

[8] Kassam AB, Gardner PA, Mintz A, Snyderman CH, Carrau RL, Horowitz M. Endoscopic endonasal clipping of an unsecured superior hypophyseal artery aneurysm. Technical note. J Neurosurg. 2007; 107(5):1047–1052

[9] Gardner PA, Tormenti MJ, Pant H, Fernandez-Miranda JC, Snyderman CH, Horowitz MB. Carotid artery injury during endoscopic endonasal skull base surgery: incidence and outcomes. Neurosurgery. 2013; 73(2) Suppl Operative:ons261–ons269, discussion ons269–ons270

[10] Hoh BL, Carter BS, Budzik RF, Putman CM, Ogilvy CS. Results after surgical and endovascular treatment of paraclinoid aneurysms by a combined neurovascular team. Neurosurgery. 2001; 48(1):78–89, discussion 89–90

[11] Barami K, Hernandez VS, Diaz FG, Guthikonda M. Paraclinoid carotid aneurysms: surgical management, complications, and outcome based on a new classification scheme. Skull Base. 2003; 13(1):31–41

[12] Iihara K, Murao K, Sakai N, et al. Unruptured paraclinoid aneurysms: a management strategy. J Neurosurg. 2003; 99(2):241–247

[13] Silveira RL, Gusmão S, Pinheiro N, Andrade GC. Aneurisma paraclinóideo: técnica cirúrgica e resultados em 51 pacientes. Arq Neuropsiquiatr. 2004; 62 2A:322–329

[14] Khan N, Yoshimura S, Roth P, et al. Conventional microsurgical treatment of paraclinoid aneurysms: state of the art with the use of the selective extradural anterior clinoidectomy SEAC. Acta Neurochir Suppl (Wien). 2005; 94 Suppl 94:23–29

[15] Liu Y, You C, He M, Cai BW. Microneurosurgical management of the clinoid and paraclinoid aneurysms. Neurol Res. 2008; 30(6):552–556

[16] Raco A, Frati A, Santoro A, et al. Long-term surgical results with aneurysms involving the ophthalmic segment of the carotid artery. J Neurosurg. 2008; 108(6):1200–1210

[17] Xu BN, Sun ZH, Jiang JL, et al. Surgical management of large and giant intracavernous and paraclinoid aneurysms. Chin Med J (Engl). 2008; 121(12):1061–1064

[18] Fulkerson DH, Horner TG, Payner TD, et al. Endovascular retrograde suction decompression as an adjunct to surgical treat- ment of ophthalmic aneurysms: analysis of risks and clinical out- comes. Neurosurgery. 2009; 64(3) Suppl:107–111

[19] Eliava SS, Filatov YM, Yakovlev SB, et al. Results of microsurgical treatment of large and giant ICA aneurysms using the retrograde suction decompression (RSD) technique: series of 92 patients. World Neurosurg. 2010; 73(6): 683–687

[20] Sharma BS, Kasliwal MK, Suri A, Sarat Chandra P, Gupta A, Mehta VS. Outcome following surgery for ophthalmic segment aneurysms. J Clin Neurosci. 2010; 17(1):38–42

[21] Son HE, Park MS, Kim SM, Jung SS, Park KS, Chung SY. The avoidance of microsurgical complications in the extradural anterior clinoidectomy to paraclinoid aneurysms. J Korean Neurosurg Soc. 2010; 48(3):199–206

[22] Xu BN, Sun ZH, Romani R, et al. Microsurgical management of large and giant paraclinoid aneurysms. World Neurosurg. 2010; 73(3):137–146, discussion e17, e19

[23] Nanda A, Javalkar V. Microneurosurgical management of ophthalmic segment of the internal carotid artery aneurysms: single-surgeon operative experience from Louisiana State University, Shreveport. Neurosurgery. 2011; 68(2):355–370, discussion 370–371

[24] Colli BO, Carlotti CG, Jr, Assirati JA, Jr, Abud DG, Amato MCM, Dezena RA. Results of microsurgical treatment of paraclinoid carotid aneurysms. Neurosurg Rev. 2013; 36(1):99–114, discussion 114–115

[25] Lai LT, Morgan MK. Outcomes for unruptured ophthalmic segment aneurysm surgery. J Clin Neurosci. 2013; 20(8):1127–1133

[26] Matano F, Tanikawa R, Kamiyama H, et al. Surgical treatment of 127 paraclinoid aneurysms with multifarious strategy: Factors related with outcome. World Neurosurg. 2016; 85:169–176

[27] Zabramski JM, Kiriş T, Sankhla SK, Cabiol J, Spetzler RF. Orbitozygomatic craniotomy. Technical note. J Neurosurg. 1998; 89(2):336–341

[28] Youssef AS, Willard L, Downes A, et al. The frontotemporal-orbitozygomatic approach: reconstructive technique and outcome. Acta Neurochir (Wien). 2012; 154(7):1275–1283

[29] Kopitnik TA, Batjer HH, Samson DS. Combined transsylvian-subtemporal exposure of cerebral aneurysms involving the basilar apex. Microsurgery. 1994; 15(8):534–540

[30] Fernandez-Miranda JC, Gardner PA, Rastelli MM, Jr, et al. Endoscopic endonasal transcavernous posterior clinoidectomy with interdural pituitary transposition. J Neurosurg. 2014; 121(1):91–99

[31] Kassam AB, Prevedello DM, Thomas A, et al. Endoscopic endonasal pituitary transposition for a transdorsum sellae approach to the interpeduncular cistern. Neurosurgery. 2008; 62(3) Suppl 1:57–72, discussion 72–74

[32] Sanai N, Tarapore P, Lee AC, Lawton MT. The current role of microsurgery for posterior circulation aneurysms: a selective approach in the endovascular era. Neurosurgery. 2008; 62(6):1236–1249, discussion 1249–1253

[33] Lawton MT. Seven Aneurysms. Tenets and Techniques for Clipping. New York, NY: Thieme; 2011

[34] Vaz-Guimaraes F, Rastelli MM, Jr, Fernandez-Miranda JC, Wang EW, Gardner PA, Snyderman CH. Impact of dynamic endoscopy and bimanual-binarial dissection in endoscopic endonasal surgery training: A laboratory investigation. J Neurol Surg B Skull Base. 2015; 76(5) B5:365–371

[35] Hadad G, Bassagasteguy L, Carrau RL, et al. A novel reconstructive technique after endoscopic expanded endonasal approaches: vascular pedicle nasoseptal flap. Laryngoscope. 2006; 116(10):1882–1886

[36] Morera VA, Fernandez-Miranda JC, Prevedello DM, et al. "Far-medial" expanded endonasal approach to the inferior third of the clivus: the transcondylar and transjugular tubercle approaches. Neurosurgery. 2010; 66(6) Suppl Operative:211–219, discussion 219–220

[37] Vaz-Guimaraes Filho F, Wang EW, Snyderman CH, Gardner PA, Fernandez-Miranda JC. Endoscopic endonasal "far-medial" transclival approach: Surgical anatomy and technique. Op Tech in Otolaryngol.. 2013; 24:222–228

[38] Froelich S, Cebula H, Debry C, Boyer P. Anterior communicating artery aneurysm clipped via an endoscopic endonasal approach: technical note. Neurosurgery. 2011; 68(2) Suppl Operative:310–316, discussion 315–316

[39] Kassam AB, Mintz AH, Gardner PA, Horowitz MB, Carrau RL, Snyderman CH. The expanded endonasal approach for an endoscopic transnasal clipping and aneurysmorrhaphy of a large vertebral artery aneurysm: technical case report. Neurosurgery. 2006; 59(1) Suppl 1:E162–E165, discussion E162–E165

[40] Kitano M, Taneda M. Extended transsphenoidal approach to anterior communicating artery aneurysm: aneurysm incidentally identified during macroadenoma resection: technical case report. Neurosurgery. 2007; 61(5) Suppl 2: E299–E300, discussion E300

[41] Enseñat J, Alobid I, de Notaris M, et al. Endoscopic endonasal clipping of a ruptured vertebral-posterior inferior cerebellar artery aneurysm: technical case report. Neurosurgery. 2011; 69(1) Suppl Operative:E121–E127, discussion E127–E128

[42] Germanwala AV, Zanation AM. Endoscopic endonasal approach for clipping of ruptured and unruptured paraclinoid cerebral aneurysms: case report. Neurosurgery. 2011; 68(1) Suppl Operative:234–239, discussion 240

[43] Drazin D, Zhuang L, Schievink WI, Mamelak AN. Expanded endonasal approach for the clipping of a ruptured basilar aneurysm and feeding artery to a cerebellar arteriovenous malformation. J Clin Neurosci. 2012; 19(1): 144–148

[44] Somanna S, Babu RA, Srinivas D, Narasinga Rao KV, Vazhayil V. Extended endoscopic endonasal transclival clipping of posterior circulation aneurysms-an alternative to the transcranial approach. Acta Neurochir (Wien). 2015; 157 (12):2077–2085

[45] Yildirim AE, Divanlioglu D, Karaoglu D, Cetinalp NE, Belen AD. Purely endoscopic endonasal clipping of an incidental anterior communicating artery aneurysm. J Craniofac Surg. 2015; 26(4):1378–1381

[46] Sundt TJ. Results of surgical management. In: Brown C, ed. Surgical Techniques for Saccular and Giant Intracranial Aneurysms. Baltimore, MD: Williams & Wilkins; 1990:19–23

[47] Peerless S, Hernesniemi JA, Drake C. Posterior circulation aneurysms. In: Wilkins R, Rengachary SS, eds. Neurosurgery. New York, NY: McGraw-Hill; 1996:2341–2356

[48] Morcos J, Heros RC. Distal basilar artery aneurysm: Surgical techniques. In: Batjer HH, Caplan L, Friberg L, Greenlee RJ, Kopitnik TJ, Young W, eds. Cerebrovascular Disease. Philadelphia, PA: Lippincott-Raven; 1997:1055–1077

[49] Samson D, Batjer HH, Kopitnik TA, Jr. Current results of the surgical management of aneurysms of the basilar apex. Neurosurgery. 1999; 44(4):697–702, discussion 702–704

[50] Kitazawa K, Tanaka Y, Muraoka S, et al. Specific characteristics and management strategies of cerebral artery aneurysms: report of eleven cases. J Clin Neurosci. 2001; 8(1):23–26

[51] Seifert V, Raabe A, Stolke D. Management-related morbidity and mortality in unselected aneurysms of the basilar trunk and vertebrobasilar junction. Acta Neurochir (Wien). 2001; 143(4):343–348, discussion 348–349

[52] D'Ambrosio AL, Kreiter KT, Bush CA, et al. Far lateral suboccipital approach for the treatment of proximal posteroinferior cerebellar artery aneurysms: surgical results and long-term outcome. Neurosurgery. 2004; 55(1):39–50, discussion 50–54

[53] Gonzalez LF, Alexander MJ, McDougall CG, Spetzler RF. Anteroinferior cerebellar artery aneurysms: surgical approaches and outcomes–a review of 34 cases. Neurosurgery. 2004; 55(5):1025–1035

[54] Honda M, Tsutsumi K, Yokoyama H, Yonekura M, Nagata I. Aneurysms of the posterior cerebral artery: retrospective review of surgical treatment. Neurol Med Chir (Tokyo). 2004; 44(4):164–168, discussion 169

[55] Lozier AP, Kim GH, Sciacca RR, Connolly ES, Jr, Solomon RA. Microsurgical treatment of basilar apex aneurysms: perioperative and long-term clinical outcome. Neurosurgery. 2004; 54(2):286–296, discussion 296–299

[56] Al-khayat H, Al-Khayat H, Beshay J, Manner D, White J. Vertebral artery-posteroinferior cerebellar artery aneurysms: clinical and lower cranial nerve outcomes in 52 patients. Neurosurgery. 2005; 56(1):2–10, discussion 11

[57] Krisht AF, Krayenbühl N, Sercl D, Bikmaz K, Kadri PA. Results of microsurgical clipping of 50 high complexity basilar apex aneurysms. Neurosurgery. 2007; 60(2):242–250, discussion 250–252

[58] Lai L, Morgan MK. Surgical management of posterior circulation aneurysms: Defining the role of microsurgery in contemporary endovascular era. In: Signorelli F, ed. Explicative Cases of Controversial Issues in Neurosurgery. Shanghai: InTech, 2012:235–256

[59] Singh RK, Behari S, Kumar V, Jaiswal AK, Jain VK. Posterior inferior cerebellar artery aneurysms: Anatomical variations and surgical strategies. Asian J Neurosurg. 2012; 7(1):2–11

[60] Shi X, Qian H, Singh KCKI, et al. Surgical management of vertebral and basilar artery aneurysms: a single center experience in 41 patients. Acta Neurochir (Wien). 2013; 155(6):1087–1093

[61] McLaughlin N, Martin NA. Extended subtemporal transtentorial approach to the anterior incisural space and upper clival region: experience with posterior circulation aneurysms. Neurosurgery. 2014; 10 Suppl 1:15–23, discussion 23–24

[62] Nanda A, Sonig A, Banerjee AD, Javalkar VK. Microsurgical management of basilar artery apex aneurysms: a single surgeon's experience from Louisiana State University, Shreveport. World Neurosurg. 2014; 82(1–2):118–129

[63] Lehto H, Niemelä M, Kivisaari R, et al. Intracranial vertebral artery aneurysms: Clinical features and outcomes of 190 patients. World Neurosurg. 2015; 84(2):380–389

[64] Nair P, Panikar D, Nair AP, Sundar S, Ayiramuthu P, Thomas A. Microsurgical management of aneurysms of the superior cerebellar artery - lessons learnt: An experience of 14 consecutive cases and review of the literature. Asian J Neurosurg. 2015; 10(1):47

[65] Fischer G, Oertel J, Perneczky A. Endoscopy in aneurysm surgery. Neurosurgery. 2012; 70(2) Suppl Operative:184–190, discussion 190–191

21 Evacuation of Intraparenchymal Hemorrhage: Moderator

Daniel R. Felbaum, Kevin M. McGrail, and Vikram V. Nayar

Summary

This chapter explores open versus minimally invasive approaches to treating spontaneous intracerebral hemorrhage (ICH). We focus on the juxtaposition between open surgical hematoma evacuation and endoscopically controlled resection. The socioeconomic and health care burden of ICH is unassailable. While interventions for ischemic strokes have grown exponentially and cemented their position in stroke management, the treatment of hemorrhagic stroke remains controversial. Two questions dominate the debate about whether and how to intervene surgically: (1) Does removal of the blood improve patient outcomes? (2) Does a less invasive approach reduce negative effects caused by a more invasive approach? The use of less invasive approaches has obscured the answer to the first question in trials performed to date. Herein, we describe how surgical intervention for spontaneous ICH can reduce mass effect and secondary injury to surrounding neurovascular structures and how the use of the endoscope can significantly minimize the surgical footprint in hematoma evacuation without increasing morbidity.

Keywords: intraparenchymal hemorrhage, endoscopic, microsurgical, evacuation, hematoma

21.1 Moderator

21.1.1 Introduction

Spontaneous intracerebral hemorrhage (ICH) continues to be a disease with devastating consequences. ICH constitutes 10 to 15% of all strokes, and it is associated with a higher morbidity than ischemic disease or cerebral aneurysm rupture.[1,2] Annual incidence ranges from 10 to 30 per 100,000 people.[3,4] Reported mortality rates are as high as 34 and 59% at 3 and 12 months, respectively.[3,5,6] Independent risk factors correlated with a worse prognosis include age older than 80 years, intraventricular hemorrhage, low score on the Glasgow Coma Scale (GCS), and hematoma volume over 30 mL.[7]

Medical treatments have not been shown to improve outcomes in ICH.[3,8,9,10] As a result, a variety of surgical treatments have been developed for ICH.[11,12,13,14,15] Open surgical treatments include craniotomy with hematoma evacuation and decompressive craniectomy. Minimally invasive treatments include endoscopic hematoma evacuation and stereotactic catheter placement, for aspiration and thrombolysis. The indications for surgery, and the choice of surgical treatment, remain subjects of controversy.[16]

21.1.2 Evolution of Treatment Options

Several early studies have compared open surgical evacuation of ICH with medical management.[13,14,17,18] The first randomized trial comparing endoscopic hematoma evacuation with medical management was published in 1989. For subcortical hematomas,

endoscopic evacuation decreased mortality. On the other hand, patients with thalamic or basal ganglia hematomas did not benefit from endoscopic clot removal.[15]

In 2005, results from the Surgical Trial in Intracerebral Hemorrhage (STICH) were published. Patients were randomized to early surgery or initial medical management. There was no statistically significant difference in mortality or functional outcome between the two groups. A subgroup analysis showed a potential benefit of surgery for patients with lobar hemorrhages extending close (1 cm or less) to the cortical surface.[11] The STICH II trial enrolled only patients with superficial lobar hemorrhages, and found no significant difference in outcomes between patients assigned to surgery and those assigned to medical management. Overall, in the largest clinical trials, early surgical intervention has not provided a statistically significant benefit for patients with supratentorial ICH.

The STICH trials' conclusions may not apply to all patients with supratentorial ICH. For a patient to be included in the trials, the surgeon had to be uncertain about the optimal treatment. Moreover, both STICH and STICH II had high crossover rates of patients from the nonsurgical arm to surgical intervention.

The surgical indications for cerebellar hemorrhage are better defined. Generally accepted criteria for cerebellar hematoma evacuation are hemorrhage size over 3 cm in diameter, brainstem compression, cisternal compression, or hydrocephalus.[19,20,21,22,23,24]

Several minimally invasive techniques for intraparenchymal clot removal have been developed, including stereotactic aspiration and instillation of thrombolytic agents.[25,26,27,28,29,30] For stereotactic aspiration, patients are placed in a stereotactic frame, and after placement of a burr hole, a catheter is placed in the hematoma and aspiration is performed.[13,29,31] Some studies describe administration of a fibrinolytic agent into the cavity.[26,27,30,32,33] The advent of frameless stereotaxy has allowed catheter placement with modern intraoperative navigation systems.[26,34,35,36,37,38]

In endoscopic surgery, an endoscope with various working ports is passed through a cylindrical tube to access the hematoma. Various instruments for endoscopic surgery have been described: a steel sheath, a transparent sheath, a bullet-shaped sheath, an expandable sheath, a 3-in-1 endoscope, an endoscope with an ultrasound aspiration device, and a balanced irrigation–suction system.[34,35,37,38,39,40,41,42,43,44,45,46,47,48,49,50,51,52] Other recent technological advances include sonothrombolysis, a modern endoport, and a suction/debridement system suited for endoscopes.[34,53,54,55,56]

Proponents of endoscopic clot evacuation argue that iatrogenic injury to brain tissue is avoided because brain retraction is minimized. This hypothetical advantage of endoscopy is highlighted in the treatment of deep-seated hematomas, rather than subcortical hematomas. Stereotactic navigation can be used to choose an optimal trajectory for the endoscope that would avoid eloquent brain tissue.[38] When compared with

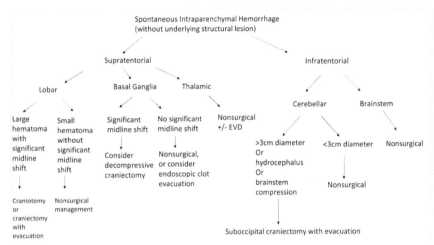

Fig. 21.1 Decision-making algorithm for treatment of intracerebral hemorrhage.

craniotomy, the skin incision and bone opening are typically smaller in endoscopic surgery, which may or may not translate into a difference in operative risks.

An advantage of open surgery is the ability to obtain hemostasis in the cavity with standard bimanual techniques, often with the use of an operative microscope. Open surgery may be optimal for the removal of organized hematomas. Microsurgical techniques are well suited for the resection of vascular or neoplastic lesions that may be detected during hematoma evacuation. Furthermore, craniotomy permits a direct intraoperative assessment of brain swelling, and allows a decompressive craniectomy to be performed when needed.

While several studies have compared minimally invasive surgery to craniotomy for clot evacuation, evidence supporting one technique over another remains weak. In the ongoing Minimally Invasive Surgery Plus rt-PA for Intracerebral Hemorrhage Evacuation (MISTIE) phase III trial, patients with ICH are randomized to medical management or to minimally invasive surgery, which entails stereotactic catheter aspiration of the hematoma, followed by tPA administration into the cavity.[27,30] A related trial, Intraoperative CT-guided Endoscopic Surgery for ICH (MISTIE-ICES), is also being conducted.[57] In the 2015 guidelines, the American Heart Association/ American Stroke Association concludes that the effectiveness of minimally invasive clot evacuation, by endoscopy or by stereotactic catheter aspiration, remains uncertain.[16] The same guidelines indicate that decompressive craniectomy may reduce mortality for patients with supratentorial ICH, in the setting of significant midline shift, coma, or medically refractory elevated ICP.

21.1.3 Decision-Making Algorithm

We propose the following algorithm for making initial treatment decisions, for patients with spontaneous intraparenchymal hemorrhage without an underlying vascular lesion or neoplasm (▶ Fig. 21.1).

21.1.4 Final Thoughts

For intraparenchymal hematomas that extend close to the cortical surface, it is our opinion that endoscopy does not increase the safety of hematoma evacuation, compared with craniotomy

using an operating microscope. The incision in cerebral or cerebellar cortex is similar, whether an endoscope or a microscope is used. With either endoscopic or open techniques, the use of brain retractors can be avoided, because the most superficial aspect of the hematoma is close to the cortex. Open craniotomy may be safer than endoscopy for several reasons: compared with the use of endoscopic instruments, bimanual microsurgical techniques may allow for better hemostasis after clot removal, facilitate better removal of fibrotic and organized hematomas, permit treatment of underlying vascular or neoplastic lesions when encountered, and provide direct assessment of brain swelling and the need for decompressive craniectomy.

The majority of intraparenchymal hematomas that require surgical evacuation are large lobar or cerebellar hematomas. Both of these types of hematomas typically extend close to the cortical surface. We generally employ craniotomy or craniectomy, with the use of the operating microscope, for their evacuation. Intraoperative ultrasonography helps determine the optimal site for cortical incision.

The advantage of endoscopy lies in its capability of accessing deep-seated hematomas with minimal trauma to the overlying brain. Basal ganglia hemorrhage can be approached by passing an endoscope along a trajectory through noneloquent brain. While basal ganglia hemorrhages are generally managed without surgery, ongoing and future research may provide support for endoscopic evacuation. The important question to be answered is whether endoscopic clot evacuation is superior to nonsurgical management in these patients. If it is, then endoscopy may expand the role of surgical intervention, to patients with deep-seated basal ganglia hemorrhage.

References

[1] Caplan LR. Intracerebral haemorrhage. Lancet. 1992; 339(8794):656–658

[2] Broderick JP, Brott T, Tomsick T, Miller R, Huster G. Intracerebral hemorrhage more than twice as common as subarachnoid hemorrhage. J Neurosurg. 1993; 78(2):188–191

[3] Qureshi AI, Tuhrim S, Broderick JP, Batjer HH, Hondo H, Hanley DF. Spontaneous intracerebral hemorrhage. N Engl J Med. 2001; 344(19):1450–1460

[4] Labovitz DL, Halim A, Boden-Albala B, Hauser WA, Sacco RL. The incidence of deep and lobar intracerebral hemorrhage in whites, blacks, and Hispanics. Neurology. 2005; 65(4):518–522

[5] Weimar C, Weber C, Wagner M, et al. German Stroke Data Bank Collaborators. Management patterns and health care use after intracerebral hemorrhage. a cost-of-illness study from a societal perspective in Germany. Cerebrovasc Dis. 2003; 15(1–2):29–36

[6] Flaherty ML, Haverbusch M, Sekar P, et al. Long-term mortality after intracerebral hemorrhage. Neurology. 2006; 66(8):1182–1186

[7] Hemphill JC, III, Bonovich DC, Besmertis L, Manley GT, Johnston SC. The ICH score: a simple, reliable grading scale for intracerebral hemorrhage. Stroke. 2001; 32(4):891–897

[8] Tellez H, Bauer RB. Dexamethasone as treatment in cerebrovascular disease. 1. A controlled study in intracerebral hemorrhage. Stroke. 1973; 4(4):541–546

[9] Poungvarin N, Bhoopat W, Viriyavejakul A, et al. Effects of dexamethasone in primary supratentorial intracerebral hemorrhage. N Engl J Med. 1987; 316 (20):1229–1233

[10] Yu YL, Kumana CR, Lauder IJ, et al. Treatment of acute cerebral hemorrhage with intravenous glycerol. A double-blind, placebo-controlled, randomized trial. Stroke. 1992; 23(7):967–971

[11] Mendelow AD, Gregson BA, Fernandes HM, et al. STICH investigators. Early surgery versus initial conservative treatment in patients with spontaneous supratentorial intracerebral haematomas in the International Surgical Trial in Intracerebral Haemorrhage (STICH): a randomised trial. Lancet. 2005; 365 (9457):387–397

[12] Mendelow AD, Gregson BA, Rowan EN, Murray GD, Gholkar A, Mitchell PM, STICH II Investigators. Early surgery versus initial conservative treatment in patients with spontaneous supratentorial lobar intracerebral haematomas (STICH II): a randomised trial. Lancet. 2013; 382(9890):397–408

[13] Zuccarello M, Brott T, Derex L, et al. Early surgical treatment for supratentorial intracerebral hemorrhage: a randomized feasibility study. Stroke. 1999; 30 (9):1833–1839

[14] Batjer HH, Reisch JS, Allen BC, Plaizier LJ, Su CJ. Failure of surgery to improve outcome in hypertensive putaminal hemorrhage. A prospective randomized trial. Arch Neurol. 1990; 47(10):1103–1106

[15] Auer LM, Deinsberger W, Niederkorn K, et al. Endoscopic surgery versus medical treatment for spontaneous intracerebral hematoma: a randomized study. J Neurosurg. 1989; 70(4):530–535

[16] Hemphill JC, III, Greenberg SM, Anderson CS, et al. American Heart Association Stroke Council, Council on Cardiovascular and Stroke Nursing, Council on Clinical Cardiology. Guidelines for the Management of Spontaneous Intracerebral Hemorrhage: a Guideline for Healthcare Professionals from the American Heart Association/American Stroke Association. Stroke. 2015; 46 (7):2032–2060

[17] Juvela S, Heiskanen O, Poranen A, et al. The treatment of spontaneous intracerebral hemorrhage. A prospective randomized trial of surgical and conservative treatment. J Neurosurg. 1989; 70(5):755–758

[18] Morgenstern LB, Frankowski RF, Shedden P, Pasteur W, Grotta JC. Surgical treatment for intracerebral hemorrhage (STICH): a single-center, randomized clinical trial. Neurology. 1998; 51(5):1359–1363

[19] Da Pian R, Bazzan A, Pasqualin A. Surgical versus medical treatment of spontaneous posterior fossa haematomas: a cooperative study on 205 cases. Neurol Res. 1984; 6(3):145–151

[20] van Loon J, Van Calenbergh F, Goffin J, Plets C. Controversies in the management of spontaneous cerebellar haemorrhage. A consecutive series of 49 cases and review of the literature. Acta Neurochir (Wien). 1993; 122(3–4):187–193

[21] Kirollos RW, Tyagi AK, Ross SA, van Hille PT, Marks PV. Management of spontaneous cerebellar hematomas: a prospective treatment protocol. Neurosurgery. 2001; 49(6):1378–1386, discussion 1386–1387

[22] Kobayashi S, Sato A, Kageyama Y, Nakamura H, Watanabe Y, Yamaura A. Treatment of hypertensive cerebellar hemorrhage: surgical or conservative management? Neurosurgery. 1994; 34(2):246–250, discussion 250–251

[23] Salvati M, Cervoni L, Raco A, Delfini R. Spontaneous cerebellar hemorrhage: clinical remarks on 50 cases. Surg Neurol. 2001; 55(3):156–161, discussion 161

[24] Raco A, Caroli E, Isidori A, Salvati M. Management of acute cerebellar infarction: one institution's experience. Neurosurgery. 2003; 53(5):1061–1065, discussion 1065–1066

[25] Teernstra OPM, Evers SM, Lodder J, Leffers P, Franke CL, Blaauw G, Multicenter randomized controlled trial (SICHPA). Stereotactic treatment of intracerebral hematoma by means of a plasminogen activator: a multicenter randomized controlled trial (SICHPA). Stroke. 2003; 34(4):968–974

[26] Vespa P, McArthur D, Miller C, et al. Frameless stereotactic aspiration and thrombolysis of deep intracerebral hemorrhage is associated with reduction

of hemorrhage volume and neurological improvement. Neurocrit Care. 2005; 2(3):274–281

[27] Mould WA, Carhuapoma JR, Muschelli J, et al. MISTIE Investigators. Minimally invasive surgery plus recombinant tissue-type plasminogen activator for intracerebral hemorrhage evacuation decreases perihematomal edema. Stroke. 2013; 44(3):627–634

[28] Hattori N, Katayama Y, Maya Y, Gatherer A. Impact of stereotactic hematoma evacuation on medical costs during the chronic period in patients with spontaneous putaminal hemorrhage: a randomized study. Surg Neurol. 2006; 65 (5):429–435, discussion 435

[29] Niizuma H, Shimizu Y, Yonemitsu T, Nakasato N, Suzuki J. Results of stereotactic aspiration in 175 cases of putaminal hemorrhage. Neurosurgery. 1989; 24(6):814–819

[30] Morgan T, Zuccarello M, Narayan R, Keyl P, Lane K, Hanley D. Preliminary findings of the minimally-invasive surgery plus rtPA for intracerebral hemorrhage evacuation (MISTIE) clinical trial. Acta Neurochir Suppl (Wien). 2008; 105:147–151

[31] Kandel EI, Peresedov VV. Stereotaxic evacuation of spontaneous intracerebral hematomas. J Neurosurg. 1985; 62(2):206–213

[32] Deinsberger W, Lang C, Hornig C, Boeker DK. Stereotactic aspiration and fibrinolysis of spontaneous supratentorial intracerebral hematomas versus conservative treatment: a matched-pair study. Zentralbl Neurochir. 2003; 64 (4):145–150

[33] Kim IS, Son BC, Lee SW, Sung JH, Hong JT. Comparison of frame-based and frameless stereotactic hematoma puncture and subsequent fibrinolytic therapy for the treatment of supratentorial deep seated spontaneous intracerebral hemorrhage. Minim Invasive Neurosurg. 2007; 50(2):86–90

[34] Dye JA, Dusick JR, Lee DJ, Gonzalez NR, Martin NA. Frontal bur hole through an eyebrow incision for image-guided endoscopic evacuation of spontaneous intracerebral hemorrhage. J Neurosurg. 2012; 117(4):767–773

[35] Miller CM, Vespa P, Saver JL, et al. Image-guided endoscopic evacuation of spontaneous intracerebral hemorrhage. Surg Neurol. 2008; 69(5):441–446, discussion 446

[36] Barlas O, Karadereler S, Bahar S, et al. Image-guided keyhole evacuation of spontaneous supratentorial intracerebral hemorrhage. Minim Invasive Neurosurg. 2009; 52(2):62–68

[37] Nishihara T, Morita A, Teraoka A, Kirino T. Endoscopy-guided removal of spontaneous intracerebral hemorrhage: comparison with computer tomography-guided stereotactic evacuation. Childs Nerv Syst. 2007; 23(6):677–683

[38] Beynon C, Schiebel P, Bösel J, Unterberg AW, Orakcioglu B. Minimally invasive endoscopic surgery for treatment of spontaneous intracerebral haematomas. Neurosurg Rev. 2015; 38(3):421–428

[39] Nishihara T, Nagata K, Tanaka S, et al. Newly developed endoscopic instruments for the removal of intracerebral hematoma. Neurocrit Care. 2005; 2 (1):67–74

[40] Bakshi A, Bakshi A, Banerji AK. Neuroendoscope-assisted evacuation of large intracerebral hematomas: introduction of a new, minimally invasive technique. Preliminary report. Neurosurg Focus. 2004; 16(6):e9

[41] Hsieh PC, Cho DY, Lee WY, Chen JT. Endoscopic evacuation of putaminal hemorrhage: how to improve the efficiency of hematoma evacuation. Surg Neurol. 2005; 64(2):147–153, discussion 153

[42] Chen CC, Chung HC, Liu CL, Lee HC, Cho DY. A newly developed endoscopic sheath for the removal of large putaminal hematomas. J Clin Neurosci. 2009; 16(10):1338–1341

[43] Cho DY, Chen CC, Chang CS, Lee WY, Tso M. Endoscopic surgery for spontaneous basal ganglia hemorrhage: comparing endoscopic surgery, stereotactic aspiration, and craniotomy in noncomatose patients. Surg Neurol. 2006; 65 (6):547–555, discussion 555–556

[44] Yamamoto T, Nakao Y, Mori K, Maeda M. Endoscopic hematoma evacuation for hypertensive cerebellar hemorrhage. Minim Invasive Neurosurg. 2006; 49 (3):173–178

[45] Kuo L-T, Chen CM, Li CH, et al. Early endoscope-assisted hematoma evacuation in patients with supratentorial intracerebral hemorrhage: case selection, surgical technique, and long-term results. Neurosurg Focus. 2011; 30(4):E9

[46] Ochalski P, Chivukula S, Shin S, Prevedello D, Engh J. Outcomes after endoscopic port surgery for spontaneous intracerebral hematomas. J Neurol Surg A Cent Eur Neurosurg. 2014; 75(3):195–205, discussion 206

[47] Almenawer SA, Crevier L, Murty N, Kassam A, Reddy K. Minimal access to deep intracranial lesions using a serial dilatation technique: case-series and review of brain tubular retractor systems. Neurosurg Rev. 2013; 36(2):321–329, discussion 329–330

[48] Nishihara T, Teraoka A, Morita A, Ueki K, Takai K, Kirino T. A transparent sheath for endoscopic surgery and its application in surgical evacuation of

spontaneous intracerebral hematomas. Technical note. J Neurosurg. 2000; 92 (6):1053–1055

[49] Nagasaka T, Tsugeno M, Ikeda H, Okamoto T, Inao S, Wakabayashi T. Early recovery and better evacuation rate in neuroendoscopic surgery for spontaneous intracerebral hemorrhage using a multifunctional cannula: preliminary study in comparison with craniotomy. J Stroke Cerebrovasc Dis. 2011; 20 (3):208–213

[50] Nagasaka T, Inao S, Ikeda H, Tsugeno M, Okamoto T. Inflation-deflation method for endoscopic evacuation of intracerebral haematoma. Acta Neurochir (Wien). 2008; 150(7):685–690, discussion 690

[51] Orakcioglu B, Uozumi Y, Unterberg A. Endoscopic intra-hematomal evacuation of intracerebral hematomas: a suitable technique for patients with coagulopathies. Acta Neurochir Suppl. 2011; 112:3–8

[52] Waran V, Vairavan N, Sia SF, Abdullah B. A new expandable cannula system for endoscopic evacuation of intraparenchymal hemorrhages. J Neurosurg. 2009; 111(6):1127–1130

[53] Przybylowski CJ, Ding D, Starke RM, Webster Crowley R, Liu KC. Endoport-assisted surgery for the management of spontaneous intracerebral hemorrhage. J Clin Neurosci. 2015; 22(11):1727–1732

[54] Ding D, Przybylowski CJ, Starke RM, et al. A minimally invasive anterior skull base approach for evacuation of a basal ganglia hemorrhage. J Clin Neurosci. 2015; 22(11):1816–1819

[55] Fiorella D, et al. Minimally invasive evacuation of parenchymal and ventricular hemorrhage using the Apollo system with simultaneous neuronavigation, neuroendoscopy and active monitoring with cone beam CT. J Neurointerv Surg. 2014:1–6

[56] Newell DW, Shah MM, Wilcox R, et al. Minimally invasive evacuation of spontaneous intracerebral hemorrhage using sonothrombolysis. J Neurosurg. 2011; 115(3):592–601

[57] Vespa PM, Martin N, Zuccarello M, Awad I, Hanley DF. Surgical trials in intracerebral hemorrhage. Stroke. 2013; 44(6) Suppl 1:S79–S82

22 Evacuation of Intraparenchymal Hemorrhage: Microscope

Nimer Adeeb, Justin Moore, Ajith J. Thomas, and Christopher S. Ogilvy

Summary

Evacuation of intraparenchymal hemorrhage has been traditionally treated with open microsurgical techniques. In this chapter, we discuss the advantages technical nuances of microsurgical treatment approaches versus novel endoscopic approaches.

Keywords: intraparenchymal hemorrhage, endoscopic, microsurgical, evacuation, hematoma

22.1 Open/Microscopic Perspective

22.1.1 Case Report

History

A 74-year-old Hispanic female with a known history of left-sided migraine awoke during the night with a severe headache. The headache was left sided, but was of greater severity and of different quality from her usual migraine attacks. It was associated with nausea and vomiting. The patient was transferred to the emergency department by her daughter.

Physical Examination

On initial examination, the patient was conscious and oriented to time, place, and person. She was anxious and diaphoretic. Her blood pressure was 187/73, heart rate was 66 bpm, respiratory rate was 18 bpm, and temperature was 97 °F.

On neurological examination, the patient was able to relate the history without difficulty. However, she was unable to name certain objects and body parts (e.g., watch and thumb). She had a right homonymous hemianopsia and right hemisensory neglect, without subjective visual disturbance. Cranial nerves (I–XII) were intact. Upper and lower limb neurological examination revealed normal muscle bulk and tone and no pronator drift bilaterally. Her motor power was 5/5 bilaterally in both the upper and lower extremities and all reflexes were present (3 +), with a negative Babinski sign. There was no tremor, clonus, or asterixis noted. Sensory examination showed no gross deficits; however, a right-sided hemisensory neglect was identified. Cerebellar examination was unremarkable. Gait could not be assessed. Her initial National Institutes of Health Stroke Scale (NIHSS) was 7.

An urgent computed tomography (CT) scan of the brain revealed a 5.5 × 3.0 cm left occipital intracerebral hemorrhage (ICH) with a circumferential area of hypodensity. There was 6 mm of midline shift to the right and almost complete effacement of the left occipital horn. There was no evidence of frank herniation or hydrocephalus (▶ Fig. 22.1).

Follow-up examination showed a progressive decrease in the patient's level of consciousness with an evolving right-sided hemiparesis. Urgent repeat CT imaging showed 10 mm of midline shift (▶ Fig. 22.2). In the light of clinical and radiological progression, the patient was taken for emergent surgical evacuation of the hematoma.

Operative Management and Technical Nuances

The patient was taken emergently to the operative room for left occipital craniotomy. She was placed in a right lateral position. Her head was turned toward the floor and held rigid in the three-point Mayfield fixation. The left occipital region was prepared and draped in the usual sterile fashion. A horseshoe-shaped incision was created and scalp bleeding controlled using bipolar forceps and RANEY clips. The scalp flap was

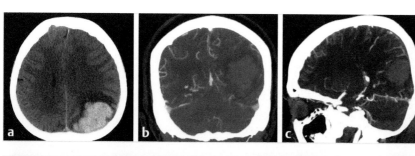

Fig. 22.1 Initial computed tomography **(a)** axial, **(b)** coronal, and **(c)** coronal scan showing left occipital intracerebral hemorrhage with midline shift.

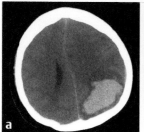
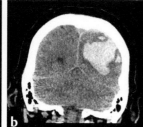
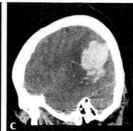

Fig. 22.2 Repeat computed tomography **(a)** axial, **(b)** coronal, and **(c)** coronal scan showing evolving intracerebral hemorrhage and increase in the midline shift.

reflected inferiorly and multiple burr holes were made around the planned craniotomy, just to the left of the sagittal sinus. The craniotome was used to complete the craniotomy. The bone flap was elevated without difficulty. The dura was moderately tense and was opened in a cruciate fashion with careful attention paid to avoid injuring dural bridging veins and venous lakes on the medial aspect of the craniotomy. The hematoma could be seen presenting to the cortical surface. Under loupe magnification, the bipolar forceps with irrigation were used to open the cortex at the point of hematoma presentation. Resection of the hematoma was performed circumferentially around the clot cavity using a no. 7 sucker and generous warm saline irrigation. Eventually, the clot was gently removed in large pieces using a tumor forceps. Bleeding vessels were coagulated using bipolar forceps. The brain was now relaxed and the cavity was lined with Surgicel and Surgiflo to achieve hemostasis. The wound was then irrigated with warm saline and the dura was closed using 4–0 Nurolon suture in a watertight fashion. Tacking sutures were placed around the craniotomy to minimize the risk of epidural hematoma. The bone flap was placed over Gelfoam and Surgicel overlaying the dura, using a microplating screw system. The wound was copiously irrigated with antibiotic solution, and the galea was closed using interrupted 2–0 buried Vicryl sutures following which the skin was closed using a running 3–0 Nylon suture in an unlocked fashion. The wound was dressed sterilely. The patient was taken to the intensive care unit in stable condition.

Postoperative Period

In the immediate postoperative period, the patient was intubated, but was opening eyes to noxious stimulus and following commands on both sides. She had right hemianopia, but her pupils were reactive bilaterally and there was no ophthalmoplegia. Motor power was 2/5 in the right upper and lower limbs and 4/5 on the left. A weaker withdrawal response to stimulus was elicited on the right side when compared to the left. A postoperative CT scan showed near-complete evacuation of the hematoma. Midline shift improved to 3 mm (▸ Fig. 22.3).

Follow-Up

On follow-up visit at 3-months, the patient was alert and oriented to time, place, and person. She still suffered from right homonymous hemianopsia. Her muscle power was 5/5 bilaterally in both upper and lower extremities. There was no sensory deficit. Cranial nerves were intact. Gait and balance were normal. She had a modified Rankin score of 1. CT scan showed complete resolution of the midline shift (▸ Fig. 22.4).

22.1.2 Open Microsurgical Approach versus Endoscope Approach

Advantages of the open approach in this case included the following:
- Very rapid; the time from positioning to clot removal was approximately 20 minutes.
- The ability to optimize the cortectomy, particularly as the region includes the eloquent visual cortex and associated areas. An open approach allows identification and preservation of superficial cortical veins and avoidance of venous sinus and sinus lakes.
- It provided the option of leaving the bone flap off if the patient had developed progressive brain edema intraoperatively.
- It allowed visual identification of where the hematoma comes to the surface of the brain, thereby minimizing transgression of intact cortex.
- The ability to use of the microscope allows a highly magnified view with excellent illumination, while avoiding loss of cavity visualization should brisk hemorrhage be encountered, a concern given the patient's neurological deterioration.
- The patient's presentation is suspicious and the possibility of an underlying lesion should be entertained in this patient given the atypical location and lack of a history of hypertension. An open approach with the use of the microscope allows the surgeon to implement a full repertoire of surgical techniques should an underlying lesion be encountered.

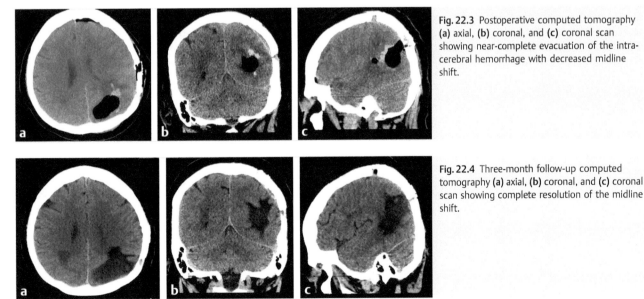

Fig. 22.3 Postoperative computed tomography (a) axial, (b) coronal, and (c) coronal scan showing near-complete evacuation of the intracerebral hemorrhage with decreased midline shift.

Fig. 22.4 Three-month follow-up computed tomography (a) axial, (b) coronal, and (c) coronal scan showing complete resolution of the midline shift.

22.1.3 Patient Selection

Open craniotomy for evacuation of hematoma can be used in treatment of patients with the following:

- Large superficial hematoma, particularly those who might develop edema, thus allowing the possibility of craniectomy.
- Atypical hemorrhages that suggest an underlying lesion.
- Hemorrhages associated with a known underlying pathology.
- Patients at high risk of intraoperative bleeding or rebleeding, such as those with early presentation (within 7 hours), or on anticoagulation or antiplatelet agents.

22.1.4 Complication Avoidance

- The open approach allows for easy and rapid response to hemorrhage with the benefit that sudden acute hemorrhage does not cause the surgeon to lose visualization of the surgical field. This is particularly useful in patients on anticoagulation. The microscope allows 3D stereo-optic binocular vision with improved depth perception and excellent illumination.
- It is important to identify and preserve cortical veins as loss of these veins can lead to brain edema and possible infarction in a patient who potentially already has brain edema. An open approach allows identification and avoidance of these structures.
- The availability of changing the magnification and depth quickly is useful for minimizing injuries and rapidly responding to new hemorrhage.
- The open approach allows access for an assistant if problems arise (such as a second sucker).
- Optimal location of cortectomy, ideally at the point where the hematoma can be seen on the surface of the brain or at a point that allows the least transgression of cortical tissue, will help minimize injury to intact cortical parenchyma.

22.1.5 Literature Review

ICH is associated with significant morbidity and mortality. Up to 30% of patients die within 30 days, and many others survive with a poor neurological outcome.[1] The main aim of surgery is to reduce mass effect on the brain by clot removal, which helps reverse progressive brain edema, remove hematoma breakdown products that may initiate inflammatory changes and secondary injury and improve cerebral perfusion to the surrounding viable brain tissue, or the penumbra.[2,3] However, the effectiveness of surgical treatment remains controversial. Studies comparing surgical versus medical treatment have shown no significant benefit in clinical outcomes after surgery.[4] Similar results were also reported in the International Surgical Trial in Intracerebral Haemorrhage (STICH) trial. This trial was designed to look at patients in whom there was equipoise between surgery and medical treatment and thus did not include patients for whom surgery was thought to be of definite benefit. In a subanalysis of patients in the initial STICH trial, a potential benefit was seen in those who had superficial hematomas evacuated, with surgery providing an 8% absolute benefit and 29% relative benefit in Glasgow Outcome Score (GOS).[3] This finding provided the impetus for a second study, "STICH II." Although early surgical evacuation (< 12 hours) suggested a trend toward better clinical outcomes (41 vs. 38%) and lower mortality rate

(18 vs. 24%) at 6 months, these findings were not of statistical significance. Interestingly, 21% of patients in the conservative group had delayed surgical treatment, which led to improved outcomes and this may have confounded the overall results.[5]

Despite these controversial findings, early surgical evacuation of superficial hematoma remains a possible treatment strategy for neurosurgeons in selected patients using either an open craniotomy or an endoscopic approach. Current data suggest that surgery is not advised for small deep-seated hematoma, or in large hematomas affecting the whole hemisphere, particularly in elderly patients who present in a poor neurological state.[1] However, in selected patients with small hematomas and progressive neurological deterioration, surgery is often recommended and can be lifesaving.

Many clinicians consider large cerebellar hematomas to be a distinct condition, with a distinct natural history, often being associated with obstruction of cerebrospinal fluid (CSF) flow or brainstem mass effect and surgery is often considered the first-line treatment for this condition. Witsch et al suggested surgical treatment for patient with a GCS less than 13 or hematomas greater than 3 cm.[6] On the other hand, if the cerebellar hematoma is small (< 3 cm) and the dominant pathology is hydrocephalus from CSF flow obstruction, an external ventricular device (EVD) can be placed, followed by close monitoring of the hematoma.[1,2,4] The American Stroke Association recommends surgical treatment for those patients with cerebellar hemorrhage who have a deteriorating neurological condition or evidence of brainstem compression or hydrocephalus.

Most surgical trials have used craniotomy as the surgical treatment for evacuation of hematoma. Auer et al conducted the first clinical trial in comparing endoscopic versus conservative treatment. They found that endoscopic evacuation of the hematoma within 24 hours resulted in 40% of patients having minimal or no disability at 6 months, compared with 25% of patients treated conservatively.[7] Two clinical trials are now being conducted to reevaluate the benefit of endoscopic surgery and validate those findings.[2] Endoscopic treatment might provide a benefit in deep-seated hematomas. However, in superficial hematomas, an appropriately performed open surgical approach, utilizing a minimal craniotomy, can provide the advantage of direct visualization of the hematoma projection to the cortical surface, which in turn allows minimal transgression of intact parenchyma, visualization of surface veins and arteries, and thus allows these structures to be protected throughout the case, allows direct and rapid hemostatic maneuvers to be employed in the event of uncontrolled hemorrhage, and can also enable treatment of potential underlying lesions that were not readily apparent on imaging. For deep-seated hematomas, if open surgery is contemplated, imaging guidance can be employed to enable the optimal trajectory to be planned to access the hematoma while avoiding eloquent brain structures. The operative microscope or microsurgical glasses can be used in certain cases to provide a magnified view, which is advantageous for adequate hemostasis and satisfactory hematoma removal. After forming a minimal cortectomy, thin retractors can be directed to the hematoma using a stereotactic probe. Once in the hematoma cavity, the microscope can be used to visualize the walls of the cavity. Parts of the hematoma can be removed with forceps while avoiding new bleeding in the margin zones.

The optimal timing for surgical evacuation of hematomas is not clear. The published studies have used different time frames, including 12,[5,8] 24,[3,9,10] 48,[9] and 72 hours,[11] but found this was not a significant influence on clinical outcomes when comparing surgery to conservative treatment. Wang et al divided patients into three groups: the ultra-early (< 7 hours), the early (7–24 hours), and delayed (> 24 hours) treatment groups. The authors suggested that surgical treatment of those in the early group (7–24 hours) provided the optimal balance between the rehemorrhage risk (high in the ultra-early group) and the eventual outcome. In the ultra-early and early stages, both the perioperative and long-term outcomes of surgical treatment were superior to that of medical treatment.[12]

22.1.6 Clinical Pearls

- For any ICH, medical management is important, particularly if surgery also occurs. Reverse any anticoagulation medication, treat coagulopathy, and aim for a blood pressure of less than 160 mm Hg.[13]
- Atypical hemorrhages, with possible underlying lesion, even though not seen on imaging should be considered candidates for open surgery, to enable a rapid change in surgical plan should an underlying lesion be detected. The Secondary Intra-cerebral Hemorrhage (SICH) score can be a useful screening test for calculating the probability of an underlying lesion.[14]
- Generous irrigation while using the bipolar forceps is critical for obtaining adequate hemostasis of the hematoma cavity.
- Open surgery enables visual identification of venous structures and cortical arteries, which can then be protected, often by covering them with a damp cottonoid.
- If there is significant hemorrhage with potential for significant cerebral edema, open surgery enables the possibility of decompressive craniectomy for intracranial pressure control.
- Placement of gentle retraction can be useful in large hematomas, particularly when they extend under a shelf of intact cortex. Using a strip of Bicol under the retractor protects underlying brain, improves hemostasis, and is not as bulky as cottonoids.
- At the conclusion of hemostasis, ask the anesthetic team to bring the blood pressure back to the patient's baseline. These helps confirm adequate hemostasis has been achieved.

References

[1] Reichart R, Frank S. Intracerebral hemorrhage, indication for surgical treatment and surgical techniques. Open Crit Care Med J. 2011; 4:68–71

[2] Vespa PM, Martin N, Zuccarello M, Awad I, Hanley DF. Surgical trials in intracerebral hemorrhage. Stroke. 2013; 44(6) Suppl 1:S79–S82

[3] Mendelow AD, Gregson BA, Fernandes HM, et al. STICH investigators. Early surgery versus initial conservative treatment in patients with spontaneous supratentorial intracerebral haematomas in the International Surgical Trial in Intracerebral Haemorrhage (STICH): a randomised trial. Lancet. 2005; 365 (9457):387–397

[4] Fernandes HM, Gregson B, Siddique S, Mendelow AD. Surgery in intracerebral hemorrhage. The uncertainty continues. Stroke. 2000; 31(10):2511–2516

[5] Mendelow AD, Gregson BA, Rowan EN, Murray GD, Gholkar A, Mitchell PM, STICH II Investigators. Early surgery versus initial conservative treatment in patients with spontaneous supratentorial lobar intracerebral haematomas (STICH II): a randomised trial. Lancet. 2013; 382(9890):397–408

[6] Witsch J, Neugebauer H, Zweckberger K, Jüttler E. Primary cerebellar haemorrhage: complications, treatment and outcome. Clin Neurol Neurosurg. 2013; 115(7):863–869

[7] Auer LM, Deinsberger W, Niederkorn K, et al. Endoscopic surgery versus medical treatment for spontaneous intracerebral hematoma: a randomized study. J Neurosurg. 1989; 70(4):530–535

[8] Morgenstern LB, Demchuk AM, Kim DH, Frankowski RF, Grotta JC. Rebleeding leads to poor outcome in ultra-early craniotomy for intracerebral hemorrhage. Neurology. 2001; 56(10):1294–1299

[9] Juvela S, Heiskanen O, Poranen A, et al. The treatment of spontaneous intracerebral hemorrhage. A prospective randomized trial of surgical and conservative treatment. J Neurosurg. 1989; 70(5):755–758

[10] Zuccarello M, Brott T, Derex L, et al. Early surgical treatment for supratentorial intracerebral hemorrhage: a randomized feasibility study. Stroke. 1999; 30 (9):1833–1839

[11] McKissock W, Richardson A, Taylor J. Primary intracerebral haematoma: a controlled trial of surgical and conservative treatment in 180 unselected cases. Lancet. 1961; 2:221–226

[12] Wang YF, Wu JS, Mao Y, Chen XC, Zhou LF, Zhang Y. The optimal time-window for surgical treatment of spontaneous intracerebral hemorrhage: result of prospective randomized controlled trial of 500 cases. Acta Neurochir Suppl (Wien). 2008; 105:141–145

[13] Anderson CS, Huang Y, Wang JG, et al. INTERACT Investigators. Intensive blood pressure reduction in acute cerebral haemorrhage trial (INTERACT): a randomised pilot trial. Lancet Neurol. 2008; 7(5):391–399

[14] Delgado Almandoz JE, Schaefer PW, Goldstein JN, et al. Practical scoring system for the identification of patients with intracerebral hemorrhage at highest risk of harboring an underlying vascular etiology: the Secondary Intracerebral Hemorrhage Score. AJNR Am J Neuroradiol. 2010; 31 (9):1653–1660

23 Evacuation of Intraparenchymal Hemorrhage: Endoscope

Sheri K. Palejwala and Peter Nakaji

Summary

The role of spontaneous intracerebral hematoma evacuation remains a highly contentious subject among neurosurgeons. Early trials showed no clear benefit for surgical hematoma evacuation over maximal medical management; however, several smaller studies and subgroup analyses implied a benefit when minimal viable brain tissue is disrupted. The application of the endoscope to hematoma evacuation has decreased the surgical footprint of the procedure and has improved visualization of clot removal and control of actively bleeding vessels. Several studies have shown patient improvement after surgical evacuation of both lobar and deeper-seated hemorrhages using the endoscope. With quick efforts aimed at evacuating hematomas in carefully selected patients, especially those with clinical deficits and evidence of mass effect, even large or deep hematomas can be successfully evacuated using the endoscope.

Keywords: clot evacuation, endoscopic surgery, intracerebral hemorrhage, minimally invasive surgery, neuroendoscopy, stroke

23.1 Endoscopic Perspective

23.1.1 Early Clinical Trials of Intracerebral Hematoma Evacuation

The largest randomized controlled trial for intracerebral hematoma (ICH) evacuation to date, the International Surgical Trial in Intracerebral Hemorrhage (STICH), included more than 1,000 patients with spontaneous intraparenchymal cerebral hemorrhage who were randomized to either surgical evacuation within 24 hours of randomization or to conservative management. The results published in 2005 showed no benefit in overall survival or functional recovery with surgical evacuation.[1] Post hoc analyses of the STICH data indicated that patients with superficial lobar hematomas, particularly those without intraventricular extension or hydrocephalus, had a significantly more favorable outcome compared to patients with deep-seated hemorrhages.[2,3] One proposition to explain this result is that, during the surgical approach, viable tissue on the cortical surface, as well as small traversing vessels and perforators, could be damaged during hematoma evacuation.[3] STICH II was conducted to test this theory. A total of 601 patients with superficial lobar hemorrhages, but without intraventricular hemorrhage, were randomized to early surgical management or to best medical management, with the option of surgical crossover.[4]

STICH I and II taught us clearly that not all patients benefit from ICH evacuation over conservative management. The post hoc analyses implied that patients with superficial lobar hemorrhages, without intraventricular hemorrhage or hydrocephalus, would likely have had improved outcomes with surgical evacuation over medical management alone; yet these differences did not reach statistical significance with randomization in STICH II.[4] Nevertheless, it is clear that some patients with spontaneous ICH stand to benefit from surgical evacuation. Some factors to consider in patient selection are the length of time between ictus and surgery and the type of surgical approach. Specifically, most patients in the STICH trials were treated with open craniotomies, which were believed to contribute, in part, to the lack of a significant survival advantage realized in the surgical group.[4]

23.1.2 Minimally Invasive Approaches to ICH Evacuation

The Minimally Invasive Surgery and Recombinant Tissue-type Plasminogen Activator for Intracerebral Hemorrhage Evacuation (MISTIE) trial was developed to test the hypothesis that minimally invasive approaches could improve clinical outcomes in patients undergoing ICH evacuation by minimizing the surgical footprint.[5,6] The preliminary study enrolled 25 patients, with a 3:1 randomization to minimally invasive surgery with recombinant tissue-type plasminogen activator or medical management, respectively, and published the results for the first 21 patients. The study showed significant clot reduction with stereotactic aspiration and instilment of recombinant tissue-type plasminogen activator, as well as a decrease in perilesional edema; however, the correlation to clinical improvement was questionable.[5,6,7]

In a meta-analysis, Zhou and colleagues evaluated both stereotactic minimally invasive and endoscopic approaches for hematoma evacuation. They found decreased death and dependency in noncomatose patients with moderately sized hemorrhages (25–40 mL) that were evacuated within 72 hours of ictus, in comparison to patients who were comatose on presentation, presented with hematoma greater than 40 mL, and underwent delayed evacuation (>72 hours from ictus).[8] A subgroup analysis concluded that stereotactic approaches were superior to endoscopy, although the combination of the two modalities was not adequately studied, whereas medical management had improved outcomes over open craniotomies.[8] Again, this finding is believed to be due to the destruction of viable tissue along the surgical corridor toward the hematoma.[4,9,10]

23.1.3 Evolution of Endoscopy

The movement toward minimizing approach-related viable brain tissue damage while maximizing clot removal to decrease mass effect lent itself to the application of endoscopy in ICH removal. In 1989, Auer et al[11] published results of a randomized controlled trial with 100 patients assigned to endoscopic evacuation or medical treatment. In comparison to medically treated patients, endoscopic surgery patients demonstrated an improvement in functional outcome and mortality with sub-cortical hemorrhages of 10 to 50 mL and in mortality for deeper-seated hemorrhages. In keeping with other large multicenter trials, no benefit was found for endoscopic surgery versus medical management in comatose patients or in those with thalamic or putaminal hemorrhages.[11] Another retrospective study of 68 patients evaluated endoscopic clot removal while decreasing the time from ictus to surgery; all operations were performed within 12 hours of ictus, and 84% were performed within 4 hours of ictus. Results showed significantly decreased mortality and morbidity, as well as high rates of hematoma evacuation, in comparison to previously published studies.[12] Endoscopic hematoma evacuation applied to deeper and larger hemorrhages has also shown favorable results, with outcomes comparable to those of open evacuation while minimizing operative time, blood loss, and length of stay in intensive care units.[13,14] In one series, neuroendoscopic surgery ($n = 43$) allowed for a more complete evacuation and more robust immediate clinical improvement for deep-seated hemorrhages compared with those for patients undergoing craniotomy for ICH ($n = 23$).[15] Most recently, the Intraoperative Stereotactic Computed Tomography-Guided Endoscopic Surgery (ICES) trial for ICH demonstrated the efficacy of stereotactic endoscopy in hematoma evacuation in 20 patients, with a reduction in morbidity sustained at 1-year postrandomization compared to a medical control cohort ($n = 36$) from the MISTIE trial.[16]

The key benefit of the endoscope in spontaneous ICH evacuation, in addition to its minimal profile, is improved visualization for both clot removal and identification and control of bleeding vessels.[17] The chief drawback of endoscopic surgery for this condition is the need for experience and facility with use of the endoscope; this drawback is increasingly being overcome now that the endoscope has become a widely used modality in multiple facets of neurosurgery. Several studies have shown the benefit of minimally invasive and endoscopic approaches over open craniotomies and medical management for treating patients with spontaneous ICH.[8,9,15,17,18]

23.1.4 Other Minimally Invasive Approaches to Treating Spontaneous ICH

In pursuit of the trend of minimizing the surgical footprint, several devices have been developed for removing lesions while minimizing damage to viable brain tissue along the surgical corridor. The Apollo device (Penumbra Inc., Alameda, CA) is an aspiration-irrigation system that was used in 29 patients with spontaneous ICH evacuation and produced a statistically significant increase in the amount of hematoma evacuated (mean volume of hematoma decreased 54.1 ± 39.1%; $p < 0.001$), but with a higher-than-average mortality rate.[19] Similarly, the Myriad device (NICO Corp., Indianapolis, IN) was used in conjunction with BrainPath (NICO Corp.) on 39 patients at 11 centers. It demonstrated a statistically significant improvement in postoperative Glasgow Coma Scale scores ($p < 0.001$) and a clot reduction rate of ≥ 90% in 72% of patients. Furthermore, the design of the dilator and smooth obturator is hypothesized to decrease disruption of viable tissue along the surgical corridor,

leaving the surrounding parenchyma without contusion or other visual markers of surgical trauma. More importantly, however, the patients achieved a high rate of functional independence, which highlights the importance of more complete hematoma evacuation, with decreased invasiveness and improved visualization.[20]

23.1.5 Timing of Intracerebral Hemorrhage Evacuation Surgery

The timing of hematoma evacuation has been a consistent variable across trials and has served as an undeniable confounder when studying the outcomes of clot removal. For example, STICH I required patients randomized to surgery to undergo hematoma evacuation within 24 hours of randomization, irrespective of timing from ictus or presentation.[1] The median time to hematoma evacuation from ictus was 21 hours in STICH II; however, no significant changes in outcomes were noted.[4] A smaller study found improved outcomes in noncomatose patients with moderately sized subcortical hemorrhages over medical management when craniotomy was performed within 8 hours of ictus.[21] In contrast, ultra-early clot evacuation, performed within 4 hours of ictus with open craniotomy, was found to have worse outcomes, largely attributed to a 40% rehemorrhage rate versus 12% in the 12-hour ictus-to-surgery group.[22]

23.1.6 Case Illustration

A 54-year-old woman presented to an outside facility with acute-onset dense left hemiparesis, facial droop, dysarthria, and a 19-mL right putaminal hemorrhage (▶ Fig. 23.1a). Upon arrival at our tertiary care center, she underwent repeat imaging that revealed a 32% interval increase in her hemorrhage (▶ Fig. 23.1b). Because of the size of the hematoma, its progressive increase in size, the associated mass effect, and her neurologic deficit, the decision was made to proceed with minimally invasive endoscopic-assisted hematoma evacuation. On the basis of the configuration of the hemorrhage, a MISTIE type A (anterior-to-posterior linear trajectory) was chosen (▶ Fig. 23.1c).[16] Under stereotactic neuronavigation, a small bur hole was created in the skull through an eyebrow incision, and an endoscope was inserted along the long axis of the clot until its posterior aspect was reached. The hematoma was aspirated with continuous irrigation, using a single pass without lateral manipulation of the endoscope to minimize trauma to the cortex. ▶ Fig. 23.2 demonstrates the intraoperative configuration of the equipment that was used. Postoperative imaging indicated near-complete hematoma evacuation, but repeat postoperative imaging showed partial reaccumulation of hematoma without significant mass effect or midline shift (▶ Fig. 23.3a and b, respectively). ▶ Fig. 23.3c, d shows the residual hematoma and impact of the trajectory on magnetic resonance imaging. At 1- and 6-month follow-up (▶ Fig. 23.4a and b, respectively), the patient had persistent dense left hemiparesis that left her largely wheelchair bound, and imaging revealed stable encephalomalacia.

A few technical nuances must be kept in mind when performing an endoscopic evacuation of an ICH. The surgeon has

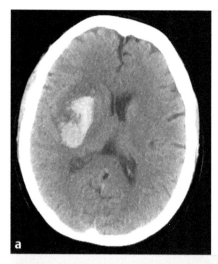 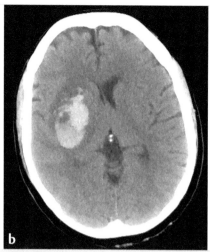 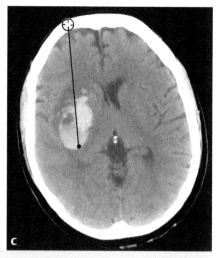

Fig. 23.1 **(a)** Preoperative axial noncontrast computed tomogram of the head showing an initial 19-mL right putaminal hematoma and **(b)** repeat imaging revealing growth to a 25-mL hematoma with **(c)** superimposed navigation trajectory. (Used with permission from Barrow Neurological Institute, Phoenix, AZ.)

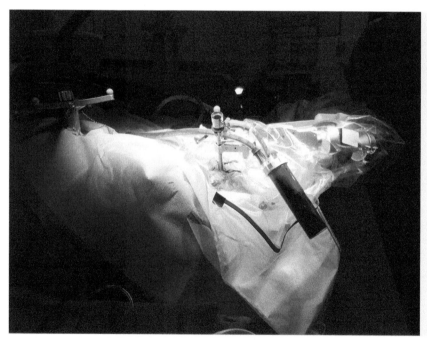

Fig. 23.2 Intraoperative view of the Frazee endoscope held in place with a Mitaka holding arm (Mitaka USA, Inc., Denver, CO), with blood aspirated under controlled wall suction into a Lukens trap (Baxter Healthcare, Deerfield, IL). (Used with permission from Barrow Neurological Institute, Phoenix, AZ.)

relatively poor visualization during the endoscopic procedure, as the endoscope is in the center of a hematoma. Irrigation is necessary to maintain some degree of visualization, but too much can be detrimental. Additionally, the goal of the surgery should not be to completely remove the hematoma, but rather to reduce mass effect and to coagulate only actively bleeding vasculature. Nonbleeding vessels in the cavity should be left alone, as they are often perforating vessels en passage. Overzealous clot removal and extensive motion of the endoscope can result in damage to otherwise intact neighboring structures, as well as potential damage to essential adjacent neurovascular structures, thereby perpetuating and propagating neural damage. The goal of surgery in this patient was not necessarily to reverse her neurologic deficit, but rather to reduce the mass effect of the growing hematoma and to preserve the patient's mental status.

23.1.7 Patient Selection for ICH Endoscopic Evacuation

As highlighted by the case illustration, the few indications for stereotactic endoscopic hematoma evacuation include hemorrhages with clinical deficit and mass effect and/or increasing size. Both large and deep-seated hemorrhages can be safely addressed with endoscopy without additional detriment to surrounding structures.

Surgical intervention for a spontaneous ICH can reduce mass effect and secondary injury to surrounding neurovascular structures. Additionally, use of the endoscope can substantially minimize the surgical footprint in hematoma evacuation without increasing the morbidity found with open approaches. Ultimately, as with any intervention, patient selection is of paramount importance, especially with respect to each patient's

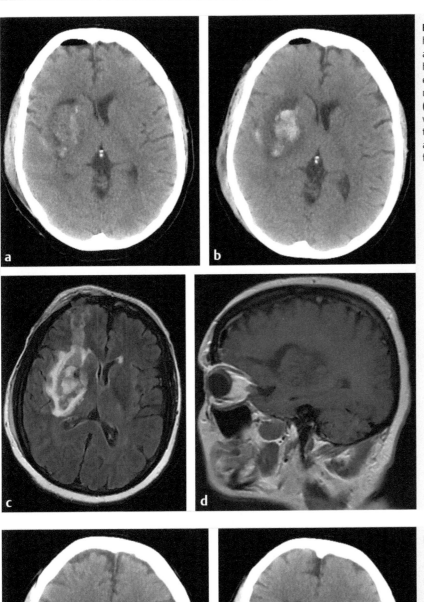

Fig. 23.3 (a) Postoperative axial noncontrast head computed tomogram (CT) taken immediately after surgery showing right basal ganglia hematoma evacuation and reduction of mass effect. (b) CT obtained 2 hours later shows partial reaccumulation of the hematoma. Postoperative (c) axial T2-weighted and (d) sagittal T1-weighted magnetic resonance images show a type A tract of the endoscope along the long access of the hematoma. (Used with permission from Barrow Neurological Institute, Phoenix, AZ.)

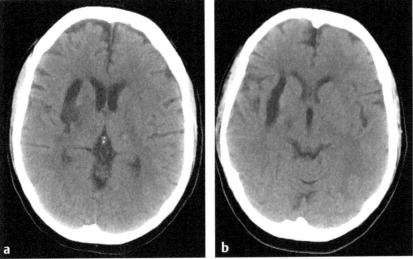

Fig. 23.4 Axial noncontrast computed tomography images of the head performed (a) at 1-month follow-up and (b) at 6-month follow-up show chronic encephalomalacia in the right basal ganglia. (Used with permission from Barrow Neurological Institute, Phoenix, AZ.)

unique pathological anatomy. In select patients, minimally invasive techniques, such as stereotactic endoscopic-assisted approaches, can be used to remove spontaneous ICHs, which can lead to clinical improvement. Although this endoscopic procedure remains controversial, we believe that the current use of endoscopic or minimally invasive surgery is preferable to open, traditional craniotomy for clot evacuation.

References

[1] Mendelow AD, Gregson BA, Fernandes HM, et al. STICH investigators. Early surgery versus initial conservative treatment in patients with spontaneous supratentorial intracerebral haematomas in the International Surgical Trial in Intracerebral Haemorrhage (STICH): a randomised trial. Lancet. 2005; 365 (9457):387–397

[2] Broderick JP. The STICH trial: what does it tell us and where do we go from here? Stroke. 2005; 36(7):1619–1620

[3] Bhattathiri PS, Gregson B, Prasad KS, Mendelow AD, Investigators S, STICH Investigators. Intraventricular hemorrhage and hydrocephalus after spontaneous intracerebral hemorrhage: results from the STICH trial. Acta Neurochir Suppl (Wien). 2006; 96:65–68

[4] Mendelow AD, Gregson BA, Rowan EN, Murray GD, Gholkar A, Mitchell PM, STICH II Investigators. Early surgery versus initial conservative treatment in patients with spontaneous supratentorial lobar intracerebral haematomas (STICH II): a randomised trial. Lancet. 2013; 382(9890):397–408

[5] Morgan T, Zuccarello M, Narayan R, Keyl P, Lane K, Hanley D. Preliminary findings of the minimally-invasive surgery plus rtPA for intracerebral hemorrhage evacuation (MISTIE) clinical trial. Acta Neurochir Suppl (Wien). 2008; 105:147–151

[6] Mould WA, Carhuapoma JR, Muschelli J, et al. MISTIE Investigators. Minimally invasive surgery plus recombinant tissue-type plasminogen activator for intracerebral hemorrhage evacuation decreases perihematomal edema. Stroke. 2013; 44(3):627–634

[7] Fiorella D, Mocco J, Arthur A. Intracerebral hemorrhage: the next frontier for minimally invasive stroke treatment. J Neurointerv Surg. 2016; 8(10):987–988

[8] Zhou X, Chen J, Li Q, et al. Minimally invasive surgery for spontaneous supratentorial intracerebral hemorrhage: a meta-analysis of randomized controlled trials. Stroke. 2012; 43(11):2923–2930

[9] Zhou H, Zhang Y, Liu L, et al. A prospective controlled study: minimally invasive stereotactic puncture therapy versus conventional craniotomy in the treatment of acute intracerebral hemorrhage. BMC Neurol. 2011; 11:76

[10] Barnes B, Hanley DF, Carhuapoma JR. Minimally invasive surgery for intracerebral haemorrhage. Curr Opin Crit Care. 2014; 20(2):148–152

[11] Auer LM, Deinsberger W, Niederkorn K, et al. Endoscopic surgery versus medical treatment for spontaneous intracerebral hematoma: a randomized study. J Neurosurg. 1989; 70(4):530–535

[12] Kuo LT, Chen CM, Li CH, et al. Early endoscope-assisted hematoma evacuation in patients with supratentorial intracerebral hemorrhage: case selection, surgical technique, and long-term results. Neurosurg Focus. 2011; 30(4):E9

[13] Yamashiro S, Hitoshi Y, Yoshida A, Kuratsu J. Effectiveness of endoscopic surgery for comatose patients with large supratentorial intracerebral hemorrhages. Neurol Med Chir (Tokyo). 2015; 55(11):819–823

[14] Wang WH, Hung YC, Hsu SP, et al. Endoscopic hematoma evacuation in patients with spontaneous supratentorial intracerebral hemorrhage. J Chin Med Assoc. 2015; 78(2):101–107

[15] Nagasaka T, Tsugeno M, Ikeda H, Okamoto T, Inao S, Wakabayashi T. Early recovery and better evacuation rate in neuroendoscopic surgery for spontaneous intracerebral hemorrhage using a multifunctional cannula: preliminary study in comparison with craniotomy. J Stroke Cerebrovasc Dis. 2011; 20 (3):208–213

[16] Vespa P, Hanley D, Betz J, et al. ICES Investigators. ICES (Intraoperative Stereotactic Computed Tomography-Guided Endoscopic Surgery) for brain hemorrhage: a multicenter randomized controlled trial. Stroke. 2016; 47(11):2749–2755

[17] Rennert RC, Signorelli JW, Abraham P, Pannell JS, Khalessi AA. Minimally invasive treatment of intracerebral hemorrhage. Expert Rev Neurother. 2015; 15 (8):919–933

[18] Cho DY, Chen CC, Chang CS, Lee WY, Tso M. Endoscopic surgery for spontaneous basal ganglia hemorrhage: comparing endoscopic surgery, stereotactic aspiration, and craniotomy in noncomatose patients. Surg Neurol. 2006; 65 (6):547–555, discussion 555–556

[19] Spiotta AM, Fiorella D, Vargas J, et al. Initial multicenter technical experience with the Apollo device for minimally invasive intracerebral hematoma evacuation. Neurosurgery. 2015; 11 Suppl 2:243–251, discussion 251

[20] Labib MA, Shah M, Kassam AB, et al. The safety and feasibility of image-guided BrainPath-mediated transsulcul hematoma evacuation: a multicenter study. Neurosurgery. 2017; 80(4):515–524

[21] Pantazis G, Tsitsopoulos P, Mihas C, Katsiva V, Stavrianos V, Zymaris S. Early surgical treatment vs conservative management for spontaneous supratentorial intracerebral hematomas: a prospective randomized study. Surg Neurol. 2006; 66(5):492–501, discussion 501–502

[22] Morgenstern LB, Demchuk AM, Kim DH, Frankowski RF, Grotta JC. Rebleeding leads to poor outcome in ultra-early craniotomy for intracerebral hemorrhage. Neurology. 2001; 56(10):1294–1299

24 Approaches to Brainstem Cavernous Malformations: Microscope

Hasan A. Zaidi and Robert F. Spetzler

Summary

Brainstem cavernous malformations are deep-seated, low-flow vascular lesions that are surrounded by important nuclei and tracts. Surgical resection of these lesions were once considered impossible. Over the last few decades, a greater understanding of brainstem anatomy, combined with novel approaches and surgical tools, has allowed surgeons safe and effective access to these lesions. In our experience, we have found that safe and effective resection of brainstem cavernomas requires a detailed understanding of the brainstem safe entry zones. For lesions within the pons, the lateral medullary zone accessed through a retrosigmoid craniotomy under microscopic magnification provides a true and tested approach. In this chapter, we summarize and describe our institutional experience in the surgical management of these lesions.

Keywords: brainstem, cavernous malformation, microsurgical, resection, safe entry zones

24.1 Microsurgical Perspective

24.1.1 Introduction

The brainstem contains a complex and interconnected web of nuclei and fibers within a small cross-sectional area. For well into the 20th century, intrinsic brainstem lesions were considered inoperable because many in the neurosurgical community believed this region was intolerant of surgical manipulation and dissection. As surgical tools improved along with a greater understanding of the microsurgical anatomy of the brainstem, some pioneering neurosurgeons, such as Lassiter et al in 1971, began to advocate surgical intervention for lesions previously considered inoperable.[1] The development of high-resolution neuroimaging and the introduction of image guidance to the neurosurgical community allowed the surgical treatment of brainstem lesions to become reproducible, reliable, and safe. The current ability to successfully treat these lesions is largely due to the aggregation of multiple advances in various disciplines over the last century. Nowhere are these approaches more efficacious in improving the quality of life than in patients who harbor brainstem cavernous malformations. Surgical approaches to these lesions require a detailed knowledge of the main safe entry zones to the brainstem. These zones contain relatively few eloquent structures and perforating blood vessels; as a result, they permit access to the lesion while minimizing the risk of permanent neurological morbidity. The safe entry zone used always dictates the preferred surgical approach for any given lesion. For lesions located within the pons or medulla, this almost always necessitates a posterolateral entry point.[2]

24.1.2 Case Example of a Contentious Pathology

History/Physical Examination

A 34-year-old woman presented to our institute with a 2-week history of right arm and leg weakness, tingling, balance difficulties, dysarthria, headache, diplopia, and dysphagia. She had no clinically relevant past medical history and was otherwise healthy. On neurological examination, she was found to have dense right-sided hemiparesis, a right facial droop, dysarthria, and poor left palatal elevation, but was otherwise neurologically intact. Magnetic resonance imaging revealed a well-circumscribed ventral pontine mass at the level of the internal auditory canal slightly eccentric to the left (▶ Fig. 24.1). A posterolateral approach via the lateral pontine brainstem safe entry zone was judged to be the ideal entry point to access this brainstem lesion. Although the lesion came closest to the surface anteriorly, it was believed that a ventral approach to this mass would place the patient's corticospinal tracts and basilar perforating vessels at risk of iatrogenic injury because the pyramids were deviated ventromedially by the lesion. In addition, when an anterior approach is used, the basilar artery perforators are often draped over areas of the anticipated myelotomy. Approaching lesions in this anatomical position via the lateral

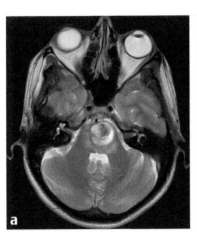
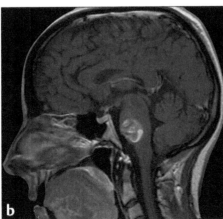

Fig. 24.1 **(a)** Preoperative axial T2-weighted magnetic resonance imaging demonstrates an expansile ventral pontine mass at the level of the internal auditory canal and **(b)** midclivus on sagittal T1-weigted unenhanced imaging. (Used with permission from Barrow Neurological Institute, Phoenix, AZ.)

pontine zone reduces the risk of injury to the pyramids and, at this level of the mid-pons, lesions are best approached using a left retrosigmoid craniotomy.[2] After thorough discussion of the risks and benefits of surgery, the patient elected to undergo microsurgical resection of this lesion.

Intraoperative Management

The patient was placed in the prone position, and after obtaining baseline somatosensory evoked potentials and monitoring of cranial nerves V through XI, the head was rotated and flexed to the right side to provide access to the left periauricular region. The stereotactic computer-guided optical navigation system was registered using contours of the scalp, and accuracy was confirmed using known anatomical landmarks. It is imperative that image guidance is accurate because the surgeon relies on this to plan the trajectory with the shortest route to the lesion through normal brainstem. After identifying and marking the transverse and sigmoid sinuses using stereotactic navigation, a straight skin incision was performed two fingerbreadths behind the earlobe. The myofascial layer was exposed and elevated, revealing the occipitomastoid suture and the mastoid. A generous retromastoid craniotomy was then performed to expose the anterior edge of the posterior sigmoid sinus as well as the inferior edge of the transverse sinus (▶ Fig. 24.2). The dura was then opened using a V-shaped incision based at the sigmoid sinus. Next, wide, sharp dissection of arachnoid adhesions allowed for brain relaxation and created adequate working space and the release of cerebrospinal fluid from the cerebellopontine cisterns. The arachnoid membrane around the trigeminal, facial,

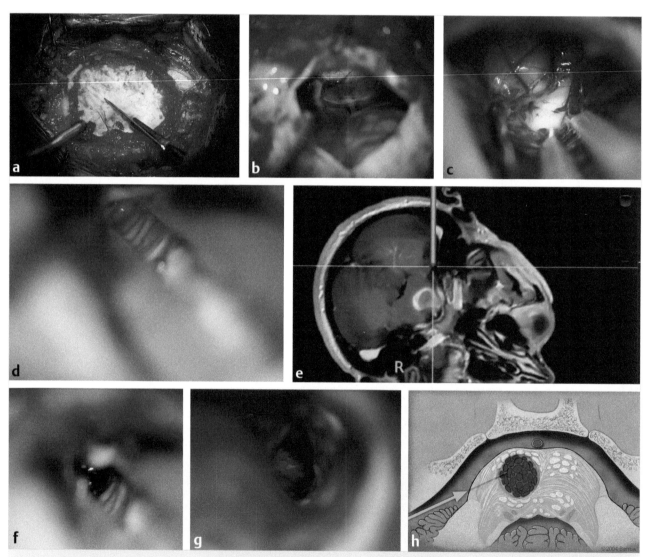

Fig. 24.2 (a) A left retrosigmoid craniotomy was performed to approach this lesion with (b) wide dissection of the arachnoid membrane to allow for maximal brain relaxation. (c) The lateral pontine zone at the level of the cranial nerve VII to VIII complex was identified and widely dissected. (d) The brainstem was entered using lighted bipolar electrocautery to improve light penetration within a deep and narrow surgical corridor after (e) intraoperative stealth guidance confirmed the ideal trajectory to the lesion. (f) The lesion was resected piecemeal, and (g) the resection cavity was circumferentially explored to confirm gross total resection of the brainstem cavernous malformation. (h) Illustration demonstrating the ideal trajectory for entry into an anteriorly situated cavernoma in the pons as in this case illustration. The entry point via the lateral pontine safe entry zone allows entry into the brainstem lateral to the motor fibers with the least possible transgression of neural tissue. (Used with permission from Barrow Neurological Institute, Phoenix, AZ.)

and vestibulocochlear nerves was sharply cut to allow exposure to identify the middle cerebellar peduncle and lateral pons. These structures provide the landmarks necessary to identify the three brainstem safe entry zones to access lesions of the ventral pons. In this particular case, given that the lesion was located relatively inferiorly in the pons, we believed that the lateral pontine zone would provide the safest trajectory through the brainstem. An entry point was planned at the level of the middle cerebellar peduncle, projecting through a point in the brainstem between the brainstem exit zones of cranial nerves VII and IX and into the center of the mass. The stereotactic navigation system was used to precisely determine the shortest trajectory to the lesion, and the middle cerebellar peduncle was entered using sharp dissection (▶ Fig. 24.2). Gentle retraction of the white matter tracts was performed until the lesion was accessed, with special attention paid to cranial nerve monitoring output, especially of cranial nerves V, VII, and VIII, in order to ensure these brainstem nuclei were not disturbed during the approach. Lighted bipolar forceps (Kogent Surgical, Chesterfield, MO) provided greater light penetration within a deep, narrow surgical corridor. When the target was reached, there was immediate release of subacute blood as a result of the previous hemorrhage. A hematoma creates a potential working space to allow the surgeon to resect the cavernous malformation piecemeal while imposing little trauma on the surrounding brainstem. It also creates a wide corridor that allows the surgeon to inspect the resection cavity for any residual lesion. After ensuring gross total resection of the mass, the dural and overlying musculocutaneous layers were closed in a standard watertight fashion.

Surgical Outcomes

The patient was successfully extubated in the operating room and transferred to the neurosurgical intensive care unit. Over the next 48 hours, her preoperative symptoms improved significantly, including the dysarthria and the facial droop. Her right-sided strength also improved, with motor examination results of 4+/5 in both upper and lower extremities. She developed no new motor or cranial nerve deficits, and she had intact hearing and normal facial sensation in the V1 through V3 distribution. She continued to suffer from balance difficulty and diplopia, which had been present preoperatively, and was given glasses with an eye patch. Immediate postoperative imaging demonstrated gross total resection of the brainstem cavernoma (▶ Fig. 24.3). She was discharged to inpatient rehabilitation therapy on postoperative day 14. At her most recent follow-up examination, she had made a significant improvement in her motor examination, with only trace weakness in her right side and some improvement in her imbalance and diplopia. She continued to wear her eye patch glasses for her diplopia. She experienced no perioperative or postoperative complications.

Between 1985 and 2014, the senior author (R.F.S.) performed microsurgical resection of brainstem cavernous malformations in a total of 397 adult patients, which represents the largest known experience in the world.[3] The male-to-female ratio was 40% male to 60% female. Of the 397 patients, 273 (69%) patients had lesions located within the pons: 59 pontomedullary (15%), 178 pontine (45%), and 36 pontomesencephalic (9%; ▶ Table 24.1). All lesions were resected using a microsurgical approach, without the aid of endoscopic visualization or ventral endonasal approaches. Between 42 and 53% of patients with pontine lesions had resolution of some or all of their preoperative symptoms, whereas 25 to 39% of patients had experienced a new postoperative cranial nerve deficit or motor nerve deficit at last follow-up. New cranial nerve neuropathies accounted for the majority of these new deficits (58%), and were often well tolerated by patients. Perioperative complications were also acceptable, with 4 (1%) perioperative mortalities and 28 (7.1%) patients with a cerebrospinal fluid leak requiring intervention. The incidence of neurological and approach-related complications improved steadily over time as the senior author's experience with the surgical and perioperative management of these lesions improved.

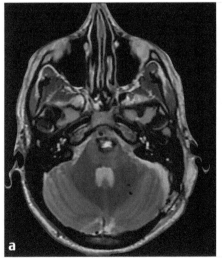
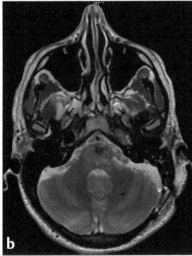

Fig. 24.3 (a) Postoperative axial T2-weighted magnetic resonance image confirms gross total resection of the pontine cavernous malformation, with (b) identification of the entry into the lateral pontine safe entry zone. (Used with permission from Barrow Neurological Institute, Phoenix, AZ.)

Table 24.1 Patient demographics and long-term follow-up of brainstem cavernous malformation patients: clinical and radiographic outcomes

BSCM location	Patients no. (%)	Mean age at admission (y)	% male/ % female	Lesion size (cm)	Clinical follow-up (mo)	Resolution of some or all pre-op symptoms no. (%)	New permanent post-op deficits no. (%)	Post-op rehemorrhage rate
Medullary	47 (12)	42.7	38/62	1.13 ± 0.43	41.7 ± 49.7	30 (64)	13 (28)	6 (13)
Pontomedullary	59 (15)	39.8	34/66	1.55 ± 0.64	30.9 ± 42.0	30 (51)	21 (36)	4 (7)
Pontine	178 (45)	42.8	42/58	1.88 ± 0.69	37.2 ± 45.9	95 (53)	69 (39)	16 (9)
Pontomesencephalic	36 (9)	40.3	56/44	2.37 ± 0.98	38.8 ± 52.0	15 (42)	9 (25)	3 (8)
Mesencephalic	77 (19)	43.3	36/64	1.80 ± 0.92	29.4 ± 35.0	35 (45)	28 (36)	4 (5)
Total	397 (100)	42.2	40/60	1.77 ± 0.79	35.5 ± 44.5	205 (52)	140 (35)	33 (8)

Abbreviations: BSCM, brainstem cavernous malformation; post-op, postoperative; pre-op, preoperative.
Source: Modified from Zaidi et al.[3]

24.1.3 Advantages of Microsurgical Approaches over Endoscopic Approaches

Cavernous malformations are angiographically occult, low-flow, and low-pressure vascular lesions, and 20% of all intracranial cavernous malformations are found in the brainstem. These lesions have a high propensity to bleed, either intralesionally or extralesionally. Repetitive hemorrhagic events create a progressive pattern of neurological decline, and many patients do not return to their prehemorrhage baseline. Resection of brainstem cavernous malformations represent one of the most complicated and potentially perilous operations performed by neurosurgeons. However, successful resection of these lesions can provide durable and potentially curable treatment of these lesions with long-lasting improvement in patients' quality of life. Successful execution of this procedure requires not only the necessary tools and a team-based effort, but also knowledge of important brainstem entry zones. The common thread among these approaches is that they rely on zones in the brainstem that (1) are relatively devoid of vascular perforators, (2) are relatively devoid of important brainstem nuclei and descending motor fiber bundles, and (3) have only a small chance of placing sensory nerves at risk of injury, which is often well tolerated (▶ Fig. 24.4, ▶ Fig. 24.5). These zones all take advantage of posterior or posterolateral exposures and avoid any ventral exposures, which are fraught with complications. For ventral pontine lesions, three well-characterized posterolateral brainstem safe entry zones are available: the peritrigeminal zone, the supratrigeminal zone, and the lateral pontine zone.[3] The peritrigeminal zone is located anterior to cranial nerve V, lateral to the corticospinal tract, and anterior to the motor and sensory nuclei of the trigeminal nerve. This approach avoids injury to the tracts of cranial nerves VI, VII, and VIII, which project inferiorly and are located posterior to the trigeminal nuclei.[4] The supratrigeminal zone is located just above the trigeminal root entry zone on the middle cerebellar peduncle.[2,5] The lateral pontine zone, as described in this case example, is found at the junction between the middle cerebellar peduncle and the pons and between the trigeminal and the facial–vestibulocochlear complex root entry zones.[6]

In our experience, ventral brainstem entry points to the pons provided by endoscopic endonasal approaches place important descending fibers at higher risk of injury. Injury to important descending corticospinal tracts can result in motor deficits that are often less well-tolerated by patients and have a greater impact on overall function and quality of life. Furthermore, due to the ventral location of the basilar artery, there is often greater risk of injury to basilar perforators because they often drape over ventral brainstem entry points. By even exposing these ventral microperforators, there is higher risk of iatrogenic injury from exposure to light from the endoscope or inadvertent manipulation, which can lead to vasospasm. For these reasons, we do not employ ventral brainstem exposures to access these lesions in our practice.

In addition to the poor brainstem entry points available via a ventral exposure, endoscopic endonasal approaches to the brainstem carry numerous inherent disadvantages compared to the microscopic approach. Brainstem lesions necessitate absolute surgical freedom and surgical dexterity in order to successfully execute the approach and resect mass-occupying lesions. Microsurgical approaches maximize both of these factors, and have been a true and time-tested method for well over three decades. Endoscopic approaches are ideal for lesions that involve *only* the soft tissue or bony structures *without involving the brain parenchyma* because surgical dexterity is not at a premium in order to effectively resect these lesions. Once intramedullary lesions are resected using the endonasal approach, the inherent instrument conflict within a narrow and deep surgical corridor does not allow one to maximize surgical dexterity. Increasing surgical exposure in order to allow more room for endonasal instruments does not increase this dexterity to any significant degree and may place the patient at higher risk of postoperative morbidity such as anosmia or cerebrospinal fluid leaks/meningitis. Furthermore, inadvertent iatrogenic vascular injury cannot be adequately managed using an endonasal approach, where the basilar artery is confrontationally exposed. This is the direct opposite situation for microsurgical approaches, where the tools and instruments needed for repair of vascular injury are readily available and familiar to the microneurosurgeon.

24.1.4 Patient Selection

Patient selection is key to achieving good surgical outcomes while mitigating potential complications.[7] Unlike other lesions, brainstem cavernomas displace rather than invade the surrounding brain, and conservative management of these lesions will naturally result in improvement of symptoms over time, until the next hemorrhagic event. Risk of surgical intervention

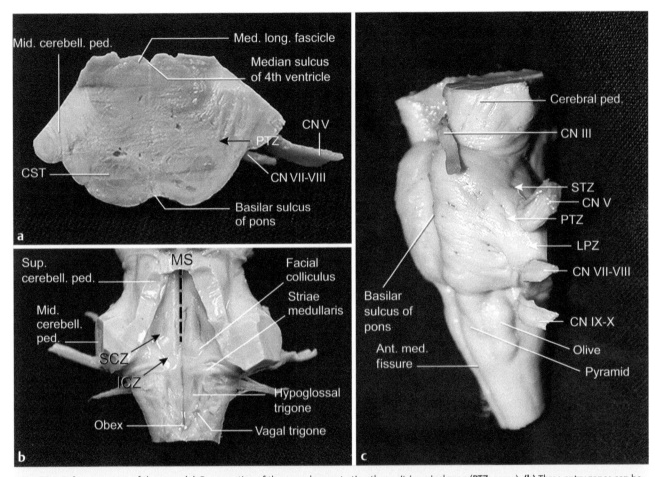

Fig. 24.4 Safe entry zones of the pons. **(a)** Cross-section of the pons demonstrating the peritrigeminal zone (PTZ; *arrow*). **(b)** Three entry zones can be used to approach the rhomboid fossa: the supracollicular zone (SCZ; *arrow*), the infracollicular zone (ICZ; *arrow*), and the median sulcus of the fourth ventricle (MS; *dashed line*). **(c)** The safe entry zones (*arrows*) for excising lateral and anterolateral pontine lesions: the supratrigeminal zone (STZ), the PTZ, and the lateral pontine zone (LPZ). Ant. med., anterior median; CST, corticospinal tract; med. long., medial longitudinal; mid. cerebell., middle cerebellar; ped., peduncle; sup. cerebell., superior cerebellar. (Adapted from Cavalcanti et al.[2])

must be balanced with the inherent risk of hemorrhage of brainstem cavernous malformations, which is reported to be from 0.25 to 2.3% per year.[7] Many authors suggest that infratentorial cavernomas have a higher rate of hemorrhage than previously reported, but due to the relative rarity of these lesions, the cause for this higher rate is unknown.[7] Surgical resection of cavernous malformations can result in new deficits related to the approach, and manipulation of the brainstem often mimics a hemorrhagic event that tends to improve over time. For this reason, we extensively counsel the patient on the risk of new neurological deficits after surgery, with the hope that these symptoms will improve over time and with the goal of preventing future bleeding episodes.[7]

Several factors are known to predict improved functional recovery after microsurgical resection of brainstem cavernomas, including younger age, smaller lesion size, lack of prior hemorrhage, and good preoperative functional status.[8,9,10] Grading scales have also been previously described to assist in identifying demographic and radiographic parameters that predict outcome after surgical intervention. These parameters include patient age, lesion size, presence of a developmental venous anomaly, extension of lesion across the midline, and acuity of hemorrhage. Lesions that approach the brain surface provide a natural corridor to resect brainstem cavernous malformations. However, the degree of brain overlying the potential entry point may be misleading in magnetic resonance images, and special attention to safe brainstem entry zones must still be taken into account.

The acuity of hemorrhage and the timing of intervention remain controversial. Some authors have suggested that delaying surgical resection after a recent intralesional or extralesional hemorrhage may allow the brain to "cool off" and rebound before surgical resection is performed.[3] As with any other mass-occupying lesion, evidence suggests that early resection after a hemorrhagic event may improve surgical outcomes.[3] Our group recently reviewed our experience with early intervention after a recent hemorrhage, and we found that patients treated within 6 weeks of hemorrhage experienced improved clinical outcomes compared to those treated more than 6 weeks after hemorrhage.[3] As demonstrated in the case example, early surgical intervention in the presence of a clot creates a natural working window to allow the surgeon to inspect the cavity in order to ensure gross total resection of the mass. For this reason, we have found that, paradoxically, resection of brainstem cavernous malformations in the acute phase is actually technically less challenging.

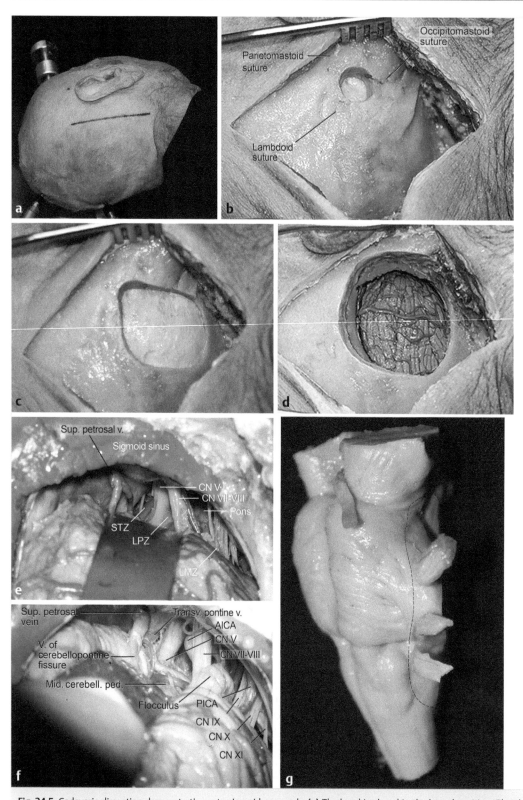

Fig. 24.5 Cadaveric dissection demonstrating retrosigmoid approach. **(a)** The head is placed in the lateral position. The skin incision is usually placed two fingerbreadths behind the pinna. **(b)** A bur hole is drilled just cranial to the asterion, on the parietomastoid suture. **(c)** The craniotomy is started in a **C**-shaped line. The posterior edge of the sigmoid sinus, as well as the transverse–sigmoid junction, is skeletonized. **(d)** The dura is opened and the cerebellar surface is exposed. **(e)** The microsurgical dissection starts along the petrosal surface of the cerebellum, reaching the cerebellopontine cistern. This approach also provides access to the supratrigeminal (STZ) and the lateral pontine (LPZ) safe entry zones, but provides a suboptimal angle of attack for the peritrigeminal zone. **(f)** Lesions abutting the middle cerebellar peduncle or the lateral pontine surface can be resected using this route. **(g)** The area of exposure on the lateral brainstem (*shaded area*) produced by the retrosigmoid approach. AICA, anterior inferior cerebellar artery; LPZ, lateral pontine zone; mid. cerebell. ped., middle cerebellar peduncle; PICA, posterior inferior cerebellar artery; STZ, supratrigeminal zone; sup., superior; transv., transverse; v, vein. (*cont.*)

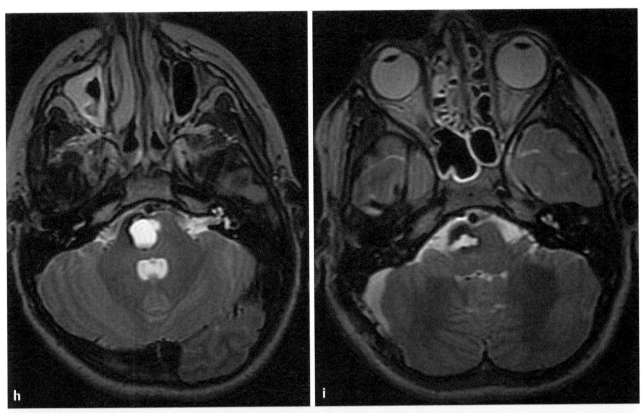

Fig 24.5 (*cont.*) Cadaveric dissection demonstrating retrosigmoid approach. **(h,i)** A pontomedullary cavernous malformation in a 10-year-old boy was approached via a retrosigmoid approach through the lateral medullary zone. (Adapted from Cavalcanti et al.[2])

24.1.5 Complication Avoidance

As our experience with treating brainstem cavernous malformations has grown, our current practice has evolved from relying on large extensive skull base approaches to more tailored and precise approaches to these lesions. These large exposures increase the risk of perioperative surgical morbidity and complications, and are largely unnecessary for the great majority of pontine lesions. Despite this evolution, the same surgical principles apply, including wide surgical exposure to allow for maximal light penetration and visualization, maximizing surgical freedom, and minimal use of brain retraction. We use a modified version of the 2-point method in order to plan surgery. This consists of creating a line connecting a point in the center of the lesion and a point at which the lesion comes closest to the surface of the brainstem. This line is then extrapolated to the calvarial surface and dictates the craniotomy and exposure. As in our case example, an eccentric anterior pontine lesion using a 2-point method would suggest a lateral transpetrous approach. However, with a modified extended retrosigmoid approach and wide arachnoid dissection, a similar trajectory as illustrated in this case can be achieved. In our experience, this approach does not compromise patient safety and reduces approach-related morbidity. For patients with anterolateral brainstem lesions, an orbitozygomatic approach can allow safe access lateral to the cerebellar peduncle.

24.1.6 Technical Nuances/Clinical Pearls

Several important technical nuances are necessary in order to safely approach and resect brainstem cavernous malformations. First, we routinely monitor somatosensory evoked potentials, motor evoked potentials, and cranial nerves adjacent to the area of the anticipated corticectomy. We do not use more extensive invasive physiological monitoring, such as motor mapping, because we believe that a detailed understanding of neuroanatomy is of paramount importance, and these images do not provide any new information. Lateral entry points using the aforementioned brainstem safe entry points are always used. We always use the smallest cortical opening possible, just large enough to accommodate bipolar forceps and a suction device. As demonstrated in the case illustration, we have found that lighted bipolar forceps and suction devices allow greater light penetration into the small resection cavity and tremendously aid the surgeon in inspecting for any residual lesion. After the corticectomy has been made, the fibers within the brainstem are dissected in a vertical, rather than a horizontal, orientation in order to stretch the brainstem fibers without disrupting them. This maneuver allows the entry into the brainstem to be well tolerated by the patient, even in the case of deep-seated intrinsic lesions.

Operative computer image guidance is of great importance for safely and effectively approaching these lesions. It assists the surgeon in situations where the cavernous malformation does not reach the pial surface, and there is no hemosiderin staining to help determine the ideal brainstem entry point. Image guidance is also useful when brainstem cavernous malformation surgery requires a transtentorial trajectory in supracerebellar infratentorial approaches for midbrain cavernous malformations.

References

[1] Lassiter KR, Alexander E, Jr, Davis CH, Jr, Kelly DL, Jr. Surgical treatment of brain stem gliomas. J Neurosurg. 1971; 34(6):719–725

[2] Cavalcanti DD, Preul MC, Kalani MY, Spetzler RF. Microsurgical anatomy of safe entry zones to the brainstem. J Neurosurg. 2016; 124(5):1359–1376

[3] Zaidi HA, Mooney MA, Levitt MR, Dru AB, Abla AA, Spetzler RF. Impact of timing of intervention among 397 consecutively treated brainstem cavernous malformations. Neurosurgery. 2017; 81(4):620–626

[4] Recalde RJ, Figueiredo EG, de Oliveira E. Microsurgical anatomy of the safe entry zones on the anterolateral brainstem related to surgical approaches to cavernous malformations. Neurosurgery. 2008; 62(3) Suppl 1:9–15, discussion 15–17

[5] Hebb MO, Spetzler RF. Lateral transpeduncular approach to intrinsic lesions of the rostral pons. Neurosurgery. 2010; 66(3) Suppl Operative:26–29, discussion 29

[6] Baghai P, Vries JK, Bechtel PC. Retromastoid approach for biopsy of brain stem tumors. Neurosurgery. 1982; 10(5):574–579

[7] Abla AA, Lekovic GP, Turner JD, de Oliveira JG, Porter R, Spetzler RF. Advances in the treatment and outcome of brainstem cavernous malformation surgery: a single-center case series of 300 surgically treated patients. Neurosurgery. 2011; 68(2):403–414, discussion 414–415

[8] Li D, Hao SY, Jia GJ, Wu Z, Zhang LW, Zhang JT. Hemorrhage risks and functional outcomes of untreated brainstem cavernous malformations. J Neurosurg. 2014; 121(1):32–41

[9] Chotai S, Qi S, Xu S. Prediction of outcomes for brainstem cavernous malformation. Clin Neurol Neurosurg. 2013; 115(10):2117–2123

[10] Pandey P, Westbroek EM, Gooderham PA, Steinberg GK. Cavernous malformation of brainstem, thalamus, and basal ganglia: a series of 176 patients. Neurosurgery. 2013; 72(4):573–589, discussion 588–589

25 Approaches to Brainstem Cavernous Malformations: Endoscope

Srikant Chakravarthi, Juanita Celix, Sammy Khalili, Melanie Fukui, Jonathan Jennings, Martin Corsten, Richard Rovin, and Amin Kassam

Summary

Cavernous malformations of the brainstem can result in symptoms from intralesions or extralesional hemorrhage. Surgical intervention has traditionally involved open posterior or posterolateral microsurgical techniques. In this chapter, we describe endoscopic ventromedial approaches as well as safe surgical corridors to brainstem cavernous malformations.

Keywords: brainstem, cavernous malformations, vascular malformation, cavernous angiomas, endoscopic, expanded endonasal

25.1 Endoscopic Perspective

25.1.1 Case Example

History and Patient Presentation

In an effort to better illustrate the concept of the endoscopic approach to the clivus, we review a case of a 39-year-old male who presented to our neurosurgical service with a sudden onset of headache and right arm weakness. Magnetic resonance imaging (MRI) subsequently revealed a hyperintense signal enhancement within the ventral pons, consistent with a cavernous malformation (cavernoma; ▶ Fig. 25.1**a, b**). Over the next several days, the patient developed rapid somatotopic neurological deterioration, including further worsening of his right upper motor neuron facial, followed by arm and leg weakness. This was followed by complete right-sided hemiplegia, facial nerve paralysis, abducens nerve palsy, and significant dysphagia and drooling. Despite the administration of mannitol and Decadron, the patient experienced further deterioration. His bulbar function had deteriorated to the point of consideration of tracheostomy and percutaneous feeding tube. The decision was made to proceed with surgical resection. In order to decide on a suitable surgical corridor to access this lesion, a diffusion tensor imaging MRI (DTI-MRI) with high-resolution tractography was obtained, which demonstrated displacement of the corticospinal tracts posterolaterally (▶ Fig. 25.1**c**). Due to the position of these tracts, a decision was made to access the lesion via an anteromedial ventral corridor, specifically the expanded endoscopic endonasal approach (EEA).

Intraoperative Management

The surgery was performed in two stages. Intraoperative neurophysiological monitoring and neuronavigation was used throughout both stages. The first stage consisted of creation of a right-sided posteriorly based Hadad–Bassagaisteguy nasoseptal flap (NSF). A right-sided maxillary antrostomy was then undertaken in order to store the NSF within the maxilla during the clivectomy and resection phases. This protected the flap during drilling. A lateral wall flap was also raised on the contralateral side to increase the amount of vascularized tissue available for reconstruction given the extensive exposure, and in particular,

the internal carotid artery (ICA) transposition that was eventually required. It is imperative to cover the ICA with vascularized tissue whenever possible following transposition and removal of the overlying bone. A posterior septectomy was then performed. A reverse flap was raised from the left side to reconstruct the denuded right anterior septum. The vomer was then removed and a wide bilateral sphenoidotomy was created. Furthermore, the nasopharyngeal mucosa was resected and the longus capitis muscle was removed, exposing the craniocervical junction. Using a high-speed drill with a 4-mm coarse hybrid drill bit, a wide bilateral clivectomy was created. Having completed the exposure, this marked the end of stage 1. Thus, the NSF and lateral wall flap were placed along the ventral skull base, including the region of the clivus.

The second stage began the following day, with re-elevation of the NSF and lateral wall flaps, which were again rotated into their respective maxillary sinuses. During the analysis of the preoperative CT angiography (CTA)/diffusion-weighted imaging (DWI)/tractography imaging, it was noted that there was a very small paramedian window between the posteromedially located basilar artery and the anterolaterally located left ICA. The ICA is in a more anterior sagittal plane; however, in the coronal plane the ability to work between them can be restrictive. Therefore, to augment this working corridor, the left ICA, especially at the level of the petroclival carotid segment, was skeletonized and translocated laterally. This was accomplished using the technique we have described previously,[1] but the sequence is described in brief here. The key first step is isolation of the vidian nerve, which is drilled and traced posteriorly in the 3 o'clock to the 9 o'clock position fashion.[2] This is followed by locating the junction of the foramen lacerum and the petrous segment of the ICA. Next, the Eustachian tube and torus tubarius is isolated and transected to expose the subpetrous portion of the ICA. The cartilage of the torus tubarius is now followed superiorly until it blends with the cartilage of the foramen lacerum. This marks the inferomedial boundary of the ICA. At this point, the bone over the ICA is egg shelled and removed. Finally, Meckel's diverticulum is exposed and the overlying bone is removed to allow for a lateral displacement of the ICA.[3]

Following this, the previous panclivectomy was reexamined and the two exposures were then connected. Neuronavigation was used to confirm the position and level of the pontine cavernous malformation. As a part of the routine opening of the pontine dura, venous bleeding was encountered but was successfully controlled with bipolar cauterization, hemostatic packing, and patience. Upon examining the surface of the pons, a clear demarcation of the region of the cavernoma could not be identified. The presumed location of the cavernoma was identified using navigation. The basilar was identified and now the untethered left ICA was mobilized laterally in order to expand the working corridor. A small perforator-free region was identified. Based on the preplanned trajectory, due to the posterolateral displacement of the corticospinal tracts, a small

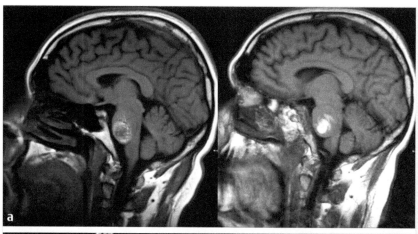

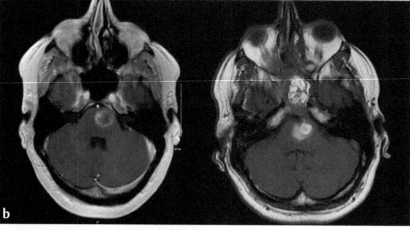

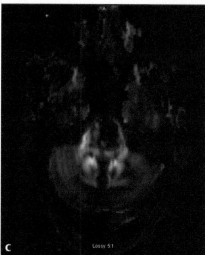

Fig. 25.1 **(a)** Sagittal T1-weighted magnetic resonance imaging (MRI) demonstrating a heterogeneously T1 hyperintense lesion in the ventral pons. Signal characteristics suspicious for a cavernous malformation. **(b)** Axial MRI T1-weighted imaging of the same lesion as in **(a)**. **(c)** Color directionally encoded DTI (diffusion tensor imaging) demonstrating signal void in the left ventral pons represents the cavernous malformation. Note the contralateral corticospinal tract in its normal projection fiber orientation (*blue*) and the posterolateral displacement and transverse rotation of the ipsilateral corticospinal tract, thereby appearing *red*. Note the thinned out ventral cerebellar peduncle fibers on the ipsilateral side.

anterior pontotomy was made in this corridor. It should be noted that at this paramedian level, the primary intrapontine fiber tracts are those of the cerebellar peduncle. While these fibers travel horizontally, we still prefer to make the pontotomy vertically. This is because if for some reason we have traveled to the deep underlying corticospinal tracts, traveling vertically will spread these critical fibers, rather than transect them.

Upon entering the pons, the cavernous malformation was in fact located anteriorly. Circumferential dissection was undertaken and the lesion was removed. Based on tractography, and the posterolaterally located corticospinal tracts, a decision was made to leave a small portion of the hematoma in front of these tracts (▶ Fig. 25.2).

Surgical Outcome

Postoperatively, the patient gradually experienced resolution of his neurological signs and symptoms. Interestingly, this occurred in a remarkable somatotopic fashion: the upper motor neuron facial weakness, right hand, right arm, right foot, and finally the right leg. The patient eventually recovered complete motor strength power graded at 5/5. With respect to the cranial

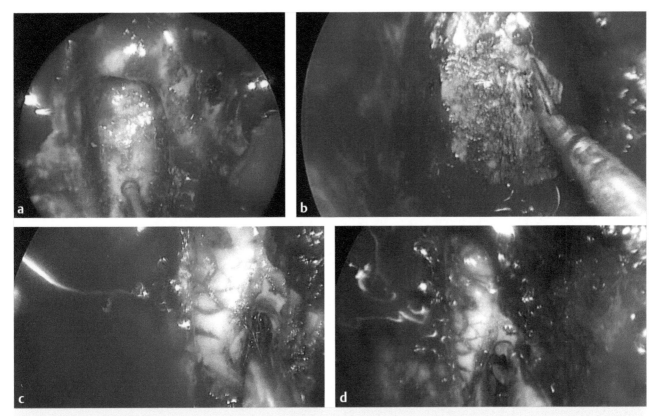

Fig. 25.2 (a) Intraoperative endoscopic view demonstrating resection and drilling of the clivus in between the two paraclival carotid arteries and below the sella. (b) Intraoperative endoscopic view showing the paramedian dural opening of the clival dura. (c) Intraoperative endoscopic view demonstrating the paramedian ventral pontotomy. Note the vertical orientation and dissection through the ventrally located cerebellar peduncle fibers and location of the underlying cavernoma. (d) Intraoperative endoscopic view demonstrating resection of cavernoma intrinsic to the left paramedian pons.

nerves, the recovery occurred with IX, X, and XII followed by the abducens nerve. Follow-up scans showed a small residual clot posteriorly (▶ Fig. 25.3), and the patient's 1-year follow-up displayed no evidence of rehemorrhage and there was complete resolution of preoperative deficits.

25.1.2 Consideration of the Endoscopic Approach

In considering approaches to skull base, we have found it useful organize a modular set of corridors, starting from the outside inward:

- *External corridor*: soft-tissue envelope and osseous framework from the skin to the dura.
- *Internal corridor*: the intradural space, that is, cistern, vasculature, or parenchyma between the dura and the pathological target.
- *Precision zone*: immediate neurovascular structures adjacent to the target, usually the cranial nerves or white matter tracts and local vasculature.

In general, the skull base can be accessed using four primary external corridors or approaches: anteromedial, anterolateral, lateral, and posterolateral. We have described this modular skull base approach as 360-degree surgery.[4,5] Over the last decade, we have strongly advocated for choosing the appropriate corridor, largely depending on the location of the pathology in

relation to the precision zone and, in particular, the cranial nerves. This, by extension, includes careful consideration of white matter tracts for resection of intraparenchymal lesions. Explicitly stated, in the majority of cases, mobilization of most soft-tissue envelopes are tolerated and overlying bone can be drilled. Furthermore, arteries can in general be transposed and manipulated. However, based on our perspective, the guiding principle behind corridor-based surgery is that transgressing the plane of nerves should be avoided whenever possible, as they represent the most vulnerable structures that can impact long-term quality of life for the patient (▶ Fig. 25.4a, b). Pathologies that arise from the ventral skull base, including meningiomas, chondrosarcomas, and chordomas, grow basally (or medially) and in turn often displace nerves laterally along their dorsal perimeter. With respect to lesions that are intraparenchymal, we consider the critical white matter tracts as essentially endophytic cranial nerves—that is, they represent discrete fiber bundles that carry afferent and efferent information along the central nervous system.

With respect to the external corridor of the clivus, we have previously categorized the ventral clivus into three segments, that is, upper, middle, and lower with their respective cisterns: interpeduncular, prepontine, and premedullary. We consider the anteromedial ventral external corridor, that is, expanded endonasal approach, viable for lesions located within these three segments of the clivus as long as the lesion is medial to the cranial nerves that are located in the respective cisterns of

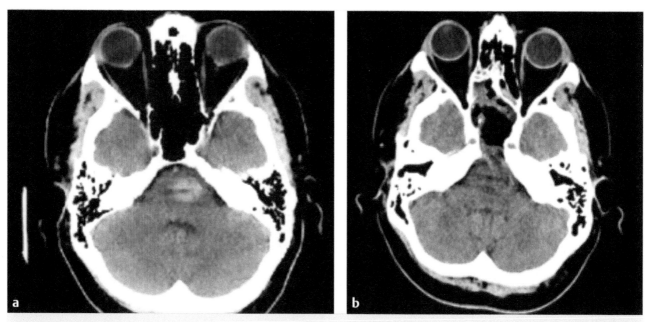

Fig. 25.3 Preoperative **(a)** and postoperative **(b)** axial computed tomography sections demonstrate transclival EEA approach with total resection of cavernous malformation. Note no residual high attenuation to indicate residual cavernoma or postoperative hemorrhage.

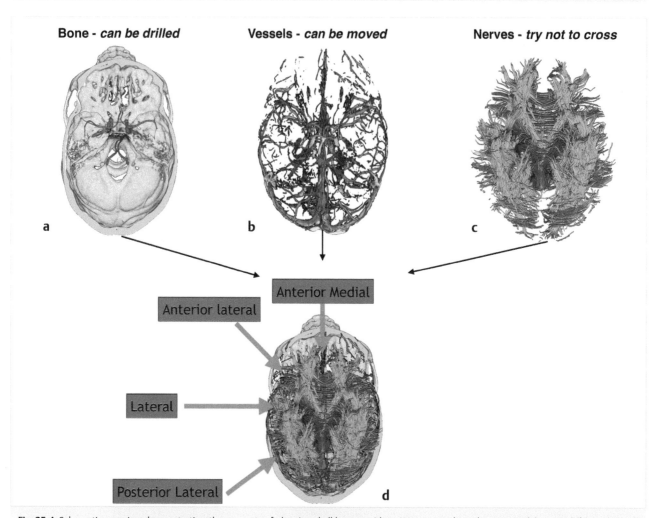

Fig. 25.4 Schematic overview demonstrating the concepts of planning skull base corridors. We can combine the osseous **(a)**, arterial **(b)**, and neural **(c)** constructs for each patient and build a 3D anatomical and surgically usable framework to decide the proper working corridor **(d)**.

these segments, that is, the 3rd, 6th, and 12th cranial nerves, respectively.

In order to approach either intradural or extradural lesions of the clivus or posterior fossa, midline panclival or modular segmental (upper, mid, or lower third) transclival approaches can be implemented (▸ Fig. 25.5); we have extensively described this previously.[6,7] In addition, some craniopharyngiomas and pituitary adenomas can descend from the sellar and suprasellar areas into the interpeduncular cistern behind the upper third of the clivus, and therefore require a modular transclival approach for complete resection. It should be noted that lesions of the upper third may require a pituitary transposition.[8] While technically challenging, we have found this to provide unprecedented exposure to the ventral portion of the interpeduncular cistern and anterior portion of the third ventricle in the precision zone below the chiasm and medial to the oculomotor nerves (▸ Fig. 25.6).

In general, lesions of the ventral brain stem are generally not amenable to any form of surgical approach. However, in the case of exophytic and encapsulated lesions, as in this case, surgery in the interpontine parenchyma was a reasonable consideration. The critical neurovascular contents in this precision zone represent the basilar artery and perforators medially, the ICA anterolaterally (as noted in the anterior sagittal plan), and the corticospinal tracts and abducens nerve posteriorly.

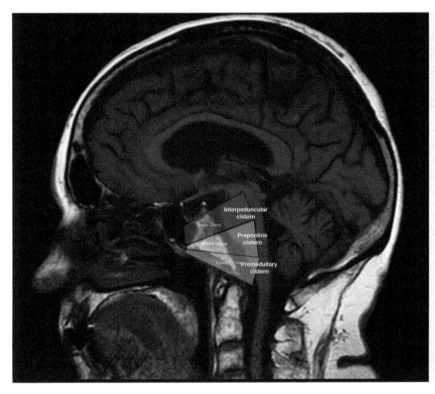

Fig. 25.5 Sagittal view demonstrating the three segments of the clivus. Upper third (*red*) extends from the sella to Dorello's canal, middle third (*blue*) extends from Dorello's canal to the jugular foramen, and lower third (*green*) extends from the jugular foramen to the craniocervical junction. The upper third, middle third, and lower third of the clivus provide access to the interpeduncular, prepontine, and premedullary cisterns, respectively.

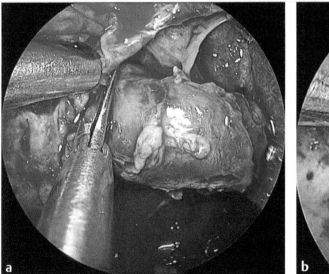
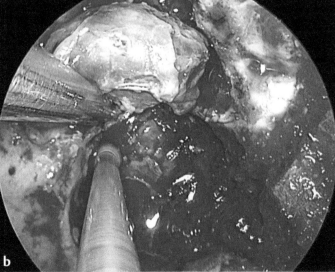

Fig. 25.6 Intraoperative endoscopic view demonstrating **(a)** isolation and transection of the right paramedian pituitary ligaments and **(b)** an intradural pituitary transposition with drilling of the dorsum sella and upper-third of the clivus.

Of these constituents, we felt the required corridor within the pons should minimize disruption of the abducens nerve, and corticospinal tract as they represent the primary determinants of permanent long-term morbidity. Given the topographic location of these structures in the precision zone, we felt that the ICA (and to a lesser extent the basilar artery) could be mobilized, the cerebellar peduncle dissected, and the corticospinal tract and abducens nerve should not be manipulated as they are the least tolerant to interaction. Given the posterolateral location of these key determinants, an orthogonal ventromedial internal corridor via an endonasal approach to the clivus and pons was selected.

In summary, based on our experience, we have come to the realization that bone can generally be drilled with little consequences and arteries can be moved with little morbidity. However, cranial nerves, and by extension white matter tracts, do not tolerate manipulation and create long-term disabilities. Therefore, in our decision algorithm in selecting operative corridors, we generally utilize the following governing rules of manipulation: soft tissue before bone, before arteries, and before nerves, and white matter tracts. By their nature, many lesions of the skull base will displace cranial nerves and tract fibers laterally. This often allows a direct, relatively safe ventromedial access to the lesion in question. Another advantage is in the case of dural-based lesions, such as clival meningiomas. It is often of importance to "devascularize" the dura early during the surgery to facilitate tumor resection.

25.1.3 The Physics of Optics

While a detailed discussion of the physics of optical systems are beyond the scope of this chapter, it is important to briefly discuss some key concepts that not only are imperative in selecting the appropriate corridor, but also have actually defined the way we undertake skull base approaches, and in particular, the external corridors required to deliver light and magnification. Conventional stereoscopic microscopes (CS-m) have a high numerical aperture (NA) that allows them to acquire light from a broad range or angle and requires them to converge this to a narrow focal point to generate the needed resolution. This creates an "ice-cream cone" effect and by definition requires a relatively large proximal external corridor to create adequate resolution at a funneled distal precision zone. This high NA by definition also creates spectral distortions lateral to any peripheral portion of the field of view (FoV) that is away from the central focal point, and in turn this distortion is directly proportional to the degree of magnification. Explicitly, the usable (centrally resolved and focused) FoV is some smaller subset of the viewable (which includes the centrally focused and peripherally distorted and blurred portions of an image) FoV with the difference being proportional to the degree of magnification applied.

In contrast, the endoscope has a lower NA, thereby delivering more parallel light and reducing the lateral spectral distortion. This thereby delivers a wider portion of the viewable FoV as a usable (focused) image. In essence, this creates a focal *plane* as opposed to a focal *point*. However, the lower NA transmits the light and image in a manner that reduces the depth of field (DoF) in comparison to CS-m. This reduced depth perception is easily recovered in endoscopy by dynamically moving the endoscope in the z-axis. This is possible in corridors such as the paranasal sinuses. We have for nearly two decades strongly advocated for dynamic endoscopic surgery, as opposed to using a traditional endoscopic holder.[9] When this is combined with the haptic feedback and proprioception of bimanual dissection, relative local positioning, which is the imperative for all 3D perception, allows for complex spatial tasks, such as carotid and pituitary transposition, as well as, brain stem perforator dissection.[8,10]

The real value of this larger and less distorted comparative FoV became evident when it was leveraged with the resolution of high-definition (HD) monitors coupled with HD cameras. The physics of optics of endoscopy now, in turn, leverages the external anteromedial corridors to leverage the paranasal sinuses to create the optimal image resolution. In addition, at the same time, we are able to reduce the soft-tissue requirements in order to capture and deliver the required light and magnification.

25.1.4 Considerations of the Microscopic Anteromedial Corridor

While beyond the scope of this chapter, it should be clearly understood that while the physics of the endoscope allow for visual optimization in the anteromedial corridor, the NA with its reduced DoF becomes a significant barrier in the anterolateral, lateral, and posterolateral corridors. The ability to dynamically move within the corridor of the paranasal sinuses allows for 3D perception and delivers a superior FoV. In contrast, the essential dynamic movement required becomes very hazardous when accessing internal corridors, which contain anatomically rich areas, such as cisterns and parenchyma associated with anterolateral and posterolateral corridors.

It should be noted that although the DoF with CS-m can be larger at low magnification, at the required higher magnification to generate a usable and resolvable intraoperative FoV, or volume of view to provide the surgeon with contextual data, it can be extremely limited using traditional microscopes and the associated convergence of light. Visualization in the anteromedial transsphenoidal corridor, in particular, can be quite limited within these deep dark surgical cavities. With the endoscopic, delivery of more parallel light does help in this regard. However, it is still limited by the fact that the endoscope needs to enter the nasal passages and the required dynamic movement within the physical boundaries of this external corridor can be encumbering.

Therefore, after nearly two decades, we have come to the conclusion that in the 360-degree skull base surgery, the use of the CS-m, or more recently, the Robotically Operated Video Optical Telescopic-microscope (ROVOT-m, Synaptive Medical Corporation, Toronto, Canada), is more suitable for the lateral (anterolateral and posterolateral) and the posterior external and internal skull base corridors. Currently, the endoscope, however, is optimal for accessing the ventral anteromedial corridor.

During the evolution of skull base surgery, there was a progressive, natural evolution of the initial anterior, lateral, and posterior external corridors to compensate for the NA of the microscope in an attempt to allow for visualization of lesions that are located more medially and ventral to the brainstem, such as within the prepontine or premedullary cisterns. Traditional attempts to reach these medial internal corridors have been simply to extend the external corridors more medially.

Explicitly, this involves drilling the osseous framework of the petrous bone with mobilization of the respective segment of the ICA. As previously described, this can be quite manageable from an external corridor perspective. If the lesion extends medially within their respective cisterns and in the precision zone, the appropriate cranial nerves now come under jeopardy. Specifically, lesions extending into the medial interpeduncular cistern now create small windows using the posterolateral external and internal corridors between the oculomotor nerve and the posterior cerebral artery. In the case of the prepontine cistern, this is now in between the superior cerebellar artery, basilar artery, and cranial nerves V to VIII. Finally, the premedullary cistern requires working between cranial nerves VI to XII and the anteroinferior cerebellar artery, posteroinferior cerebellar artery, and basilar and vertebral arteries.

Due to the efforts and limitations to develop more ventral trajectories, removal of additional medial bone became necessary, thereby giving birth to the presigmoid and anterior and posterior petrosectomies. Further efforts to develop more ventral approaches led to the development of the transcranial, extended transsphenoidal, and transoral route as the ventral external corridor approach. Several disadvantages limited the generalizability of these external corridors to the ventral skull base. In particular, the transoral external soft-tissue envelopes require disruption of the oropharynx and palate with manipulation of Passavant's ridge and the function of the constrictors that can lead to significant swallowing and velopalatine morbidity. In addition, the approaches have not been proven to be effective for intradural lesions, due to CSF leak and infection rates. The differences between the endonasal and transoral approaches are represented by the inherent differences in bacterial load and pathogens associated with the respective soft-tissue envelope. The oropharynx has a logarithmically larger and more virulent pathogen load in comparison to the nasopharynx. In addition, the learning curve of the EEA associated with construction of local pedicle-based vascularized flaps was resolved over the mid-2000s and led to the routine use of the NSF and lateral wall flap.[11,12] In fact, the infection rates were less than 2% in 1,000 consecutive cases performed by the senior author (A.K.).[13]

The transoral approach is also limited in its ability to expose the craniocervical junction and the lower third of the clivus. To access more superior segments of the middle and upper third of the clivus, additional transfacial and sublabial external corridors have been developed to overcome the limitations of this external corridor to deliver convergent light and magnification with a microscope. Efforts to extend the transnasal transsphenoidal corridor also proved to be subject to the same limitations.[14] Certainly the transracial more extensive soft-tissue external corridors have helped in providing more convergent light on the CS-m and bimanual dissection of the middle and upper third of the clivus. However, over the past decade the endoscope has progressively obviated the need for microscopic transnasal corridors. The often cited argument of the absence of 3D perception has been mitigated as increasingly more complex procedures, such as aneurysm repairs and vascular tumor dissections, have increasingly been performed via the expanded EEA. However, it should be noted that EEAs also have limitations in their caudal extensions based on the external transnasal corridor. We have explicitly described that only lesions above the nasopalatine line can be addressed via an EEA.[2,6,7,15]

25.1.5 Patient Selection

From the senior author's personal experience, which is now approaching 2,000 EEAs, it is critical to emphasize that EEA cannot be considered as the only route to the clivus. Over the past two decades, the senior author has employed all of the described corridors to the clivus based on the anatomic nuances of the lesion and the optical limitations. The decision-making process outlined earlier is based primarily on an "inside-out decision algorithm" with the following precedence in the decision algorithm: white matter tracts/cranial nerves followed by vessels followed by osseous followed by external soft-tissue envelopes. Specifically, the precision zone and the relative plane of the cranial nerve, and, by extension, the white matter tract, determine the internal (*intradural*) corridor and the eventual external (*extradural*) soft-tissue envelope is a function of this consideration coupled with the optics used. We have found that the endoscopic endonasal anteromedial approach can be utilized for a majority of lesions of the clivus. We have not found specific lesional characteristics to be prohibitive, but rather the experience of the surgeon to be a greater barrier. If the surgeon is not experienced with EEA, then considerations of vascularity of the lesion and density should be considered. We have previously published a learning curve that is recommended.[4] The one caveat to this rule that we caution the surgeon against is the treatment of intradural dermoid and epidermoid tumors, as we believe the avascular nature of these lesions can allow inoculation of the cavity with nasopharyngeal pathogens that can be difficult to eradicate despite adequate CSF closures.

25.1.6 Complication Avoidance

Selecting the optimal corridor represents the most critical step in avoiding long-term morbidity that ultimately affects the patient's quality of life. While the external corridors have short- and medium-term impact, significant cranial nerve or white matter tract injury can create permanent disabilities. Therefore, we believe that corridor selection is the most critical factor in complication avoidance. In the following section, we will review relevant nuances and technical considerations to reduce the most common complications encountered within each of the respective components of the corridors.

External Corridors

In the case of endonasal surgery, we will consider the external corridor, including soft tissue of the paranasal sinuses and osseous framework of the paranasal sinuses to the level of dura, and review the major complications and nuances to avoid them.

Cerebrospinal Fluid Leak

Unlike conventional skull base approaches, in the case of EEA, the reconstruction phase begins prior to the approach phase. Specifically, the specific vascularized flap needs to be decided upon and raised. To protect the pedicle, in general, the flap is raised from the contralateral side of ICA that needs to be transposed. For the clivus, the NSF can be short in its ability to reach down a deep cavity and this can be effectively replaced or augmented by the lateral wall flap (▸ Fig. 25.7).

Bimanual Dissection

Next, in the exposure it is important to consider removal of the inferior turbinate to reach the lower third of the clivus and the middle turbinate to reach the middle and upper thirds. This, combined with posterior septectomy, provides for an external corridor that facilitates bimanual dissection. It is equally important to reduce all of the septa within the cavity creating a smooth flat cavity permitting unencumbered movement. Perhaps the most important consideration in this regard is the creation of a "cavity and a half" in entering the external corridor. Exoscopes, such as microscopes, remain outside the cavity and do not require the same degree of exposure within the corridor. Endoscopes, on the other hand, enter the cavity and require physical space within the external corridor. Thus, the external corridor consists of a half cavity, for the endoscope, consisting of an adjacent superior sinus relative to the full working cavity representing the sinus. This allows for bimanual dissection.

Anosmia

When creating the upper extent of the external corridor, it is important to not extend the septectomy too far superiorly in order to preserve olfaction.

Venous Bleeding

In removing the osseous component of the external corridor, several considerations need to be taken into account. To access

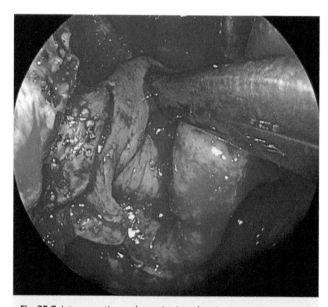

Fig. 25.7 Intraoperative endoscopic view showing reconstruction with a nasoseptal flap.

the upper third of the clivus and interpeduncular cistern, the dorsum sella and posterior clinoids have to be removed. During this phase, venous bleeding is common and is managed with hemostatic packing. The technique to perform this is beyond the scope of this chapter and the reader is referred to our previous descriptions.[4]

Internal Carotid Artery Injury

It is imperative when performing the clivectomy that the anatomic boundaries of the ICA are respected as they mark the lateral boundaries of the clivectomy. Key anatomic landmarks for each segment of the clivus are noted below:

- *Upper third*: medial opticocarotid recesses.
- *Middle third*: "medial pterygoid wedge" and the vidian artery.
- *Lower third*: Eustachian tube.

We have previously described these boundaries and presented detailed anatomic descriptions to identify them.[16,17,18] In fact, we have defined the two critical planes for endonasal skull base surgery based on the ventral course of the ICA: the sagittal plane (between the ICAs) and the coronal plane laterally. There are several key points that are worth reiterating:

- The vidian nerve needs to be respected as a critical landmark to identify the medial to inferior border of the petrous and paraclival ICA segments.
- The ICA is most vulnerable at its two most ventral and medial projections: the paraclinoidal segment at the level of the medical opticocarotid recess (mOCR) and the petroclival genu at the level of the foramen lacerum.
- During transection of the Eustachian tube, the petrous portion of the ICA is at significant risk and the scissors must be held in a horizontal plane parallel to the horizontal ICA.
- A course hybrid drill should be used and cutter drills should be avoided at all costs. The drilling should be continued until the overlying bone is egg shelled and can be flaked off. Kerrison punches should be minimized as much as possible. The periosteum of the bone and the adventitia of the ICA can be fused and the artery can be easily lacerated.
- In order to allow for lateral displacement, all of the bone lateral to the artery must be removed, especially the lingular process, which attaches to the sphenomandibular ligament.
- The artery must be completely covered with a vascularized flap at the end of the procedure to avoid dehiscence in delayed fashion due to exposure.

Osseous Instability

During removal of the lower third of the clivus, it is important to not violate the plane of the hypoglossal canal. This not only protects the hypoglossal nerve, but also precludes drilling of the lateral portion of the Occiput-C1 joint (occipital-condylar joint), thus reducing the risk of cervical instability.

Postoperative Crusting

Finally, it is very important to cover all of the denuded bone with vascularized tissue during the reconstruction to minimize postoperative crusting. This is also true for the donor site of the NSF that is covered with reverse anterior-based pedicle flap.[19]

Internal Corridors

Venous Bleeding

The space in between the periosteal and meningeal layer of the dura represents a rich venous basilar plexus. We have found that bipolar coagulation is somewhat effective; judicious use of the targeted hemostatic agents is most effective. Occasionally, this will require doing the procedure in two stages. At the level of the venous gulf, particular care should be taken to avoid overpacking and compressing the abducens nerve.

Cranial Nerves

Oculomotor

The third cranial nerve is most commonly injured in its cisternal segment as it can be tightly adherent to the arachnoid and the tumor capsule. The best way to avoid this is by undertaking an adequate exposure that allows for bimanual sharp dissection. In our experience, this requires a pituitary transposition rather than working between a small suprasellar window between the pituitary stalk, ICA, and chiasm as many others have advocated.[8]

Abducens Nerve

Understanding the course of the abducens nerve is critical. It originates just above the vertebrobasilar junction (VBJ). We have previously published that the floor of the sphenoid sinus is a critical landmark to locate the VBJ.[20] The sixth nerve then runs obliquely in the cistern and in between the two dural layers until it reaches the venous gulf where it bends laterally to form the horizontal genu. Therefore, the initial dural opening should be below the VBJ and the sixth nerve is identified and located within the cistern. The nerve is tracked under direct visualization or electrical stimulation until it enters the meningeal layer of the dura. Care is taken not to extend the dural opening lateral at this point. Heat from the bipolar can be a significant source of thermal injury.

Hypoglossal Nerve

In general, with respect to the hypoglossal canal, the supratubercular groove provides a good surrogate landmark to protect against injury.

Cerebrospinal Fluid Leak

Reconstruction of the internal corridor is critical. We perform a two-layer anatomic reconstruction starting with arachnoid using an inlay of collagen implant with a dural substitute. This is immediately followed by a vascularized flap when feasible. We prefer not to place biologics (sealants), bone grafts, and/or titanium substitute in between as they delay neovascularization and prevent osseous capillary integration of the flap. It is imperative that the flap makes complete contact everywhere with bone and no air gaps are left. If they are, the flap will quickly migrate in search for bone, contracting away from the boundary of the defect, creating delayed CSF leaks. If for some reason we cannot get complete coverage, wherein the flap cannot make continuous contact with the bone and still cover the margins of the defect, then judicious layering to build volume between the inlay graft and the flap can be used to cover the air gap. We do use lumbar drains for 72 hours for intramural civil lesions as we feel that in general we open more than two cisterns, thereby creating a high-flow leak.

Precision Zone

As discussed previously, accessing lesions of the clevis begins with selecting the optimum corridor. Additionally, restricting the dissection to the epiphytic lesions and avoiding intraparenchymal lesions are important. If intraparenchymal dissection is needed, then we generally restrict this to the pons only, as an anterior paramedian pontotomy will somatotopically require manipulation of the cerebellar peduncle, which is reasonably well tolerated. As previously pointed out, we can identify a perforator-free window and perform the pontotomy in a vertical direction despite the horizontal orientation of the peduncle fibers. We believe this is more likely to protect the more critical fibers of the vertically running predecussation corticospinal tracts located immediately posteriorly. The initial pontotomy is made above the VBJ to avoid injury to the sixth nerve.

25.1.7 Evidence and Conclusion

Over the two decades, endoscopic endonasal surgery has seen rapid advancement and evolution in its applications to skull base surgery. Initially, approaches were generally reserved only for the sellar and suprasellar lesions—most commonly being removal of pituitary tumors. We initially coined the term expanded endonasal approach in the late 1990s to embody a global collective effort by pioneers, such as Cappabianca, Frank, Stammberger, Stamm, Pesquini, Castelnuovo, and many others, that expanded approaches vertically along the clivus,[6,21] introduced the concept of the midline, transsphenoidal approach to clival and paraclival lesions, and even described the access to the ventral brainstem. More recently, in an effort to describe in more detail the approaches to middle cranial fossa and posterior fossa tumors, Prevedello et al (2010) elucidated the anatomic and surgical nuances needed for effective endonasal corridor-based surgery.[4,22]

As a corollary to this, several studies have demonstrated the safety and effectiveness of expanded EEAs to the clivus. One review conducted by Cutler et al[23] expounded on the excellent visualization, which we believe represents the difference in the physics of optics associated with endoscope previously discussed, provided in this region using the endoscope and the ability to achieve near or subtotal resections of moderately sized tumors. Fraser at al[24] commented that the transclival approach was less invasive and more direct in resection of midline clival chordomas. This is related to a greater preservation of the tissue envelope of the needed external corridor to deliver optics. In addition, following our initial resection of a ventral brain stem cavernoma in 2010, a similar case of an endoscopic transclival resection of a brainstem cavernoma was reported by Linsler and Oertel.[25] Their surgical resection also led to a successful resection with no postoperative neurological complications. CSF leak was minimal as the cranial defect was secured with a pedicled, vascularized NSF.[23,24,25]

In essence, the endonasal transclival approach provides the most direct access to lesions of the ventral brainstem, especially that of the pons. In all, the technological advancement associated with expanded endoscopic endonasal skull base surgery, including trajectory-planned, CT-DTI co-registered neuronavigation, access, and resection, has greatly improved the endoscopic approach to the clivus, resulting in a safe alternative for patients. However, we caution the reader that this represents simply one more tool in the armamentarium of the contemporary skull base surgery. We strongly urge the reader to respect the algorithm we have provided in deciding on the applicability of this approach, as it represents one of four corridors to the skull base. There has been a rapid evolution of the imaging technology that is increasing the conspicuity of the cranial nerves and white matter within an osseous and vascular framework. We are hopeful that this evolution continues as it is necessary to provide anatomic objectivity in making critical decisions that have long-term implications for our patients.

25.2 Disclosures

Amin Kassam reports involvement in Synaptive Medical (consultant), KLS Martin (consultant), and Medtronic (advisory board). Srikant Chakravarthi, Juanita Celix, Sammy Khalili, Melanie Fukui, Jonathan Jennings, Martin Corsten, and Richard Rovin have nothing to disclose.

References

[1] Labib MA, Prevedello DM, Carrau R, et al. A road map to the internal carotid artery in expanded endoscopic endonasal approaches to the ventral cranial base. Neurosurgery. 2014; 10 Suppl 3:448–471, discussion 471

[2] Kassam AB, Gardner PA, Snyderman CH, Carrau RL, Mintz AH, Prevedello DM. Expanded endonasal approach, a fully endoscopic transnasal approach for the resection of midline suprasellar craniopharyngiomas: a new classification based on the infundibulum. J Neurosurg. 2008; 108(4):715–728

[3] Kassam AB, Prevedello DM, Carrau RL, et al. The front door to meckel's cave: an anteromedial corridor via expanded endoscopic endonasal approach-technical considerations and clinical series. Neurosurgery. 2009; 64(3) Suppl: ons71–ons82, discussion ons82–ons83

[4] Kassam AB, Prevedello DM, Carrau RL, et al. Endoscopic endonasal skull base surgery: analysis of complications in the authors' initial 800 patients. J Neurosurg. 2011; 114(6):1544–1568

[5] Pirris SM, Pollack IF, Snyderman CH, et al. Corridor surgery: the current paradigm for skull base surgery. Childs Nerv Syst. 2007; 23(4):377–384

[6] Kassam A, Snyderman CH, Mintz A, Gardner P, Carrau RL. Expanded endonasal approach: the rostrocaudal axis. Part I. Crista galli to the sella turcica. Neurosurg Focus. 2005a; 19(1):E3

[7] Kassam A, Snyderman CH, Mintz A, Gardner P, Carrau RL. Expanded endonasal approach: the rostrocaudal axis. Part II. Posterior clinoids to the foramen magnum. Neurosurg Focus. 2005b; 19(1):E4

[8] Kassam AB, Prevedello DM, Thomas A, et al. Endoscopic endonasal pituitary transposition for a transdorsum sellae approach to the interpeduncular cistern. Neurosurgery. 2008; 62(3) Suppl 1:57–72, discussion 72–74

[9] Carrau RL, Kassam AB, Snyderman CH. Pituitary surgery. Otolaryngol Clin North Am. 2001; 34(6):1143–1155, ix

[10] Kassam AB, Mintz AH, Gardner PA, et al. The expanded endonasal approach for an endoscopic transnasal clipping and aneurysmorrhaphy of a large vertebral artery aneurysm: technical case report. Neurosurgery. 2006; 59(1 Suppl 1):ONSE162–ONSE165; discussion ONSE162-5

[11] Fortes FSG, Carrau RL, Snyderman CH, et al. The posterior pedicle inferior turbinate flap: a new vascularized flap for skull base reconstruction. Laryngoscope. 2007; 117(8):1329–1332

[12] Kassam AB, Thomas A, Carrau RL, et al. Endoscopic reconstruction of the cranial base using a pedicled nasoseptal flap. Neurosurgery. 2008; 63(1) Suppl 1:ONS44–ONS52, discussion ONS52–ONS53

[13] Kono Y, Prevedello DM, Snyderman CH, et al. One thousand endoscopic skull base surgical procedures demystifying the infection potential: incidence and description of postoperative meningitis and brain abscesses. Infect Control Hosp Epidemiol. 2011; 32(1):77–83

[14] Al-Mefty O, Kadri PAS, Hasan DM, Isolan GR, Pravdenkova S. Anterior clivectomy: surgical technique and clinical applications. J Neurosurg. 2008; 109 (5):783–793

[15] Almeida JP, De Albuquerque LA, Dal Fabbro M, et al. Endoscopic skull base surgery: evaluation of current clinical outcomes. J Neurosurg Sci. 2015

[16] Kassam AB, Vescan AD, Carrau RL, et al. Expanded endonasal approach: vidian canal as a landmark to the petrous internal carotid artery. J Neurosurg. 2008; 108(1):177–183

[17] Pinheiro-Neto CD, Prevedello DM, Carrau RL, et al. Improving the design of the pedicled nasoseptal flap for skull base reconstruction: a radioanatomic study. Laryngoscope. 2007; 117(9):1560–1569

[18] Vescan AD, Snyderman CH, Carrau RL, et al. Vidian canal: analysis and relationship to the internal carotid artery. Laryngoscope. 2007; 117(8):1338–1342

[19] Hadad G, Rivera-Serrano CM, Bassagaisteguy LH, et al. Anterior pedicle lateral nasal wall flap: a novel technique for the reconstruction of anterior skull base defects. Laryngoscope. 2011; 121(8):1606–1610

[20] Barges-Coll J, Fernandez-Miranda JC, Prevedello DM, et al. Avoiding injury to the abducens nerve during expanded endonasal endoscopic surgery: anatomic and clinical case studies. Neurosurgery. 2010; 67(1):144–154, discussion 154

[21] Kassam AB, Gardner P, Snyderman C, Mintz A, Carrau R. Expanded endonasal approach: fully endoscopic, completely transnasal approach to the middle third of the clivus, petrous bone, middle cranial fossa, and infratemporal fossa. Neurosurg Focus. 2005; 19(1):E6

[22] Prevedello DM, Pinheiro-Neto CD, Fernandez-Miranda JC, et al. Vidian nerve transposition for endoscopic endonasal middle fossa approaches. Neurosurgery. 2010; 67(2 Suppl Operative):478–484

[23] Cutler AR, Mundi JS, Solomon N, Suh JD, Wang MB, Bergsneider M. Critical appraisal of extent of resection of clival lesions using the expanded endoscopic endonasal approach. J Neurol Surg B Skull Base. 2013; 74(4):217–224

[24] Fraser JF, Nyquist GG, Moore N, Anand VK, Schwartz TH. Endoscopic endonasal transclival resection of chordomas: operative technique, clinical outcome, and review of the literature. J Neurosurg. 2010; 112(5):1061–1069

[25] Linsler S, Oertel J. Endoscopic endonasal transclival resection of a brainstem cavernoma: a detailed account of our technique and comparison with the literature. World Neurosurg. 2015; 84(6):2064–2071

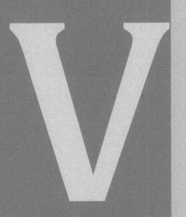

Part V

Tumors

26 Open versus Endoscopic Supracerebellar Infratentorial Approaches

Hasan A. Zaidi and Peter Nakaji

Summary

Supracerebellar infratentorial (SCIT) approaches have previously been described for various lesions in the pineal region with the use of an operating microscope to aid visualization. The deep, narrow surgical corridor and the necessity to place the patient in a sitting or prone position in most cases can result in decreased visualization, poor ergonomics for the surgeon, and increased frustration for the surgeon. The advent and popularity of the endoscope in neurosurgical procedures can be applied to the SCIT approach. We describe our experience using this relatively novel visualization technique, and we demonstrate its applicability for various lesions in both the supratentorial and infratentorial spaces. Compared to microscopic-assisted techniques, the endoscopic SCIT approach reduces surgeon fatigue, improves surgical ergonomics, and increases visualization and light penetration within a small surgical corridor.

Keywords: endoscopic, pineal region, posterior fossa, SCIT

26.1 Open Microsurgical Approaches to the Pineal Region

Microsurgical resection is the most popular treatment modality for most pineal region tumors, including metastatic tumors, meningiomas, parenchymal tumors, germ cell tumors, and large symptomatic pineal region cysts. Surgical resection is especially effective for lesions that are not radiosensitive and that have radiographic features of well-demarcated borders against the surrounding brain tissue. Gross total tumor resection can provide relief of mass effect, potentially obviating the need for permanent cerebrospinal fluid diversion surgery.[1,2] It can also provide an ample specimen for histopathologic diagnosis, decreasing the potential for a sampling error that might occur during minimally invasive tumor biopsy. For lesions that surround or invade critical neurovascular structures in the pineal region, tumor debulking has demonstrated an improved response to postoperative adjuvant radiosurgery or chemotherapy.

Open surgical approaches to pineal region disease are driven largely by the neuroanatomical relationship of the lesion to the surrounding neurovascular structures. For lesions that push the vein of Galen posteriorly, anterior approaches (e.g., posterior interhemispheric craniotomies) provide direct access to the lesion. In many situations, intrinsic pineal region tumors push the vein of Galen and its tributaries anteriorly; in these situations, many authors advocate either supracerebellar infratentorial (SCIT) or supratentorial transtentorial approaches. For lesions that involve the inferior temporal or occipital lobe, SCIT transtentorial approaches provide direct access to the lesion while obviating significant brain retraction.[3] These approaches allow for more direct access to the lesion, unobstructed by the

deep venous structures. Each approach has its own advantages and disadvantages.

26.1.1 Advantages and Disadvantages of Microsurgical SCIT Approaches

Open microsurgical SCIT approaches are advantageous for most neurosurgeons, largely because of the neurosurgeon's familiarity with the surgical instruments and operating room setup.[4,5] The surgical team does not require specialized training to prepare the operating room for surgery. Unlike endoscopic SCIT approaches, which require the use of specialized instruments and an unfamiliar operating room setup with endoscopes and video towers, microscopic SCIT approaches use the same tools available for standard craniotomies and microsurgical dissection. Furthermore, endoscopic SCIT approaches require two surgeons to work simultaneously: an assistant surgeon to hold the endoscope and a primary surgeon to perform the intracranial dissection.[6] This two-surgeon setup is not necessary with microscopic SCIT approaches that allow the primary surgeon to complete all the necessary surgical tasks alone. At many nonacademic institutions, or even at some academic teaching hospitals, establishing and coordinating a team effort to perform endoscopic SCIT approaches requires a considerable degree of training and effort, which may not be logistically possible.

26.1.2 Surgical Approaches and Technical Nuances

The open microsurgical SCIT approach to the pineal region is performed with the patient in either a sitting or a prone position. With the patient in the sitting position, gravity retraction of the cerebellar hemispheres increases the potential working space for the surgeon and, in many cases, obviates the need for fixed retraction. However, there are several disadvantages to the sitting microscopic SCIT approach. First, the patient has a higher risk of developing a venous air embolism with the potential for catastrophic hemodynamic or cerebrovascular complications. Therefore, all patients require extensive preoperative and intraoperative evaluation, including bubble echocardiograms, precordial Doppler monitoring, and a right atrial central-line placement during surgical resection to detect and treat air embolism. Second, open SCIT approaches using the sitting position place the surgeon's hands in midair for a prolonged period of time, increasing the risk of surgeon fatigue during the resection of large tumors. This fatigue can limit the degree and safety of tumor resection, as the surgeon's hands are not ergonomically positioned for several hours. To avoid these limitations, many skull base centers advocate the use of prone positioning during microsurgical SCIT approaches. This position allows the surgeon's hands to rest comfortably during the entire course of

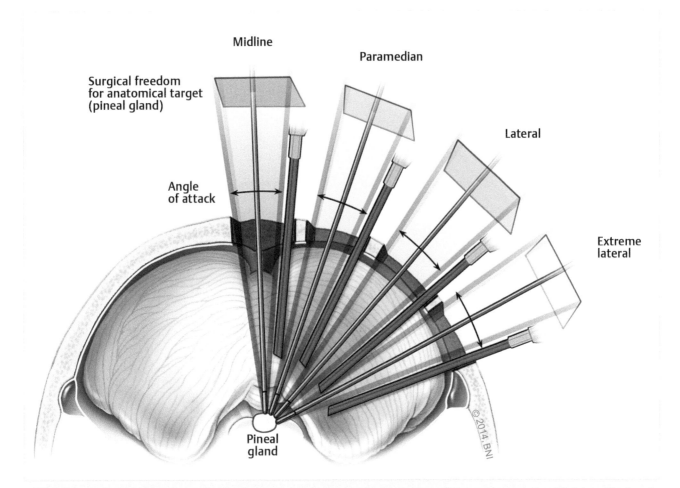

Fig. 26.1 Various supracerebellar infratentorial approaches have been described, including the midline (*purple*), paramedian (*blue*), lateral (*teal*), and far lateral (*green*) approaches. (Used with permission from Barrow Neurological Institute, Phoenix, AZ.)

the resection. However, abdominal compression of the patient on the operating room table and the considerable neck flexion necessary to optimize the angle of attack during positioning result in substantial venous outflow obstruction. Reduced venous outflow results in a fuller cerebellum and a reduction in the size of the potential working space for the surgeon, with a concomitant venous engorgement and increased risk of significant blood loss. Therefore, surgeons who use the prone position for microsurgical SCIT approaches rely more on fixed cerebellar retraction, which has an increased risk of retraction-related injury.

Microscopic SCIT approaches necessitate a generous vertical midline incision in the posterior scalp, followed by a wide suboccipital craniotomy exposing the torcula and transverse sinuses and permitting upward retraction of the posterior edge of the tentorium to allow access to the supracerebellar space. Over the last few decades, many authors have transitioned to minimizing the craniotomy and incision, because wide bilateral exposure of the suboccipital region does not substantially improve operative visualization and places the patient at undue risk of iatrogenic injury to the sinuses during exposure. Nonetheless, a generous craniotomy is still necessary in open microsurgical approaches to allow adequate light penetration and

better maneuverability of instruments deep within the narrow surgical corridor.

Various SCIT approaches have been described, including the midline approach, and the paramedian, lateral, and extreme lateral approaches (▶ Fig. 26.1). At our institution, we advocate off-midline SCIT approaches, rather than a midline SCIT approach, to avoid exposure-related injury to the torcula and the sacrifice of major tentorial bridging veins that are often encountered in the midline. Off-midline approaches also permit better visualization of the pineal region around the peak of the culmen of the cerebellum in the midline, which routinely obstructs the view in midline approaches.

Walter Dandy first described the posterior interhemispheric approaches to pineal region pathology. Although the posterior interhemispheric approach is ideal for lesions that push the vein of Galen posteriorly, it requires the exposure and retraction of midline interhemispheric veins adjacent to the central sulcus. Furthermore, the retraction of the occipital lobes places the primary visual cortex under an increased risk of retraction-related injury. Similarly, transtentorial variants, which allow access to pineal region lesions that push the venous structures anteriorly, place dural tributaries within the tentorium at increased risk of injury with the potential for large blood loss.

For these reasons, these approaches are less often used at our institution.

26.2 Endoscopic Approaches to the Pineal Region

Endoscopically controlled SCIT approaches to the pineal region are a relatively novel method to reach lesions located in the pineal region, superior cerebellum, or inferior occipital or temporal lobes.[7,8] This method applies many of the same concepts used in endoscopic endonasal approaches to the skull base, and it is a natural transition for surgeons who are adept at endonasal skull base surgery. This technique provides superior visualization of the intracranial contents, while affording a smaller incision and craniotomy. It takes advantage of the natural airspace created between the cerebellum and the tentorium, which is a relatively safe corridor into the pineal and supracerebellar spaces and to various transtentorial regions. Various lesions can be treated using the endoscopic visualization technique, with several groups demonstrating efficacy in resecting pineal cysts, germinal tumors, and parenchymal tumors. The endoscope improves visualization and illumination, and it reduces the fatigue of the surgeon because of improved comfort during lesion resection, which may help reduce approach-related morbidity.

26.2.1 Patient Selection

Microscopic SCIT approaches are a well-established and powerful method to access various lesions. However, the long and deep surgical corridor requires the surgeon to increase the degree of traction on the cerebellum and tentorium (1) to improve illumination of the surgical bed by allowing light from an extracranial source to penetrate deep within the surgical cavity, (2) to reduce instrument conflict, and (3) to reduce the likelihood that surgical instruments will obstruct the surgeon's microscopic view of the surgical bed. Furthermore, lesions with extensive supratentorial extension are outside the surgeon's line of sight, which forces the surgeon to rely on tactile feedback rather than on direct visualization during the dissection of important neurovascular structures. These limitations of the traditional microscopic visualization technique for SCIT approaches increase the risk of retraction-related injury and iatrogenic injury during the manipulation of important neurovascular structures. However, with the endoscopic visualization technique, both the light source and the lens are located within the intracranial vault. Doing so allows the surgeon to directly and clearly visualize intracranial pathology during surgical dissection without requiring significant cerebellar retraction. For lesions with extensive supratentorial extension, angled endoscopic visualization potentially reduces the risk of iatrogenic injury by providing the surgeon with a wider field of view.

26.2.2 Positioning

A safe access zone is necessary to provide a working space to place an endoscope. All patients who undergo an endoscopic SCIT approach at our institution are placed in a sitting or semi-sitting position (▶ Fig. 26.2). Simple positioning techniques, combined with wide arachnoid dissection and generous use of intravenous mannitol, expand the infratentorial space. In rare instances, when a patient has full cerebellar hemispheres or a large mass-occupying lesion, lumbar drainage further aids cerebellar relaxation and creates a potential working space for the endoscope. The sitting position also allows the primary surgeon and the assistant holding the endoscope to stand with their instruments and arms in a more natural position during the course of the procedure. Video screens that project the microscope's video output are placed directly across from the primary surgeon, and an additional "slave" screen is placed directly opposite the assistant. These subtle, but important, advantages to patient positioning and operating room setup for the endoscopic SCIT approach allow both surgeons to be comfortable during the resection, improving ergonomics, and potentially reducing surgeon fatigue. Finally, placing the patient in the sitting position reduces venous outflow obstruction, decreases bleeding during surgical manipulation, and allows blood products to drain freely away from the surgical field.

The sitting approach presents several disadvantages of which one must be cognizant. First, and as previously mentioned, the sitting position places the patient at the risk of developing a venous air embolism if the sinuses or large dural or bony venous tributaries are violated during the approach. During the preoperative testing phase, all patients must undergo a cardiac bubble echocardiogram to confirm the absence of a patent foramen ovale. At our institution, the presence of a patent foramen ovale contraindicates the use of a sitting position for surgeries requiring an endoscopic SCIT approach. Second, if an emergent conversion to a traditional open microscopic approach becomes necessary when the patient is in the sitting position, it places the arms of both surgeons in an ergonomically unfavorable position.

26.2.3 Surgical Exposure

Preoperatively, all patients undergo high-resolution, 1-mm thin-cut gadolinium contrast-enhanced magnetic resonance imaging (▶ Fig. 26.3), which is loaded on an image guidance platform and registered after patient positioning. The neuronavigation system enables the surgeon to precisely locate the transverse sinus and torcula, thereby allowing a smaller incision and improving safety. At our institution, we perform all craniotomies off-midline, approximately 2 to 3 cm lateral to the torcula, starting at the level of the transverse sinus and extending downward. A 2.5 × 1.5 cm keyhole craniotomy is performed that exposes the inferior aspect of the transverse sinus and the upper aspect of the cerebellum (▶ Fig. 26.4). Although microscopic approaches necessitate the full exposure of the transverse sinus to mobilize the transverse sinus up and away from the operative field to allow for greater light penetration, the process of unroofing the transverse sinus and exposing it to light from the microscope increases the risk of iatrogenic injury or thrombosis. However, an endoscopic approach does not require the full exposure of the transverse sinus, since the light source is located within the cranial vault and the upward mobilization of the transverse sinus does not affect the degree of illumination of the operative corridor (▶ Fig. 26.5). Unlike microscopic techniques, endoscopic approaches afford smaller craniotomies that do not compromise visualization, but they may result in increased instrument conflict and surgeon

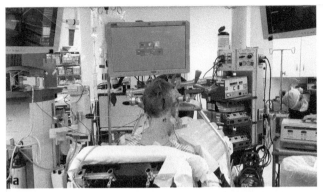
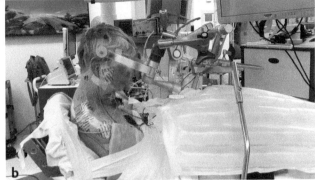
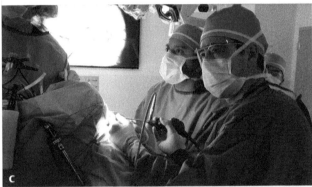
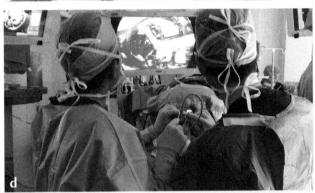

Fig. 26.2 A patient is placed in a sitting position for an endoscopic supracerebellar infratentorial transtentorial approach. **(a)** The video monitors are placed directly across from the patient to allow the surgeon to comfortably view the screen. **(b)** The neck of the patient is maximally flexed to allow the tentorium to be as parallel to the floor as possible. This positioning increases the potential working space by allowing the cerebellum to fall away using gravity retraction. **(c)** During the course of the surgical resection, both the primary surgeon and the assistant surgeon are standing and **(d)** can comfortably view the video monitor. (Used with permission from Barrow Neurological Institute, Phoenix, AZ.)

frustration. However, the application of basic endoscopic principles helps improve surgical freedom.

The endoscope is held by an assistant and introduced to the upper outer corner of the craniotomy, opposite the surgeon's dominant hand (▶ Fig. 26.5). Placing the endoscope in this position optimizes the primary surgeon's dexterity and maneuverability. For lesions located in the midline, a left-sided craniotomy is preferable when the surgeon is right handed. After a cruciate or curvilinear incision, cerebrospinal fluid is aggressively drained and mannitol is administered to relax the cerebellum and increase the potential working space. The surgeon's knowledge of anatomy is paramount to a safe and effective surgical resection. It is aided by adapters using the neuronavigation system that can be connected to the endoscope to provide real-time triangulation of the endoscope tip within the cranial vault during the course of surgical resection.

26.2.4 Surgical Technique

Using direct visualization of the intracranial anatomical structures, the surgeon should advance the endoscope at 90 degrees to the calvarial surface and should ultimately remove it using the same trajectory. Large "sweeping" motions can result in shearing of the bridging veins outside the line of sight of the endoscope, with major bleeding and/or cerebellar contusions occurring during exposure. Additionally, the endoscope should be a dynamic visualization tool. As the primary surgeon introduces surgical dissection instruments and suction, it is imperative for the assistant holding the endoscope to remove it from

the cranial vault and to advance it back into the cranium, while following the instruments to the surgical target. Doing so permits the primary surgeon to prevent instruments from inadvertently injuring superficial neurovascular structures outside the line of sight. With a microscopic approach, these maneuvers are not necessary, and many microscopically trained neurosurgeons may find the endoscopic technique time consuming, uncomfortable, and tedious. However, we have found that with a team-based approach following general neuroendoscopic principles, these maneuvers become second nature and do not increase the length of surgical procedures.

Once the endoscope is advanced, standard microsurgical principles can be followed to effectively proceed with the exposure and the resection of the lesion (▶ Fig. 26.6). Large bridging veins obstructing the surgical view can be coagulated using standard bipolar instruments and cut sharply. In our experience, endoscopic visualization does not require specialized bipolar or microdissection instruments other than those typically used in standard open microsurgical procedures. For access to the pineal region, the endoscope can be further advanced following a trajectory parallel to the tentorium. For tumors in the supratentorial space that are accessed using the endoscopic SCIT transtentorial route, angled endoscopes can help the surgeon to visualize around sharp corners, especially with lesions extending far up the temporal or occipital lobes. It is critical to be able to visualize the tip of the dissector being introduced into the intracranial space at all times and to use a protective moist cottonoid patty to guard against inadvertent injury to the cerebellum (▶ Fig. 26.7). One common complaint

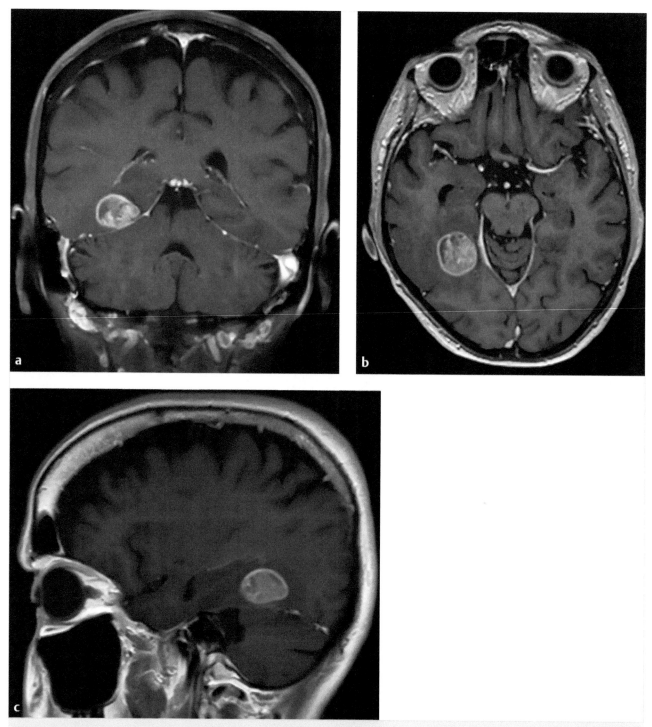

Fig. 26.3 A 53-year-old female patient presented with persistent headaches and intermittent confusion but was otherwise neurologically intact. **(a)** Coronal, **(b)** axial, and **(c)** sagittal preoperative gadolinium-enhanced magnetic resonance images demonstrate a mass in the left inferior temporal lobe overlying the tentorium. A transcortical approach to the lesion would place the visual fibers at risk, and a subtemporal approach would necessitate significant temporal lobe retraction to access the lesion. The patient elected to undergo an endoscopic supracerebellar infratentorial transtentorial approach to this lesion. (Used with permission from Barrow Neurological Institute, Phoenix, AZ.)

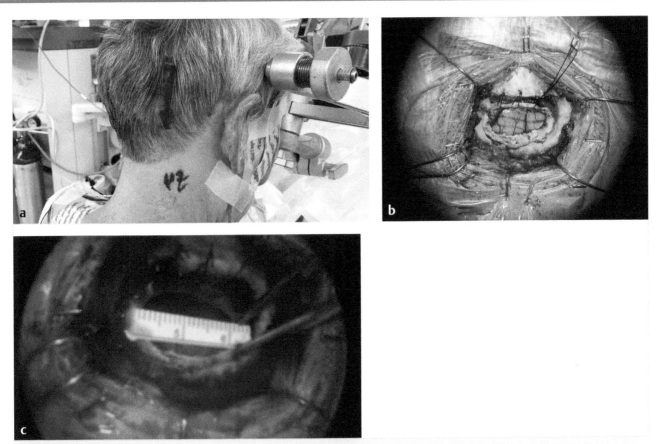

Fig. 26.4 **(a)** An off-midline incision is planned, approximately 2 to 3 cm lateral to the torcula, starting at the level of the transverse sinus and extending downward. **(b,c)** A 2.5 × 1.5-cm keyhole craniotomy is performed, exposing the inferior aspect of the transverse sinus and the upper aspect of the cerebellum. (Used with permission from Barrow Neurological Institute, Phoenix, AZ.)

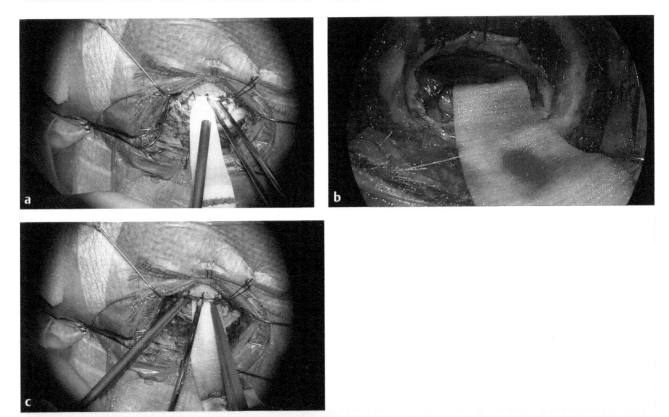

Fig. 26.5 **(a)** An overhead view and **(b)** an endoscopic view demonstrate the placement of moist Cottonoid patties to protect the cerebellar cortex during the course of surgery. **(c)** The endoscope is held by an assistant surgeon and introduced to the upper outer corner of the craniotomy opposite the surgeon's dominant hand. This placement optimizes the primary surgeon's dexterity and maneuverability. (Used with permission from Barrow Neurological Institute, Phoenix, AZ.)

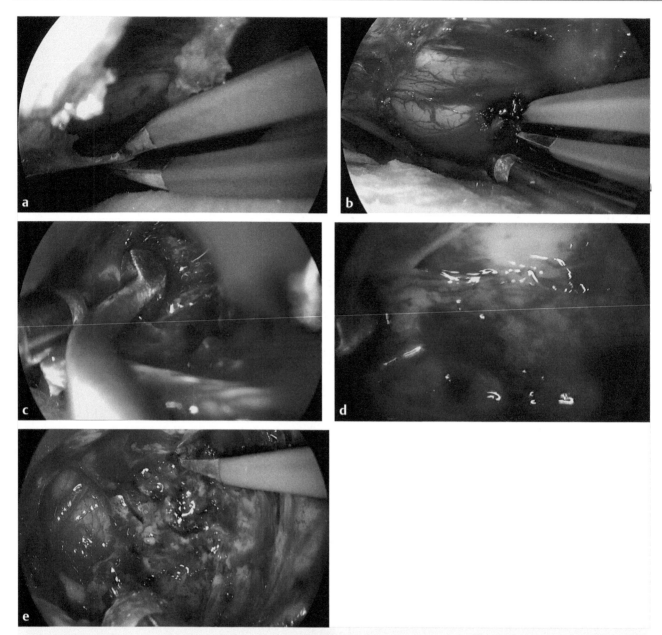

Fig. 26.6 **(a)** The tentorium is opened using a combination of bipolar electrocautery and sharp microsurgical dissection. Aside from the endoscope, no additional tools are necessary other than those in the standard microsurgical dissection set. **(b)** Bipolar electrocautery is used to perform a cortisectomy, and **(c)** standard dissection tools are used for piecemeal resection of the tumor. **(d)** The endoscope is advanced to the surgical cavity to better identify the border between tumor and normal brain tissue. **(e)** Angled endoscopes can be advanced to the surgical cavity to inspect the resection bed and ensure that there is no residual disease. (Used with permission from Barrow Neurological Institute, Phoenix, AZ.)

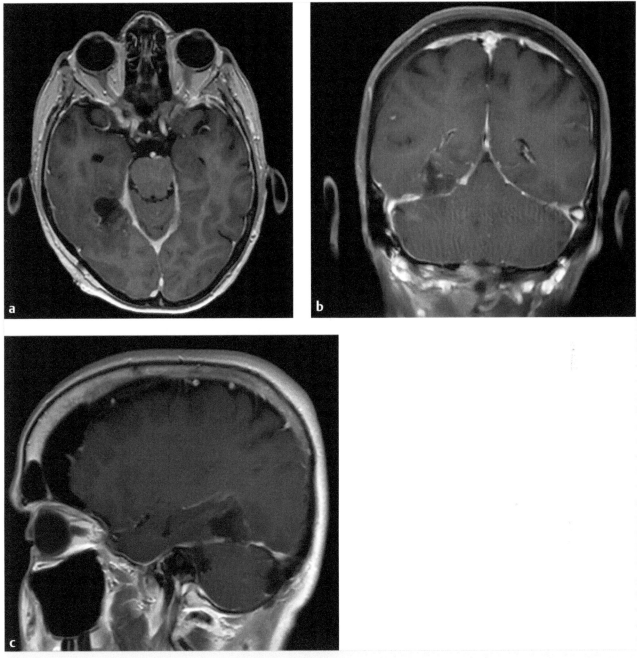

Fig. 26.7 **(a)** Axial, **(b)** coronal, and **(c)** sagittal postoperative gadolinium-enhanced magnetic resonance images demonstrate gross total tumor resection. Final pathologic examination confirmed a high-grade glioma. The patient awoke with no visual field deficits, and she was otherwise neurologically intact. She was discharged home on postoperative day 1. (Used with permission from Barrow Neurological Institute, Phoenix, AZ.)

from open microscopic surgeons is that the endoscope does not allow for "fluid" instrument movements as a result of frequent instrument conflict. However, we have found that surgical fluidity and dexterity can dramatically improve when the assistant surgeon is adept at moving the endoscope out of the way of the primary surgeon. To reach this stage requires a team-based approach, with substantial trial-and-error development of the process because of the steep learning curve.

26.3 Conclusion

A common challenge of skull base surgery is to effectively and safely perform microneurosurgery in a deep operative corridor. The SCIT method represents one such challenging approach: a small working space that requires microdissection of important neurovascular structures. The endoscope is a relatively novel tool that provides panoramic views, improved illumination from the placement of the light source within the surgical cavity, and angled viewing around corners. The use of the endoscope as the primary visual tool can improve surgical outcomes by enhancing intraoperative visualization, alleviating surgeon fatigue through the use of more ergonomically sound patient positioning, and reducing approach-related morbidity. Although the SCIT approach is associated with a steep learning curve, familiarity with endoscopic instruments and a coordinated team-based approach will likely result in improved patient outcomes.

References

[1] Abay EO, II, Laws ER, Jr, Grado GL, et al. Pineal tumors in children and adolescents. Treatment by CSF shunting and radiotherapy. J Neurosurg. 1981; 55 (6):889–895

[2] Sebag-Montefiore DJ, Douek E, Kingston JE, Plowman PN. Intracranial germ cell tumours: I. Experience with platinum based chemotherapy and implications for curative chemoradiotherapy. Clin Oncol (R Coll Radiol). 1992; 4 (6):345–350

[3] Stein BM. The infratentorial supracerebellar approach to pineal lesions. J Neurosurg. 1971; 35(2):197–202

[4] Vishteh AG, David CA, Marciano FF, Coscarella E, Spetzler RF. Extreme lateral supracerebellar infratentorial approach to the posterolateral mesencephalon: technique and clinical experience. Neurosurgery. 2000; 46(2):384–388, discussion 388–389

[5] Ogata N, Yonekawa Y. Paramedian supracerebellar approach to the upper brain stem and peduncular lesions. Neurosurgery. 1997; 40(1):101–104, discussion 104–105

[6] Pople IK, Athanasiou TC, Sandeman DR, Coakham HB. The role of endoscopic biopsy and third ventriculostomy in the management of pineal region tumours. Br J Neurosurg. 2001; 15(4):305–311

[7] Gore PA, Gonzalez LF, Rekate HL, Nakaji P. Endoscopic supracerebellar infratentorial approach for pineal cyst resection: technical case report. Neurosurgery. 2008; 62(3) Suppl 1:108–109, discussion 109

[8] Uschold T, Abla AA, Fusco D, Bristol RE, Nakaji P. Supracerebellar infratentorial endoscopically controlled resection of pineal lesions: case series and operative technique. J Neurosurg Pediatr. 2011; 8(6):554–564

27 Intraparenchymal Brain Tumors: Moderator

Chikezie Eseonu, Jordina Rincon-Torroella, and Alfredo Quinones-Hinojosa

Summary

Resection of brain tumors has evolved from unaided open surgical resection to high-magnification microsurgical resection. The advent of the endoscope has demonstrated improved illumination with panoramic visualization for ventral skull base lesions. Several groups have now applied the principles of ventral skull base endoscopic techniques for supratentorial intraparenchymal brain tumors. In this chapter, we discuss the advantages and disadvantages of the endoscopic versus microsurgical approaches for intraparenchymal brain tumors.

Keywords: microscope, endoscope, intraparenchymal tumor, controversy, tubular retraction

27.1 Moderator

27.1.1 Introduction

Over the last several decades, the resection technique for intraparenchymal brain tumors has evolved. The operating room has seen the introduction of the microscope, functional magnetic resonance imaging (fMRI), and diffusion tensor imaging (DTI) to identify eloquent cortical function and white matter tracts and to improve tumor resection while reducing morbidity. For the last few decades, the microscope has predominantly been used to resect intraparenchymal primary or metastatic lesions.[1,2] Stereotactic image guidance has improved the precision of these surgeries; however, for tumors that do not present to the pial surface, a corticectomy and dissection through the white matter tract is needed before the tumor can be reached.[2,3] Once the subcortical tumor is reached, it can be difficult to visualize the tumor and the surrounding structures during the operation with the operating microscope.[1] The endoscope presents a surgical option that has the potential to gain better access to deep subcortical lesions, while minimizing the amount of damage to the surrounding brain tissue (▶ Fig. 27.1). Traditionally, the endoscope has been used to approach lesions in natural body cavities, such as the ventricular system; however, over the last decade, endoscopic approaches have been used to resect intraparenchymal lesions.[1]

This chapter explores the microscopic and endoscopic surgical approaches for intraparenchymal tumors, exploring the evolution of the approaches and evaluating the utility of both techniques.

27.1.2 Evolution of Surgical Treatment Options

Removal of brain tumors was first documented in 1879, after Scottish surgeon William Macewen performed the first brain tumor resection.[4] Throughout the late 19th and early 20th centuries, surgeons continued to conduct brain tumor surgery with basic tools, such as chisels and curettes.[5,6] The surgical

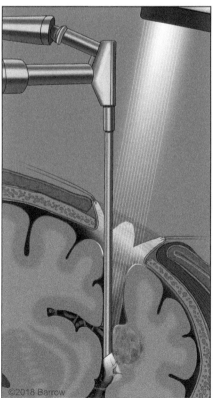
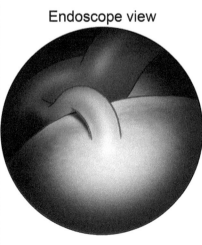

Endoscope view

Fig. 27.1 Illustration showing access to deep subcortical tissue with better illumination (inset) than with microsurgical visualization. (Used with permission from Barrow Neurological Institute, Phoenix, AZ.)

©2018 Barrow

microscope entered the neurosurgical field in 1957 when it was used to remove a neurilemoma in a 5-year-old patient.[7] Since that time, the operating microscope has seen significant improvement, regarding magnification and illumination of the operative field, making it an integral part of most neurosurgical operations.[7]

In order to improve the visualization of the operative field with the microscope, the use of a retractor system is often employed to create a visual corridor that exposes a lesion. Common blade retractors for intracranial tumors include the Leyla, Budde Halo, and Greenberg systems.[8] Prolonged retraction, however, can lead to injury to the surrounding brain parenchyma via prolonged compression of the cerebral vasculature by the retractor, which causes ischemia to the brain tissue.[9,10] Although advances in the retractor systems, such as flexible arms, have reduced retractor-induced insults, they still pose a problem in neurosurgical cases.[11,12,13]

In the 1980s, Kelly et al first described the use of a stereotactic, 20-mm-diameter, cylindrical retractor that aimed to provide a small corridor with less retraction for the operating microscope.[2,14,15] Over the last three decades, these cylindrical retractors, as well as tubular retractors, or ports, have allowed for safe dilation of brain parenchyma to access deep lesions. In addition, transparent versions of the port system allow for better visualization of the surgical corridor.[3,8]

With modified retractors reducing parenchymal damage, surgeons sought additional ways to limit retraction injury. In 1980, stereotactic endoscopy through a conduit was beginning to be used, with the endoscope being mounted on a fixed stereotactic frame.[16,17] Otsuki et al would later describe stereotactic endoscopy through a conduit made from a guide tube in 1990.[18] This guide tube was also attached to a stereotactic frame, which lacked the mobility to address large tumors at various angles. Other variations of the fixed tubular retraction system were later developed (i.e., Vycor Viewsite Brain Access System [VBAS]); however, only small lesions were able to be completely resected because of the small diameter of the surgical space provided by the tubular system.[3,16,17,18,19,20]

In 2003, Kassam et al bypassed this surgical space limitation by using a bimanual technique that adjusted the tubular system throughout the surgery in order to aid with the resection.[2] During these procedures, they used frameless image guidance with an endoscope and port, or dilatable conduit. This method allowed for changes in the angle of the port and endoscope, which provided multiple views of the tumor, via a single cannulation with a small corticectomy.[2] In order to optimize the endoscopic approach, the endoscopic port must cannulate to the deepest portion of the tumor (resection occurs from deep to superficial, as oppose to microscopic methods). By removing the endoscopic dilator after cannulation, a potential space is created between the endoscopic conduit and the tumor that allows for a pressure gradient where the extracavitary tumor will begin to deliver itself into the port, which will help with tumor resection (▶ Fig. 27.2).[2]

Advancements in the tubular retractor systems (i.e., NICO BrainPath) have been developed that have more atraumatic tips, which allow for better white matter dissection with less tissue damage from displacement. In addition, neuronavigation can be affixed to the tubular system to aid in obtaining the optimal trajectory. These advancements could be applied to both the microscopic and endoscopic approaches (▶ Fig. 27.3).

Within the last decade, the development of a telescope-based exoscope system has been used in open cranial surgery for tumor surgery.[21,22] In addition to the operating microscope and endoscope, the exoscope consists of an operating telescope, light source, camera head, and video display that can produce high-quality images with a wide field of view. The exoscope can sit far away from the surgical site, similar to the operating microscope, and allows for passage of instruments under the scope that is not possible with the endoscope.[21] Since the exoscope camera head can be rotated 360 degrees, the image

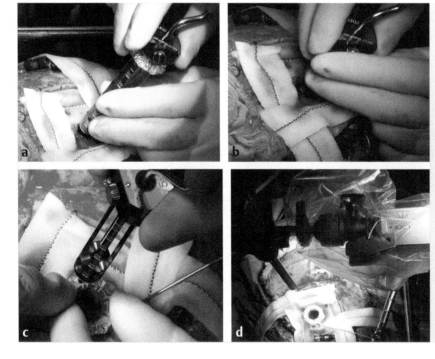

Fig. 27.2 Port-assisted surgical planning using an endoscope. **(a)** Planning of trajectory and angulation with neuronavigation inserted within the tubular retractor. **(b)** Advancement of the tubular retractor. **(c)** Removal of internal dilator. **(d)** The endoscope is being adjusted to visualize the contents of the tubular retractor.

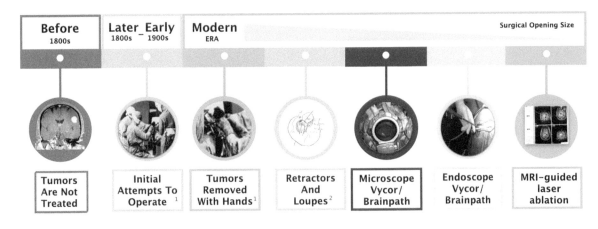

Timeline Treatment of Intraparenchymal Brain Tumors

| Before 1800s | Later 1800s – Early 1900s | Modern ERA | | | | Surgical Opening Size |

| Tumors Are Not Treated | Initial Attempts To Operate [1] | Tumors Removed With Hands [1] | Retractors And Loupes [2] | Microscope Vycor/ Brainpath | Endoscope Vycor/ Brainpath | MRI-guided laser ablation |

1. Harvey Cushing during a first attempt of Brain Tumor surgery. From Santiago Ramon y Cajal and Harvey Cushing two localizers of neuroscience and neurosurgery. Zachery, Benob CJ, Pendleton C, Russ G, Cohen, Gadol AA. Quinones- Hinojosa A. World Neurosurg. 2011 Nov;76(5):464–76. doi: 10.1016/j.wneu.2011.04.001

2. Dr. Harvey Cushing's intra-operative illustration of his approach to third ventricle drainage with retractors and loupes. From Harvey Cushing's use of a transplanted human skin to treat hydrocephalus in an infant in the early 1900s. Historical vignette. Pendleton C1, Zada HA, Jallo G, Cohen- Gadol AA. Quinones- Hinojosa A. J Neurosurg Pediatr. 2010 May;5(5):525–7. doi: 10.3171/2009.12.PEDS09286.

Fig. 27.3 Timeline of the evolution of brain tumor resection.

display on the monitor can be adjusted to match the position of the surgeon relative to the anatomy. The small size of the exoscope (weighing about 1.5 lb) can be easily positioned for an operation and transported from site to site, compared to the operating microscope that is bulky and can often take up a large amount of the operating room.[22] The system is also less expensive than the standard operating microscope that can range from $200 to 450,000.[21] The exoscope has had little use clinically for intraparenchymal tumors given the difficulty of maneuverability of the scope holder intraoperatively as well as the lack of stereopsis, or depth perception.[21,22]

27.1.3 Advantages and Disadvantages of the Two Approaches

The development of endoscopy for intraparenchymal tumors gave surgeons two options for resecting intraparenchymal lesions. The open microscopic and endoscopic approaches each possess their advantages and disadvantages when resecting these types of tumors.

Imaging

The microscope allows for high-definition imaging that can be viewed in three dimensions. This view, however, is limited to the line of sight of the surgeon and can have poor illumination at deeper depths.[1] Alternatively, the endoscope presents a high-definition image with good illumination and visualization at depths. The angled scopes for the endoscopes allow for a surgeon to see beyond of the line of sight when evaluating a resection cavity for residual tumor.[1,2] The images obtained from the endoscope are in two dimensions due to loss of binocular vision. This 2D view can be supplemented by changing the angles of view and proprioceptive feedback with the scope to provide a degree of depth perception, and new trials of 3D endoscopes are being developed.[1,8]

Technique

The open microscopic technique allows for the use of a two-handed microsurgical resection, by a single surgeon. Since the microscope is utilized throughout many applications in neurosurgery, the learning curve for its use on intraparenchymal tumors is less steep. There is also no need for cleaning the microscope lens during a procedure.

The endoscope requires two surgeons in order for a two-handed resection technique to be implemented. If a fixation stand is used for the endoscope, then one surgeon can use the two-handed technique, but will require constant adjustment of the endoscope, which can lengthen the procedure time.[8] There is also a steep learning curve for the use of the endoscope, and the scope will often need to be cleaned and defogged during the operation.[8]

Craniotomy

The size of the craniotomy and corticectomy for a microscopic approach depends on the lesion, but is often larger with microscopic approaches that do not utilize a port retraction system. White matter tracts can often be transected during the microscopic procedure, which can lead to surgical morbidity.[2] For temporal and frontal lobe lesions, a large frontotemporal craniotomy is normally done for microscopic procedures. The large myocutaneous flaps can cause postoperative temporal and orbital swelling that often requires an extradural drain.[1]

The endoscopic approach often requires a small craniotomy. For temporal tumors, the temporalis muscle is incised instead of elevated, causing minimal swelling of the orbital or temporal region. The access corridor is a small 1- to 1.5-cm corticectomy, regardless of the size of the tumor, and no retractor device is needed.[1] The endoscopic approach avoids transecting white matter fascicles by using an endoscopic dilator in the trajectory to the tumor, creating a parafascicular approach to the target lesion.[2] With such small incisions, no extradural drain is needed, although there is a risk of inadvertent widening of the access corridor from scope manipulation.[1]

Retraction

For the microscopic approach, blade retraction or tubular retraction can be used. Blade retractors allow for the surgeon to work at a far working distance with wide visualization of the operative field, but can have traumatic placement that causes damage on the white matter tracts and can lead to postoperative encephalomalacia.

The tubular retractors can be used with both microscopic and endoscopic approaches, are less traumatic on the brain tissue, and provide circumferential retraction. There is a learning curve with using tubular retraction systems. The working corridor for these tubular retractors is more narrow than blade retractors and often must use neuronavigation to help create an appropriate trajectory. For specific tubular retractors, such as the VBAS, only the Greenberg retractors are able to attach to this system.[3] A wide corticectomy is often needed to insert the tubular retractor and the narrow working channel can make it difficult to obtain hemostasis during a tumor resection.

The endoscopic approach can also use peel-away catheters that minimize the extent of retraction on the brain; however, these provide minimal visualization and are reserved for intraventricular lesions or highly cystic parenchymal masses.

Location

The microscopic approach is used for intraparenchymal lesions in all intracranial locations, especially superficial lesions, while the endoscopic approach is used for subcortical intraparenchymal lesions, particularly deep lesions in the temporal, frontal, cerebellar, and intraventricular regions. Cystic lesions allow for a suitable access corridor for the endoscope, providing surgical space following the draining of the cyst.[1]

27.1.4 Decision-making Algorithm Including Nonsurgical Management

Overall decision-making for which surgical approach is best for intraparenchymal tumors requires consideration of location, size, and histology of the lesion.[23]

Tumor Location

Determining whether the location of the tumor is superficial or deep is the first step to determine appropriate management of the lesion. Superficial lesions that are less than 3 cm from the surface of the brain can often be resected with standard open microsurgical methods.[8] For deeper tumors that have overlying white matter fascicles that would need to be transected in order to create a corridor for tumor resection, more minimally invasive techniques are needed.[2] Care must also be taken with the deeper lesions that do not have clear margins between the tumor and the regular brain, as increased white matter manipulation is more common.[23]

The next decision for a deep-seated tumor that must be made is to determine if the operation will be a full resection or solely a biopsy. Open stereotactic biopsies of intraparenchymal lesions have a symptomatic hemorrhage complication rate of 1.1 to 4.35%.[24,25,26] Using an endoscope and guided navigation allows for a biopsy to be obtained under direct visualization and is able to stop bleeding from a lesion while obtaining adequate tissue.[27] This method is less invasive than a small craniotomy biopsy, and can be useful for a biopsy of potentially hemorrhagic lesions.[8,28] Tanei et al showed reduced intracranial hemorrhage after biopsies under endoscopic monitoring of gliomas and malignant lympomas.[28] The disadvantage of an endoscopic biopsy compared to an open stereotactic biopsy is that it creates a larger diameter of its trajectory, often needing a 10-mm-diameter conduit sheath that can cause brain tissue damage, compared to a stereotactic biopsy needle that is 2.5-mm diameter.[28]

Planning Surgical Trajectory

Once the tumor location is determined, the next step is to decide the surgical trajectory for the operation. Creating a corridor to access a deep-seated tumor has been historically difficult and involves a corticectomy of the surface, followed by creating a trajectory down to the lesion using a retraction device to split the white fiber tracts.[16,17,18,29] Tubular retraction devices are fixed to a frame, but allows for maneuvering, which can aid in the resection of larger tumors (▶ Fig. 27.4). However, the constant movement of the tubular system could increase the stress on the surrounding brain, possibly contributing to brain edema.[2]

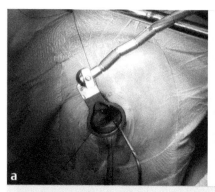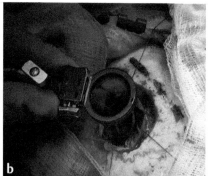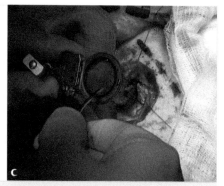

Fig. 27.4 Intraoperative maneuvering of a tubular retractor. **(a)** Tubular retractor in place with instruments being used through the corridor. **(b)** Movement of the tubular retractor to a new position. **(c)** Small movements can be done with the retractor to achieve the optimal position while achieving best visualization with suctioning.

Plaha et al utilized a 30-degree viewing angle and modified microsurgical curved instruments that allowed for better maneuvering through a small corridor and access to areas outside of the direct line of vision that would be obtained with a microscope.[1]

Utilizing fMRI and DTI with neuronavigation can aid with safe trajectory planning and detection of eloquent structures at a good sensitivity and specificity.[30] Correlation of DTI with brain mapping of the subcortical tracts with direct electrical stimulation (DES) showed a reliability of 82%, although negative tractography on DTI was shown to have some fiber tracts with DES.[31,32]

For small lesions, either a port-assisted resection or an open microsurgical resection with or without blade retraction can be used depending on the surgeon's preference. Larger tumors can utilize open microsurgery with blade retraction, or port-assisted resection. The designation of small and large tumors is arbitrarily assigned in this chapter and would be determined by the surgeon. We generally consider greater than 3 cm a large tumor.

Port-assisted Planning

A number of factors must be considered when planning a port-assisted neurosurgery including the anatomical location of the lesion and the presumed histology.[2,8] Cerebellar hemispheric lesions and cerebral lesions in the deep white matter or basal ganglia are ideal for port surgery. Deep lesions allow for good access with a port with less collateral brain tissue damage by distributing the radial retraction on the surrounding brain evenly as well as with a minimally sized craniotomy (▶ Fig. 27.4).[8]

Histology

Often, tumors that are soft and easy to suction are favored in port-assisted surgeries. These tumors often consist of high-grade gliomas and certain metastatic lesions (i.e., melanoma, breast cancer). More dense lesions (i.e., recurrent lesions with scar tissue, metastatic sarcomas, meningiomas) can present difficulties when using a port system. Using an ultrasonic aspirator with cutting features can facilitate the use of the port-assisted microscopy in those cases.[8] Hemorrhagic lesions, such as renal cell carcinoma, would not be amenable to the port-assisted endoscopic approach, as the intratumoral piecemeal resection method would be complicated by significant bleeding that could obscure the endoscopic operative field.[8]

Endoscopic Planning

When the location and histology are amenable, the endoscopic approach can be used. For endoscopic planning, the target is determined and the entry point is set on the surface of the brain using neuronavigation at a point that is considered functionally safe. The trajectory to the lesion is evaluated to determine that no eloquent structure is traversed by the trajectory.[28] The trajectory should also avoid passing through the ventricle or the sulcus, as trajectory proximity to the sulcus has been shown to cause adverse cortical complications.[33] Caution must also be taken to minimize the amount of cerebral spinal fluid loss during the procedure in order to reduce the amount of brain shift, which can alter the accuracy of the neuronavigation.[28] (▶ Fig. 27.5)

27.1.5 Final Thoughts/Expert Recommendations

Over the last few decades, the treatment for intraparenchymal tumors has evolved. Open microscopic surgery was first implemented with the use of retractors, and later there was the development of a tubular port system. The port system created a corridor that would soon allow for both the microscope and the endoscope to be utilized. Both methods can be effectively used by surgeons to resect intraparenchymal lesions, but there is a dearth of comparative outcome studies that can aid in deciding which method is most efficacious.

When evaluating the extent of resection between the two approaches, Plaha et al reported a series of 50 fully endoscopic intraparenchymal tumor resections. Seventy percent of these cases had at least a 95% resection, and 48% had gross total

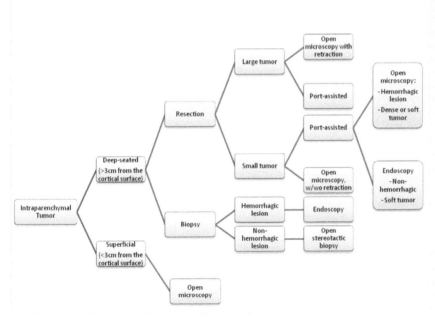

Fig. 27.5 Decision-making algorithm for intraparenchymal tumor management.

resections.[1] Kassam et al achieved total resection in 38% of their endoscopic intraparenchymal cases, and near-total resection in 28%.[2] The only comparative study between the microscopic and the endoscopic approach for intraparenchymal lesions was described by Hong et al who reported 20 patients, 5 of which had endoscopic-assisted port resections and 15 had microscopic-assisted port resections of deep-seated lesions. They found that more incomplete resections (near and subtotal) were found in 80% of endoscopic-assisted port resections, while 13% of microscopic-assisted port resections were incomplete ($p < 0.002$). Complications were found to be low and similar in both cohorts. The authors attribute the difference in extent of resection to the wider and 3D binocular view of the microscope compared to the endoscope.[8] Other studies have also shown successful microscopic-assisted port resections of brain tumors with high percentages of gross total resections.[3,34]

In regard to overall survival, Kelly found that endoscopic resection of glioblastoma was not shown to extend life compared to a microscopic resection.[35] Also, regarding length of hospitalization, Plaha et al reported a 4.8-day length of stay mean compared to a median of 5 days reported in a large study of 400 microscopic-assisted craniotomies for intra-axial brain tumors.[1,36]

The microscopic approach for intraparenchymal lesions has been a technique that has been used for decades, and early studies have shown better resection outcomes and similar neurological outcomes and complications compared to the endoscopic approach.[1,2,3,8,34,35] Preliminary findings suggest that for intraparenchymal lesions, the microsurgical approach is the preferred technique, but ultimately as surgeons become more facile with endoscopy and technology evolves, the approach to use will ultimately come down to surgeon preference.

References

[1] Plaha P, Livermore LJ, Voets N, Pereira E, Cudlip S. Minimally invasive endoscopic resection of intraparenchymal brain tumors. World Neurosurg. 2014; 82(6):1198–1208

[2] Kassam AB, Engh JA, Mintz AH, Prevedello DM. Completely endoscopic resection of intraparenchymal brain tumors. J Neurosurg. 2009; 110(1):116–123

[3] Raza SM, Recinos PF, Avendano J, Adams H, Jallo GI, Quinones-Hinojosa A. Minimally invasive trans-portal resection of deep intracranial lesions. Minim Invasive Neurosurg. 2011; 54(1):5–11

[4] Pendleton C, Ahn ES, Quiñones-Hinojosa A. Harvey Cushing and pediatric brain tumors at Johns Hopkins: the early stages of development. J Neurosurg Pediatr. 2011; 7(6):575–588

[5] Latimer K, Pendleton C, Olivi A, Cohen-Gadol AA, Brem H, Quiñones-Hinojosa A. Harvey Cushing's open and thorough documentation of surgical mishaps at the dawn of neurologic surgery. Arch Surg. 2011; 146(2):226–232

[6] Zamora-Berridi GJ, Pendleton C, Ruiz G, Cohen-Gadol AA, Quiñones-Hinojosa A. Santiago Ramón y Cajal and Harvey Cushing: two forefathers of neuroscience and neurosurgery. World Neurosurg. 2011; 76(5):466–476

[7] Uluç K, Kujoth GC, Başkaya MK. Operating microscopes: past, present, and future. Neurosurg Focus. 2009; 27(3):E4

[8] Hong CS, Prevedello DM, Elder JB. Comparison of endoscope- versus microscope-assisted resection of deep-seated intracranial lesions using a minimally invasive port retractor system. J Neurosurg. 2016; 124(3):799–810

[9] Albin MS, Bunegin L, Dujovny M, Bennett MH, Jannetta PJ, Wisotzkey HM. Brain retraction pressure during intracranial procedures. Surg Forum. 1975; 26:499–500

[10] Bennett MH, Albin MS, Bunegin L, Dujovny M, Hellstrom H, Jannetta PJ. Evoked potential changes during brain retraction in dogs. Stroke. 1977; 8 (4):487–492

[11] Zamorano L, Martinez-Coll A, Dujovny M. Transposition of image-defined trajectories into arc-quadrant centered stereotactic systems. Acta Neurochir Suppl (Wien). 1989; 46:109–111

[12] Leksell L, Lindquist C, Adler JR, Leksell D, Jernberg B, Steiner L. A new fixation device for the Leksell stereotaxic system. Technical note. J Neurosurg. 1987; 66(4):626–629

[13] Horwitz MJ. The Leyla retractor: use in acoustic neuroma and neurotologic surgery. Otolaryngology. 1978; 86(6, Pt 1):ORL-934–ORL-935

[14] Kelly PJ, Kall BA, Goerss S, Earnest F, IV. Computer-assisted stereotaxic laser resection of intra-axial brain neoplasms. J Neurosurg. 1986; 64(3):427–439

[15] Kelly PJ, Goerss SJ, Kall BA. The stereotaxic retractor in computer-assisted stereotaxic microsurgery. Technical note. J Neurosurg. 1988; 69(2):301–306

[16] Shelden CH, McCann G, Jacques S, et al. Development of a computerized microstereotaxic method for localization and removal of minute CNS lesions under direct 3-D vision. Technical report. J Neurosurg. 1980; 52(1):21–27

[17] Jacques S, Shelden CH, McCann GD, Freshwater DB, Rand R. Computerized three-dimensional stereotaxic removal of small central nervous system lesions in patients. J Neurosurg. 1980; 53(6):816–820

[18] Otsuki T, Jokura H, Yoshimoto T. Stereotactic guiding tube for open-system endoscopy: a new approach for the stereotactic endoscopic resection of intra-axial brain tumors. Neurosurgery. 1990; 27(2):326–330

[19] Greenfield JP, Cobb WS, Tsouris AJ, Schwartz TH. Stereotactic minimally invasive tubular retractor system for deep brain lesions. Neurosurgery. 2008; 63 (4) Suppl 2:334–339, discussion 339–340

[20] Jo KW, Shin HJ, Nam DH, et al. Efficacy of endoport-guided endoscopic resection for deep-seated brain lesions. Neurosurg Rev. 2011; 34(4):457–463

[21] Mamelak AN, Nobuto T, Berci G. Initial clinical experience with a high-definition exoscope system for microneurosurgery. Neurosurgery. 2010; 67 (2):476–483

[22] Mamelak AN, Danielpour M, Black KL, Hagike M, Berci G. A high-definition exoscope system for neurosurgery and other microsurgical disciplines: preliminary report. Surg Innov. 2008; 15(1):38–46

[23] Cavallo LM, Solari D, Cappabianca P. The endoscopic technique for removal of intraparenchymal lesions: a smooth passage in between brain fascicles. World Neurosurg. 2015; 83(2):155–156

[24] Chen CC, Hsu PW, Erich Wu TW, et al. Stereotactic brain biopsy: single center retrospective analysis of complications. Clin Neurol Neurosurg. 2009; 111 (10):835–839

[25] Dammers R, Haitsma IK, Schouten JW, Kros JM, Avezaat CJ, Vincent AJ. Safety and efficacy of frameless and frame-based intracranial biopsy techniques. Acta Neurochir (Wien). 2008; 150(1):23–29

[26] Yamada K, Goto S, Kochi M, Ushio Y. Stereotactic biopsy for multifocal, diffuse, and deep-seated brain tumors using Leksell's system. J Clin Neurosci. 2004; 11(3):263–267

[27] Zamorano L, Chavantes C, Moure F. Endoscopic stereotactic interventions in the treatment of brain lesions. Acta Neurochir Suppl (Wien). 1994; 61:92–97

[28] Tanei T, Nakahara N, Takebayashi S, et al. Endoscopic biopsy for lesions located in the parenchyma of the brain: preoperative planning based on stereotactic methods. Technical note. Neurol Med Chir (Tokyo). 2012; 52 (8):617–621

[29] Jacques S, Shelden CH, McCann G, Linn S. A microstereotactic approach to small CNS lesions. Part I. Development of CT localization and 3-D reconstruction techniques. No Shinkei Geka. 1980; 8(6):527–537

[30] Giussani C, Roux FE, Ojemann J, Sganzerla EP, Pirillo D, Papagno C. Is preoperative functional magnetic resonance imaging reliable for language areas mapping in brain tumor surgery? Review of language functional magnetic resonance imaging and direct cortical stimulation correlation studies. Neurosurgery. 2010; 66(1):113–120

[31] Duffau H. The dangers of magnetic resonance imaging diffusion tensor tractography in brain surgery. World Neurosurg. 2014; 81(1):56–58

[32] Leclercq D, Duffau H, Delmaire C, et al. Comparison of diffusion tensor imaging tractography of language tracts and intraoperative subcortical stimulations. J Neurosurg. 2010; 112(3):503–511

[33] Elias WJ, Sansur CA, Frysinger RC. Sulcal and ventricular trajectories in stereotactic surgery. J Neurosurg. 2009; 110(2):201–207

[34] Herrera SR, Shin JH, Chan M, Kouloumberis P, Goellner E, Slavin KV. Use of transparent plastic tubular retractor in surgery for deep brain lesions: a case series. Surg Technol Int. 2010; 19:47–50

[35] Kelly PJ. Technology in the resection of gliomas and the definition of madness. J Neurosurg. 2004; 101(2):284–286, discussion 286

[36] Sawaya R, Hammoud M, Schoppa D, et al. Neurosurgical outcomes in a modern series of 400 craniotomies for treatment of parenchymal tumors. Neurosurgery. 1998; 42(5):1044–1055, discussion 1055–1056

28 Intraparenchymal Brain Tumors: Microscope versus Endoscope

André Beer-Furlan, Daniel M. Prevedello, Christopher S. Hong, and J. Bradley Elder

Summary

Minimally invasive techniques in neurosurgery have grown in the past decade with the rationale of decreasing neurologic morbidity and possibly mortality. A specific advantage of most minimally invasive techniques used for the resection of intra-axial is limiting retractor-induced parenchymal injury associated with the use of blade or ribbon systems. In this chapter, we describe and discuss the advantages and disadvantages of endoscopic and microscopic minimally invasive port surgery based on the our experience and literature review.

Keywords: minimally invasive, endoscopic, port, surgery, cranial

28.1 Endoscopic and Port Surgery Perspective

28.1.1 Introduction

There has been a strong trend toward expanding the use of minimally invasive techniques in neurosurgery. This pattern has been particularly impressive in skull base surgery with advances in endoscopic approaches. Proponents justify these strategies because of the assumed decrease in neurologic morbidity and possibly mortality. A specific advantage of most minimally invasive techniques used for resection of intra-axial lesions is the potential to limit retractor-induced parenchymal injury associated with the use of blade or ribbon retractor systems.[1]

Fixed retraction systems that use blades for retraction can injure the brain through direct cortical and subcortical compression, as well as ischemic damage from suboptimal perfusion of local tissue.[1] Early work in a dog model suggested that a postoperative sensorimotor deficit was due to prolonged brain retraction. This conclusion was corroborated by microscopic findings showing pathologic changes in cortical tissue.[2]

Another animal model involved measuring cortical evoked potentials and laser-Doppler cerebral blood flow during subtemporal retraction in a pig. Results from this work showed that retraction pressure for 10 to 20 minutes caused a 50% decrease in the evoked potential amplitude, which improved after 5 to 10 minutes of relaxation.[3] Human studies were conducted to validate these findings. In a study of patients undergoing open cerebrovascular surgery, the pH, the partial pressure of oxygen and of carbon dioxide were measured and the results indicated the presence of ischemic changes with brain retraction.[4] Intraparenchymal microdialysis probes have also been used to demonstrate increased concentrations of lactate, glutamate, and glycerol after brain retraction, demonstrating metabolic changes consistent with parenchymal damage and injury to cellular membranes.[5]

Because of these findings, multiple attempts have been made to adjust surgical techniques to minimize brain retraction. Early investigations analyzed different retractor blade profiles in the hopes of reducing retraction injury, but despite these engineering alterations, no differences were observed in one study, comparing flat, flat with round edges, and curved blade profiles in reducing the risk of ischemic injury.[6] However, other technical aspects of the components of retractor systems—such as stereotactic frame systems, the Leyla flexible retractor arm, and cylindrical-shaped retractors, the latter of which is the basis of this study—have advanced considerably and thereby reduced retractor-induced injury.[7,8,9]

Cylindrical-shaped retractors were originally modeled after the curves of the gynecological speculum,[10] intended to progressively dilate the brain with larger-diameter cylinders to create a safe, surgical corridor for accessing deep-seated areas. Moreover, this design of a "tubular" retractor was readily compatible with existing stereotactic frame systems and could also serve as a fixed reference point for intraoperative navigation.[10,11] Current, modern versions of tubular retractors are widely utilized in minimally invasive spine surgeries, including routine diskectomies, spinal stenosis decompressions, and vertebral interbody fusions.[12,13,14,15] However, use of tubular retractors in brain surgery remains relatively uncommon, and most of the literature is comprised of individual case reports or small case series that describe the resection of deep-seated lesions.[16,17,18,19,20,21]

Recently, a new tubular retractor designed specifically for intracranial use has been integrated into our practice and referred to in this chapter as the "port." Unlike conventional tubular retractors used in spine surgery, the port is transparent and thus allows for visualization of retracted brain along the length of the entire surgical corridor. It is also compatible with most modern, frameless neuronavigation systems. A handful of previous case series have documented surgical experiences with the port utilizing both endoscope- and microscope-assisted visualization but in a surgeon preference–dependent manner.[21,22,23,24,25,26] On the other hand, we were the first group to compare endoscope-assisted to microscope-assisted port procedures for resection of deep-seated lesions in regard to extent of resection and clinical outcomes.[27] Similar comparisons, albeit unrelated to port surgery, have been made for other approaches, including those to the sella turcica, cerebellopontine angle, and posterior fossa.[28,29,30,31] In our experience, the majority of cases we now perform with port surgery utilize the microscope for operative visualization, but there are certain circumstances in which endoscope-assisted surgery may be more optimal. In this chapter, we present our cumulative experience with port surgery, as well as a systemic analysis of the literature, concerning the use of the port in accessing deep-seated areas of the brain.

28.1.2 Port Technique

At our institution, port surgery is performed with the Viewsite Brain Access System by Vycor Medical Inc. (Boca Raton, FL) for surgical access to intraparenchymal brain tumors. Currently, the Vycor port is available in four widths, as measured at the distal opening (12, 17, 21, and 28 mm) and three lengths (3, 5, and 7 cm). The port is constructed with transparent plastic, which enables the surgeon to visualize the surrounding brain along the entire length of the port. Prior to port entry, a cannula is inserted into the channel of the port to facilitate initial brain dissection and is removed after reaching the desired position of the port. Subsequently, port placement is secured via an attachment flange that can fix onto most surgical arm systems. In our experience, most cases with port surgery can be performed with the 12-mm-diameter port. In select cases, the 12-mm port may be substituted with a 17-mm port during surgery to optimize visualization.

What follows is a brief description of the general techniques utilized at our institution during port surgery for deep-seated intra-axial brain tumors. Preoperative imaging is obtained for surgical trajectory planning and includes diffusion tensor imaging (DTI) to ensure the planned trajectory does not transect white matter tracts, but instead travels parallel to white matter tracts. Skin incision is performed in a curvilinear fashion and made to accommodate a 3×3 cm craniotomy. After routine bone flap removal and opening of the dura, the optimal entry point is determined between insertion through a gyrus or sulcus, taking into consideration the presence of overlying superficial vessels. For gyral entry, the pia is incised with a 1.5-cm linear incision, followed by blunt dissection of up to 2 cm in depth before port placement or the advancement of a peel-away catheter in the direction of the lesion advanced with image guidance. For sulcal entry, the microscope is utilized to dissect a 1.5-cm-wide opening down to the fundus, carefully avoiding vascular structures. At the fundus, a linear incision is subsequently made prior to port placement using similar technique.

Selection of the proper length of the port is determined by measuring the distance from the overlying cortical opening to the far edge of the lesion. As stated earlier, the 12-mm-diameter port is always used initially but may be substituted, following

tumor debulking, with the larger 17-mm-diameter port, if deemed helpful. In our experience, use of the 21- and 28-mm-diameter ports has been unnecessary. Guidance of the port to the lesion is facilitated by fixing the navigation wand into the port channel with bone wax, with the tip of the wand located at the end of the port (▶ Fig. 28.1). Alternatively, the port can be configured with navigation capabilities with an attached navigation frame. Upon reaching the appropriate depth with the port, the navigation wand and cannula are removed, and the port is then secured to a snake retractor arm that is attached to a Mayfield head clamp. Afterward, the microscope or the endoscope is brought into the field to visualize and remove the tumor through the port.

During tumor resection, the angulation of the port may be manipulated as needed to traverse the entire width of the lesion. Utilizing the surface of the brain as a "fulcrum," small, careful movements are made to alter the angulation of the port. Likewise, the port may be inserted deeper into the lesion to reach the far edges of the tumor. Following resection of the tumor, hemostasis is achieved with standard techniques within the resection cavity and along the entire length of the surgical corridor. The port is removed, and the port trajectory is again inspected for adequate hemostasis. The craniotomy is then closed routinely.

28.1.3 Case Illustration: Endoscope-assisted Port Surgery

A 52-year-old female presented at our institution after a newly developed expressive aphasia and a right-side hemiplegia. She had recent diagnosis of breast cancer treated with mastectomy. Investigation with head computed tomography (CT) and MRI demonstrated a left-side contrast-enhancing frontal lesion immediately anterior to the motor cortex (▶ Fig. 28.2). There are also signs of blood products and significant edema on the surrounding brain parenchyma. After obtaining proper consent,

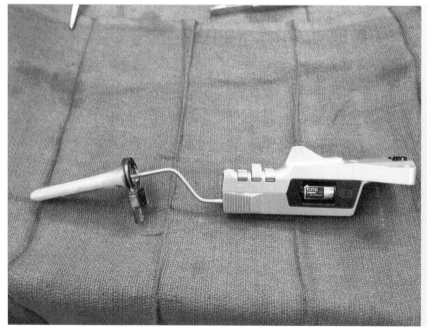

Fig. 28.1 Photograph demonstrating the image guidance device inserted inside a 12 mm × 8 mm × 7 cm Vycor port stabilized with bone wax just before insertion.

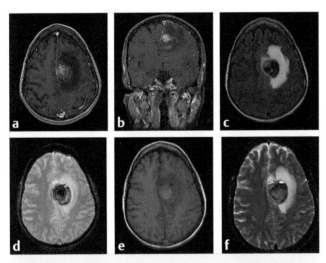

Fig. 28.2 Preoperative magnetic resonance imaging (MRI). **(a)** Axial T1-weighted (T1W) images with contrast. **(b)** Coronal T1 W images with contrast. **(c)** Axial fluid-attenuated inversion recovery (FLAIR). **(d)** Axial SWI. **(e)** Axial T1 W images without contrast. **(f)** Axial T2-weighted images. They demonstrate a left-side contrast-enhancing frontal lesion immediately anterior to the motor cortex with hemorrhagic component.

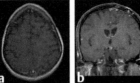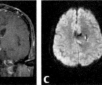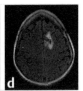

Fig. 28.3 Postoperative magnetic resonance imaging (MRI), after endoscopic assisted port surgery. **(a)** Axial T1-weighted (T1W) images with contrast. **(b)** Coronal T1 W images with contrast. **(c)** Axial diffusion-weighted imaging (DWI). **(d)** Axial fluid-attenuated inversion recovery (FLAIR). They demonstrate total resection with minimal brain manipulation.

28.1.4 Surgical Outcomes with Endoscope-assisted Port Surgery

At our institution, we have extensively utilized the endoscope for minimally invasive, transnasal approaches to the anterior skull base.[32,33,34] Building upon these experiences, we initially performed port surgery under endoscopic visualization. We detailed our early work with the endoscopic port technique describing our successful resections of the third ventricular colloid cyst, ventricular tumors, and parenchymal brain tumors.[22,23,35] Subsequently, we further reported our outcomes with endoscopic and microscopic port surgery in Hong et al.[27] In this study, the five cases operated through the endoscopic technique had the following pathology: metastasis (lung), metastasis (breast), neurocytoma, primitive neuroectodermal tumor (PNET), and glioblastoma multiforme (GBM). The locations of the tumors were in the right cerebellum (both metastases), right basal ganglia (neurocytoma and PNET), and left frontal lobe (GBM).

The 12-mm-diameter port was used in all but three cases (meningioma, melanoma metastasis, and GBM, all located in the basal ganglia), which required substitution with a larger 17-mm-diameter port. Incomplete resection was associated with the use of the endoscope. Only one case on this small series had a total resection.[27]

28.1.5 Case Illustration: Microscope-assisted Port Surgery

A 63-year-old female with no pertinent past medical history presented with 6 weeks of worsening headaches, accompanied by persistent nausea, vomiting, and a 20-lb weight loss. Her neurological examination was unremarkable. A noncontrast head CT suggested a cystic mass in the left cerebellum. Subsequently, the T1-weighted brain MRI postgadolinium contrast administration demonstrated a 4.1 × 3.0 cm complex cystic mass centered in the left cerebellar hemisphere with a lateral enhancing nodular component, measuring 2.8 × 2.0 cm in size (▶ Fig. 28.4a). The mass was causing near-complete effacement of the fourth ventricle, approximately 9 mm of midline shift, and downward herniation of the cerebellar tonsils.

The patient was subsequently taken to surgery for planned complete resection of the mass via microscope-assisted port

the patient was taken to the operating room for planned total resection via a left frontal craniotomy with intraoperative neuronavigation and use of the endoscope. A small corticectomy was made through which the port was inserted and advanced toward the lesion. Proper trajectory was confirmed by the neuronavigation wand, positioned within the lumen of the port supported by the introduction of bone wax. Subsequently, tumor debulking was achieved without complications and immediate postoperative imaging demonstrated gross total resection (GTR) with minimal evidence of the surgical corridor. Final pathology confirmed metastatic breast cancer. The immediate postoperative MRI demonstrated complete tumor resection with no additional edema on the surrounding brain and no evidence of surgery-related ischemic injury on diffusion-weighted imaging (DWI). At a 3-month follow-up visit, the patient's presenting symptoms had largely improved and imaging showed minimal brain manipulation (▶ Fig. 28.3). Endoscopic dissections were performed and varied between the 0-, 30-, and 45-degree Hopkins II rod-lens endoscopes (Karl Storz Endoscopy) measuring 4 mm × 18 cm. The endoscope was connected to a light source through a fiberoptic cable and a camera fitted with three charge-couple device sensors. The endoscope system consisted of an endoscope, a working sheath, and an obturator, all of which were accommodated by the port and still permitted the bimanual technique. There was excellent illumination of the surgical field by virtue of the endoscope's proximity to the anatomical structures. Wide-angle optics from the Hopkins II rod-lens provided high-resolution images. The angled endoscopes were used in the depth and in "around-the-corner" areas of the surgical cavity. The availability of multiple-angle endoscopes facilitated the examination of areas that would be otherwise obscured from direct straight down inspection.

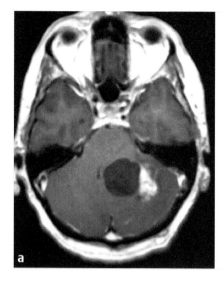 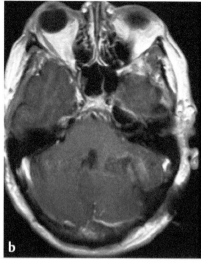

Fig. 28.4 (a) Axial cut of a T1-weighted brain magnetic resonance imaging (MRI) postgadolinium contrast administration demonstrates a 4.1 × 3.0 cm complex cystic mass with a 2.8 × 2.0 cm enhancing nodular component in the left cerebellum. (b) Axial cut of a T1-weighted brain MRI postgadolinium contrast administration, taken 2 days after surgery, demonstrates gross total resection of the lesion and decompression of the cyst. There is evidence of a minimal surgical corridor.

surgery. Using standard techniques with intraoperative neuronavigation, the dura overlying the lesion was opened via an approximate 3 × 3 cm craniotomy. After performing a small corticotomy, a 12 mm × 5 cm port was inserted under navigation guidance up to the surface of the nodular enhancing portion of the tumor. Subsequently, the OPMI Pentero 900 (Carl Zeiss Meditec AG) microscope was brought in and used for the remaining portion of the tumor resection. Blunt microsurgical dissection was used to develop a plane between tumor and surrounding cerebellar tissue. A red solid mass was noted, suggestive of hemangioblastoma. Subsequently, a longer port measuring 12 mm × 7 cm was substituted to better visualize the deeper cyst. Following drainage and decompression of the cyst, the mass was circumferentially dissected and removed in piecemeal. After achieving proper hemostasis through the port, the port was slowly removed, and closure proceeded in standard fashion. A brain MRI with contrast taken on postoperative day 2 demonstrated GTR and evidence of a minimal surgical corridor (▶ Fig. 28.4b). There was no evidence of ischemic injury on DWI. Final pathology was diagnostic of hemangioblastoma. The patient recovered uneventfully from surgery and was discharged in asymptomatic condition. She remained free of neurological complaints with no radiographic evidence of recurrence at 2-year follow-up.

28.1.6 Surgical Outcomes with Microscope-assisted Port Surgery

In the same study describing our initial experiences with endoscopic visualization during port surgery, we also described an additional 15 consecutive cases of port surgery utilizing the microscope.[27] The most common location operated on using the microscopic port technique was the basal ganglia (n = 9), followed by the cerebellum (n = 2), temporal lobe (n = 2), frontal lobe (n = 1), and parietal lobe (n = 1). The final pathologies of the resected lesions included metastases (n = 6), glioma (n = 6), meningioma (n = 1), radiation necrosis (n = 1), and hemangioblastoma (n = 1).[27]

The 12 mm × 7 cm port size was used in all cases, except one case of lung metastasis, which utilized the 12 mm × 5 cm port exclusively. Three cases, all located within the basal ganglia (meningioma, metastasis, and GBM), required an additional use of a larger diameter 17-mm port and achieved GTR. In 13 of 15 (87%) microscopic cases, GTR was achieved. In the remaining two patients, near-total resection (NTR) was obtained. In analyzing all 20 cases, incomplete resection (i.e., NTR or subtotal resection [STR]) was associated with lesion location within the basal ganglia as well as use of the endoscope.

28.1.7 Literature Review and Current Evidence

In addition to our own study,[27] others have described the success of port surgery for resection of intraparenchymal brain lesions. Herrera et al reported that in 16 cases of port surgery, including 2 intraventricular tumors and 2 deep-seated hematomas, none resulted in postoperative hematomas.[24] Nine of the 13 brain tumors achieved GTR, while the remaining 4 resulted in STR, although the details regarding lesion location and histology of the incomplete resections were not noted. Raza et al described nine adult and pediatric patients treated with port surgery, two of whom underwent excisional biopsy.[25] In the remaining seven patients, six achieved GTR with no evidence of retractor-related injury on T2-weighted MRI and DWI, while the lone case of STR, a patient with a papillary tumor of the pineal region, did exhibit radiographic evidence of white matter manipulation although without any clinical manifestations. In a separate study by the same senior authors, Recinos et al described successful resection with port surgery of deep-seated tumors in four pediatric patients, including complete resection of two gliomas, for which GTR was the preoperative goal.[26] Only one patient demonstrated radiographic evidence of white matter injury on T2-weighted MRI and DWI. Interestingly, like the case in Raza et al, this patient had also undergone resection of pineal region tumor, raising the possibility that port surgery may be nonadvantageous for approaches to the pineal region.

At our institution, we have successfully performed port surgery with the assistance of both the microscope and the endoscope. In Hong et al, we specifically sought to compare outcomes between microscope- versus endoscope-assisted visualization during port surgery.[27] As mentioned earlier in this chapter, use of the endoscope was significantly associated with incomplete resection of the target lesion. However, it is important to explain that our change to start performing port surgery primarily using the microscope was not a consequence of this study. The main aspect was the frustration during the endoscopic cases related to the lack of space offered by the presence of the endoscope inside the port and decreasing the freedom of movements.

28.1.8 Advantages/Disadvantages of the Microscopic and Endoscopic Techniques

In our opinion, there are three major advantages that the microscope confers over the endoscope during port surgery. First, modern microscopes, such as those utilized in Hong et al,[27] permit binocular, 3D visualization of the surgical field, in comparison to 2D views offered by conventional endoscopes. Improved depth perception afforded by 3D visualization is thought to improve the accuracy of surgical instrument manipulation, as supported by evidence that newer 3D endoscopes reduce operating times and shorten learning curves, compared to traditional endoscopes.[36] In addition, modern microscopes typically have an integrated double-iris diaphragm, which, depending on the size of the port, can be adjusted to afford maximum light and resolution or depth of field. Furthermore, the two-channel illumination design can modulate light brightness and prevents excessive light shadowing when illuminating deeper cavities. Second, although the smallest 12-mm-diameter port can adequately facilitate bimanual technique during endoscopic port surgery, the absence of the endoscope afforded by microscopic visualization allows for additional space within the port to accommodate more instruments and improved freedom of movements. We frequently utilize this opportunity to include a third assisting hand for further suctioning or microretracting. Third, microscopic visualization during port surgery allows for fluid and rapid manual manipulation of the port. In contrast, during endoscopic port surgery the endoscope is "fixed" to the port when using a holder and therefore must be disconnected prior to adjustment of the port. Subsequently, the port must be repositioned without direct visualization, and then reconnected to the endoscope to confirm proper placement. On the other hand, microscopic visualization permits minor adjustments of the port under direct visualization. If larger changes in the trajectory of the port are required, such as during resection of large tumors or inspection of the resection cavity, the surface of the brain can act as a "fulcrum" to adjust the angulation of the port and typically does not extend beyond 15 degrees in any direction. While the tip of the port moves the greatest distance during this movement, this is felt to be safe since the distal end of the port almost exclusively remains within the tumor bed. In contrast, attention must be paid to avoid translational movement at the fulcrum (i.e., brain surface) during port adjustment to prevent additional insult to cerebral tissues beyond the initial cortictectomy. Port entry can be continuously reassessed under direct visualization throughout surgery to ensure that the position of the port has not migrated, secondary to relaxation of the brain.

Encouraged by our findings reported in Hong et al, we no longer routinely perform port surgery with endoscope-assisted visualization alone. However, there are instances in which the endoscope may be utilized in conjunction with the microscope. In cases where a large surgical cavity remains after resection of the lesion, the endoscope may be brought into the field to inspect the surgical bed, prior to port removal, to ensure the absence of any remaining mass and to confirm suitable hemostasis. In particular, we have found that port surgery for intraventricular lesions frequently benefit from the use of endoscopic inspection after microscope-assisted port surgery.

28.1.9 Selection of Patients for Port Surgery

In our experience, the two most important factors to consider when considering patients for port surgery are location of the lesion and presumed histology. Regarding anatomic location, the best candidates for port surgery include tumors within the cerebellar hemispheres, basal ganglia, and deep cerebral white matter tracts. In contrast, we do not utilize port surgery for lesions whose deepest point is under 3 cm from the surface of the brain, as use of the port is not felt to offer any additional advantages. For lesions within the deep white matter tracts and basal ganglia, port surgery allows for a smaller craniotomy and also minimizes neurological morbidity via even, radial retraction of overlying brain tissue. The latter can be further facilitated by preoperative functional MRI and DTI to aid in planning a surgical corridor that runs parallel to white matter tracts. Utilizing this approach, we have demonstrated that port surgery could successfully resect deep-seated lesions with no evidence of ischemic injury on DWI.[27] In contrast, our experiences suggest that the advantages of port surgery differ for lesions within the cerebellar hemispheres. Although not studied as an objective outcome, we have anecdotally found that patients who underwent port surgery for resection of their posterior fossa lesions experienced less postoperative pain than those treated with traditional microsurgery, possibly due to minimization of the incision and craniotomy. As such, preoperative planning for cerebellar port surgery is focused on minimizing the extent of the surgical corridor. Likewise, there is greater emphasis on identification and avoidance of critical vessels like the transverse sinus, rather than eloquent neural structures seen with supratentorial lesions. Compared to supratentorial lesions, greater care must be taken intraoperatively to avoid cerebrospinal fluid (CSF) leakage, which may anecdotally also be an advantage of cerebellar port surgery. However, further objective study to verify this possibility is required.

As mentioned earlier, the presumed histology of the lesion is the second important factor when considering patients for port surgery. In our experience, lesions with a soft, "suckable" consistency are optimal, as suction removal of the lesion encourages the outer edges of the resection cavity to collapse into view during debulking, preventing excessive manipulation of the port. Histologies that fit this description include most metastatic tumors (i.e., breast cancer, melanoma) and high-grade gliomas. Likewise, non-neoplastic, soft lesions like hematomas may also be amenable to port surgery.[21] On the other hand, firmer tumors seem to be less amenable to port surgery and may result in increased morbidity due to the need for greater manipulation of the port. Such histologies include meningiomas, metastatic sarcomas, and lesions with significant scar tissue such as recurrent gliomas. However, in the cases where suboptimal firmer consistencies are discovered during port surgery, use of an ultrasonic aspirator and suction cutter device, such as the NICO Myriad (NICO Corporation, Indianapolis, IN), may aid in complete resection of the lesion through the port. In addition, lesions that are prone to hemorrhage during piecemeal resection, such as metastatic renal cell carcinomas, may not be best suited for port surgery, as significant bleeding may be difficult to control within the port and may significantly prolong operative time.

In our experience, tumor size is not as important of a consideration as lesion location and presumed histology in selecting patients for port surgery. Even if very large, for softer tumors, the peripheral edges will generally be coaxed into view under the pressure of surrounding normal brain, as the central portions of the lesion are resected. On the other hand, the combination of larger size and firm consistency is the least desirable for port surgery, as this would likely entail significant manipulation of the port.

Taken together, we consider lesions that are deep seated (> 3 cm from the edge of the overlying brain) and soft in consistency, based on presumed histology, to be best suited for port surgery. Utilizing this approach, none of the cases described in Hong et al required abortion of the port and conversion to open surgery or expansion of the craniotomy. That being said, we feel that it is important during port surgery to prepare the surgical field to allow for widening of the craniotomy, should it become necessary.

28.1.10 Conclusion

In conclusion, port surgery is a successful, minimally invasive method for resecting deep-seated lesions of the brain and incurs minimal neurologic morbidity. In our experience, visualization and corridor optimization is generally superior with the microscope in comparison to that provided with the endoscope inside the port. Patients best suited to port surgery include deep-seated (> 3 cm from overlying brain surface) location and histology suggestive of a soft, "suckable" consistency. As evidence continues to accumulate supporting port surgery as a safe and effective approach, future studies directly comparing outcomes between port surgery and conventional open microsurgery are needed to further refine the optimal indications for port surgery.

28.1.11 Complication Avoidance and Clinical Pearls

- Select lesions most optimal for port surgery: (1) deep-seated anatomic location (> 3 cm, measured from the deepest point of the lesion to the surface of the overlying brain) and (2) soft consistency, determined by the presumed histology.
- Utilize preoperative functional MRI and/or DTI to plan a trajectory that avoids eloquent cortex and ventricles, particularly for supratentorial lesions.
- Minimize size of the incision (particularly for cerebellar lesions) and craniotomy (3 × 3 cm) but prepare surgical field to allow for potential widening of craniotomy.

- Perform minor corticectomy or opening of the sulcus under microscopic visualization and obtain proper hemostasis.
- Firmly secure the port to the retractor arm to avoid movement that could damage normal brain tissue.
- Utilize the surface of the brain as a fulcrum to adjust angulation of the port and periodically check for gross injury at the fulcrum site.
- Utilize the operative microscope for visualization during port surgery. Following resection of the mass, an endoscope may be utilized to inspect the entirety of the surgical cavity for residual lesion and proper hemostasis.

References

[1] Spetzler RF, Sanai N. The quiet revolution: retractorless surgery for complex vascular and skull base lesions. J Neurosurg. 2012; 116(2):291–300

[2] Bennett MH, Albin MS, Bunegin L, Dujovny M, Hellstrom H, Jannetta PJ. Evoked potential changes during brain retraction in dogs. Stroke. 1977; 8 (4):487–492

[3] Andrews RJ, Muto RP. Retraction brain ischaemia: cerebral blood flow, evoked potentials, hypotension and hyperventilation in a new animal model. Neurol Res. 1992; 14(1):12–18

[4] Hoffman WE, Charbel FT, Portillo GG, Edelman G, Ausman JI. Regional tissue pO2, pCO2, pH and temperature measurement. Neurol Res. 1998; 20 Suppl 1: S81–S84

[5] Xu W, Mellergård P, Ungerstedt U, Nordström CH. Local changes in cerebral energy metabolism due to brain retraction during routine neurosurgical procedures. Acta Neurochir (Wien). 2002; 144(7):679–683

[6] Rosenørn J, Diemer NH. The influence of the profile of brain retractors on regional cerebral blood flow in the rat. Acta Neurochir (Wien). 1987; 87(3–4):140–143

[7] Horwitz MJ. The Leyla retractor: use in acoustic neuroma and neurotologic surgery. Otolaryngology. 1978; 86(6)(,)(Pt 1):ORL-934–ORL-935

[8] Leksell L, Lindquist C, Adler JR, Leksell D, Jernberg B, Steiner L. A new fixation device for the Leksell stereotaxic system. Technical note. J Neurosurg. 1987; 66(4):626–629

[9] Zamorano L, Martinez-Coll A, Dujovny M. Transposition of image-defined trajectories into arc-quadrant centered stereotactic systems. Acta Neurochir Suppl (Wien). 1989; 46:109–111

[10] Kelly PJ, Goerss SJ, Kall BA. The stereotaxic retractor in computer-assisted stereotaxic microsurgery. Technical note. J Neurosurg. 1988; 69(2):301–306

[11] Kelly PJ. Future perspectives in stereotactic neurosurgery: stereotactic microsurgical removal of deep brain tumors. J Neurosurg Sci. 1989; 33 (1):149–154

[12] Chotigavanichaya C, Korwutthikulrangsri E, Suratkarndawadee S, et al. Minimally invasive lumbar disectomy with the tubular retractor system: 4–7 years follow-up. J Med Assoc Thai. 2012; 95 Suppl 9:S82–S86

[13] Franke J, Greiner-Perth R, Boehm H, et al. Comparison of a minimally invasive procedure versus standard microscopic discotomy: a prospective randomised controlled clinical trial. Eur Spine J. 2009; 18(7):992–1000

[14] Kotwal S, Kawaguchi S, Lebl D, et al. Minimally invasive lateral lumbar interbody fusion: clinical and radiographic outcome at a minimum 2-year follow-up. J Spinal Disord Tech. 2015; 28(4):119–125

[15] Popov V, Anderson DG. Minimal invasive decompression for lumbar spinal stenosis. Adv Orthop. 2012; 2012:645321

[16] Cabbell KL, Ross DA. Stereotactic microsurgical craniotomy for the treatment of third ventricular colloid cysts. Neurosurgery. 1996; 38(2):301–307

[17] Kelly PJ, Kall BA, Goerss SJ. Computer-interactive stereotactic resection of deep-seated and centrally located intraaxial brain lesions. Appl Neurophysiol. 1987; 50(1–6):107–113

[18] Moshel YA, Link MJ, Kelly PJ. Stereotactic volumetric resection of thalamic pilocytic astrocytomas. Neurosurgery. 2007; 61(1):66–75, discussion 75

[19] Otsuki T, Jokura H, Yoshimoto T. Stereotactic guiding tube for open-system endoscopy: a new approach for the stereotactic endoscopic resection of intra-axial brain tumors. Neurosurgery. 1990; 27(2):326–330

[20] Patil AA. Free-standing, stereotactic, microsurgical retraction technique in "key hole" intracranial procedures. Acta Neurochir (Wien). 1991; 108(3–4):148–153

[21] Yadav YR, Yadav S, Sherekar S, Parihar V. A new minimally invasive tubular brain retractor system for surgery of deep intracerebral hematoma. Neurol India. 2011; 59(1):74–77

[22] McLaughlin N, Prevedello DM, Engh J, Kelly DF, Kassam AB. Endoneurosurgical resection of intraventricular and intraparenchymal lesions using the port technique. World Neurosurg. 2013; 79(2) Suppl:18.e1–18.e8

[23] Engh JA, Lunsford LD, Amin DV, et al. Stereotactically guided endoscopic port surgery for intraventricular tumor and colloid cyst resection. Neurosurgery. 2010; 67(3) Suppl Operative:ons198–ons204, discussion ons204–ons205

[24] Herrera SR, Shin JH, Chan M, Kouloumberis P, Goellner E, Slavin KV. Use of transparent plastic tubular retractor in surgery for deep brain lesions: a case series. Surg Technol Int. 2010; 19:47–50

[25] Raza SM, Recinos PF, Avendano J, Adams H, Jallo GI, Quinones-Hinojosa A. Minimally invasive trans-portal resection of deep intracranial lesions. Minim Invasive Neurosurg. 2011; 54(1):5–11

[26] Recinos PF, Raza SM, Jallo GI, Recinos VR. Use of a minimally invasive tubular retraction system for deep-seated tumors in pediatric patients. J Neurosurg Pediatr. 2011; 7(5):516–521

[27] Hong CS, Prevedello DM, Elder JB. Comparison of endoscope- versus microscope-assisted resection of deep-seated intracranial lesions using a minimally invasive port retractor system. J Neurosurg. 2015; 28:1–12

[28] Kahilogullari G, Beton S, Al-Beyati ES, et al. Olfactory functions after transsphenoidal pituitary surgery: endoscopic versus microscopic approach. Laryngoscope. 2013; 123(9):2112–2119

[29] McLaughlin N, Eisenberg AA, Cohan P, Chaloner CB, Kelly DF. Value of endoscopy for maximizing tumor removal in endonasal transsphenoidal pituitary adenoma surgery. J Neurosurg. 2013; 118(3):613–620

[30] Takemura Y, Inoue T, Morishita T, Rhoton AL, Jr. Comparison of microscopic and endoscopic approaches to the cerebellopontine angle. World Neurosurg. 2014; 82(3-4):427–441

[31] Van Rompaey J, Bush C, McKinnon B, Solares AC. Minimally invasive access to the posterior cranial fossa: an anatomical study comparing a retrosigmoidal endoscopic approach to a microscopic approach. J Neurol Surg A Cent Eur Neurosurg. 2013; 74(1):1–6

[32] Carrau RL, Prevedello DM, de Lara D, Durmus K, Ozer E. Combined transoral robotic surgery and endoscopic endonasal approach for the resection of extensive malignancies of the skull base. Head Neck. 2013; 35(11):E351–E358

[33] Kassam AB, Prevedello DM, Carrau RL, et al. Endoscopic endonasal skull base surgery: analysis of complications in the authors' initial 800 patients. J Neurosurg. 2011; 114(6):1544–1568

[34] Prevedello DM, Ebner FH, de Lara D, Ditzel Filho L, Otto BA, Carrau RL. Extracapsular dissection technique with the cotton swab for pituitary adenomas through an endoscopic endonasal approach: how I do it. Acta Neurochir (Wien). 2013; 155(9):1629–1632

[35] Ochalski PG, Fernandez-Miranda JC, Prevedello DM, Pollack IF, Engh JA. Endoscopic port surgery for resection of lesions of the cerebellar peduncles: technical note. Neurosurgery. 2011; 68(5):1444–1450, discussion 1450–1451

[36] Barkhoudarian G, Del Carmen Becerra Romero A, Laws ER. Evaluation of the 3-dimensional endoscope in transsphenoidal surgery. Neurosurgery. 2013; 73(1) Suppl Operative:ons74–ons78, discussion ons78–ons79

Part VI

Pediatrics

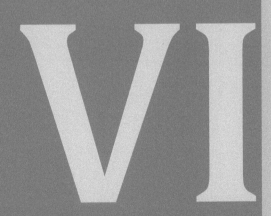

29 Surgical Management of Hypothalamic Hamartomas

Ruth E. Bristol

Summary

Hypothalamic hamartomas are nonneoplastic gray matter lesions that commonly occur in pediatric patients who present with gelastic seizures and precocious puberty. These lesions are characterized by their deep-seated location. Traditional microscopic approaches for accessing large lesions are well described. For smaller lesions located primarily within the third ventricle, our group has used minimally invasive endoscopic approaches. We find that this technique reduces approach-related morbidity without minimizing the efficacy of the procedure. In this chapter, we describe our institutional experience with the perioperative management of patients with hypothalamic hamartomas.

Keywords: endocrinopathy, epileptogenesis, gelastic epilepsy, hamartoma, hypothalamus

29.1 Introduction

Hypothalamic hamartomas (HHs) are nonneoplastic gray matter lesions, generally occurring within or below the third ventricle. The most common presentations are gelastic seizures and precocious puberty. Some correlation has been found between location and presenting symptoms, as lesions within the third ventricle are more likely to cause epilepsy.[1] Most cases are identified in childhood. Careful history taking often reveals that the symptoms have been present since an early age, sometimes since birth. Lesions are infrequently large enough to cause mass effect on adjacent structures or cerebrospinal fluid obstruction. Hamartomas do not grow disproportionately to the brain over time.

The HH tissue is inherently epileptogenic. Intraoperative recordings and single-cell in vitro recordings have demonstrated spontaneous firing from hamartoma neurons.[2] The particular type of seizures generated by this tissue is called gelastic, and these seizures respond poorly to medical therapy.

The location of the attachment of the HH determines its symptomatology. HHs have been found within the third ventricle, occupying the floor of the third ventricle, and attached along the hypothalamic infundibulum. With large lesions, it may be difficult to determine the site of attachment, or the lesions may be attached to multiple regions. HHs are classified according to the Delalande classification,[3] which is based on the location of attachment (▶ Fig. 29.1). Lesions are categorized into types I through IV: (1) pedunculated lesions below the third ventricle, (2) sessile lesions within the third ventricle, (3) lesions with combined attachment above and below the floor of the third ventricle, and (4) giant lesions. Lesions with purely infundibular attachments are more likely to result in precocious puberty than epilepsy. The particular interaction between hamartoma cells and cells of the hypophyseal system is not well understood.

29.2 Clinical Features

Gelastic epilepsy is the most common presenting symptom. The semiology most often involves laughter that is inappropriate, uncontrollable, and unprovoked by the environment. Gelastic seizures can number in the hundreds per day, and frequently last only a few seconds. However, a constant state of seizing or "status gelasticus" has been described.[4] Many patients with HH present with other seizure types and also exhibit presumed secondary epileptogenesis. The second most common type of seizure is the complex partial seizure. These seizures tend to be more responsive to medication than gelastic seizures.

The second category of presenting symptoms for HH patients is an endocrine disturbance. Precocious puberty is the most common result, but other endocrinopathies have been seen. Many patients with precocious puberty may be managed on a gonadotropin-releasing hormone agonist until an age when puberty is appropriate or until surgical resection is performed.

The frequent involvement of the mammillary bodies often results in memory deficits, and patients may experience declining

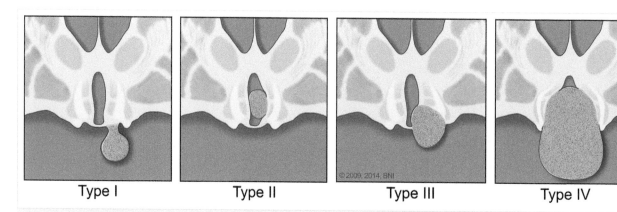

Fig. 29.1 Artist's illustration shows the Delalande classification of hypothalamic hamartomas. Type I: pedunculated lesion below the third ventricle. Type II: sessile lesion within the third ventricle. Type III: combined attachment above and below the floor of the third ventricle. Type IV: giant lesion. (Used with permission from Barrow Neurological Institute, Phoenix, AZ.)

school function as they age. Such deterioration is also considered an indication for treatment, as it offers the potential for subsequent improvement.[5] Patients who exhibit the greatest degree of impairment but have the shortest duration of seizures are the most likely to improve.

Finally, aggressive behavior and "rage attacks" are common in patients with HH. Younger patients may require restraints to maintain their safety, and older patients may have to be institutionalized because of injury to themselves and others. Fortunately, the aggression and rage related to HH invariably improve with resection.

29.3 Case Example: Endoscopic

29.3.1 History

A 13-year-old adolescent boy (patient 1) was referred to our neurosurgery center after his seizure disorder led to a diagnosis of a type 2 HH, defined as a sessile lesion within the third ventricle (▶ Fig. 29.2). In retrospect, the family recognized that he had experienced gelastic seizures from 18 months of age, characterized by an "unprovoked" laugh and automatisms. At age 4 years, he developed complex partial seizures. At age 8 years, he underwent Gamma Knife (Leksell Gamma Knife; Elekta AB, Stockholm, Sweden) radiosurgery of the lesion that resulted in initial improvement in seizure frequency, but the seizures subsequently returned. At age 11 years, he underwent a second Gamma Knife procedure, with no appreciable postoperative change in symptoms. None of several previous trials of antiepileptic medication (carbamazepine, lamotrigine, valproic acid,

levetiracetam, and topiramate) had any effect on seizure frequency. The patient had no endocrinology abnormalities. When the patient was 13 years old, he still had multiple gelastic seizures daily, and his family chose to pursue surgical resection.

29.3.2 Physical Examination

Physical examination of the patient showed that he had normal motor skills for his age. Neuropsychological evaluation revealed normal to low overall intelligence and working memory deficit. He also experienced learning difficulties in school.

29.3.3 Intraoperative Management

The patient was placed in the supine position. An incision was planned in the right frontal scalp, as directed by neuronavigation to yield the best angle into the third ventricle and toward the HH. The HH was approached endoscopically through the right lateral ventricle. A combination of grasping forceps and electrocautery was used to remove the lesion. Stereotactic guidance confirmed the margin of the lesion. No external ventricular drain was used.

29.3.4 Surgical Outcome

At 3-year follow-up, the patient had complete resolution of the gelastic seizures. He was taking no medication and had stopped having seizures. His schoolwork was slowly improving, although he continued to struggle with reading comprehension.

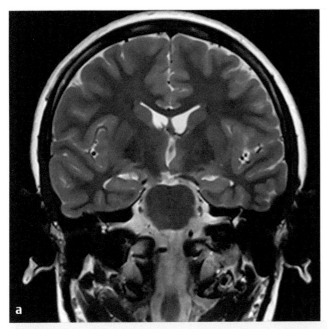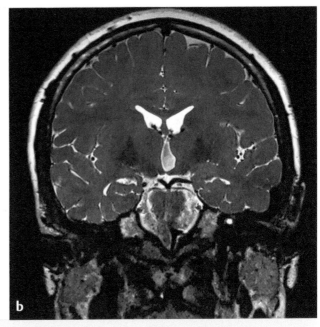

Fig. 29.2 Patient 1. **(a)** Preoperative coronal T2-weighted magnetic resonance imaging (MRI) shows a 1-cm hyperintense lesion within the third ventricle on the left, above the mammillary body, slightly displacing it. The lesion has no true attachment to the right mammillary body, as determined intraoperatively. **(b)** Two-year postoperative coronal T2-weighted MRI shows removal of the hamartoma. (Used with permission from Barrow Neurological Institute, Phoenix, AZ.)

29.4 Case Example: Open

29.4.1 History

A 4.5-year-old girl (patient 2) presented to our neurosurgery center with gelastic epilepsy that had been present since birth. She also experienced complex partial seizures that had begun when she was 3 years of age. She had no endocrinology abnormalities. Her previous medications included oxcarbazepine and topiramate. Magnetic resonance imaging (MRI) revealed a type 2 HH with bilateral thalamic attachment (▶ Fig. 29.3).

29.4.2 Physical Examination

Results of the physical examination revealed no abnormalities. Neuropsychological testing revealed low to average intelligence and weakness in word retrieval. Receptive language and repetition were within the average range. The patient had difficulties with behavioral and emotional adjustment, characterized by aggressive behavior. She became easily angered. She had difficulty with times of transition, such as arriving at school or switching to new activities.

29.4.3 Intraoperative Management

The patient was placed in the supine position with her head in a Mayfield head holder. Her head was turned 90 degrees to the right, so that the interhemispheric fissure would be parallel to the floor. Next, her head was tilted toward the left shoulder, approximately 45 degrees. A coronally oriented incision was planned just anterior to the coronal suture. A rectangular craniotomy measuring 4 cm from front to back and 3 cm from side to side was used, placed two-thirds in front of and one-third behind the coronal suture. An interhemispheric dissection was made over the right frontal lobe, and a transcallosal, interforniceal approach into the third ventricle was then used for gross total resection of the HH. Stereotactic guidance was used for the approach and to direct the extent of resection. The tumor was removed with the assistance of microsurgical dissectors and ultrasonic aspiration. No external ventricular drain was placed intraoperatively.

29.4.4 Surgical Outcome

At 3-year follow-up, the patient was seizure free and off all medication. Neuropsychological testing revealed improvement from the preoperative state in overall intellectual function, although short-term memory continued to be weak. Cognitive function was stronger at the 3-year follow-up than it had been at the 1-year follow-up. The patient had some verbal and visual skills that measured in the above-average range, but her memory continued to be impaired and she was still emotionally labile.

29.5 Advantages and Disadvantages of the Endoscopic Approach

With recent improvements in intraoperative optics, lighting, and resection techniques, small HH lesions or lesions with small attachments are amenable to endoscopic resection. Lesions that are entirely within the third ventricle, or that make up the floor of the ventricle, are most suitable for endoscopic resection. If a lesion extends laterally within the suprasellar

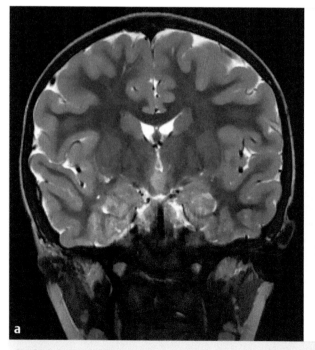
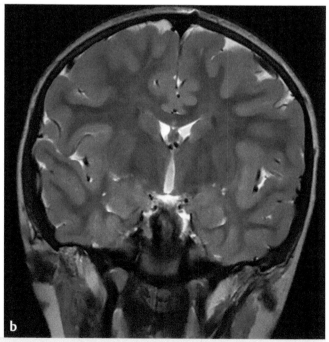

Fig. 29.3 Patient 2. **(a)** Preoperative coronal T2-weighted magnetic resonance imaging (MRI) shows a type 2 hypothalamic hamartoma with bilateral thalamic attachment. **(b)** One-year postoperative coronal T2-weighted MRI shows complete resection of the lesion. (Used with permission from Barrow Neurological Institute, Phoenix, AZ.)

cistern, it will not be reachable from a single transventricular endoscopic approach. Size remains a significant limitation to neuroendoscopy. We do not recommend attempted resection of lesions larger than 1.5 cm in size. However, neuroendoscopy can be useful as a second stage in resecting large lesions that have been incompletely resected via another approach.

The patient is positioned supine with the head in the neutral position. Stereotactic guidance is used to determine the optimal trajectory through the foramen of Monro to the base of the lesion. The ventricle contralateral to the attachment of the lesion is entered using a bur hole and an endoscopic sheath. After the foramen of Monro is traversed, the lesion can be visualized along the contralateral wall (▶ Fig. 29.4). Operating from the ipsilateral side is not recommended because of difficulty in achieving the appropriate angle to detach the lesion. Initial resection should be aimed at the base of the lesion to disconnect it from the hypothalamus. If this attachment is left until the end of the resection, it can be difficult to achieve a satisfactory resection. HHs are favorable targets for resection because they are hypovascular and have a consistency that is easily removed piecemeal with endoscopic pituitary rongeurs. The rongeur is positioned parallel to the wall of attachment and is pressed gently into the lesion while being closed. Gently twisting the rongeur will then remove the lesion from the surrounding tissue, and the rongeur can be withdrawn. After the lesion is collected, the rongeur is advanced again. The use of two rongeurs in an alternating fashion expedites the resection. After disconnection has been conducted across the base, the lesion is removed, often in one or a few large pieces. The advent of suction and cutting devices that fit through an endoscope has improved efficiency, and laser coagulation with thulium can be

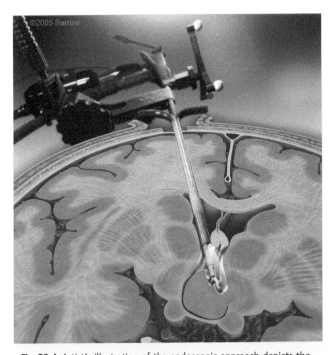

Fig. 29.4 Artist's illustration of the endoscopic approach depicts the stereotactic navigation system and the micromanipulator on the endoscope. The trajectory is contralateral to the lesion attachment. The endoscope is advanced through the foramen of Monro to visualize the third ventricular mass. (Used with permission from Barrow Neurological Institute, Phoenix, AZ.)

used instead of rongeurs. Similarly, after the gross bulk of the lesion has been removed, an aspiration device or laser can be used to shave the wall if there is suspected residual HH. External pneumatic, or locking, arms and endoscope "micromanipulators," which attach between the endoscope and the pneumatic arm, facilitate tumor resection and reduce the human error inherent in holding a scope for a prolonged period. Although this approach should reduce the risk of memory loss, the rate of permanent memory loss is about 8% in both open and endoscopic series.[6]

Advantages of endoscopic resection of HHs include a faster recovery, a shorter hospital stay, and a lower surgical complication rate. The main disadvantage is the size restriction. Until endoscopic aspirating devices are more readily available, it is inadvisable to approach a lesion larger than 1.5 cm. Most of the resection is conducted with micropituitary rongeurs, thereby removing only a fraction of a millimeter with each bite. In addition, lesions located more posteriorly in the third ventricle can be more difficult to visualize through the foramen and can place the fornix at greater risk.

29.6 Advantages and Disadvantages of the Open Approach

29.6.1 Lesions within the Third Ventricle

The transcallosal interforniceal approach to HHs was first described in 2001 by Jeffrey Rosenfeld[7,8] and was further developed by Harold Rekate and the Barrow Neurological Institute team in 2003. Although the transcallosal approach remains a common and direct route for open surgical resection, advances in endoscopy and laser thermoablation have offered more minimally invasive approaches over the past 5 to 10 years.

The interforniceal approach affords full visualization of the third ventricle, and the use of a variety of resection methods. The patient is positioned supine, with the head turned 90 degrees so that the falx is parallel to the floor. Intraoperative stereotactic guidance is used to identify the midline of the corpus callosum, and an interforniceal dissection is made into the third ventricle. The tumor is visualized in the wall of the third ventricle. Standard tumor resection techniques, including the use of microdissectors and ultrasonic aspiration, are used. The drawback of this approach is potential injury to the delicate forniceal structures with the risk of memory loss. Children appear to tolerate this dissection better than adults.[9] An alternate approach, of splitting the choroidal fissure or operating through an enlarged foramen of Monro, may be possible in certain patients. In a combined approach, a standard interhemispheric approach to the lateral ventricle can be used, and the endoscope can then be advanced through the foramen of Monro. This approach is useful in patients with small ventricles for whom pure endoscopy is not ideal.[10]

29.6.2 Lesions below the Third Ventricle

Lesions below the floor of the third ventricle require resection via a pterional or an orbitozygomatic approach. In patients younger than 10 years, the orbitozygomatic approach is generally not needed, and a standard pterional approach will suffice. The pterional approach affords protection of vascular structures, the pituitary stalk, and the chiasm. Caution is required in dissecting between perforating vessels from the carotid and anterior cerebral arteries. One drawback is poor visualization of the ipsilateral attachment to the mammillary body and hypothalamus. For this reason, surgical resection is planned from the contralateral side.

29.7 Other Approaches

Stereotactic radiosurgery provides a more minimally invasive treatment option. We have found that efficacy frequently requires 12 to 18 months, or even as long as 24 months, whereas some reports in the medical literature encourage waiting as long as 3 years.[11] As a result, this modality is reserved for patients with milder or less frequent symptoms, or for those who are stable with conservative therapy. As with the endoscopic approach, radiosurgery also has a size limitation. Patients with lesions larger than 3 cm are not considered candidates for radiosurgery. Lesions are also excluded if they are immediately adjacent to the optic tracts or chiasm. Another minimally invasive approach is stereotactic laser thermoablation, which has been used more for smaller lesions or for those with an attachment point amenable to approach via a straight line from the surface. The size of the lesion created by the thermal probe must be planned carefully with respect to adjacent structures. Lesions can be treated with radiosurgery when the base of attachment is large enough to accommodate the laser, but not so sessile that the margins cannot be reached.

Other types of treatment have also been used for the management of HHs. These include radiofrequency ablation,[12] vagus nerve stimulation, deep brain stimulation,[13] and interstitial radiosurgery. Alternative surgical approaches include subfrontal or "eyebrow" craniotomy. Many of these alternatives have been reported in small series only. Morbidity appears similar to that of standard treatments.

29.8 Patient Selection

The team-guided decision to intervene in a patient with an HH should be made on a case-by-case basis. Patients with many gelastic events per day, or in whom the frequency of seizures has progressed, are generally considered candidates for surgery. Similarly, precocious puberty and other endocrine disturbances that are unresponsive to medical treatment are also indications for intervention. Finally, the evidence is clear that patients with severe behavioral problems often improve significantly after HH resection. A series of four patients treated solely for unmanageable behavior problems (e.g., paroxysms of rage, behavior threatening to others) showed dramatic improvement after surgery.[14] At this time, there are no clear contraindications to surgery. As always, the risk of surgical intervention must be carefully weighed and discussed with the family and care team. The endoscopic approach is most appropriate for smaller lesions within the third ventricle, whereas open surgical approaches are used to treat lesions larger than 1.2 cm or with significant extension below the third ventricle.

29.9 Diagnosis and Neuroimaging

The diagnosis of HH is typically made with MRI, as HHs have a characteristic appearance on MRIs. They are usually hyperintense on T2-weighted MRIs and hypointense to isointense on T1-weighted MRIs. Associated cysts are not uncommon but rarely have contrast enhancement. The following MRI sequences are recommended for optimal diagnosis:
1. 3D T1-weighted MRI 1-mm isotropic voxels.
2. Sagittal T1-weighted MRI: minimum echo time (TE); 3-mm slice, 0.5-mm gap; field of view (FOV) 20 cm.
3. Sagittal T2-weighted (fast-spin echo [FSE]) MRI: 2-mm slice, no gap; FOV 20 cm.
4. Coronal T2-weighted (FSE) MRI: 2-mm slice, no gap; FOV 16 cm.
5. Coronal T1-weighted MRI: 3D spoiled gradient recalled echo (SPGR); 2-mm slice; FOV 24 cm: reconstructed for axial.
6. Axial T2-weighted (FSE) MRI: routine brain.

The coronal T2-weighted (FSE) MRI sequence is better for identifying HHs because the tissue stands out more than normal brain on this sequence.

As of this writing, functional MRI, diffusion tensor imaging, and positron emission tomography have not yet provided information that has changed diagnosis or management. A correlation between the glial and the neuronal fraction has been found with magnetic resonance spectroscopy. Lesions with a larger glial component tend to be more hyperintense on T2-weighted MRIs.[15] Although many lesions appear to be attached bilaterally, we frequently find a true attachment on only one side, with the lesion abutting the contralateral side. This detail is not always distinguishable radiographically.

29.10 Complication Avoidance

As with all intraventricular endoscopy, the baseline risks of entering the ventricular system must be addressed. Risk is increased with small ventricles, without the use of stereotactic navigation, and when landmarks cannot be identified. Stereotactic navigation is recommended for all HH resections, which mitigates most of the risk inherent in ventricular entry. If the foramen of Monro is large and visible on coronal T2-weighted MRIs, then small ventricles should not be a deterrent.

When a pneumatic arm is used to hold the endoscope, malfunction of the arm must also be considered a potential risk. Movements of the pneumatic arm that are jerky or unpredictable can pose a substantial risk in this location. In the event of failure of the arm, an assistant may be used to hold the endoscope.

With all approaches, the indistinct border between the tumor and the hypothalamus is clearly the greatest challenge in all types of HH treatment. Because the tumor tissue itself is grossly identical to the surrounding hypothalamus, there are few anatomical means for determining the appropriate extent of resection. The presence of mammillary bodies is helpful, but these are usually on the far side of the lesion and are therefore encountered late in the dissection. We have found that the identification of small perforating vessels often indicates the margin, although they do not always correlate with complete resection of T2-weighted hyperintense material on MRIs. Stereotactic guidance is useful in this regard. The presence of shift is rarely limiting in these cases. Over-resection leads to worsened postoperative complications, particularly endocrinologic adverse effects such as obesity. Under-resection decreases efficacy with respect to seizure control. Giant lesions frequently require multimodality treatment with any combination of the available surgical approaches.

Failure to alleviate seizures because of incomplete resection is one of the most frequent complications. Such failure emanates from the inability to differentiate HH tissue from normal hypothalamic tissue. Residual tissue visible on MRIs may indicate the need for a repeat or a different surgical approach.

Endocrinologic adverse effects are also common. Up to 60% of patients may experience weight gain, and 34% may experience other hormonal derangements.[9] Transient memory deficits are common, with 14% of patients reporting memory deficits in the immediate postoperative period. Postoperative memory deficits typically improve to a permanent loss of 8%, which is similar to the rate for open surgical groups. Injuries to the mammillary bodies or fornices are most common. Many lesions may exhibit attachment along the tract, rather than at a discrete point, which increases risk. Every attempt should be made to limit injury to a unilateral mammillothalamic tract to maximize preservation of memory. This tract must be considered when planning a second approach in a patient who may already have experienced some anatomical damage.

The proximity of HHs to the prepontine cistern, and to the perforating vessels therein, is another source of infrequent complications. Injury in this region may affect brainstem and thalamic perforators, resulting in stroke and hemiparesis. Patients with this complication have varying degrees of recovery.

Postoperative hydrocephalus is less common in endoscopic approaches than in open approaches. As discussed previously, preoperative hydrocephalus should be addressed with appropriate drainage.

29.11 Postoperative Management

Most postoperative management is performed by the intensive care unit (ICU) and endocrine care teams. Many patients develop transient diabetes insipidus (DI), which will be long term or permanent for a few patients. Part of this deficit often involves a "triple-phase" response, in which the patient will first exhibit DI, then transition to the syndrome of inappropriate antidiuretic hormone before swinging back to DI. In most patients, this triple phase occurs within 5 to 7 days of surgery. Strict fluid management is essential to avoid severe hypernatremia or hyponatremia and its associated adverse effects. Deficits in hormones (thyroid, growth, stress, and sex) are often not observed for several months postoperatively. We advocate preoperative and postoperative neuropsychological assessment. The postoperative assessment is usually completed 3 to 6 months after surgery.

29.12 Outcome and Prognosis

In the largest reported series of endoscopically resected HHs ($n = 90$), 7 patients (8%) required additional procedures.[16]

In contrast, 26 of 165 patients (15.8%) treated by other means required additional procedures. Up to 49% of patients who underwent endoscopic resection experienced complete seizure cessation in the first 20 months of follow-up. This percentage decreased to around 29% over the long term (mean, 58 months).[9] Seizure reduction was reported in 55 to 91% of patients, which compares favorably with the 54% rate of initial complete cessation in patients treated with open approaches. Many of the endocrinopathies and memory deficits are temporary and improve significantly with time.[17] The mean hospital stay was 4.1 days in patients who had endoscopic resection and 7.7 days for patients treated using open approaches.

29.13 Technical Nuances and Clinical Pearls

- Side of approach: Entry into the third ventricle from the contralateral side facilitates dissection of the attachment of the lesion. This applies primarily to endoscopic approaches. However, in the case of a bilaterally attached lesion, entry should be contralateral to the largest attachment.
- Stereotactic guidance: Intraoperative stereotactic guidance is useful for determining the most appropriate trajectory to reach the lesion and to enter the small lateral ventricles for both open and endoscopic cases. Margins of resection can also be determined before closure.
- Cerebrospinal fluid diversion: In patients with preoperative ventriculomegaly, a ventriculostomy is recommended. However, in the absence of prior hydrocephalus, it is not required. Young children (< 3 years) are more prone to the development of pseudomeningoceles, which can impair bone healing. Temporary diversion of cerebrospinal fluid can be helpful in preventing this problem.
- Intraoperative MRI: Because of the difficulty in assessing HH margins grossly, these lesions are excellent candidates for the use of intraoperative MRI.
- Endoscopic tumor removal: Several devices have been developed to remove tissue through the endoscope. They use suction, sonication, rotary cutting, or a combination of techniques. HHs are ideal for these devices because of their low blood supply and thicker texture.

29.14 Literature Review for the Endoscopic Approach

Our review of the medical literature on HHs revealed that institutions are at various stages of utilization and acceptance of the currently available technologies. Many centers are focusing more on laser thermoablation techniques[18,19] or endoscopy. Some centers favor a combination approach.[6,20]

Intraventricular neuroendoscopy provides a more minimally invasive approach to the resection of HHs. Small lesions are ideal for endoscopic resection because of their minimal vascularity and soft texture. The average hospital stay is shorter for patients who undergo endoscopic resection than it is for patients who undergo open surgical resections, with comparable seizure control rates. The rate of pseudomeningocele formation and the rate of healing complications are both lower for the endoscopic approach. Further advances in endoscopic technology will likely improve the removal technique, expanding the number of patients with lesions amenable to resection.

References

[1] Abla AA, Shetter AG, Chang SW, et al. Gamma Knife surgery for hypothalamic hamartomas and epilepsy: patient selection and outcomes. J Neurosurg. 2010; 113 Suppl:207–214

[2] Steinmetz PN, Wait SD, Lekovic GP, Rekate HL, Kerrigan JF. Firing behavior and network activity of single neurons in human epileptic hypothalamic hamartoma. Front Neurol. 2013; 4:210

[3] Delalande O, Fohlen M. Disconnecting surgical treatment of hypothalamic hamartoma in children and adults with refractory epilepsy and proposal of a new classification. Neurol Med Chir (Tokyo). 2003; 43(2):61–68

[4] Ng YT, Rekate HL. Emergency transcallosal resection of hypothalamic hamartoma for "status gelasticus." Epilepsia. 2005; 46(4):592–594

[5] Wethe JV, Prigatano GP, Gray J, Chapple K, Rekate HL, Kerrigan JF. Cognitive functioning before and after surgical resection for hypothalamic hamartoma and epilepsy. Neurology. 2013; 81(12):1044–1050

[6] Ng YT, Rekate HL, Prenger EC, et al. Endoscopic resection of hypothalamic hamartomas for refractory symptomatic epilepsy. Neurology. 2008; 70 (17):1543–1548

[7] Rosenfeld JV, Harvey AS, Wrennall J, Zacharin M, Berkovic SF. Transcallosal resection of hypothalamic hamartomas, with control of seizures, in children with gelastic epilepsy. Neurosurgery. 2001; 48(1):108–118

[8] Rosenfeld JV. The evolution of treatment for hypothalamic hamartoma: a personal odyssey. Neurosurg Focus. 2011; 30(2):E1

[9] Drees C, Chapman K, Prenger E, et al. Seizure outcome and complications following hypothalamic hamartoma treatment in adults: endoscopic, open, and Gamma Knife procedures. J Neurosurg. 2012; 117(2):255–261

[10] Roth J, Bercu MM, Constantini S. Combined open microsurgical and endoscopic resection of hypothalamic hamartomas. J Neurosurg Pediatr. 2013; 11 (5):491–494

[11] Régis J, Scavarda D, Tamura M, et al. Gamma Knife surgery for epilepsy related to hypothalamic hamartomas. Semin Pediatr Neurol. 2007; 14(2):73–79

[12] Fujimoto Y, Kato A, Saitoh Y, et al. Stereotactic radiofrequency ablation for sessile hypothalamic hamartoma with an image fusion technique. Acta Neurochir (Wien). 2003; 145(8):697–700, discussion 700–701

[13] Khan S, Wright I, Javed S, et al. High frequency stimulation of the mamillothalamic tract for the treatment of resistant seizures associated with hypothalamic hamartoma. Epilepsia. 2009; 50(6):1608–1611

[14] Ng YT, Hastriter EV, Wethe J, et al. Surgical resection of hypothalamic hamartomas for severe behavioral symptoms. Epilepsy Behav. 2011; 20(1):75–78

[15] Amstutz DR, Coons SW, Kerrigan JF, Rekate HL, Heiserman JE. Hypothalamic hamartomas: correlation of MR imaging and spectroscopic findings with tumor glial content. AJNR Am J Neuroradiol. 2006; 27(4):794–798

[16] Wait SD, Abla AA, Killory BD, Nakaji P, Rekate HL. Surgical approaches to hypothalamic hamartomas. Neurosurg Focus. 2011; 30(2):E2

[17] Freeman JL, Zacharin M, Rosenfeld JV, Harvey AS. The endocrinology of hypothalamic hamartoma surgery for intractable epilepsy. Epileptic Disord. 2003; 5(4):239–247

[18] Wilfong AA, Curry DJ. Hypothalamic hamartomas: optimal approach to clinical evaluation and diagnosis. Epilepsia. 2013; 54 Suppl 9:109–114

[19] Buckley R, Estronza-Ojeda S, Ojemann JG. Laser ablation in pediatric epilepsy. Neurosurg Clin N Am. 2016; 27(1):69–78

[20] Calisto A, Dorfmüller G, Fohlen M, Bulteau C, Conti A, Delalande O. Endoscopic disconnection of hypothalamic hamartomas: safety and feasibility of robot-assisted, thulium laser-based procedures. J Neurosurg Pediatr. 2014; 14 (6):563–572

30 Craniosynostosis Surgery: Moderator

Amy Lee and Richard G. Ellenbogen

Summary

Craniosynostosis, or the premature fusion of one of more cranial sutures, and early fusion lead to abnormal skull growth of the cranial vault and skull base. The main indications for surgical treatment of craniosynostosis include making adequate space for normal brain growth and to provision the best aesthetic outcome, which helps alleviate any psychosocial impact it may have in the future. The last century has produced several iterations in the treatment of craniosynostosis. In this chapter, we discuss the endoscopic versus microsurgical approaches in the treatment of craniosynostosis.

Keywords: craniosynostosis, minimally invasive, pediatric, endoscopic

30.1 Moderator

30.1.1 Introduction

Craniosynostosis, or the premature fusion of one of more cranial sutures, affects 1 in every 2,000 to 2,500 live births.[1,2] Early fusion leads to abnormal skull growth of the cranial vault and skull base. The direction of abnormal growth depends on the suture involved. The sagittal suture is the most common suture involved (53–60% of all cases). It is followed by coronal synostosis (17–29%; unicoronal synostosis presents twice as frequently as bicoronal synostosis; ▶ Fig. 30.1), metopic synostosis (4–10%), and then lambdoid synostosis (< 2% of cases).[3] The etiology of nonsyndromic craniosynostosis is not completely understood, and it is likely due to a combination of genetic and external factors that result in premature fusion of the suture.

Although early anatomists appreciated the cranial sutures and deformities of the skull, it was not until the late 1700s when Sommerling noted the role of the sutures in skull growth and abnormal head shape as a consequence of premature fusion.[4,5] Later, Otto and Virchow made similar observations about normal skull growth occurring perpendicular to the plane of the suture. Virchow's landmark paper in 1851 described restriction of growth adjacent to a prematurely fused suture and compensatory growth along nonfused sutures in a direction parallel to the involved suture to accommodate for brain growth.[4,6,7] This principle is known as "Virchow's law." Just over a century later, Moss tried to unify all types of craniosynostosis by proposing that the primary mechanism behind skull deformity began at the skull base.[8] This theory was disproven when surgeries that removed the fused suture not only improved skull deformities, but also improved abnormalities at the cranial base.[9] He did, however, recognize when describing the "functional matrix theory" that the active growth of the brain dictated the growth of the skull.

These contributions and others have expanded our understanding of the cranial sutures and the effects of premature fusion on the growing skull and have shaped the evolution of surgical treatment from suturectomies and strip craniectomies to the more complex cranial vault reconstructions and endoscopic techniques we use today.

30.1.2 Evolution of Surgical Treatment Options

In 1890, Lannelongue performed the first strip craniectomy in Paris.[10] Shortly thereafter, in 1892 in San Francisco, Lane performed the first strip craniectomy with bilateral parietal bone strips for sagittal synostosis.[11] Unfortunately, the patient died of anesthetic complications 14 hours postoperatively. These surgeries soon fell out of favor due to high mortality rates and poor patient selection, but by the 1940s, strip craniectomies and suturectomies became widely accepted again. It was during this time that early intervention was noted to have better cosmetic and functional outcomes, and reossification in older children became an apparent complication leading to multiple procedures with little benefit.[4]

By the 1950s, advancements in anesthesia, blood transfusion, and surgical technique at high-volume centers made craniosynostosis surgery very safe.[4] For the next several decades, the limitations of strip craniectomies were becoming recognized, particularly in the treatment of children with late diagnoses. The need for immediate deformity correction inspired surgeons to develop innovative techniques for complex cranial vault remodeling. In the 1970s, Jane et al developed the pi procedure for treatment of sagittal synostosis.[12] Efficacy and safety of these procedures led to the involvement of craniofacial surgeons like Paul Tessier, who pioneered modern techniques that have significantly improved cosmetic outcomes.[13] Since then, modifications of the pi procedure for sagittal synostosis and procedures such as fronto-orbital advancement for metopic and coronal synostosis have become the most commonly used open techniques. But some drawbacks of extensive open calvarial remodeling persist. Open procedures are associated with long operative times, significant blood loss requiring transfusion, and longer hospital stays.[14]

In 1998, Jimenez and Barone first described the endoscope-assisted craniectomy technique for treatment of craniosynostosis. They reported significant benefits over open cranial vault reconstruction when performed within the first 6 months of life.[15,16] Postoperatively, infants require wearing custom-made molding helmets to reshape their growing skull.[17] The endoscopic-assisted craniectomy was adopted by many centers as a viable alternative to the open procedure, and it has been shown to decrease blood loss, transfusion requirements, operative times, and hospital stays.[17,18,19,20,21,22] The method described by Jimenez and Barone relies on a wide vertex (4–6 cm) craniectomy of the sagittal suture with biparietal and bitemporal "barrel-stave," or wedge, osteotomies.[15,17,18] More recently, a second endoscopic-assisted approach by Ridgway et al recommends less bone removal with a narrow vertex strip craniectomy

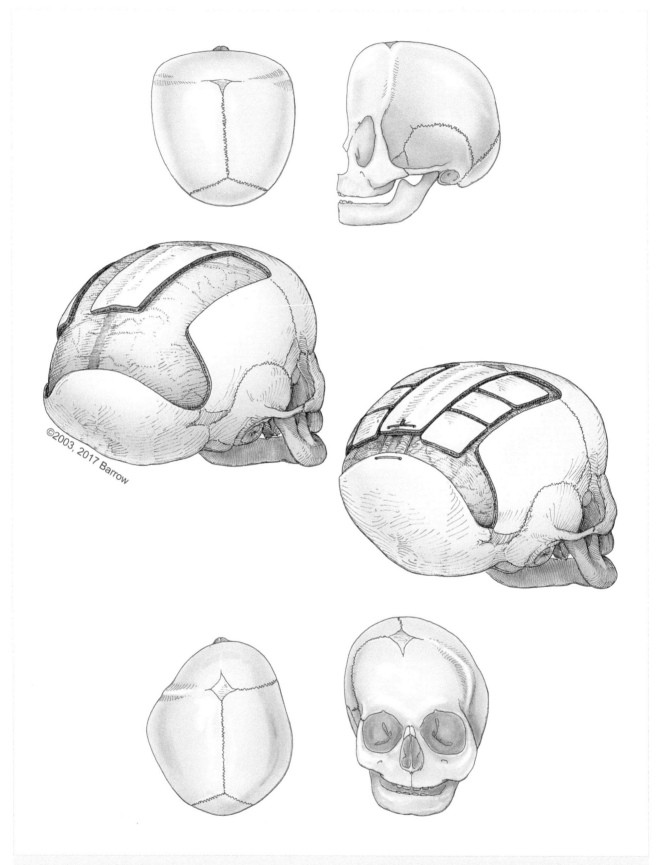

Fig. 30.1 Illustration of bicoronal and unicoronal synostosis. (Used with permission from Barrow Neurological Institute, Phoenix, AZ.)

(~2 cm).[23] A comparison study of both endoscopic-assisted methods by Dlouhy et al have produced similar results between the two procedures, with fewer procedural steps and less operative time using the narrow vertex approach.[16]

30.1.3 Decision-making Algorithm

The main indications for surgical treatment of craniosynostosis include making adequate space for normal brain growth and to provision the best aesthetic outcome, which helps alleviate any psychosocial impact it may have in the future. Previous studies have shown elevated intracranial pressure (ICP; > 15 mm Hg) in 8 to 13% of patients with single suture synostosis.[24] Since there is no reliable way to determine which patients will develop problems from craniosynostosis, early intervention is advocated for all patients.

The decision regarding performance of the open versus the endoscopic technique depends on several variables: age of the patient, the suture that is fused, the severity of the deformity, the surgeon's familiarity with both techniques, and family preference. Age of the patient is the most important determinant for the endoscopic approach to optimize surgical outcome. Early presentation takes advantage of the thinness of the bone that can be cut with heavy scissors during the procedure, and it gives the best opportunity for molding the head shape correctly. All endoscopic-assisted surgeries are best performed under the age of 6 months, but more severe asymmetry, often seen in unicoronal synostosis, is best treated under the age of 3 months.

The endoscopic technique is appealing to some families due to the limited scar, less blood loss, shorter operative time, and shorter hospital stay, but wearing a helmet for 23 hours a day for up to a year of age, with frequent travel time involved to maintain the proper fit of the helmet, may be daunting for some families. Despite the higher risk of blood transfusion, larger scar, and longer operative time, some families choose the open procedure because they find comfort in its proven longevity, and they prefer the convenience of a completed therapy after the surgery. In our center, both procedures are performed and the decision-making is a complex mixture of parental preference and appropriate patient selection. Clearly, family preference weighs heavily into the decision-making when the patient is a suitable candidate for either procedure. Additionally, the open technique should also be reserved if reoperation is necessary for suboptimal results of the endoscopic procedure. The outcome of both procedures is relatively similar when the best patients are selected for each and the surgical team is experienced in both the surgical procedure and postprocedure care.

Nonsurgical management of craniosynostosis is not ideal. However, mild deformities in children with late diagnoses may be considered for conservative nonoperative management. However, monitoring is advised because skull deformity severity does not uniformly correspond to neurodevelopmental outcomes.[25] These nonoperatively managed patients should be followed until 6 to 7 years of age or longer, specifically until the most rapid brain and skull growth is nearly complete.

30.1.4 Final Thoughts/Expert Recommendations

The last century has produced several iterations in the treatment of craniosynostosis. However, given the wide variability in management, good outcome measures for the spectrum of procedures and neurodevelopmental outcomes are lacking. Children with nonsyndromic synostosis often live normal lives with good long-term outcomes after surgery by both the open and endoscopic techniques. The procedures yield similar outcomes when patients are properly selected and the operative teams are experienced in the technical aspects of the procedure and postoperative management. The selection criterion, like for most operations, is a major part of the art in managing this condition by a skilled craniofacial team. Furthermore, we feel the craniofacial centers that offer both procedures often are in the best position to achieve the best outcomes for each procedure. It is important to recognize that regardless of whether one chooses the endoscopic or open procedure, both require multidisciplinary care provided by pediatric neurosurgeons, craniofacial plastic surgeons, pediatricians, geneticist, pediatric nurses, and ophthalmologists. Because of the complexity of their management, referral to craniofacial centers of excellence is recommended.

References

[1] Warren SM, Proctor MR, Bartlett SP, et al. Parameters of care for craniosynostosis: craniofacial and neurologic surgery perspectives. Plast Reconstr Surg. 2012; 129(3):731–737

[2] Di Rocco F, Arnaud E, Renier D. Evolution in the frequency of nonsyndromic craniosynostosis. J Neurosurg Pediatr. 2009; 4(1):21–25

[3] Shillito J, Jr, Matson DD. Craniosynostosis: a review of 519 surgical patients. Pediatrics. 1968; 41(4):829–853

[4] Mehta VA, Bettegowda C, Jallo GI, Ahn ES. The evolution of surgical management for craniosynostosis. Neurosurg Focus. 2010; 29(6):E5

[5] Sommering Sv. Vom Baue des Menschlichen Korpers. Frankfurt am Main: Varrentrapp und Wenner; 1801

[6] Virchow R. Uber den Cretinismus, namentlich in Franken, und uber pathologische Schadelformen. Verh Phys Med Gesell Wurzburg.. 1851; 2:230–271

[7] Andersson H, Gomes SP. Craniosynostosis. Review of the literature and indications for surgery. Acta Paediatr Scand. 1968; 57(1):47–54

[8] Moss ML. The pathogenesis of premature cranial synostosis in man. Acta Anat (Basel). 1959; 37:351–370

[9] Marsh JL, Vannier MW. Cranial base changes following surgical treatment of craniosynostosis. Cleft Palate J. 1986; 23 Suppl 1:9–18

[10] Lannelongue M. De la craniectomie dans la microcephalie. Compt Rend Seances Acad Sci.. 1890; 50:1382–1385

[11] Lane L. Pioneer craniectomy for relief of mental imbecility due to premature sutural closure and microcephalus. JAMA. 1892; 18:49–50

[12] Jane JA, Edgerton MT, Futrell JW, Park TS. Immediate correction of sagittal synostosis. J Neurosurg. 1978; 49(5):705–710

[13] Tessier P. Relationship of craniostenoses to craniofacial dysostoses, and to faciostenoses: a study with therapeutic implications. Plast Reconstr Surg. 1971; 48(3):224–237

[14] Tunçbilek G, Vargel I, Erdem A, Mavili ME, Benli K, Erk Y. Blood loss and transfusion rates during repair of craniofacial deformities. J Craniofac Surg. 2005; 16(1):59–62

[15] Jimenez DF, Barone CM. Endoscopic craniectomy for early surgical correction of sagittal craniosynostosis. J Neurosurg. 1998; 88(1):77–81

[16] Dlouhy BJ, Nguyen DC, Patel KB, et al. Endoscope-assisted management of sagittal synostosis: wide vertex suturectomy and barrel stave osteotomies versus narrow vertex suturectomy. J Neurosurg Pediatr. 2016; 25 (6):674–678

[17] Jimenez DF, Barone CM, Cartwright CC, Baker L. Early management of craniosynostosis using endoscopic-assisted strip craniectomies and cranial orthotic molding therapy. Pediatrics. 2002; 110(1, Pt 1):97–104

[18] Jimenez DF, Barone CM. Endoscopy-assisted wide-vertex craniectomy, "barrel-stave" osteotomies, and postoperative helmet molding therapy in the early management of sagittal suture craniosynostosis. Neurosurg Focus. 2000; 9(3):e2

[19] Jimenez DF, Barone CM. Multiple-suture nonsyndromic craniosynostosis: early and effective management using endoscopic techniques. J Neurosurg Pediatr. 2010; 5(3):223–231

[20] Shah MN, Kane AA, Petersen JD, Woo AS, Naidoo SD, Smyth MD. Endoscopically assisted versus open repair of sagittal craniosynostosis: the St. Louis Children's Hospital experience. J Neurosurg Pediatr. 2011; 8(2):165–170

[21] Vogel TW, Woo AS, Kane AA, Patel KB, Naidoo SD, Smyth MD. A comparison of costs associated with endoscope-assisted craniectomy versus open cranial vault repair for infants with sagittal synostosis. J Neurosurg Pediatr. 2014; 13 (3):324–331

[22] Berry-Candelario J, Ridgway EB, Grondin RT, Rogers GF, Proctor MR. Endoscope-assisted strip craniectomy and postoperative helmet therapy for treatment of craniosynostosis. Neurosurg Focus. 2011; 31(2):E5

[23] Ridgway EB, Berry-Candelario J, Grondin RT, Rogers GF, Proctor MR. The management of sagittal synostosis using endoscopic suturectomy and postoperative helmet therapy. J Neurosurg Pediatr. 2011; 7(6):620–626

[24] Renier D, Sainte-Rose C, Marchac D, Hirsch JF. Intracranial pressure in craniostenosis. J Neurosurg. 1982; 57(3):370–377

[25] Starr JR, Lin HJ, Ruiz-Correa S, et al. Little evidence of association between severity of trigonocephaly and cognitive development in infants with single-suture metopic synostosis. Neurosurgery. 2010; 67(2):408–415, discussion 415–416

31 Craniosynostosis Surgery: Microscope and Endoscope

Syed Hassan Akbari, Kamlesh Patel, and Matthew D. Smyth

Summary

Craniosynostosis, or the premature closure of one or multiple sutures of the cranial vault, is associated with increase intracranial pressure and cosmetic abnormalities. While open cranial vault reconstruction has been predominantly used for correction of craniosynostosis, endoscopic correction has recently become more popular. After presenting clinical examples of the two treatment modalities, this chapter discusses the differences between these approaches, highlighting differences in preoperative, operative, and postoperative characteristics.

Keywords: Craniosynostosis, minimally invasive, pediatric, endoscopic

31.1 Open and Endoscopic Perspective

31.1.1 Introduction

Craniosynostosis refers to the premature closure of one or more sutures of the cranial vault during development. In 1851, Virchow described the classic head growth patterns associated with each suture involved. He postulated that normal skull growth occurs in a plane perpendicular to a given suture, while growth occurs parallel to the affected suture in craniosynostosis.[1] Years later, Delashaw amended Virchow's law to state that bone plates connected by a fused suture will act as a single bone plate with compensatory growth along sutures in line with the synostotic suture.[2] Early fusion of the sutures affects the cranial vault and skull base and has been implicated in pathologies of brain development and growth.

Craniosynostosis has an incidence of 1 in every 2,500 live births.[3] Based on the affected sutures, a series of characteristic head shapes may result, from brachycephaly to scaphocephaly to trigonocephaly (▶ Table 31.1).[1,4,5,6] Multiple gene mutations and external factors have been implicated in nonsyndromic cases.[3,7,8,9,10] Craniosynostosis has also been implicated in a variety of craniofacial syndromes including Crouzon,[11] Pfeiffer,[12] Apert,[13] and Saethre–Chotzen syndromes.[14]

Table 31.1 Prevalence and characteristic head shape for various forms of synostosis.

Sutures affected	Head shape	Prevalence (%)
Sagittal	Scaphocephaly	53–60
Unilateral coronal	Anterior plagiocephaly	11–19
Metopic	Trigonocephaly	10–20
Bilateral coronal	Brachycephaly	6–10
Lambdoid	Posterior plagiocephaly	2
Pansynostosis	Oxycephaly	Rare

The primary goals of surgery are to correct skull shape and to ensure adequate space for normal brain growth. Historically, patients underwent suturectomies in treatment of craniosynostosis. This was largely abandoned in the early 20th century due to high mortality.[15] In the late 20th century, open calvarial vault reconstruction procedures gained popularity and continue to be a large proportion of the neurosurgeon's armamentarium today. However, with recent advances in endoscopy, neuroendoscopic suturectomy is gaining popularity as a minimally invasive technique for correcting synostosis in infancy.[16] The fundamental goal of surgery differs between the open and endoscopic approaches. While the open calvarial vault reconstruction aims to immediately correct and reconstruct the skull, the goal of endoscopic surgery is to excise and release the fused suture(s), and harness normal radial brain growth to drive a slow correction. A custom molding helmet is critical to guiding and normalizing skull shape.[16] Even with now nearly 20 years of experience using this minimally invasive approach, there still exists significant controversy in the treatment of this complex disease.[16,17] While a large number of studies have established the safety and efficacy of the endoscopic approach, there still exists a significant level of skepticism that has slowed the adoption of this approach at many craniofacial centers.[16]

31.1.2 Case Presentation

While open and endoscopic synostosis repair can be achieved in all categories of synostosis, the subsequent case presentations will emphasize sagittal synostosis strategies as this is the most common form of synostosis.

Case 1: Open Surgical Management

Patient History and Workup

LT was a 3-year-old adopted boy who was noted to have an abnormal head shape. The patient was born at full term via vaginal delivery. He was otherwise healthy and meeting his milestones. The patient's head circumference was 53.5 cm. On examination, he appeared scaphocephalic with a biparietal diameter of 136 mm and an anteroposterior (AP) diameter of 186 mm. His cephalic index was 73.0. The patient underwent imaging and preoperative photos revealed sagittal synostosis with scaphocephaly (▶ Fig. 31.1). Because of the patient's advanced age, open synostosis repair was discussed with the family who elected to proceed with surgery.

Operative Technique

The patient was placed in the Mayfield (Integra LifeSciences Corporation, Plainsboro, NJ) head holder, supine with the head slightly flexed with no rotation. A coronally oriented zigzag incision was designed and the hair clipped. Local anesthetic

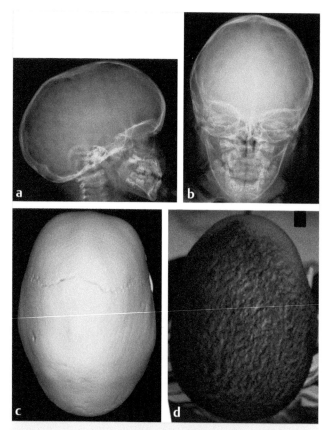

Fig. 31.1 A 3-year-old boy with sagittal synostosis. (a) Lateral and (b) anteroposterior (AP) X-ray revealing scaphocephaly and sagittal synostosis. (c) 3D reconstruction of CT scan showing sagittal synostosis and scaphocephaly. (d) Preoperative photograph revealing scaphocephaly.

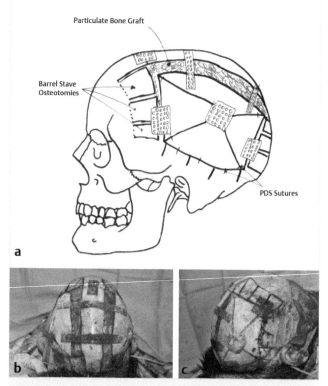

Fig. 31.2 Intraoperative images and diagrams. (a) Intraoperative diagram of a 3-year-old patient undergoing open repair of sagittal synostosis. (b,c) Intraoperative photographs of sagittal synostosis repair.

was applied along the proposed incision line. The patient was prepped and draped. Preoperative antibiotics, dexamethasone, and tranexamic acid were administered. The incision was made sharply with further dissection achieved with electrocautery. Subperiosteal dissection was performed anterior to the brow and posteriorly to the lambdoid suture. Osteotomies were designed with two large parietal pieces with markings posterior to the coronal suture and anterior to the lambdoid suture above the squamosal suture. A central 2.5-cm strip encompassing the sagittal suture was preserved. The bone segments were then removed using the Midas Rex drill to create a series of burr holes and the footplate attachment used to create the craniectomies. Blunt dissection of the dura anteriorly across the coronal suture and posteriorly beyond the lambdoid sutures was performed. A series of parallel barrel stave osteotomies (BSO) were then made anteriorly as well as posteriorly and laterally (▶ Fig. 31.2). These allowed panels of bone to be elevated. The inner surface of the parietal bone segments was morselized to create particulate bone graft using the D'Errico drill bit. Attention was then turned to contouring the bone segments, which were affixed using 2–0 PDS suture and absorbable plates. Bone graft was used to fill in cranial defects and fixed with Tisseel. A Jackson–Pratt drain was inserted. Closure of the scalp was performed with 3–0 Monocryl interrupted suture for the galea and 4–0 plain for the skin edges. Bacitracin and

Xeroform were applied to the incision as well as a head wrap. The patient received 210 mL of packed red blood cells. Estimated blood loss was 175 mL. Surgical time was 215 minutes. The patient was extubated and admitted to the pediatric intensive care unit (ICU). Postoperatively, the biparietal diameter was 152 mm and the AP diameter was 186 mm with a cephalic index of 82.0 and a head circumference of 54.0 cm.

Perioperative Course

The patient did well in the ICU. A postoperative hemoglobin/hematocrit was 9.0/26.0. Dexamethasone was continued postoperatively. A hemoglobin/hematocrit on postoperative day 1 was 8.1/22.7. A blood transfusion of 2 units packed red blood cells was given with a response to 10.3/28.8. No other transfusions were given through the patient's stay. The patient was transferred to the floor on postoperative day 1. The head wrap was removed on postoperative day 2. Steroids were tapered over the next 3 days. The patient tolerated oral diet and was at his neurological baseline. The drain was removed on postoperative day 3, and the patient was discharged.

Follow-Up

At 1-year follow-up, the patient was doing well. His head circumference was 54.4 cm with a cephalic index of 79.0. A follow up CT scan and photograph were obtained at this visit (▶ Fig. 31.3). At 2-year follow up, the biparietal diameter was 147 mm with an AP diameter of 186 mm and a cephalic index of 79.0. The head circumference was 54.9 cm.

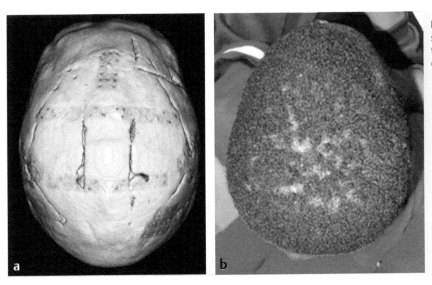

Fig. 31.3 One-year follow-up images after open sagittal synostosis repair. (a) 3D CT reconstruction and (b) photograph showing improvement of cephalic index.

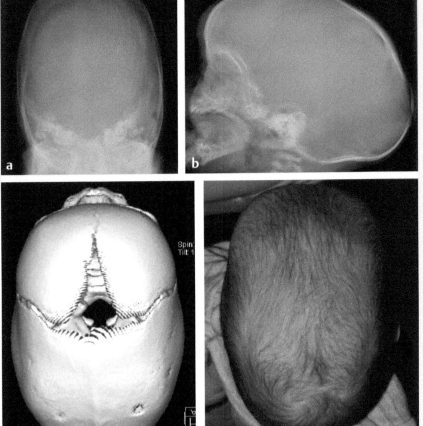

Fig. 31.4 A 1.5-month-old infant with craniosynostosis. (a) Anteroposterior (AP) skull X-ray revealing fused sagittal suture. (b) Lateral X-ray revealing scaphocephaly. (c) 3D reconstruction of computed tomography (CT) scan revealing fused sagittal suture and scaphocephaly. (d) Preoperative photograph showing scaphocephaly.

Case 2: Endoscopic Surgical Management

Patient History and Workup

MR was a 6-week-old infant referred to plastic and neurosurgery by his primary care physician for concerns of head shape. The patient was born at term via C-section. He was otherwise healthy and developing normally. The patient's head circumference was 40 cm (96th percentile). On examination, the patient appeared scaphocephalic with a biparietal width of 98 mm and AP dimension of 148 mm. The patient's cephalic index was 66. The patient underwent imaging and preoperative photos revealing sagittal synostosis (▶ Fig. 31.4). Treatment options were discussed, and the family elected for the endoscopic approach.

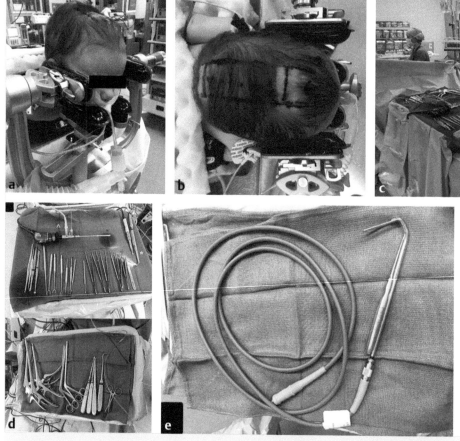

Fig. 31.5 Intraoperative photographs from an endoscopic repair of sagittal synostosis. **(a)** Patient placed in the sphinx position in the Doro head holder after intubation. The vertex is placed as the superior-most aspect of the operative field. **(b)** Coronally oriented incisions are marked to span approximately 1 cm on either side of the affected suture. The midpoint between the anterior and posterior incisions is made to be the midpoint of the suture. Incisions are placed behind the hairline. **(c)** The patient is prepped and draped. Surgical instruments are placed above the operating table with monopolar cautery and the endoscope tower in close proximity. **(d)** Typical arrangement of instruments utilized in the endoscopic approach. The endoscope is attached to the Endo-Scrub (^). The lighted Aufricht retractor (*) assists in visualizing epidural dissection, craniectomy, and bleeding craniectomy edges requiring cauterization. **(e)** The lighted Aufricht retractor.

Operative Technique

The patient was placed in the sphinx position in the Doro (Pro Med Instruments, Freiburg, Germany) head holder (▶ Fig. 31.5a). The anterior fontanelle was marked, as well as posterior lambda. A horizontal incision 2.5 cm in length was marked just posterior to the anterior fontanelle and another anterior to the lambda (▶ Fig. 31.5b). Local anesthesia was infiltrated at these sites. The patient was prepped and draped, preoperative antibiotics given, and sharp dissection was used to advance to the galea (▶ Fig. 31.5c, d). Subgaleal dissection was used to connect the two incisions. The pericranium was then coagulated and the Midas Rex drill (Medtronic, Inc., Jacksonville, FL) with a high-speed acorn drill bit was used to create a burr hole on one side of each access incision. Curettes and Kerrison punches were used to widen the craniectomy across midline. Penfield dissectors were used to extend the craniectomy to the posterior aspect of the anterior fontanelle and posteriorly to lambda. Dry endoscopy was performed using a rigid endoscope affixed to a standard endoscopy tower for visualization, which was coupled to the Endo-Scrub (Medtronic, Inc.)

for maintaining the endoscopic visual field. The endoscope and/ or the Aufricht lighted retractor (Electro Surgical Instrument, Co, Rochester, MN; ▶ Fig. 31.5e) was then introduced into the epidural space and used from anterior to posterior to dissect the dura from the overlying bone. Paramedian osteotomies were then made using bone scissors to 2.5 cm width. The bone edges were rapidly cauterized with suction monopolar cautery set at 50 W. FloSeal (Baxter Healthcare Corporation, Deerfield, IL) was applied to the craniectomy defect and the incisions were closed with Monocryl for the galea and skin edges with a superficial layer of skin adhesive. No drain was placed. Estimated blood loss was 20 mL. Operative time was 47 minutes. The patient did not receive any transfusions intraoperatively. He was extubated and was admitted to the floor.

Perioperative Course

The patient did well on the floor. A postoperative hemoglobin/ hematocrit was 8.2/22.6. No transfusions were given. The patient tolerated oral diet and remained at his neurologic baseline. He was discharged on postoperative day 1.

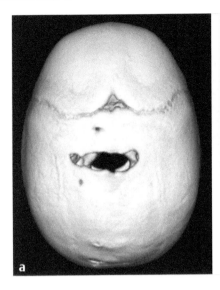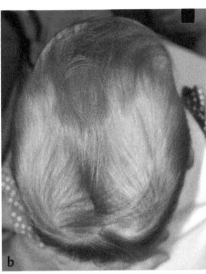

Fig. 31.6 A 12-month-old infant status post endoscopic sagittal suturectomy. **(a)** 3D reconstruction of CT scan with improvement in cephalic index. **(b)** Postoperative photograph.

Follow-Up

Helmet therapy was initiated soon after discharge. The patient was seen at 2-week follow-up with a biparietal diameter of 105 mm, an AP diameter of 145 mm, and a cephalic index of 72. At 6 weeks, biparietal diameter was 109 mm and AP diameter was 147 mm with a cephalic index of 73. At 7.5 months, the cephalic index was 77.4. The head circumference had improved to 46 cm (76th percentile). Helmet therapy was continued until the patient was 1 year of age, at which point a follow-up computed tomography (CT) scan and photograph were obtained (▶ Fig. 31.6). A total of four helmets were used.

Additional Situations: Technical Pearls of Nonsagittal Endoscopic Synostosis Repair

Endoscopic repair is an option for all categories of synostosis, with some variations. Patients with coronal and metopic synostoses are positioned supine with the head elevated to minimize blood loss, and lambdoid synostoses are positioned in the prone position. The small incisions are typically placed over the center of the fused suture while respecting the hairline. The sutures are resected using rongeurs and scissors, with endoscopic assistance to confirm the epidural spaces are dissected from the overlying bone. Postoperative management, transfusion thresholds, and helmeting techniques are similar to those used in endoscopic sagittal synostosis cases.

31.1.3 Comparison between Open and Endoscopic Approaches

Patient Selection and Demographics

Patient Selection

The diagnosis of craniosynostosis involving a variety of different sutures can often be made based on clinical history and examination alone, but the head shape must be differentiated from benign positional plagiocephaly. Skull radiographs may be helpful in showing fused sutures. Recently, 3D CT has been used to provide information regarding overall head shape in addition to the involved suture, but it should be used judiciously due to effects of CT exposure on the developing brain.

Intracranial pressure elevation is another indication for surgery and can be seen in 4 to 14% of single-suture patients compared to as much as 67% in those where multiple sutures are involved.[18,19,20] Renier et al found elevated intracranial pressure in 12% of unilateral coronal synostosis, 8% of sagittal synostosis, and 6% of metopic synostosis patients, with higher incidence of elevated pressure in older patients and those with multiple fused sutures. He also found lower cognitive ability correlating with higher intracranial pressure.[19] Baird et al reported on 17 patients who underwent craniofacial repair of synostosis and found a reduction in postoperative signs and symptoms of elevated intracranial pressure.[21] Additional studies have demonstrated improvement of IQ scores, papilledema, and behavior following reconstruction.[19,22,23]

Age

In general, endoscopic surgery is performed in a younger population. Endoscopic suturectomy is typically performed in patients at roughly 2 to 6 months of age[24,25] when brain growth is a significant driver of skull growth. Helmets are usually used postoperatively to help further mold the postoperative skull during the rapid phase of infant brain growth. Open vault reconstructions are typically performed in an older population from 4 to 12 months and are almost universally the treatment of choice in patients older than 1 year.[26] At this point, brain growth has a lesser impact on skull growth. Additionally, the skull is too thick to perform an endoscopic procedure at this age. Thus, a more definitive correction of the cranial vault is required. Age is a particularly important factor additionally because of the smaller circulating blood volume at younger ages.

Cost and Familial Stress

Endoscope-assisted craniectomy is also associated with decreased cost compared to cranial vault remodeling. Vogel et al assessed 42 patients who underwent open reconstruction compared to endoscopic surgery for sagittal synostosis and found endoscopic surgery with helmet therapy was approximately $20,000 cheaper than open surgery ($37,200 vs. 57,000).[24] Gociman et al found a near-halving of cost for metopic synostosis ($12,400 compared to 33,000).[27] Chan et al reviewed 57 patients undergoing surgical repair for synostosis of varying sutures and found a similar cost reduction ($24,400 vs. 42,700).[28] Interestingly, Kim et al administered the Parenting Stress Index-Short Form to patient families undergoing open and endoscopic repair of craniosynostosis and found a significant reduction in total stress in families undergoing endoscopic repair.[29] Thus, endoscopic repair with helmet therapy for craniosynostosis represents a cost-effective low-stress surgical option for synostosis repair.

Perioperative Management

Operative Factors

Intraoperative blood loss and the need for possible transfusion are of particular concern for patients undergoing synostosis repair. This is especially true for open cranial vault reconstruction where some studies have shown an intraoperative blood loss between 25 and 500% of a patient's blood volume[30] and in some studies a near universal transfusion rate.[31] Some in the past would transfuse blood loss intraoperatively cubic centimeter for cubic centimeter.[32] There have been some recent efforts to reduce the need for intraoperative blood transfusion. One study found that using Cell Saver was associated with a significant decrease in the rate of homologous blood transfusions.[30] Dadure et al tried utilizing tranexamic acid (TXA) and found that the volume of transfused red cells was reduced by 85% intraoperatively and by 57% in the perioperative period in those receiving TXA compared to those who did not receive TXA. Additionally, the percentage of children receiving transfusions was significantly reduced from 70 to 37%.[33] Goobie et al found decreased blood loss and lower transfusion rates in a double-blind placebo-control trial of TXA in patients undergoing suture repair.[34] Recently, Harroud et al postulated a contribution of intraoperative hemodilution in the rates of intraoperative anemia and found a near 30% reduction in transfusion with the administration of furosemide.[35] While lower hemoglobin parameters are generally accepted,[36] there is still a substantial risk of exposing the patient to erythrocytes during these surgeries despite best efforts. Endoscopic therapy presents a useful alternative with significantly decreased blood loss. Chan et al showed a near-200-mL decrease in estimated blood loss and 140-mL decrease in transfused blood.[28] Vogel et al found similar results for patients undergoing sagittal synostosis correction with a 90% decrease in transfusion rate and near-200-mL decrease in blood loss.[24] Berry-Candelario et al found a mere 4.6% transfusion rate among 173 patients undergoing endoscopic repair.[37] Finally, Shah et al found similar results in their cohort of sagittal synostosis patients.[38] Recently, a single-center review of all synostosis patients from the last 10 years showed a significant reduction in blood loss and transfusions in the endoscopically treated group.[39] Specifically, they found a near-250-mL reduction in blood loss, a 90% reduction in intraoperative transfusions, and a 35% reduction in postoperative transfusions. A lower hemoglobin level is generally tolerated in the endoscopic group as long as patients are asymptomatic compared to the open group in which continued postoperative blood loss is common and necessitates more conservative transfusion parameters.[38,40] Endoscope-assisted craniosynostosis repair seems to decrease the need for perioperative blood transfusions, thus reducing the risk of transfusion-related

complications. In the authors' practice, TXA and blood transfusions are routinely started at the beginning of open synostosis cases. Postoperative hemoglobin and hematocrit levels are checked in the evening of postoperative day 0 and checked again on postoperative day 1 with a transfusion threshold of a hematocrit less than 25%. Endoscopic cases are started with emergency-release blood available, while a type and cross are pending. These cases typically have an estimated blood loss around 30 to 40 mL and require transfusions in less than 5% of cases. A postoperative hemoglobin and hematocrit are checked 4 hours postoperatively with a transfusion threshold of a hematocrit less than 18%.

In addition to blood loss and transfusions, exposure to anesthetic agents is of particular importance to the neurosurgeon. Cumulative exposure to anesthetic agents has been associated with poor neurodevelopmental outcomes.[41,42,43] Therefore, reducing operative times is of particular concern in the pediatric population. Various studies have shown a statistically significant decrease in operative time in those treated with endoscopic suturectomy compared to open calvarial vault reconstruction. These studies typically show a near halving of operative time.[24,28,38,39] Reduction in operative time is important as it may reduce the effect of anesthesia on neurodevelopment.

The endoscope-assisted approach originally relied on wide vertex craniectomies of the sagittal suture in addition to biparietal and bitemporal "barrel stave" or wedge osteotomies as initially described by Jimenez and Barone.[44,45,46] However, endoscope-assisted narrow (~2 cm) strip vertex craniectomies have been described by Ridgway et al.[37,47] Both approaches utilize similar postoperative helmet therapy. Recently, Dlouhy et al conducted an age-matched retrospective study analyzing 14 patients undergoing wide vertex suturectomy and BSO (WVS + BSO) versus 14 patients undergoing narrow vertex suturectomy (NVS).[48] They found that the two approaches did not have significant differences in 1-year postoperative cephalic index, estimated blood loss, complications, postoperative hemoglobin, or transfusion requirements. Additionally, the time to reach the final postoperative cephalic index was similar in both groups. However, there was a significant reduction in operative time from 83.4 minutes in the WVS + BSO group to 59.0 minutes in the NVS group. This suggests that the two approaches yield similar outcome with a decrease in anesthesia risk in the NVS group, leading to a shift to NVS at the authors' institution.

Postoperative Management and Cosmetic Result

The postoperative course for patients undergoing open vault reconstruction is vastly different from those undergoing endoscopic surgery. The average hospital stay for patients undergoing open surgery was 3.9 to 4.9 days compared to 1.1 to 1.4 days in the endoscopic group.[24,28,37,38] This relates to a decreased complication rate, decreased transfusion need, reduced postoperative swelling, and ultimately translates into decreased hospital cost. In the authors' practice, patients undergoing open vault reconstruction will have a Jackson–Pratt drain and head wrap placed intraoperatively and spend at least the first day in the ICU. These patients are then transferred to the floor for an additional 2 to 3 days. Dressings and drains are typically left in place until the second postoperative day with prophylactic antibiotics used until the drain is removed. Discharge medications will often include narcotic pain relievers. This compares to those undergoing the endoscopic procedure who will be admitted to the floor overnight without a drain or head wrap and are discharged the following day with acetaminophen and ibuprofen. Follow-up is arranged in 3 to 4 weeks postoperatively for both approaches, but multiple orthotist visits are scheduled for the endoscopic patients, initially every other week and then monthly until about 12 months of age.

One important consideration in patient selection for endoscopic suturectomy is compliance with helmet therapy. While open calvarial reconstruction leads to an immediate change in shape without a reliance on brain growth, endoscopic surgery excises the affected suture and requires brain growth and helmet therapy to further affect head shape. In the authors' experience, helmet therapy is initiated in the first week after surgery. The average time of helmet therapy ranges from 6 to 11 months.[24,25,28,40,47] Sixty-two percent of patients required a second helmet and 10% required a third helmet with an average of 2.31 helmets needed per patient.[24,28,40] Chan et al found a noncompliance rate of 17%,[28] while Shah et al found a similar noncompliance rate of 15%.[38] Noncompliance seems to negatively impact aesthetic result from surgery.[40] A significant factor in noncompliance relates to multiple early postoperative visits to either the craniofacial surgical team or the orthotic company. Open reconstruction patients had a mean of 1.62 visits in the first postoperative year compared to 3.76 visits in the endoscopic group, not including visits to an orthotist. Honeycutt commented that multiple long-distance trips were prohibitive for patients and, in some cases, led to the selection of open surgery.[40] Another factor is patient intolerance of helmets, which may lead to reformation of synostosis and later open surgery.[49] In the authors' experience, potential noncompliance with helmet therapy is a contraindication for endoscopic surgery.

Cephalic index (ratio of maximum cranial width to maximum head length) is the most common quantitative measure used to evaluate both severity and outcome. Dvoracek et al described the limitations of this measurement as temporal protrusion in patients with sagittal synostosis moves the location of maximum head width (euryon) to a more caudal location.[50] Normal values for cephalic index are typically 75 to 80%. Shah et al found similar correction rates between endoscopic and open cases.[38] In other studies, excellent results in the cephalic index were achieved in 87% of patients with endoscopic repair of sagittal synostosis,[51] with equivalence to open procedures based on 3D photographs taken years postoperatively.[52] Additionally, Ghenbot et al found a mean 12% correction in the cephalic index between open and endoscopic groups with no significant difference in cephalic index or cranial vault volume between the two groups.[53] For coronal synostosis, the same group found a significant correction in vertical dystopia, midsagittal plane deviation, nasal and sagittal craniofacial deviation, and supraorbital rim advancement in those undergoing endoscopic repair.[54,55] Another study looked at various factors and found the two operative approaches were similar in supraorbital symmetry and lower facial depth, while the endoscopic approach yielded better facial symmetry in midline deviation, nasal tip deviation, and middle facial depth.[56] Additionally, MacKinnon et al found that patients had better ophthalmological outcomes, decreased amblyopia and astigmatism, and fewer

strabismus correction surgeries in a sample of patients undergoing endoscopic repair versus those undergoing open fronto-orbital advancement.[57] For bilateral coronal synostosis, studies have reported similar improvements in head circumference, vertical dystopia, nasal deviation, and cephalic index.[58,59] With respect to lambdoid synostosis, one study found similar postoperative results between open and endoscopic approaches with respect to posterior fossa deflection angle, petrous ridge angle, mastoid cant angle, and external acoustic meatus displacement.[60] Finally, for metopic synostosis, multiple studies have shown a similar equivalence between the two groups. Nguyen et al found improvement in trigonocephaly for both groups using the bilateral zygomaticofrontal sutures to glabella angle and interfrontal angle with no difference between the groups.[61] Meanwhile, other studies used laser scanning to evaluate the metopic angle or postoperative photographs and CT scans and found a significant correction using the endoscopic approach.[27,62]

Operative Complications

Common operative complications include surgical infections and wound complications. Early reports from open reconstruction showed an infection rate of approximately 1.6%.[63] This rate has largely held stable ranging between 0.5 and 2%.[38,64] Of particular importance in the endoscopic group is wound breakdown secondary to helmet therapy. Chan et al found a 5.7% rate of wound breakdown in patients undergoing endoscopic treatment with helmets. These complications are easily treated with brief respite from helmet therapy with standard wound care. None required reoperation.[28] Shah et al found a 2.4% rate of wound defects in the open group requiring reoperation, while one patient in the endoscopic group required a reoperation at age 5 years for a persistent vertex defect treated with mesh cranioplasty.[38] Usually patients undergoing endoscopic repair nearly completely reossify by the end of helmet therapy. However, Honeycutt also found significant postoperative skull defects requiring therapy, one so far treated with autologous cranioplasty and synthetic bone.[40] A study of 328 patients found a 1.4 and 1.3% reoperation rate for cranial defects for endoscopic and open treatment, respectively, in addition to a 0.6% rate of reoperation for chronic wound dehiscence in the open group.[39]

Dural lacerations are also of particular concern. In their series of open repair, Boop et al had a 3.5% dural laceration rate, all of which were primarily repaired intraoperatively and did not lead to postoperative morbidity.[32] Seruya et al reported a 0.5% rate of cerebrospinal fluid (CSF) leak.[64] In a study of 328 patients treated for craniosynostosis, Han et al found an intraoperative durotomy rate of 3.6 and 7.8% in the nonsyndromic endoscopic and open groups, respectively, all of which were treated primarily and none of which required reoperation.[39] Meanwhile, Honeycutt reports in his endoscopic series a 2.7% rate of dural laceration, one requiring an additional scalp incision to repair with an underlying clinically insignificant cortical laceration and the other associated with brisk bleeding secondary to its proximity to the sinus, which was incompletely repaired without sequelae. In their cohort of patients treated for bilateral coronal synostosis, Rottgers et al had a 5.6% rate of CSF leak.[58] Finally, Aryan et al reported the unique complication after endoscopic sagittal synostosis repair of a dural laceration leading to the development of a leptomeningeal cyst that required surgical repair.[65] Overall, it appears that the two surgical approaches have similar rates of dural lacerations, which infrequently require surgical intervention.

Another potential complication is the reformation of synostosis or reoperation for poor cosmetic result. A recent informal survey even suggests that reoperation rates may be underrepresented in the literature.[49] Yarbrough et al found a delayed synostosis rate of 2.1 and 1.7% in the open and endoscopic groups, respectively.[66] The patients who had undergone open surgery developed new sagittal synostosis compared to coronal synostosis in the endoscopic group. Three out of Ridgway et al's 56 (5.36%) patients undergoing endoscopic suturectomy for sagittal synostosis required reoperations for recurrent or new synostosis.[47] Sivakumar et al reported a unique case of postoperative pansynostosis in a patient initially treated with endoscopic repair of sagittal synostosis in the setting of inconsistent helmet compliance and poor follow-up.[67] Meanwhile, Jenkins et al reported a similar event of pansynostosis after endoscopic sagittal suturectomy in the setting of helmet compliance.[68] Each of the two patients in the above reports required an open cranial vault reconstruction. A retrospective review of 100 patients who underwent endoscopic repair showed a reoperation rate of 7%.[69] Six of these patients developed multisuture synostosis, and four showed signs of papilledema on follow-up ophthalmological examination. Six of the patients underwent fronto-orbital advancement, while one underwent calvarial vault reconstruction followed by fronto-orbital advancement. All required ICU admissions and intraoperative red blood cell transfusions. The numbers of involved sutures, syndromic cases, and postoperative ICU admission were significantly associated with the need for reoperation. Intracranial hypertension and aesthetic results also form significant proportions of reoperations. In a series of 212 patients undergoing open reconstruction, Seruya et al found a 10.8% reoperation rate, 52.2% of which were due to signs and symptoms of intracranial hypertension.[64] The rest were secondary to poor aesthetic results (30%), recurrent or new synostosis (13%), and persistent calvarial defects (4%). It is hypothesized that postoperative constriction of the calvarial vault may contribute to elevation of intracranial pressure In Han et al's cohort, 0.71% of endoscopically treated patients and 1.94% of open reconstruction patients underwent reoperation for poor aesthetic result.[39] Meanwhile, Honeycutt's cohort showed a reoperation rate of 4.11% for aesthetic result.[40] Finally, Rottgers et al's cohort of bilateral coronal synostosis had a 33% reoperation rate, mostly in the syndromic subset of patients.[58] All reported reoperations utilized the open method. These studies allude to the possibility of using open reconstruction for more complicated cases of pan- or multisuture synostosis, syndromic patients, or as a salvage technique after failed endoscopic intervention.

Other less frequent complications, including sinus injury,[40] venous air embolism,[69,70,71,72] growing skull fracture,[49] hematoma, and contusion,[39,64] have been reported in the literature for endoscopic and open surgery. All except for sinus injury seem to appear more commonly in those undergoing open surgery compared to endoscopic. Additionally, a recent study argued that patients undergoing open vault reconstruction attained higher intelligence quotient and achievement scores compared to those undergoing endoscopic repair.[73] However, this study was unable to obtain preoperative scores among other methodological issues.[74] Therefore, more information is needed to assess the effect of surgical method on neuropsychological development. Finally, an informal study among craniofacial surgeons in North America indicated that there were potentially some unreported complications including reoperation for recurrent synostosis.[49] The study also highlighted some major unreported complications to endoscopic surgery, including a single death, severe postoperative bleeding requiring lengthy hospitalization and transfusion, and a sagittal sinus injury leading to cardiac arrest and infarction.[49] While these three complications are regrettable, the results were from an informal survey and does not emphasize that these three events are out of the thousands of operations performed across the continent at the surveyed institutions. What the survey does emphasize, however, is that patient selection and proper family-informed consent are essential factors in selection of treatment approach. It also highlights the need for additional research, including the effect of suturectomy size, factors that predict resynostosis, and the effect of surgeon experience.

Neosuture Formation

A unique phenomenon more commonly reported with endoscopic suturectomy is bone growth that ultimately forms radiographically normal-appearing sutures and persistent craniectomy gap patency.[75,76,77,78,79] Neosuture rates range from 16.7 to 23.9%. At this point, it is unclear what role neosuture formation plays in the long-term postoperative course of craniosynostosis. More studies are currently needed to understand this phenomenon.

31.1.4 Clinical Pearls

The treatment options for craniosynostosis have evolved from traditional open calvarial vault reconstruction with or without front-orbital advancement to now include endoscopic suturectomy with helmet therapy.

- Appropriate patient selection ensures maximal benefit from either treatment option with the least risk, as both options have equivalent clinical outcomes with unique morbidity profiles.
- The endoscopic technique is associated with decreased operative time, blood loss, transfusions, hospital stay, and cost.
- Endoscope-assisted NVS gives similar results with decreased anesthetic risk compared to the endoscope-assisted WVS + BSO approach.
- Helmet compliance is an important factor affecting outcome from the endoscopic technique and warrants a detailed conversation with the family in determining the operative approach.
- Complications from either approach include infection, wound breakdown, dural laceration, resynostosis, intracranial hypertension, sinus injury, venous air embolism, hematoma, contusion, and reoperation for poor aesthetic result.
- The endoscopic approach is ideal for young nonsyndromic patients with single-suture synostosis who will be compliant with helmet therapy, while the open approach should be reserved for older patients, complicated or multisuture synos-

tosis, syndromic patients, patients who are likely to be non-compliant with helmet therapy, or those who failed with the endoscopic approach.

References

[1] Virchow R. Uber den Cretinismus, namentlich in Franken, und uber pathologische Schadelformen. Verh Phys Med Gesell Wurzburg.. 1851; 2:230–271

[2] Delashaw JB, Persing JA, Broaddus WC, Jane JA. Cranial vault growth in craniosynostosis. J Neurosurg. 1989; 70(2):159–165

[3] Warren SM, Proctor MR, Bartlett SP, et al. Parameters of care for craniosynostosis: craniofacial and neurologic surgery perspectives. Plast Reconstr Surg. 2012; 129(3):731–737

[4] Di Rocco F, Arnaud E, Renier D. Evolution in the frequency of nonsyndromic craniosynostosis. J Neurosurg Pediatr. 2009; 4(1):21–25

[5] Shillito J, Jr, Matson DD. Craniosynostosis: a review of 519 surgical patients. Pediatrics. 1968; 41(4):829–853

[6] Shuper A, Merlob P, Grunebaum M, Reisner SH. The incidence of isolated craniosynostosis in the newborn infant. Am J Dis Child. 1985; 139(1):85–86

[7] Ciurea AV, Toader C. Genetics of craniosynostosis: review of the literature. J Med Life. 2009; 2(1):5–17

[8] Carmichael SL, Ma C, Rasmussen SA, Honein MA, Lammer EJ, Shaw GM, National Birth Defects, Prevention Study. Craniosynostosis and maternal smoking. Birth Defects Res A Clin Mol Teratol. 2008; 82(2):78–85

[9] Seto ML, Hing AV, Chang J, et al. Isolated sagittal and coronal craniosynostosis associated with TWIST box mutations. Am J Med Genet A. 2007; 143A (7):678–686

[10] Mefford HC, Shafer N, Antonacci F, et al. Copy number variation analysis in single-suture craniosynostosis: multiple rare variants including RUNX2 duplication in two cousins with metopic craniosynostosis. Am J Med Genet A. 2010; 152A(9):2203–2210

[11] Cohen MM, Jr, Kreiborg S. Birth prevalence studies of the Crouzon syndrome: comparison of direct and indirect methods. Clin Genet. 1992; 41(1):12–15

[12] Winter RM. Pfeiffer syndrome. Am J Med Genet. 1994; 49(3):357–359

[13] Lajeunie E, Cameron R, El Ghouzzi V, et al. Clinical variability in patients with Apert's syndrome. J Neurosurg. 1999; 90(3):443–447

[14] Reardon W, Winter RM. Saethre-Chotzen syndrome. J Med Genet. 1994; 31 (5):393–396

[15] Jacobi A. Non nocere. Med Rec. 1894; 45:609–618

[16] Proctor MR. Endoscopic craniosynostosis repair. Transl Pediatr. 2014; 3 (3):247–258

[17] Doumit GD, Papay FA, Moores N, Zins JE. Management of sagittal synostosis: a solution to equipoise. J Craniofac Surg. 2014; 25(4):1260–1265

[18] Gault DT, Renier D, Marchac D, Jones BM. Intracranial pressure and intracranial volume in children with craniosynostosis. Plast Reconstr Surg. 1992; 90 (3):377–381

[19] Renier D, Sainte-Rose C, Marchac D, Hirsch JF. Intracranial pressure in craniostenosis. J Neurosurg. 1982; 57(3):370–377

[20] Blount JP, Louis RG, Jr, Tubbs RS, Grant JH. Pansynostosis: a review. Childs Nerv Syst. 2007; 23(10):1103–1109

[21] Baird LC, Gonda D, Cohen SR, et al. Craniofacial reconstruction as a treatment for elevated intracranial pressure. Childs Nerv Syst. 2012; 28(3):411–418

[22] Cohen SR, Dauser RC, Newman MH, Muraszko K. Surgical techniques of cranial vault expansion for increases in intracranial pressure in older children. J Craniofac Surg. 1993; 4(3):167–176, discussion 174–176

[23] Siddiqi SN, Posnick JC, Buncic R, et al. The detection and management of intracranial hypertension after initial suture release and decompression for craniofacial dysostosis syndromes. Neurosurgery. 1995; 36(4):703–708, discussion 708–709

[24] Vogel TW, Woo AS, Kane AA, Patel KB, Naidoo SD, Smyth MD. A comparison of costs associated with endoscope-assisted craniectomy versus open cranial vault repair for infants with sagittal synostosis. J Neurosurg Pediatr. 2014; 13 (3):324–331

[25] Delye HH, Arts S, Borstlap WA, et al. Endoscopically assisted craniosynostosis surgery (EACS): the craniofacial team Nijmegen experience. J Craniomaxillofac Surg. 2016; 44(8):1029–1036

[26] Iyengar RJ, Klinge PM, Chen WS, Boxerman JL, Sullivan SR, Taylor HO. Management of craniosynostosis at an advanced age: controversies, clinical findings, and surgical treatment. J Craniofac Surg. 2016; 27(5):e435–e441

[27] Gociman B, Agko M, Blagg R, Garlick J, Kestle JR, Siddiqi F. Endoscopic-assisted correction of metopic synostosis. J Craniofac Surg. 2013; 24(3):763–768

[28] Chan JW, Stewart CL, Stalder MW, St Hilaire H, McBride L, Moses MH. Endoscope-assisted versus open repair of craniosynostosis: a comparison of perioperative cost and risk. J Craniofac Surg. 2013; 24(1):170–174

[29] Kim D, Pryor LS, Broder K, et al. Comparison of open versus minimally invasive craniosynostosis procedures from the perspective of the parent. J Craniofac Surg. 2008; 19(1):128–131

[30] Jimenez DF, Barone CM. Intraoperative autologous blood transfusion in the surgical correction of craniosynostosis. Neurosurgery. 1995; 37(6):1075–1079

[31] Faberowski LW, Black S, Mickle JP. Blood loss and transfusion practice in the perioperative management of craniosynostosis repair. J Neurosurg Anesthesiol. 1999; 11(3):167–172

[32] Boop FA, Chadduck WM, Shewmake K, Teo C. Outcome analysis of 85 patients undergoing the pi procedure for correction of sagittal synostosis. J Neurosurg. 1996; 85(1):50–55

[33] Dadure C, Sauter M, Bringuier S, et al. Intraoperative tranexamic acid reduces blood transfusion in children undergoing craniosynostosis surgery: a randomized double-blind study. Anesthesiology. 2011; 114(4):856–861

[34] Goobie SM, Meier PM, Pereira LM, et al. Efficacy of tranexamic acid in pediatric craniosynostosis surgery: a double-blind, placebo-controlled trial. Anesthesiology. 2011; 114(4):862–871

[35] Harroud A, Weil AG, Turgeon J, Mercier C, Crevier L. Association of postoperative furosemide use with a reduced blood transfusion rate in sagittal craniosynostosis surgery. J Neurosurg Pediatr. 2016; 17(1):34–40

[36] Bonfield CM, Sharma J, Cochrane DD, Singhal A, Steinbok P. Minimizing blood transfusions in the surgical correction of craniosynostosis: a 10-year single-center experience. Childs Nerv Syst. 2016; 32(1):143–151

[37] Berry-Candelario J, Ridgway EB, Grondin RT, Rogers GF, Proctor MR. Endoscope-assisted strip craniectomy and postoperative helmet therapy for treatment of craniosynostosis. Neurosurg Focus. 2011; 31(2):E5

[38] Shah MN, Kane AA, Petersen JD, Woo AS, Naidoo SD, Smyth MD. Endoscopically assisted versus open repair of sagittal craniosynostosis: the St. Louis Children's Hospital experience. J Neurosurg Pediatr. 2011; 8(2):165–170

[39] Han RH, Nguyen DC, Bruck BS, et al. Characterization of complications associated with open and endoscopic craniosynostosis surgery at a single institution. J Neurosurg Pediatr. 2016; 17(3):361–370

[40] Honeycutt JH. Endoscopic-assisted craniosynostosis surgery. Semin Plast Surg. 2014; 28(3):144–149

[41] Diaz LK, Gaynor JW, Koh SJ, et al. Increasing cumulative exposure to volatile anesthetic agents is associated with poorer neurodevelopmental outcomes in children with hypoplastic left heart syndrome. J Thorac Cardiovasc Surg. 2016; 152(2):482–489

[42] Ing C, Wall MM, DiMaggio CJ, et al. Latent class analysis of neurodevelopmental deficit after exposure to anesthesia in early childhood. J Neurosurg Anesthesiol. 2016

[43] Ing C, DiMaggio C, Whitehouse A, et al. Long-term differences in language and cognitive function after childhood exposure to anesthesia. Pediatrics. 2012; 130(3):e476–e485

[44] Jimenez DF, Barone CM. Endoscopic craniectomy for early surgical correction of sagittal craniosynostosis. J Neurosurg. 1998; 88(1):77–81

[45] Jimenez DF, Barone CM. Endoscopy-assisted wide-vertex craniectomy, "barrel-stave" osteotomies, and postoperative helmet molding therapy in the early management of sagittal suture craniosynostosis. Neurosurg Focus. 2000; 9(3):e2

[46] Jimenez DF, Barone CM, McGee ME, Cartwright CC, Baker CL. Endoscopy-assisted wide-vertex craniectomy, barrel stave osteotomies, and postoperative helmet molding therapy in the management of sagittal suture craniosynostosis. J Neurosurg. 2004; 100(5) Suppl Pediatrics:407–417

[47] Ridgway EB, Berry-Candelario J, Grondin RT, Rogers GF, Proctor MR. The management of sagittal synostosis using endoscopic suturectomy and postoperative helmet therapy. J Neurosurg Pediatr. 2011; 7(6):620–626

[48] Dlouhy BJ, Nguyen DC, Patel KB, et al. Endoscope-assisted management of sagittal synostosis: wide vertex suturectomy and barrel stave osteotomies versus narrow vertex suturectomy. J Neurosurg Pediatr. 2016; 25(6):674–678

[49] Kung TA, Vercler CJ, Muraszko KM, Buchman SR. Endoscopic strip craniectomy for craniosynostosis: do we really understand the indications, outcomes, and risks? J Craniofac Surg. 2016; 27(2):293–298

[50] Dvoracek LA, Skolnick GB, Nguyen DC, et al. Comparison of traditional versus normative cephalic index in patients with sagittal synostosis: measure of scaphocephaly and postoperative outcome. Plast Reconstr Surg. 2015; 136 (3):541–548

[51] Jimenez DF, Barone CM. Endoscopic technique for sagittal synostosis. Childs Nerv Syst. 2012; 28(9):1333–1339

[52] Le MB, Patel K, Skolnick G, et al. Assessing long-term outcomes of open and endoscopic sagittal synostosis reconstruction using three-dimensional photography. J Craniofac Surg. 2014; 25(2):573–576

[53] Ghenbot RG, Patel KB, Skolnick GB, Naidoo SD, Smyth MD, Woo AS. Effects of open and endoscopic surgery on skull growth and calvarial vault volumes in sagittal synostosis. J Craniofac Surg. 2015; 26(1):161–164

[54] Jimenez DF, Barone CM. Endoscopic technique for coronal synostosis. Childs Nerv Syst. 2012; 28(9):1429–1432

[55] Jimenez DF, Barone CM. Early treatment of coronal synostosis with endoscopy-assisted craniectomy and postoperative cranial orthosis therapy: 16-year experience. J Neurosurg Pediatr. 2013; 12(3):207–219

[56] Tan SP, Proctor MR, Mulliken JB, Rogers GF. Early frontofacial symmetry after correction of unilateral coronal synostosis: frontoorbital advancement vs endoscopic strip craniectomy and helmet therapy. J Craniofac Surg. 2013; 24(4):1190–1194

[57] MacKinnon S, Proctor MR, Rogers GF, Meara JG, Whitecross S, Dagi LR. Improving ophthalmic outcomes in children with unilateral coronal synostosis by treatment with endoscopic strip craniectomy and helmet therapy rather than fronto-orbital advancement. J AAPOS. 2013; 17(3):259–265

[58] Rottgers SA, Lohani S, Proctor MR. Outcomes of endoscopic suturectomy with postoperative helmet therapy in bilateral coronal craniosynostosis. J Neurosurg Pediatr. 2016; 18(3):281–286

[59] Jimenez DF, Barone CM. Multiple-suture nonsyndromic craniosynostosis: early and effective management using endoscopic techniques. J Neurosurg Pediatr. 2010; 5(3):223–231

[60] Zubovic E, Woo AS, Skolnick GB, Naidoo SD, Smyth MD, Patel KB. Cranial base and posterior cranial vault asymmetry after open and endoscopic repair of isolated lambdoid craniosynostosis. J Craniofac Surg. 2015; 26(5):1568–1573

[61] Nguyen DC, Patel KB, Skolnick GB, et al. Are endoscopic and open treatments of metopic synostosis equivalent in treating trigonocephaly and hypotelorism? J Craniofac Surg. 2015; 26(1):129–134

[62] Erşahin Y. Endoscope-assisted repair of metopic synostosis. Childs Nerv Syst. 2013; 29(12):2195–2199

[63] Breugem CC, van R Zeeman BJ. Retrospective study of nonsyndromic craniosynostosis treated over a 10-year period. J Craniofac Surg. 1999; 10(2):140–143

[64] Seruya M, Oh AK, Boyajian MJ, et al. Long-term outcomes of primary craniofacial reconstruction for craniosynostosis: a 12-year experience. Plast Reconstr Surg. 2011; 127(6):2397–2406

[65] Aryan HE, Meltzer HS, Gerras GG, Jandial R, Levy ML. Leptomeningeal cyst development after endoscopic craniosynostosis repair: case report. Neurosurgery. 2004; 55(1):235–237, discussion 237–238

[66] Yarbrough CK, Smyth MD, Holekamp TF, et al. Delayed synostoses of uninvolved sutures after surgical treatment of nonsyndromic craniosynostosis. J Craniofac Surg. 2014; 25(1):119–123

[67] Sivakumar W, Goodwin I, Blagg R, et al. Pancraniosynostosis following endoscopic-assisted strip craniectomy for sagittal suture craniosynostosis in the setting of poor compliance with follow-up: a case report. J Med Case Reports. 2015; 9:64

[68] Jenkins GH, Smith NR, McNeely PD. Pancraniosynostosis following endoscope-assisted strip craniectomy and helmet orthosis for sagittal suture craniosynostosis in a nonsyndromic patient. J Neurosurg Pediatr. 2013; 12(1):77–79

[69] Meier PM, Goobie SM, DiNardo JA, Proctor MR, Zurakowski D, Soriano SG. Endoscopic strip craniectomy in early infancy: the initial five years of anesthesia experience. Anesth Analg. 2011; 112(2):407–414

[70] Felema GG, Bryskin RB, Heger IM, Saswata R. Venous air embolism from Tisseel use during endoscopic cranial vault remodeling for craniosynostosis repair: a case report. Paediatr Anaesth. 2013; 23(8):754–756

[71] Tobias JD, Johnson JO, Jimenez DF, Barone CM, McBride DS, Jr. Venous air embolism during endoscopic strip craniectomy for repair of craniosynostosis in infants. Anesthesiology. 2001; 95(2):340–342

[72] Faberowski LW, Black S, Mickle JP. Incidence of venous air embolism during craniectomy for craniosynostosis repair. Anesthesiology. 2000; 92(1):20–23

[73] Hashim PW, Patel A, Yang JF, et al. The effects of whole-vault cranioplasty versus strip craniectomy on long-term neuropsychological outcomes in sagittal craniosynostosis. Plast Reconstr Surg. 2014; 134(3):491–501

[74] Derderian CA, Heppner C, Cradock MM, et al. The effects of whole-vault cranioplasty versus strip craniectomy on long-term neuropsychological outcomes in sagittal craniosynostosis. Plast Reconstr Surg. 2015; 136(1):114e–115e

[75] Agrawal D, Steinbok P, Cochrane DD. Reformation of the sagittal suture following surgery for isolated sagittal craniosynostosis. J Neurosurg. 2006; 105(2) Suppl:115–117

[76] Kinsella CR, Jr, Cray JJ, Cooper GM, Pollack IF, Losee JE. Parasagittal suture after strip craniectomy. J Craniofac Surg. 2011; 22(1):66–67

[77] Sauerhammer TM, Seruya M, Ropper AE, Oh AK, Proctor MR, Rogers GF. Craniectomy gap patency and neosuture formation following endoscopic suturectomy for unilateral coronal craniosynostosis. Plast Reconstr Surg. 2014; 134(1):81e–91e

[78] Shillito J. A new cranial suture appearing in the site of craniectomy for synostosis. Radiology. 1973; 107(1):83–88

[79] Salehi A, Ott K, Skolnick GB, et al. Neosuture formation after endoscope-assisted craniosynostosis repair. J Neurosurg Pediatr. 2016; 18(2):196–200

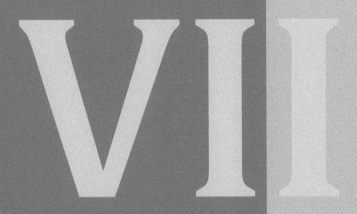

32 Cervical Diskectomy/Foraminotomy: Moderator

Luis M. Tumialán

Summary

In this discussion of *open microsurgical versus endoscopic approaches for a cervical diskectomy/foraminotomy*, the controversy regarding an endoscopic versus open microsurgical posterior cervical foraminotomy has essentially been nullified by Dr. Hartl and his colleagues (Chapter 33) and Drs. Kasliwal and Fessler (Chapter 34). Both chapters describe a paraspinal transmuscular approach to the posterior cervical spine using a table-mounted minimal access port through which this procedure is performed. A minimal access posterior cervical operation, whether visualized with an endoscope or a microscope, is associated with less blood loss, shorter hospital stays, decreased risk of infection, and less postoperative pain than a midline open approach. Thus, the controversy discussed here is not whether a minimal access approach to the posterior cervical spine is preferable to a midline open approach, but rather the subtleties of the minimal access technique itself, such as a sitting or a prone position, an endoscope or a microscope for visualization, fluoroscopy or image guidance for localization, and optimal diameter of the port. Surgeons who use the minimal access posterior cervical foraminotomy have several options to consider, which the authors saliently present. Overall, the benefit to patients with a single-level unilateral radiculopathy can be fully realized with a minimally invasive motion-preserving outpatient procedure with either technique presented by the authors.

Keywords: cervical radiculopathy, minimally invasive, motion preservation

32.1 Moderator

32.1.1 Introduction

The rubric of this book on controversies in neuroendoscopy has the moderator begin with an introduction regarding the pathology in question. In this chapter, the controversy about an endoscopic versus an open microsurgical posterior cervical foraminotomy has essentially been nullified by what the supposedly opposing authors have presented with regard to endoscopic and microscopic approaches. Dr. Hartl and his colleagues (Chapter 33) and Drs. Kasliwal and Fessler (Chapter 34) describe the use of a paraspinal transmuscular approach to the posterior cervical spine and the use of a table-mounted minimal access port through which this procedure is performed. Although many spine surgeons would agree that there is little difference between a minimal access lumbar diskectomy and an open microdiskectomy, with ample literature to support that position, such a comparison becomes more tenuous in the cervical spine.

The complexity of the musculature in the posterior cervical spine has the potential to cause significant blood loss from the exposure, immediate and considerable postoperative discomfort, and long-term atrophy when the posterior cervical spine is approached through the midline. Whereas a minimal access posterior cervical foraminotomy is a well-tolerated outpatient

procedure, an open midline posterior cervical foraminotomy tends not to be. A minimal access posterior cervical operation, whether visualized with an endoscope or a microscope, is associated with less blood loss, shorter hospital stays, decreased risk of infection, and less postoperative pain than a midline open approach. The abundant surgical literature cited by both groups of authors suggests that there is little controversy in this statement. Thus, we have reached a point in the evolution of the management of unilateral cervical radiculopathy that the controversy is not whether a minimal access approach to the posterior cervical spine is preferable to a midline open approach. Perhaps for the posterior cervical foraminotomy, the controversy now resides in the subtleties of the minimal access technique. Therefore, the moderation of this chapter focuses on the subtleties of the minimal access cervical foraminotomy: positioning, localization, visualization, and diameter of the port.

32.1.2 Decisions in Performing a Minimal Access Cervical Foraminotomy

Positioning: Sitting versus Prone

Fessler has long been a proponent of the sitting position for a posterior cervical foraminotomy. The argument is a sound one: the sitting position allows for adequate venous drainage from the epidural venous plexus and thereby minimizes blood loss. Fessler has been able to build this concept into his program with considerable investment and acceptance from our colleagues in anesthesia, who have their own concerns regarding venous air embolism. The use of a central venous catheter placed into the right atrium and precordial Doppler monitoring are mentioned as options. However, the authors explain that these adjuncts are not routinely used in their practice. Hartl and his colleagues are more accepting of the realities of the anesthetic limitations and, although they mention the sitting position, the prone position seems to be their preference.

Early in the author's experience with posterior cervical foraminotomy procedures, the author attempted to incorporate the sitting position as recommended by Fessler. The main limitation that was encountered had nothing to do with the patient or the actual mechanics of positioning. The resistance came from an obvious aversion to this position from the author's colleagues in anesthesia. It became readily apparent to the author that a sitting position would be a difficult one to maintain while minimizing the patient's time under anesthesia and optimizing efficiency. Furthermore, in outpatient settings, especially in an ambulatory surgery center, the placement of a central venous line and precordial Doppler monitoring out of concern for a potential venous air embolus are simply incompatible with the clinical setting.

Regardless of the position chosen, the cervical spine should be in a neutral position to optimize venous drainage. A flexed position of the neck should be avoided. Even in the prone position, patients can be placed in the reverse Trendelenburg position to minimize engorgement of the cervical epidural venous plexus and to optimize venous drainage. In the author's practice, the prone position with reverse Trendelenburg has become the accepted position, but at times the author does encounter the circumstance of vigorous epidural venous bleeding and cannot help but wonder whether the sitting position would have precluded it.

Localization: Fluoroscopy versus Image Guidance

Fluoroscopy has been the mainstay of visualization for securing the minimal access port in both the cervical and the lumbar spine since the development of the minimal access port. Kasliwal and Fessler describe the use of fluoroscopy in this technique. The rise of computer-assisted navigation introduces yet another option for localization of the level. Hartl and colleagues have adopted this technique. The obvious advantages of the latter approach include the elimination of ionizing radiation to the surgeon and the operating room team. There are also potential disadvantages, such as the radiation dose administered to the patient. Although it is a one-time dose, that dose far exceeds the dose of a few fluoroscopic images. The second disadvantage is accuracy. Unlike the lumbar spine, which is less likely to have significant drift during a procedure, the cervical spine that hangs between a Mayfield head holder and chest rolls is analogous to a suspension bridge. After registration of the intraoperative computed tomogram, the downward pressure on the cervical spine with each sequential dilator will have an impact on the accuracy of computer-assisted navigation. As with a suspension bridge, greater movement will occur at the mid-cervical region and less movement will occur toward the areas of support (i.e., the Mayfield head holder and the chest rolls). A potential role for this technology may in fact be localization of the lower segments, especially C7–T1, which may not be directly visualized on lateral fluoroscopic imaging.

The final disadvantage of computer-assisted navigation again relates to the clinical location of the procedure. As minimal access surgery moves more to the outpatient setting, the cost associated with computer-assisted navigation becomes untenable for ambulatory surgery centers and outpatient hospitals.

For the outpatient posterior cervical foraminotomy with diskectomy, it is difficult at this time to replace fluoroscopy for localizing the level and placing the minimal access port. Concern about radiation exposure may be valid in transpsoas approaches or percutaneous instrumentation, but during a posterior cervical foraminotomy, where only three or four images may be required to secure a minimal access port, radiation exposure should not be a principal concern. However, a patient of a certain body habitus may be difficult to image, especially at the cervicothoracic junction. The amount of shoulder traction necessary to facilitate that visualization on a lateral fluoroscopic image may result in brachial plexus neuropraxia. Computer-assisted navigation in that circumstance has potential value and warrants consideration.

Visualization: Endoscope versus Microscope

The next area of controversy in the minimal access posterior cervical foraminotomy is the type of visualization used to perform the procedure itself. Fessler has popularized the use of the endoscope, which requires a specific skill set. Hartl and colleagues have described the use of an operating microscope. The author is certain that Fessler and his colleagues do not necessarily view the disadvantages of the endoscope as listed by Hartl et al as true disadvantages. The absence of direct visualization of neurovascular structures does not change the capacity to actually view the bony structures themselves and accomplish the decompression. Perhaps the proximity of the camera to the exiting nerve root, capable of being seen only through an endoscope, may actually serve as an advantage. The main form of hemostasis in this type of foraminotomy tends to be a hemostatic matrix and a cottonoid, both of which work identically whether viewed through a microscope or an endoscope; this makes the supposition of superiority of vascular control with a microscope over an endoscope a difficult position to maintain. Using a minimal access port forces the surgeon's mind to reconstruct the anatomy at depth. That mental reconstruction must take place without the midline structures serving as a reference whether an endoscope or a microscope is used.

Diameter of the Minimal Access Port

The final topic that merits comment regarding the minimally invasive posterior cervical foraminotomy, but that is not specifically discussed by either group of authors, is the diameter of the minimal access port. Selection of the diameter is less an area of controversy and more an area of the surgeon's preference; however, in the author's experience, the diameter of the port has implications for the postoperative course of the patient. As this procedure has migrated almost entirely to the outpatient setting, minimal discomfort becomes an essential ingredient to the patient feeling comfortable going home after this procedure. Kasliwal and Fessler discuss the use of an 18-mm access port in their surgical technique, whereas no specific diameter is mentioned by Hartl and colleagues. It stands to reason that a smaller diameter will correlate with less postoperative discomfort, which is consistent with the author's experience in reducing the port diameter for this procedure.

When that principle is invoked, the smallest diameter that will encompass the requisite anatomy for the decompression should be used for a posterior cervical foraminotomy. In this circumstance, the requisite anatomy may be defined by the distance from pedicle to pedicle and by access to the canal medial to the pedicle and the foramen lateral to the pedicle (▶ Fig. 32.1). The distance from pedicle to pedicle in the cervical spine is seldom more than 12 mm, or less in those cases when the patient has advanced spondylosis. The diameter of a cervical pedicle is typically less than 5 mm. Having 2 mm of access to the canal medial to the pedicle and 2 mm of access to the foramen lateral to the pedicle would require at least 9 to 10 mm of exposure. By this definition, the requisite anatomy for a posterior cervical foraminotomy may be encompassed with a 14-mm-diameter port. If a port with this diameter is placed precisely over the cervical pedicle as demonstrated in ▶ Fig. 32.1, then access to the entire requisite anatomy for a comprehensive decompression of the nerve root can be readily accomplished (▶ Fig. 32.2). Precise placement of a 14-mm-diameter port is imperative.

There is little question that the diameter of the access port affects postoperative recovery. The author has noted a difference in the postoperative discomfort of patients in whom he has used a 16-mm minimal access port instead of a 14-mm access port because of the size of the disk herniation or the

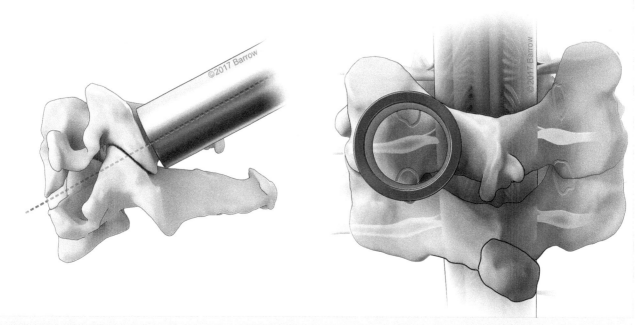

Fig. 32.1 Left: Artist's rendition of the cervical foramen with the distance between the pedicles defining the rostral caudal dimensions of the foramen. Right: These dimensions establish the basis for the diameter of a minimal access port. (Used with permission from Barrow Neurological Institute, Phoenix, AZ.)

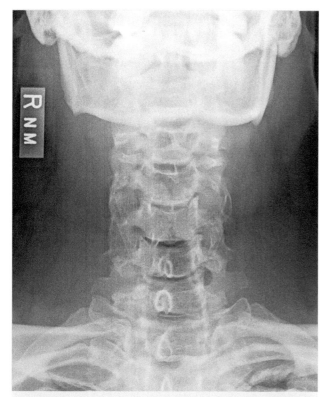

Fig. 32.2 Postoperative anteroposterior cervical radiograph demonstrating the bony work of a C7 foraminotomy. Note the foraminotomy is centered over the top of the C7 pedicle and spans from pedicle to pedicle with several millimeters of access on either side of the pedicle. (Used with permission from Barrow Neurological Institute, Phoenix, AZ.)

patient's body habitus. The noticeable decrease in postoperative discomfort with a 14-mm access port that the author observed has allowed a reliable transition to an outpatient setting for this procedure, with patients typically going home within an hour after the procedure.

32.1.3 Conclusion

The complexity of the posterior cervical musculature makes a muscle-stripping midline approach difficult to match a precisely placed minimal access port. As a result, the posterior cervical foraminotomy has now become firmly established as a minimal access procedure. The agreement by this chapter's authors on this point shifts the controversy on this procedure away from endoscopy versus open microsurgery. The reality is that the midline approach has an increasingly scarce role and is unlikely to be used by the next generation of surgeons.

Surgeons who use the minimal access posterior cervical foraminotomy have several options to consider, which the authors in Chapters 33 and 34 saliently present. A sitting position or a prone position, an endoscope or a microscope, and fluoroscopy or image guidance are all viable alternatives for this procedure. The overall benefit to patients with a single-level unilateral radiculopathy can be fully realized with a minimally invasive motion-preserving outpatient procedure with either technique presented by the authors.

33 Cervical Diskectomy/Foraminotomy: Microscope

Roger Hartl, Rodrigo Navarro-Ramirez, and Tim Heiland

Summary

Posterior cervical diskectomy and foraminotomy is an effective method to treat cervical radiculopathy without the need for instrumentation. In this chapter, we describe the surgical considerations and technical nuances of microsurgical techniques to treat cervical disc pathology. We also describe distinct advantages of microsurgical techniques over novel endoscopic techniques for cervical discectomy.

Keywords: cervical, posterior, foraminotomy, microsurgical, open

33.1 Microsurgical Perspective

33.1.1 Introduction

Frykholm et al in 1951 described the surgical anatomy of the cervical spine with emphasis on the posterior "laminoforaminotomy" approach, also known as the posterior cervical foraminotomy (PCF). This approach avoids the risk of vascular, airway, or esophageal lesion and helps preserve mobility of the cervical spine by minimizing the muscle, ligament, and osseous disruption. This is counterbalanced by the risk of postoperative neck pain and muscle spasms. However, nowadays, minimally open/tubular approaches may reduce the incidence of the aforementioned postoperative events.[1,2,3,4]

33.1.2 Case Example

History

A 26-year-old male presented with left arm and shoulder pain after doing pushups. The pain persisted for 6 weeks despite over-the-counter pain medication treatment and physical therapy for 4 weeks. At the time when surgery was suggested, he also presented with left deltoid and left hand weakness. Those symptoms were worse with lifting or reaching. Magnetic resonance imaging (MRI) demonstrated a C6–C7 left paracentral/foraminal-extruded disk that compressed the left C7 nerve root, without radiological evidence of central cord compression (▶ Fig. 33.1).

Physical Examination

Neurological examination revealed proximal weakness of the left hand, deltoid muscle 2/5, and biceps 3/5, and reflexes were normal. He also complained of dropping objects and being unable to open bottles with the left hand.

Intraoperative Management

Patients undergoing posterior laminoforaminotomy can be positioned either prone or sitting. This decision depends on the surgeon's preference and the resources available for transeso-phageal and central-line monitoring. Intraoperative monitoring

of motor evoked potentials and electromyogram (EMG) is recommended. Nowadays, most of the surgeons are more familiar and comfortable with the prone positioning. In such case, the patient is placed over a radiolucent table/frame and fixed with either a Mayfield or a Gardner–Wells head holder. Traction of the head or shoulder depression is also to be decided on a case-by-case fashion (▶ Fig. 33.2).

X-ray localization is mandatory, despite the decision to performing the surgery via a conventional midline or lateral trans-muscular access. We have been able to incorporate real-time navigation using an intraoperative computed tomography (CT; ▶ Fig. 33.2c). In this manner, the lateral skin incision and trans-muscular approach is meant to provide an excellent exposure without extensive muscle detachment and surgical bleeding.

Performing the procedure using either microscope magnification or surgical loupes is always encouraged. A high-speed burr through a 15-mm tube is used to drill the lamina and medial aspect of the superior facet (up to 50%) until the bone is thinned down and then removed with a 1-mm Kerrison punch or "flicked off" with a 3–0 curette.

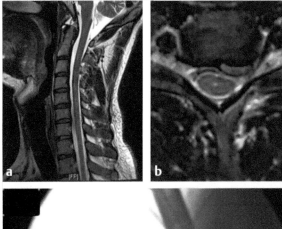

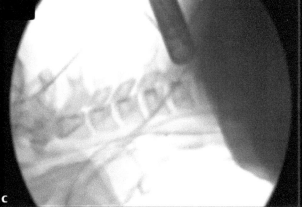

Fig. 33.1 A 26-year-old male presented with left arm and shoulder pain. A preoperative **(a)** sagittal and **(b)** axial T2-weighted magnetic resonance imaging (MRI) demonstrates a C6–C7 left paracentral/foraminal-extruded disk that contacts the left C7 nerve root but without central cord compression. **(c)** A cervical lateral X-ray demonstrates no spondylolisthesis.

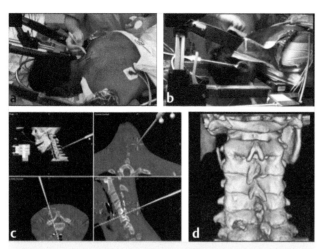

Fig. 33.2 The patient was positioned **(a)** prone intraoperatively with **(b)** a fixed shoulder retractor and tongs were used in order to aid in visualization of the C6–C7 vertebral bodies. **(c)** Intraoperative neuronavigation provides targeted trajectory to access the C6–C7 foramen. **(d)** Postoperative computed tomography (CT) 3D reconstruction demonstrates width of foraminotomy without facet disruption.

If a diskectomy is intended, the disk space should be approached through the exiting nerve root axilla. Careful upward mobilization of the nerve root can be safely performed, but central cord manipulation should be avoided. Using Gelfoam (Pfizer, New York, NY) soaked in procoagulant preparation almost always ensures hemostasis; bipolar coagulation can be used, but it is not always recommended. The fascia is then closed in a watertight fashion, and the skin is closed in the usual standard fashion.[1,2,5]

33.1.3 Surgical Outcomes

Generally, the literature indicates that for PCF immediate symptom improvement ranges from 82 to 100%. Improvement in radiculopathy symptoms is 91.4% at short-term evaluation/discharge and drops to 85% at 4-year follow-up.[3] On the other hand, reoperation rate is observed to be between 5 and 9.9%. Same level reoperation rate was only 6.6%. Reoperations were more common and in a shorter period of time on those patients who presented with radicular symptoms + neck pain. Among those patients who required a reoperation, this was not necessarily correlated with adjacent segment pathology.[2,3]

33.1.4 Advantages of Open Microsurgical Approach for the Case Illustration

PCF through a microsurgical mini-open transtubular approach has been preferred for young patients, athletes, and those in whom preserved range of motion is intended. Patients with high risk of nonunion through a conventional anterior cervical approach and fusion are also good candidates for a PCF.

Anatomical indications for this PCF include lateral or foraminal nerve root compression and lateral soft disk herniations that fail to be treated conservatively. Finally, cost-analysis studies have demonstrated that PCF is also appealing compared to the anterior approach.

33.1.5 Disadvantage of the Endoscope

Several disadvantages have been identified when performing endoscopic spine surgical procedures, similar to the limitations identified when performing PCF. Most of these disadvantages are inherent to the optics of the hardware and the endoscope itself, which can lead to indirect visualization of neural structures, limited vascular control, and limited spatial orientation due to minimal anatomical exposure. In addition, prolonged learning curve and cutting-edge equipment may be necessary to master and perform the endoscopic PCF technique.

33.1.6 Patient Selection

We consider this procedure to be optimal in patients who present with unilateral or bilateral cervical radiculopathy due to lateral osteophyte or lateral soft disk herniation that are refractory to nonoperative treatment.

33.1.7 Complication Avoidance

General complications may include nerve root damage, dural tears, cervical C5 palsy, and vascular damage.[6] Also, patients having surgery in a sitting position must be carefully monitored for air embolism, and transesophageal Doppler and central-line placement may be necessary.

Despite the use of the prone or sitting position, if a conventional midline approach is going to be performed, avoiding extensive muscle detachment will reduce postoperative pain and risk of postoperative instability.[5] In this regard, the lateral transmuscular approach may produce less mechanical instability but may increase the risk of postoperative muscle spasms. During the PCF, resection of 50% of the facet or less (▸ Fig. 33.2**d**) will reduce the risk of mechanical instability.[5] In addition, we recommend evaluating all the patients with flexion–extension films for the presence of significant cervical kyphosis. Presence of cervical kyphosis is considered a relative contraindication for this procedure.

Central disk herniations and/or calcified disks are also relative contraindications for this procedure. We encourage the use of intraoperative navigation to avoid wrong level surgery and improve pathology localization. We prefer intraoperative navigation at C6/C7 or below even if the patient is in Gardner's tongues (▸ Fig. 33.2**c**).

33.1.8 Technical Nuances

Patients presenting with significant neck pain, cervical kyphosis, or identified instability are poor candidates for PCF. Extensive facet drilling (more than 50%) will increase the risk of segment instability and mechanical failure. The pedicle below and above the indexed level should be palpable with a nerve hook after the drilling.[5]

33.1.9 Literature Review/Evidence in Favor of Microscopic Approach

There are no prospective comparative studies favoring endoscopic PCF over microscopic PCF. However, Kim et al 2009 presented a randomized, controlled trial comparing the minimally invasive tubular microscopic posterior approach with an open conventional approach but failed to demonstrate better clinical outcomes between the two techniques.[7] Recently, in 2014 Lawton et al reported long-term outcomes on endoscopic PCF. However, their data favoring endoscopic PCF must be interpreted with caution. Only one-third of the patients that had surgery were followed long term; standardized outcome measurements were reported in less than 50% of those patients.[8] In addition, as mentioned earlier, endoscopic PCF requires specific surgical hardware and a steep learning curve, and limited anatomy exposure and neurovascular control may represent a mayor downside for this technique in comparison with the conventional/tubular PCF.[9]

33.1.10 Clinical Pearls

- Perform intraoperative traction to open up the foramen and decrease the risk of nerve injury.
- We recommend using an open Jackson table.
- Use Rhoton instruments for dissection, especially if the foramen in very tight. We use Rhoton's bayonetted forceps.
- Sometimes, it might be necessary to drill a bit into the pedicle in order to create more room around the nerve root.
- Navigation use helps with pathology localization of the lower cervical segments.
- Make the skin incision a little bit bigger and use sharp dissection through the muscle fascia and finger palpation for

placement of the first dilator; that will minimize bleeding and the amount of pressure and manipulation needed to place the retractor. Meticulous hemostasis under the microscope is suggested.
- Use microscope from skin to skin.

References

[1] Caridi JM, Pumberger M, Hughes AP. Cervical radiculopathy: a review. HSS J. 2011; 7(3):265–272

[2] Härtl R, Korge A, eds. Minimally Invasive Spine Surgery: Techniques, Evidence, and Controversies. Davos-Platz, Switzerland: AOSpine; 2012

[3] Bydon M, Mathios D, Macki M, et al. Long-term patient outcomes after posterior cervical foraminotomy: an analysis of 151 cases. J Neurosurg Spine. 2014; 21(5):727–731

[4] Branch BC, Hilton DL, Jr, Watts C. Minimally invasive tubular access for posterior cervical foraminotomy. Surg Neurol Int. 2015; 6:81

[5] Zdeblick TA, Zou D, Warden KE, McCabe R, Kunz D, Vanderby R. Cervical stability after foraminotomy. A biomechanical in vitro analysis. J Bone Joint Surg Am. 1992; 74(1):22–27

[6] Clark JG, Abdullah KG, Steinmetz MP, Benzel EC, Mroz TE. Minimally invasive versus open cervical foraminotomy: a systematic review. Global Spine J. 2011; 1(1):9–14

[7] Kim KT, Kim YB. Comparison between open procedure and tubular retractor assisted procedure for cervical radiculopathy: results of a randomized controlled study. J Korean Med Sci. 2009; 24(4):649–653

[8] Lawton CD, Smith ZA, Lam SK, Habib A, Wong RHM, Fessler RG. Clinical outcomes of microendoscopic foraminotomy and decompression in the cervical spine. World Neurosurg. 2014; 81(2):422–427

[9] Ziewacz JE, Wu J-C, Mummaneni PV. Microendoscopic cervical foraminotomy and discectomy: are we there yet? World Neurosurg. 2014; 81(2):290–291

34 Cervical Diskectomy/Foraminotomy: Endoscope

Manish K. Kasliwal and Richard G. Fessler

Summary

Posterior cervical discectomy has been traditionally treated with microscopic visualization. In this chapter, we describe novel endoscopic controlled approaches to cervical disc disease. We also describe the technical nuances of this procedure as well as the advantages of endoscopic controlled approaches versus traditional microsurgical techniques.

Keywords: endoscopic, foraminotomy, minimally invasive, spine, cervical

34.1 Endoscopic Perspective

34.1.1 Case Example

Patient History

A 45-year-old male presented with a 3-month history of left neck, shoulder, and arm pain. His pain radiated along the medial forearm to his little finger. His neck disability index (NDI) was 35/100 and visual analog scale (VAS) score for neck and arm pain was 3/10 and 8/10, respectively.

Examination

The patient's neurological examination revealed 4/5 strength in the finger abduction and adduction with decreased pinprick along the medial forearm and little finger. The patient tried narcotic analgesics, massage, physical therapy, and chiropractic care with no significance, with persistent radicular pain being his predominant complaint.

Imaging

Magnetic resonance imaging (MRI) of the cervical spine demonstrated a large left-sided C7–T1 disk herniation resulting in severe foraminal stenosis (▶ Fig. 34.1).

34.1.2 Case Discussion

Cervical radiculopathy leads to neck and radiating arm pain or numbness in the distribution of a specific nerve root. Often, this radicular pain is accompanied by motor or sensory disturbances. This case represents classic presentation of a patient with cervical C8 radiculopathy. Most patients with cervical radiculopathy have a favorable prognosis. The natural history of patients with cervical radiculopathy is benign with approximately half of patients with cervical radiculopathy having good resolution of symptoms within 6 weeks of onset with varying degrees of nonoperative management.[1] Overall, nonsurgical treatment options have been shown to have up to a 90% success rate in the initial management of patients with cervical radiculopathy making urgent surgical intervention often unnecessary. A large epidemiologic study demonstrated that over a 5-year follow-up period, 31.7% of patients with symptomatic cervical radiculopathy had symptom recurrence and 26% needed surgical intervention for intractable pain, sensory deficit, or objective weakness. At final follow-up, however, nearly 90% of patients were asymptomatic or only mildly incapacitated by the pain.[2] Another study reporting the natural history of cervical radiculopathy followed 51 patients over a period of 2 to 19 years and showed that 43% of patients had no further symptoms after a few months, 29% had mild or intermittent symptoms, and 27% had more disabling pain. None of the patients with radiculopathy progressed to myelopathy during the study period.[3] The benign natural history of cervical radiculopathy can also be envisaged from the statement proposed by the Degenerative Disorders Work Group of the North American Spine Society Evidence-Based Clinical Guideline Development Committee: "It is likely that for most patients with cervical radiculopathy from degenerative disorders signs and symptoms will be self-limited and will resolve spontaneously over a variable length of time without specific treatment."[1] Considering the findings from various studies, it is completely reasonable to attempt nonoperative management, which was done in this case. However, a certain percentage of patients may not

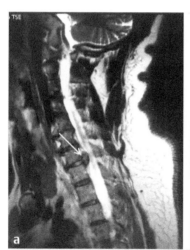
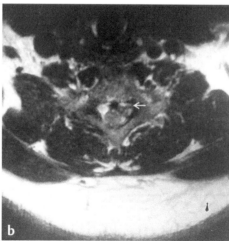

Fig. 34.1 T2-weighed sagittal (**a**) and axial (**b**) MRI scans of the cervical spine demonstrating a laterally herniated left C7–T1 disk herniation (*white arrow*) causing severe foraminal stenosis with compression of the exiting nerve root.

improve with nonoperative treatment, and in these subset of patients, surgery has been shown to result in significant improvement.[2] For patients with radiculopathy secondary to single-level disease and in whom nonoperative treatment fails and once the decision for surgical intervention has been made, the most common procedures performed include anterior cervical diskectomy and fusion (ACDF), posterior cervical foraminotomy (PCF), and cervical arthroplasty.[1,4] The discussion of pros and cons of one treatment over another is outside the domain of this debate. All have shown excellent and durable results in terms of pain relief, neurological recovery, and a very acceptable complication rate. Even though individual surgeons may have their own preferences, we prefer a minimally invasive endoscopic posterior foraminotomy with or without diskectomy if the clinical and radiological parameters correlate well. The details of our surgical technique are described in the following section.

34.1.3 Intraoperative Management

After the induction of general endotracheal anesthesia, adequate intravenous access was secured. Routine perioperative antibiotics were administered. The patient was then positioned in a semi-sitting position with a Mayfield head holder, which helps improve visualization and decrease blood loss (▶ Fig. 34.2). After the patient had been positioned in the semi-sitting position, utmost care was directed toward ensuring that the cervical spine and neck musculature were not kinked or held in an unfavorable position. During positioning, the table is progressively flexed and placed into Trendelenburg to bring the patient into a semi-sitting position so that the head is flexed but not rotated and the long axis of the cervical spine is perpendicular to the floor. The neck, chin, and chest were allowed to be loose and free of compression. Use of a central venous pressure catheter placed into the right atrium and precordial Doppler monitoring in anticipation of blood loss and possible venous air embolus is optional. We do not use this routinely due to the brevity and minimal blood loss of the operation. The fluoroscopic C-arm was then brought into the surgical field so that real-time lateral fluoroscopic images could be obtained (▶ Fig. 34.2). We routinely use intraoperative somatosensory and motor evoked potential monitoring of the dermatome operated on as well as of distal distributions to examine spinal cord integrity. We prefer to avoid/minimize paralytic agents after induction to allow for physical intraoperative feedback of nerve root irritation and formal neurophysiologic monitoring.

A stab incision was made approximately 1 cm off midline ipsilateral to and at the level of the pathological lesion. Under fluoroscopic guidance and direct vision, the trapezius fascia was incised is incised using a Metzenbaum scissors, which are also used to bluntly dissect and spread the muscular layers until docked on to the facets. This allows for safe passage of the sequential dilating cannulas with a minimum of force. A series of dilators were then inserted sequentially through the neck soft tissues, over which an 18-mm tubular retractor was then inserted. Real-time lateral radiographic images were obtained as often as needed to ensure a proper working trajectory throughout this process. The working channel (tubular retractor) was then attached to a flexible retractor affixed to the operating table side rail and locked in position at the junction of the lamina and lateral mass. The endoscope was then attached to the tubular retractor via a circular plastic friction couple (▶ Fig. 34.3). Once the tubular retractor was set in the desired position, a Bovie cautery with a long tip was then used to remove the remaining muscle and soft tissue overlying the lateral mass and facet. A small, straight endoscopic curette was used to scrape the inferior edge of the superior lamina and the medial edge of the lateral mass/facet. This exposure was then carried beneath the lamina and facet with a small angled endoscopic curette. A small, angled endoscopic Kerrison rongeur was then used to begin the foraminotomy. Periosteal and bone bleeding was addressed with bone wax and cautery. A drill with a long endoscopic bit can also be used to further thin the medial facet and lateral mass. The laminoforaminotomy was completed when the nerve root had been well exposed along its proximal foraminal course. Additional exposure was obtained by drilling a small portion of the superomedial portion of the pedicle directly below the exiting nerve root. A nerve hook was used to mobilize the nerve root superiorly to expose the disk space and fragment. With the root retracted, the disk fragment was then removed in a standard manner with curettes and long endoscopic pituitary rongeurs. Upon completion of the diskectomy and decompression, the nerve hook was again passed along the exiting root to confirm its free passage, and a lateral fluoroscopic image is obtained. Hemostasis was obtained by bipolar cautery and gentle tamponade with

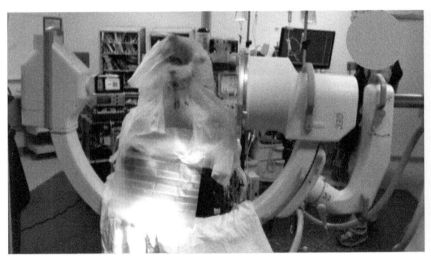

Fig. 34.2 Intraoperative photograph showing the operative semi-sitting positioning of a patient with a Mayfield head holder ensuring that the long axis of the cervical spine is perpendicular to the floor.

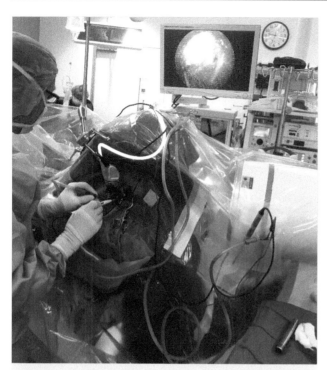

Fig. 34.3 Intraoperative picture demonstrating the setup during surgery.

thrombin-soaked Gelfoam pledgets. The area was then copiously irrigated with lactated Ringer's solution impregnated with bacitracin antibiotics. The tubular retractor and endoscope were then removed, and the fascia and skin were closed routinely. Marcaine (0.25%) was used to inject the skin edges before closure. The patient was awakened from anesthesia and taken to the postanesthesia recovery unit. The patient was discharged from the postanesthesia recovery to home after observing for 3 to 4 hours with a prescription of combination of muscle relaxants and an oral opioid for breakthrough pain. The patient had significant improvement in his left arm pain right after the surgery and has been doing very well with no symptom recurrence at 1-year follow-up with an NDI of 10 and VAS score of 1/10 for both neck and arm pain.

34.1.4 Advantages of Endoscopic Approach

The principal goal of minimal access techniques is to reduce approach-related morbidity. With the wider application of muscle-splitting tubular retractor systems and associated instruments, the application of minimally invasive techniques to posterior cervical decompressive procedures especially laminoforaminotomy with or without diskectomy has become quite popular in the past decade or so.[5,6] Although standard open approaches are effective based on clinical outcome, minimally invasive approaches have been developed to avoid the extensive subperiosteal stripping of paraspinal musculature that can result in significant postoperative pain, muscle spasm, and dysfunction in 18 to 60% of patients.[7] Preclinical, histological, serological, radiological, and clinical outcome data have shown evidence of profound iatrogenic tissue injury associated with

typical open posterior spinal approaches.[8] Any minimally access surgery must be proven to treat symptoms to the same degree as compared to open procedures, while at the same time decreasing muscular and soft-tissue trauma, reducing physiological stress to the patient, enabling maintenance of the normal biomechanics of the spine, and improving on the perioperative endpoints achieved with traditional surgeries. Minimally invasive cervical diskectomy/foraminotomy (MICD/F) has been shown to have clinical efficacy equal to that of open procedures in addition to having less blood loss, shorter hospital stay, and decreased risk of infection and postoperative pain.[5,6,7,9,10] However, there is a significant learning curve with potential of increased complications during that time period.[5,9] At our center, minimally invasive endoscopic laminoforaminotomy is performed as a same-day procedure with patients routinely discharged the same day of surgery. A shorter hospital stay compared to the open microsurgical group and a decreased infection with endoscopic laminoforaminotomy and diskectomy can translate into decreased health care burden in the era where health care cost-cutting and bundled payments are becoming the cynosure for health care administrators and providers.

34.1.5 Disadvantages of Microscopic Approach

While standard microsurgical laminoforaminotomy has a very high success rate in alleviating the radiculopathy in patients with foraminal stenosis and lateral disk herniation, the muscle dissection often needed to obtain an adequate surgical exposure has been associated with increased postoperative muscle spasm, neck pain, and recovery time.[7] A number of studies have clearly demonstrated the benefits of minimally invasive or tubular microdiskectomy/laminoforaminotomy as compared to open techniques at least in the short term mainly in duration of hospital stay, amount of postoperative narcotic use, and decreased infection rate all favoring the minimally invasive surgery (MIS) group.[5,7,9,10] Although not reported, the potential of violating adjacent facets during open laminoforaminotomy may accelerate development of adjacent segment disease.

34.1.6 Patient Selection

For patients to be candidates for open or minimally invasive laminoforaminotomy with or without diskectomy, the importance of appropriate patient selection cannot be overemphasized. Imaging should clearly demonstrate a lateral/foraminal soft disk herniation or mild/moderate spur.[5,6] In order to differentiate soft disk from calcified spur, both MR-based and computed tomography (CT) based studies may be useful; the MR scans best demonstrate the soft tissues, while the CT scans readily identify the calcification. Similarly, PCF/diskectomy should be avoided in patients with pure axial neck pain without neurologic symptoms, gross cervical instability, and symptomatic central disk herniation.

34.1.7 Complication Avoidance and Technical Nuances

Even though the procedure can be performed in the prone or semi-sitting position, the latter offers the advantages of improved fluoroscopic visualization of the cervical spine and decreased blood accumulation in the operative field. Because the guide wire can penetrate the dura in the cervical interlaminar space, its use should preferably be avoided in these cases. Use of anteroposterior radiographic images may be useful in the first few cases to guarantee proper positioning of the dilator and the working portal. While cutting the fascia with the scissors or Bovie, care should be taken not to cut muscle fibers to avoid unnecessary blood loss. Good dissection of the underlying flavum and dura from the bone defines the relevant anatomy and helps prevent incidental dural tears. It should be ensured that at least 50% of the facet complex is preserved to minimize potential postoperative instability. While performing a diskectomy in addition to the laminoforaminotomy, the importance of additional exposure obtained by drilling the superomedial portion of the pedicle directly below the exiting nerve root cannot be overemphasized.[5]

34.1.8 Literature Review/Evidence in Favor of Endoscopic Approach

PCF with or without diskectomy is an essential component of the spinal surgeon's armamentarium in the surgical treatment of symptomatic cervical radiculopathy. Even though anterior cervical procedures have recently gained increasing popularity partly because of its versatility in terms of indications, posterior cervical laminoforaminotomy remains of proven benefit, relieving symptoms in 92 to 97% of patients in appropriately selected patients with symptomatic cervical radiculopathy secondary to foraminal stenosis or lateral herniated disks.[5,6,7,11] While recent studies on MICD/F have demonstrated that efficacy is equivalent to that of open cases with blood loss, length of stay, and postoperative medication usage for pain all reduced in the MICD/F cases, there is lack of high-quality studies comparing the open versus minimally invasive approaches.[7,12] Also, the term "minimally invasive posterior foraminotomy" has been used for a variety of surgical techniques. Only the procedures performed using a tubular retractor followed by either endoscope or microscope are considered minimally invasive in this chapter.

Lidar and Salame reported a series of 32 patients who underwent MICD/F.[13] Mean operative time was 62 minutes, mean estimated blood loss 60 was mL, and average hospital stay 1.5 was days. The mean VAS for radicular pain decreased from 8 preoperatively to 4.8 immediately postoperatively and finally to 0.75 at 12-month follow-up. The same series showed a decrease in the mean preoperative VAS for neck pain from 6.75 to 5.75 immediately postoperatively and then to 0.9 at 12-month follow-up. The 36-item Short Form Questionnaire (SF-36) showed statistically significant improvements in all eight domains at 6-month follow-up.

In a randomized controlled trial, Kim and Kim performed an open PCF in 19 patients and tubular retractor–assisted PCF in 22 patients.[10] At 24-month follow-up, clinical success was achieved in 16/19 (84.2%) of the open cohort and 19/22 (86.4%) of the tubular retractor–assisted cohort according to the Odom criteria.

A prospective cohort study by Fessler and Khoo compared open ($n = 26$) or tubular retractor–based ($n = 25$) laminoforaminotomy.[5]

This study reported that minimally invasive cases had lower blood loss by 108 mL (138 vs. 246 mL), a shorter surgical time by 62 minutes (115 vs. 177 minutes), less analgesic use by 29 to 31 Eq (9–11 vs. 40 Eq), and a shorter hospital stay by 48 hours (20 vs. 68 hours) compared with open controls.

These findings were echoed in the retrospective study by Winder and Thomas comparing 65 open and 42 microscopic tubular-assisted posterior laminoforaminotomies with lower blood loss, less recovery room analgesic use, less discharge analgesic use, and a shorter hospital stay in the tubular-assisted group as compared to open controls.[14]

A recent systematic review by Clark et al reported on the results of open versus percutaneous foraminotomy.[12] While the results were biased due to that fact that most of the studies were classified as class III evidence due to lack of an adequate comparison group or substantial limitations in the cohort design with inclusion of only one randomized trial in the review, results indicate that patients undergoing percutaneous cervical laminoforaminotomy have lower blood loss by 120.7 mL (open: 173.5 mL; percutaneous: 52.8 mL; $n = 5,670$), a shorter surgical time by 50.0 minutes (open: 108.3 minutes; percutaneous: 58.3 minutes; $n = 5,882$), less inpatient analgesic use by 25.1 Eq (open: 27.6 Eq; percutaneous: 2.5 Eq; $n = 5,356$), and a shorter hospital stay by 2.2 days (open: 3.2 days; percutaneous: 1.0 days; $n = 51,472$), compared with patients undergoing open procedures.

Open versus minimally invasive techniques were compared in a recent meta-analysis by McAnany et al, which concluded that patients with symptomatic cervical radiculopathy from foraminal stenosis can be effectively managed with either a traditional open or an MIS foraminotomy with no significant difference in the pooled outcomes between the two groups.[7]

However, there were a number of limitations with the meta-analysis. Among eight enrolled studies, only one article was a comparative study between open surgery and MIS, with the others being single-arm studies! The surgical techniques utilized were also variable introducing too much heterogeneity in the meta-analysis.

To conclude, while the level of evidence demonstrating the superiority of minimally invasive foraminotomy is not very high, this technique has demonstrated equivalent or improved outcomes compared with the open technique and the benefits secondary to decreased iatrogenic disruption of the normal anatomy such as decreased blood loss, length of stay, and postoperative medication usage in a number of studies.

References

[1] Bono CM, Ghiselli G, Gilbert TJ, et al. North American Spine Society. An evidence-based clinical guideline for the diagnosis and treatment of cervical radiculopathy from degenerative disorders. Spine J. 2011; 11(1):64–72

[2] Radhakrishnan K, Litchy WJ, O'Fallon WM, Kurland LT. Epidemiology of cervical radiculopathy. A population-based study from Rochester, Minnesota, 1976 through 1990. Brain. 1994; 117(Pt 2):325–335

[3] Lees F, Turner JW. Natural history and prognosis of cervical spondylosis. BMJ. 1963; 2(5373):1607–1610

[4] Kasliwal MK, Traynelis VC. Motion preservation in cervical spine: review. J Neurosurg Sci. 2012; 56(1):13–25

[5] Fessler RG, Khoo LT. Minimally invasive cervical microendoscopic foraminotomy: an initial clinical experience. Neurosurgery. 2002; 51(5) Suppl:S37–S45

[6] Coric D, Adamson T. Minimally invasive cervical microendoscopic laminoforaminotomy. Neurosurg Focus. 2008; 25(2):E2

[7] McAnany SJ, Kim JS, Overley SC, Baird EO, Anderson PA, Qureshi SA. A meta-analysis of cervical foraminotomy: open versus minimally-invasive techniques. Spine J. 2015; 15(5):849–856

[8] Kim CW. Scientific basis of minimally invasive spine surgery: prevention of multifidus muscle injury during posterior lumbar surgery. Spine. 2010; 35 (26) Suppl:S281–S286

[9] Skovrlj B, Gologorsky Y, Haque R, Fessler RG, Qureshi SA. Complications, outcomes, and need for fusion after minimally invasive posterior cervical foraminotomy and microdiscectomy. Spine J. 2014; 14(10):2405–2411

[10] Kim KT, Kim YB. Comparison between open procedure and tubular retractor assisted procedure for cervical radiculopathy: results of a randomized controlled study. J Korean Med Sci. 2009; 24(4):649–653

[11] Henderson CM, Hennessy RG, Shuey HM, Jr, Shackelford EG. Posterior-lateral foraminotomy as an exclusive operative technique for cervical radiculopathy: a review of 846 consecutively operated cases. Neurosurgery. 1983; 13 (5):504–512

[12] Clark JG, Abdullah KG, Steinmetz MP, Benzel EC, Mroz TE. Minimally invasive versus open cervical foraminotomy: a systematic review. Global Spine J. 2011; 1(1):9–14

[13] Lidar Z, Salame K. Minimally invasive posterior cervical discectomy for cervical radiculopathy: technique and clinical results. J Spinal Disord Tech. 2011; 24(8):521–524

[14] Winder MJ, Thomas KC. Minimally invasive versus open approach for cervical laminoforaminotomy. Can J Neurol Sci. 2011; 38(2):262–267

35 Thoracic Diskectomy: Moderator

Saksham Gupta and Hasan A. Zaidi

Summary

Thoracic disc herniations are rare yet complex lesions which can result in neurological dysfunction. Traditional surgical intervention carries significant approach related morbidity. Endoscopic approaches have the advantage of reducing surgical morbidity, but carry a steep learning curve. In this chapter we introduce both open and endoscopic treatment approaches to thoracic disc herniations.

Keywords: thoracic, discectomy, endoscopic, thoracoscopic, fusion

35.1 Moderator Introduction

35.1.1 Thoracic Disk Disease

Thoracic disk herniation (TDH) is a common anomaly with a radiographic prevalence estimated to range from 11 to 37%.[1,2,3] Only 1 in a million patients annually develops symptoms, and these patients are usually young to middle-aged adults.[4] Patients with chronic disease may present with a radiculopathic thoracic back pain, myelopathy, and/or nondermatomal leg pain. Severe cases may progress to bilateral lower extremity paresis and paraplegia with autonomic dysfunction. Trauma or stressors to the back (i.e., heavy lifting) may acutely worsen the degree of herniation and thus cause more acute presentation.[5] These symptoms can often be attributed to degenerative changes of the disk itself, causing herniation into the spinal cord. It is increasingly thought that the inflammatory milieu generated by tumor necrosis factor-alpha plays a prominent role in the sensation of pain itself.[6] Surgery is indicated electively in patients refractory to conservative therapy and urgently for patients presenting with TDH that causes symptoms of cord compression.

The variable radiographic features of TDH often make surgical decision-making difficult. Computed tomography (CT) aids in visualizing the spinal bony anatomy and the herniation itself. CT also identifies the laterality and degree of calcification, which are vital in the determination of the optimal surgical approach.[7] Nuclear magnetic resonance imaging (MRI) provides a detailed view of the spinal cord and nerve roots. MRI allows for the determination of dural sac penetration and spinal cord signal change as well. CT and MRI play crucial roles in operative planning of TDH regardless of surgical approach.

The difficulty of access and visualization of TDH also presents a surgical challenge (▶ Fig. 35.1). Regardless of approach, decompressive diskectomy is preferred and offers favorable outcomes.[4,8,9] Open approaches include posterolateral, lateral, and transthoracic thoracotomy. The nontransthoracic approaches often employ costotransversectomy or transpedicular approach for access as well.[10,11] More recently, innovations in thoracoscopic devices and technique have paved the way for minimal access thoracoscopic diskectomies.[12] Novel mini-open and transternal approaches are currently being innovated as well. These diverse approaches for this complex entity have motivated robust debate into optimal surgical technique based on location, degree of calcification, and dural involvement. This determination is imperative, since injury to the spinal cord risks devastating, permanent neurologic disability. This chapter focuses on the respective benefits of traditional open and thoracoscopic approaches for TDH and summarizes these in a final recommendation.

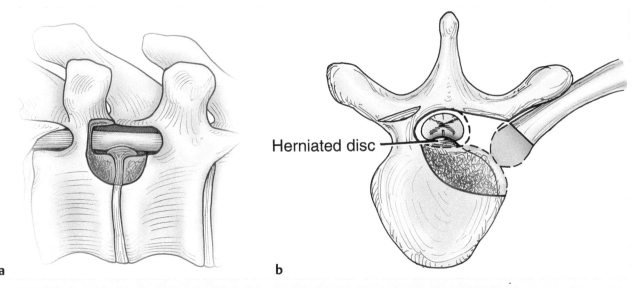

Fig. 35.1 Diagram illustrating **(a)** lateral and **(b)** axial views of a herniated thoracic disk. (Modified with permission from Rosenthal D, Dickman CA: Thoracoscopic microsurgical excision of herniated thoracic discs. J Neurosurg. 1998;89(2):224-235.)

35.1.2 Evolution of Surgical Treatment Options for Thoracic Diskectomy

The first case of simple laminectomy for TDH was performed in 1922 by Adson.[7] The first published report of TDH laminectomy was made by Young in 1946.[13] At the time, this was a relatively unknown pathology and some surgeons believed the optimal surgical management was none at all. The field of open posterior laminectomy for TDH accelerated with a landmark case series published by Love and Kiefer in 1950.[14] Noting the scant attention afforded to TDH, they published a series of 17 cases managed with laminectomy and reported favorable response in patients who presented early in their disease course and whose surgeries did not involve cord manipulation. The relative lack of knowledge about the pathology (many cases of lateral TDH continued to undergo cardiac and abdominal procedures since TDH was not considered on the differential diagnosis) and negative attitude toward laminectomy continued into the decade, however.[15] Drs. Abbott and Retter emphasized the need for a wide laminectomy, opening of the dura for medially located TDH, and dorsal root rhizotomy for compressed nerves and reported favorable outcomes in the majority of their series.[15]

As the procedure gained traction, it was noted that the open posterior procedure remained ineffective for patients with medial TDH and patients with severe neurological deficits.[16,17] Dr. Hulme at Frenchay Hospital in Bristol applied the lateral paramedian approach with extended costotransversectomy in 1960, similar to the approach used to expose vertebral bodies in Pott's disease of the spine, to provide better exposure for medial TDH and his initial results were promising.[17,18] However, this approach had questionable long-term efficacy. The transthoracic transpleural approach was innovated to meet these challenges in 1969 by Drs. Perot and Munro as well as by Dr. Ransohoff et al in two separate reports.[11,17] Critics of this approach pointed out the difficulty of intradural exploration and risk during resection near the spinal dura given the potential for TDH erosion into the dura itself. This technique was further refined by Dr. Carson et al in 1971 with the posterolateral transthoracic approach, which then gave way to an anterolateral approach by Dr. Albrand and Corkill in 1979.[4,19] The anterolateral approach for transthoracic transpleural laminectomy provided excellent visualization without the need to mobilize the spine. The lateral extracavitary approach was explored by Dr. Maiman et al in a case series of 23 patients to provide another wide, nontransthoracic approach.[20] This series demonstrated successful results, but it has been suggested that the paraspinous muscle mobilization it requires can denervate and devascularize these muscular structures.[7]

Technological improvements in video-assisted thoracoscopic surgery (VATS) opened the door for a paradigm shift toward the endoscopic approach for TDH. A thoracoscope was initially reported to treat pleural effusions by Dr. Jacobaeus in 1909.[21] While the thoracoscope provided a means for minimal access surgery, it was limited in the magnitude and quality of the image provided. The addition of a camera and image processor led to the development of VATS. Improvements in fiberoptic light transmission and image processing in the early 1990s ushered an era of rapidly growing indications for VATS; it is now commonly used for the management of many mediastinal, pleural, and pulmonary diseases including myotomy for achalasia, pleurodesis pneumothorax, and resection for lung cancer.[21] VATS has demonstrated variable success in improving outcomes for different indications, but is generally thought to reduce postoperative pain and hospitalization length. VATS has a higher upfront cost than traditional thoracotomy and whether it saves money in the long term is unknown. It also presents a challenge in surgical training with a steep learning curve.[7]

Up to the early 1990s, the thoracotomy remained the standard approach for TDH.[7] The development of VATS would soon inevitably challenge this. Indeed, Dr. Caputy et al reported the first successful use of VATS to access and perform thoracic diskectomy in a cadaver and porcine model and then in a clinical case.[22] The field thoracoscopic diskectomy has burgeoned since this first report. Novel long thoracoscopic tools aided in access to the spine itself, and rigorous clinical trials have demonstrated the efficacy of the approach. A unique difficulty for the management of TDH was intraoperative disease localization, but the integration of CT and ultrasound image guidance with VATS provides helpful 3D guidance.[23,24] Thoracoscopic-assisted mini-open surgery for TDH laminectomy is another emerging technique that is undergoing clinical testing just as combined mini-open operations have seen increasing usage for other thoracic and abdominal pathologies.[25] Finally, new approaches altogether, such as the mini-open trans-sternal approach for anterior high thoracic spine disease, continue to explore novel surgical improvements.[26]

35.1.3 Review of Open versus Endoscopic Procedures (How Many People Are Doing Either and for What?)

Surgical management of TDH has advanced rapidly with novel open procedures affording increasingly excellent visualization and new VATS technologies that provide minimal access. The open posterolateral, lateral, and transthoracic approaches still remain used today for TDH, and VATS has emerged as an excellent option as well. However, low TDH prevalence and increasing numbers of options have made well-powered comparative trials between different open procedures and VATS difficult, notwithstanding challenges in randomizing patients for surgical trials (i.e., different anatomies, different levels of operative skill, difficulty in blinding). However, new data are emerging to aid in delineating optimal approaches for specific patients. It is increasingly seen that the lateralization, calcification, dural involvement, and experience of the surgeon have implications in dictating optimal approach.

An innovation on the classic lateral extracavitary approach is the lateral extracavitary mini-thoracotomy, which was reported by Dr. Uribe et al to afford favorable outcomes while minimizing complications in a recent series of 60 patients.[27] These patients were not stratified by the location of disease or the degree of calcification, which makes it difficult to assess which patients it is appropriate for. The lateral approach continues to provide excellent access to lateral TDH with dural involvement.

Posterior approaches have also undergone recent innovation with promising results. These flexible approaches can include costotransversectomy, foraminotomy, transfacet, transpedicular, and interlaminar approaches that may be personalized for each patient's pathology.[28] A small series of posterior transdural diskectomies of 13 central TDH by Dr. Coppes et al demonstrated symptomatic reduction in all but 1 patient, with no nonreversible complications reported.[29] However, this approach does threaten the spinal cord even if not reported in this series.[29] This technique involves the usage of drill adjacent to exposed cord and fibrin glue to seal the dura.[30] A modified posterior transfacet pedicle-sparing approach with diskectomy and interbody fusion for 18 cases of TDH with central involvement was reported by Dr. Bransford et al with mixed results.[31] In particular, 6 patients required additional surgery for postoperative complications. Novel techniques and technologies have recently demonstrated promising results in favor of the posterior approach. In head-to-head comparison for a small cohort of patients receiving posterolateral or mini-open transpedicular diskectomy, patients in the latter cohort had better early postoperative Prolo scores and less blood loss.[32] Lateral TDH may be especially amenable for transfacet approach. Furthermore, endoscope-assisted posterior approach can offer adequate visualization and resection of even central calcified TDH, which is usually not amenable to the posterior approach.[33,34] Posterior transfacet decompression and diskectomy with an L-shaped osteotome was also safe and effective for a series of 27 patients with central calcified TDH reported by Dr. Zhuang et al.[35]

The open transthoracic transpleural approach remains popular for most TDH and the standard for central TDH. This approach can afford access for difficult central calcified lesions. A series of 27 cases of central calcified TDH reported by Dr. Ayhan et al showed postoperative objective improvement in about half of their series.[36] In head-to-head comparison of transthoracic, lateral, and posterolateral approaches, the transthoracic approach demonstrated improved neurological recovery, despite greater pulmonary complications.[37] Transthoracic approaches in general demonstrated increased in-hospital morbidity and mortality as well as higher cost in a large registry-based study, but this study may suffer from bias as these approaches are favored for specific anatomical features not captured by the database.[38] It has also undergone modification toward minimal access, and mini-transthoracic approach demonstrated improved efficacy over posterolateral approaches for central, large, calcified disks in comparative analysis.[39] Dr. Deviren et al have described a minimal access approach using a novel retractor system to minimize the morbidity associated with open technique.[40] It has remained popular due to the exquisite visualization it provides, but the morbidity associated with operating near vital thoracic structures has limited its usage.

Thoracoscopic microdiskectomy has presented similar outcomes to other approaches in case series. In particular, an early prospective trial by Drs. Anand and Regan showed favorable results in 100 consecutive TDH cases with thoracoscopic diskectomy.[41] The large majority of patients were satisfied by the procedure. No patients experienced major complications and the average ICU stay was only 1 day.[41] A prospective series of 167 single-level thoracoscopic diskectomy by Dr. Quint et al demonstrated favorable functional outcomes for 80% of patients and pain reduction in 79% of patients with a low major complication rate.[42] Another prospective series of 121 patients reported by Dr. Wait et al demonstrated that thoracoscopy provides clinical efficacy while minimizing morbidity, especially for smaller, anterior TDH.[43] Meta-analysis of studies of thoracoscopic

approach demonstrated similar results—a 79% complete resolution rate and 24% overall complication rate—and suggested that patients with small disease and no calcified dural attachments benefit from thoracoscopy in the hands of experienced operators. Clearly, this approach requires experience with thoracoscopic technique, but these data demonstrate potential.

Of note, giant central TDH compromises over 40% of the spinal canal on CT and presents a particularly challenging entity. These are often calcified and have dural extension. Microscopic mini-thoracotomy is a modification of traditional thoracotomy and is more technically straightforward for operators without extensive experience with thoracoscopic technique. Dr. Moran et al innovated the transthoracic mini-thoracotomy for medial giant TDH and Dr. Russo et al devised the anterior transthoracic approach for microsurgical mini-thoracotomy, both with favorable outcomes.[44, 45] These results were corroborated again by Dr. Roelz et al's series of 17 cases of retropleural mini-thoracotomy for giant central TDH, in which 76% were calcified and intradural extension was present in 35% of patients. Only 2 patients experienced transient postoperative neurological decline.[46] Mini-thoracotomy has demonstrated similar outcomes in operative length, postoperative stay, and duration of chest drain to thoracoscopy.[47] Dr. Hott et al reported that thoracoscopic approach was associated with worse functional outcomes than open thoracotomy.[48]

These trials have advanced the field and provide motivation for continued debate. Trends toward improved outcomes with open thoracotomy and mini-thoracotomy over thoracoscopy appear for large central lesions. It is difficult to discern the effect of the "learning curve" in these results. Patients with rare multilevel disease require personalized care that often hinges on open approaches for their disease as well.[49]

35.1.4 Expert Recommendation

The range of well-studied open surgical approaches for thoracic diskectomy includes posterolateral, wide lateral, and transthoracic approaches. Emerging techniques include mini-thoracotomy for these approaches and the trans-sternal approach. Thoracoscopy offers a minimal access approach to the thoracic spine as well. Based on current evidence, our recommendations are as follows. We believe posterior and posterolateral mini-open or open thoracotomy with costotransversectomy are appropriate for single-level lateral TDH with minimal central involvement and multi-level disease with no central involvement. The posterior transfacet approach is amenable for lateral TDH with spinal cord involvement. Lateral mini-open or open thoracotomy is appropriate for single-level lateral TDH with minimal central involvement, though emerging technologies may make the posterior approach a feasible option for difficult central lesions in the future. The transthoracic transpleural approach is preferred for TDH that is primarily central and requires comfort by the neurosurgeon to operate near cardiopulmonary structures and by the anesthesiologist to monitor physiological conditions for a thoracic case. Thoracoscopy is amenable for small, central disease without major calcification or spinal cord involvement, in which case the transpleural approach remains the standard. Integration of thoracoscopic simulation tasks as part of residency training and continuing medical education will allow neurosurgeons to add this technique to their repertoire and may expand indications for this approach.

References

[1] Awwad EE, Martin DS, Smith KR, Jr, Baker BK. Asymptomatic versus symptomatic herniated thoracic discs: their frequency and characteristics as detected by computed tomography after myelography. Neurosurgery. 1991; 28 (2):180–186

[2] Williams MP, Cherryman GR, Husband JE. Significance of thoracic disc herniation demonstrated by MR imaging. J Comput Assist Tomogr. 1989; 13 (2):211–214

[3] Wood KB, Garvey TA, Gundry C, Heithoff KB. Magnetic resonance imaging of the thoracic spine. Evaluation of asymptomatic individuals. J Bone Joint Surg Am. 1995; 77(11):1631–1638

[4] Carson J, Gumpert J, Jefferson A. Diagnosis and treatment of thoracic intervertebral disc protrusions. J Neurol Neurosurg Psychiatry. 1971; 34(1):68–77

[5] Le Roux PD, Haglund MM, Harris AB. Thoracic disc disease: experience with the transpedicular approach in twenty consecutive patients. Neurosurgery. 1993; 33(1):58–66

[6] Séguin CA, Pilliar RM, Roughley PJ, Kandel RA. Tumor necrosis factor-alpha modulates matrix production and catabolism in nucleus pulposus tissue. Spine. 2005; 30(17):1940–1948

[7] Burke TG, Caputy AJ. Treatment of thoracic disc herniation: evolution toward the minimally invasive thoracoscopic technique. Neurosurg Focus. 2000; 9 (4):e9

[8] Dickman CA, Rosenthal D, Karahalios DG, et al. Thoracic vertebrectomy and reconstruction using a microsurgical thoracoscopic approach. Neurosurgery. 1996; 38(2):279–293

[9] Otani K, Yoshida M, Fujii E, Nakai S, Shibasaki K. Thoracic disc herniation. Surgical treatment in 23 patients. Spine. 1988; 13(11):1262–1267

[10] Mack MJ, Regan JJ, Bobechko WP, Acuff TE. Application of thoracoscopy for diseases of the spine. Ann Thorac Surg. 1993; 56(3):736–738

[11] Ransohoff J, Spencer F, Siew F, Gage L, Jr. Transthoracic removal of thoracic disc. Report of three cases. J Neurosurg. 1969; 31(4):459–461

[12] Lesoin F, Rousseaux M, Autricque A, et al. Thoracic disc herniations: evolution in the approach and indications. Acta Neurochir (Wien). 1986; 80(1–2):30–34

[13] Young JH. Cervical and thoracic intervertebral disk disease. Med J Aust. 1946; 2(24):833–838

[14] Love JG, Kiefer EJ. Root pain and paraplegia due to protrusions of thoracic intervertebral disks. J Neurosurg. 1950; 7(1):62–69, illust

[15] Abbott KH, Retter RH. Protrusions of thoracic intervertebral disks. Neurology. 1956; 6(1):1–10

[16] Logue V. Thoracic intervertebral disc prolapse with spinal cord compression. J Neurol Neurosurg Psychiatry. 1952; 15(4):227–241

[17] Perot PL, Jr, Munro DD. Transthoracic removal of midline thoracic disc protrusions causing spinal cord compression. J Neurosurg. 1969; 31(4):452–458

[18] Hulme A. The surgical approach to thoracic intervertebral disc protrusions. J Neurol Neurosurg Psychiatry. 1960; 23:133–137

[19] Albrand OW, Corkill G. Thoracic disc herniation. Treatment and prognosis. Spine. 1979; 4(1):41–46

[20] Maiman DJ, Larson SJ, Luck E, El-Ghatit A. Lateral extracavitary approach to the spine for thoracic disc herniation: report of 23 cases. Neurosurgery. 1984; 14(2):178–182

[21] Luh SP, Liu HP. Video-assisted thoracic surgery: the past, present status and the future. J Zhejiang Univ Sci B. 2006; 7(2):118–128

[22] Caputy A, Starr J, Riedel C. Video-assisted endoscopic spinal surgery: thoracoscopic discectomy. Acta Neurochir (Wien). 1995; 134(3–4):196–199

[23] Johnson JP, Drazin D, King WA, Kim TT. Image-guided navigation and video-assisted thoracoscopic spine surgery: the second generation. Neurosurg Focus. 2014; 36(3):E8

[24] Johnson JP, Stokes JK, Oskouian RJ, Choi WW, King WA. Image-guided thoracoscopic spinal surgery: a merging of 2 technologies. Spine. 2005; 30(19):E572–E578

[25] Xu BS, Xu HW, Yuan QM, et al. Thoracic endoscopic-assisted mini-open surgery for thoracic and thoracolumbar spinal cord compression. Orthop Surg. 2016; 8(4):523–526

[26] Brogna C, Thakur B, Fiengo L, et al. Mini transsternal approach to the anterior high thoracic spine (T1-T4 vertebrae). BioMed Res Int. 2016; 2016:4854217

[27] Uribe JS, Smith WD, Pimenta L, et al. Minimally invasive lateral approach for symptomatic thoracic disc herniation: initial multicenter clinical experience. J Neurosurg Spine. 2012; 16(3):264–279

[28] Börm W, Bäzner U, König RW, Kretschmer T, Antoniadis G, Kandenwein J. Surgical treatment of thoracic disc herniations via tailored posterior approaches. Eur Spine J. 2011; 20(10):1684–1690

[29] Coppes MH, Bakker NA, Metzemaekers JD, Groen RJ. Posterior transdural discectomy: a new approach for the removal of a central thoracic disc herniation. Eur Spine J. 2012; 21(4):623–628

[30] Mehdian SM. Reviewer's comment concerning "Posterior transdural discectomy: a new approach for the removal of a central thoracic disc herniation." (doi:10.1007/s00586-011-1990-4 by H.M. Coppes et al.). Eur Spine J. 2012; 21(4):629

[31] Bransford R, Zhang F, Bellabarba C, Konodi M, Chapman JR. Early experience treating thoracic disc herniations using a modified transfacet pedicle-sparing decompression and fusion. J Neurosurg Spine. 2010; 12(2):221–231

[32] Chi JH, Dhall SS, Kanter AS, Mummaneni PV. The Mini-Open transpedicular thoracic discectomy: surgical technique and assessment. Neurosurg Focus. 2008; 25(2):E5

[33] Paolini S, Tola S, Missori P, Esposito V, Cantore G. Endoscope-assisted resection of calcified thoracic disc herniations. Eur Spine J. 2016; 25(1):200–206

[34] Wagner R, Telfeian AE, Iprenburg M, et al. Transforaminal endoscopic foraminoplasty and discectomy for the treatment of a thoracic disc herniation. World Neurosurg. 2016; 90:194–198

[35] Zhuang QS, Lun DX, Xu ZW, Dai WH, Liu DY. Surgical treatment for central calcified thoracic disk herniation: a novel L-shaped osteotome. Orthopedics. 2015; 38(9):e794–e798

[36] Ayhan S, Nelson C, Gok B, et al. Transthoracic surgical treatment for centrally located thoracic disc herniations presenting with myelopathy: a 5-year institutional experience. J Spinal Disord Tech. 2010; 23(2):79–88

[37] Mulier S, Debois V. Thoracic disc herniations: transthoracic, lateral, or posterolateral approach? A review. Surg Neurol. 1998; 49(6):599–606, discussion 606–608

[38] Yoshihara H, Yoneoka D. Comparison of in-hospital morbidity and mortality rates between anterior and nonanterior approach procedures for thoracic disc herniation. Spine. 2014; 39(12):E728–E733

[39] Arts MP, Bartels RH. Anterior or posterior approach of thoracic disc herniation? A comparative cohort of mini-transthoracic versus transpedicular discectomies. Spine J. 2014; 14(8):1654–1662

[40] Deviren V, Kuelling FA, Poulter G, Pekmezci M. Minimal invasive anterolateral transthoracic transpleural approach: a novel technique for thoracic disc herniation. A review of the literature, description of a new surgical technique and experience with first 12 consecutive patients. J Spinal Disord Tech. 2011; 24(5):E40–E48

[41] Anand N, Regan JJ. Video-assisted thoracoscopic surgery for thoracic disc disease: classification and outcome study of 100 consecutive cases with a 2-year minimum follow-up period. Spine. 2002; 27(8):871–879

[42] Quint U, Bordon G, Preissl I, Sanner C, Rosenthal D. Thoracoscopic treatment for single level symptomatic thoracic disc herniation: a prospective followed cohort study in a group of 167 consecutive cases. Eur Spine J. 2012; 21 (4):637–645

[43] Wait SD, Fox DJ, Jr, Kenny KJ, Dickman CA. Thoracoscopic resection of symptomatic herniated thoracic discs: clinical results in 121 patients. Spine. 2012; 37(1):35–40

[44] Moran C, Ali Z, McEvoy L, Bolger C. Mini-open retropleural transthoracic approach for the treatment of giant thoracic disc herniation. Spine. 2012; 37 (17):E1079–E1084

[45] Russo A, Balamurali G, Nowicki R, Boszczyk BM. Anterior thoracic foraminotomy through mini-thoracotomy for the treatment of giant thoracic disc herniations. Eur Spine J. 2012(21 Suppl 2):S212–S220

[46] Roelz R, Scholz C, Klingler JH, Scheiwe C, Sircar R, Hubbe U. Giant central thoracic disc herniations: surgical outcome in 17 consecutive patients treated by mini-thoracotomy. Eur Spine J. 2016; 25(5):1443–1451

[47] Bartels RH, Peul WC. Mini-thoracotomy or thoracoscopic treatment for medially located thoracic herniated disc? Spine. 2007; 32(20):E581–E584

[48] Hott JS, Feiz-Erfan I, Kenny K, Dickman CA. Surgical management of giant herniated thoracic discs: analysis of 20 cases. J Neurosurg Spine. 2005; 3(3):191–197

[49] Oppenlander ME, Clark JC, Kalyvas J, Dickman CA. Surgical management and clinical outcomes of multiple-level symptomatic herniated thoracic discs. J Neurosurg Spine. 2013; 19(6):774–783

36 Thoracic Diskectomy: Microscope and Endoscopic

J. Patrick Johnson, Doniel G. Drazin, Terrence T. Kim, Paul E. Kaloostian, and Samer S. Ghostine

Summary

Herniated thoracic disks are rare pathologies that can result in progressive radiculopathy, paraparesis, or paraplegia depending on the degree and configuration of thoracic disk compression on the neural elements. These lesions can be approached using traditional open microsurgical techniques from either a posterior or an anterior approach. Open microsurgical anterior approaches carry significant approach-related morbidity. Utilizing techniques and tools developed by thoracic surgeons, in the last few decades several neurosurgeons have begun to utilize endoscopic port-assisted techniques to approach these lesions. In this chapter, we discuss the advantages and disadvantages of these techniques for herniated thoracic disks.

Keywords: thoracic discectomy, myelopathy, endoscopic, video assisted thoracoscopic surgery, spinal cord compression

36.1 Introduction

Thoracic spine disk disease is a rare but quite complex surgical conundrum that has been a significant challenge to spine surgeons for many years. Disks in the spinal thoracic region are statistically infrequent and represent only 2 to 4% of all disk problems in the human spinal column. Due to the unique anatomic location and limited incidence of these relatively rare spinal disorders, most surgeons have limited experience treating such pathology. Nevertheless, over the last few decades, there has been gradual but continued improvement in techniques used to approach this complex and potentially devastating thoracic disk herniation, while minimizing neurological compromise in these patients. We will thoroughly explore the classical presentation of such patients, imaging characteristics, factors that play a role in treatment decision-making, and finally comparing the pros and cons of both an open and an endoscopic approach in treating patients with thoracic spine disk disease.

36.1.1 Clinical Presentation

Patients with thoracic degenerative disk disease can present with a myriad of clinical symptoms. Most symptomatic patients present with thoracic back pain, radiculopathy, vague nondermatomal leg pain and/or myelopathy. In severe cases, patients can present with gradual or acute paraplegia or paraparesis with associated bilateral lower extremity numbness, gait imbalance, and bowel/bladder dysfunction. Patients can present with predominantly two types of scenarios causing thoracic spine disease. The first relates to chronic thoracic degenerative disk disease with progressive deterioration and evolution of disk–osteophyte formation with or without spinal cord compression. Second, patients can present acute posttrauma classically with a soft disk herniation with or without spinal cord compression. Herein, we will limit our discussion to thoracic disk herniations that would typically cause myelopathy and require an anterior approach, open thoracotomy, or thoracoscopic approach (video-assisted thoracoscopic surgery [VATS]), and discuss the controversial aspects of these two approaches.

36.1.2 Imaging Characteristics

Diagnostic modalities for thoracic disk disease include a computed tomography (CT) scan as well as a magnetic resonance imaging (MRI) scan without contrast of the thoracic spine. CT scan is useful to identify the bony anatomy, spinal level, and landmarks of the bulging or herniated thoracic disk, including the composition of the disk itself. Determining whether the disk herniation is soft or hard (calcified) is critical toward establishing a treatment protocol for the patient. Also, a CT scan is useful for determining the laterality of the disk herniation in relation to the spinal canal. For example, a soft lateral disk herniation may be more amenable to a posterolateral approach, whereas a central calcified disk herniation would be more amenable to a transthoracic anterolateral approach. Finally, a CT scan should ideally be done to include extension up to C2 for disk herniation around T6 and above, or extension down to S1 for disk herniation from T6 and below. This would enable the surgeon and radiologist to localize precisely the spinal level(s) of the disk herniation(s), as localization is often not very simple, despite being of utmost importance. The MRI is also important in determining the relationship of the thoracic disk–osteophyte complex to the nearby spinal cord and/or nerve roots, detecting the presence of spinal cord signal change, and for assessing for penetration of the dural sac. These factors all affect surgical decision-making. Patients who cannot get an MRI given implantable metal electrodes or claustrophobia may be studied using a CT myelogram, which will show the extent of spinal cord deformation.

36.1.3 Surgical Indications for Thoracic Diskectomy

Surgical indications for thoracic diskectomy include severe and unrelenting axial back pain and thoracic radiculopathy refractory to all conservative routes such as physical therapy, epidural steroid injections, and nonsteroidal anti-inflammatory drugs for more than 3 months. Additionally, ventral thoracic disk herniation causing myelopathy is a more urgent problem that requires immediate neurosurgical attention and treatment in order to prevent permanent neurological compromise including bilateral lower extremity paralysis (paraparesis), numbness, and bowel/bladder dysfunction.

36.1.4 Localization

Localization of the exact spinal level for thoracic disk disease is crucial and oftentimes quite difficult. For large calcified disk bulges, intraoperative X-ray/C-arm may be all that is needed, as long as preoperative lateral thoracic X-rays demonstrate the disk herniation clearly. This may be made even simpler if associated vertebral body compression or deformity is present. However, this is often not the case. Another method of determining the exact spinal level is a full spinal CT scan scout image with the ability to either count down from cervical region and/or count up from S1. Alternatively, percutaneous placement of a radiopaque marker (e.g., a Guglielmi detachable coil) in the pedicle adjacent to the disk in question preoperatively can be performed using CT guidance from a dorsal approach. A lateral X-ray of the thoracic spine should be done preoperatively to make sure the coil is seen on X-ray, in order to verify that it will be seen on intraoperative X-ray. Finally, one can use modern intraoperative navigation technology such as the O arm (Medtronic) and Ziehm Navigation; these modalities, though expensive, can be quite useful intraoperatively in spinal-level localization through a single spin. Navigation is also useful intraoperatively as the surgeon progresses from rib resection to pedicle drilling and finally to the appropriate disk space.

36.1.5 Surgical Anatomy

Having a clear understanding of the thoracic spine surgical anatomy from a posterior, anterior, and lateral aspect is of great importance in providing the best care for these patients. For example, for a T7/T8 diskectomy, it is the T8 (inferior) rib that should be resected. In terms of level count, the disk space is cephalad to the pedicle. The neurovascular bundle runs on the inferior border of the rib and thus careful dissection along the inferior rib margins is critical to avoid neurovascular injury. Above T10, a complete rib resection may be needed to expose the disk space. Also, the artery of Adamkiewicz is usually on the left and between T9 and L3. Segmental vessels are located in the midportion of the vertebral body and these can be moved aside or coagulated if necessary. Finally, if the portal of entry is below T7, diaphragmatic injury can be encountered (▶ Fig. 36.1).

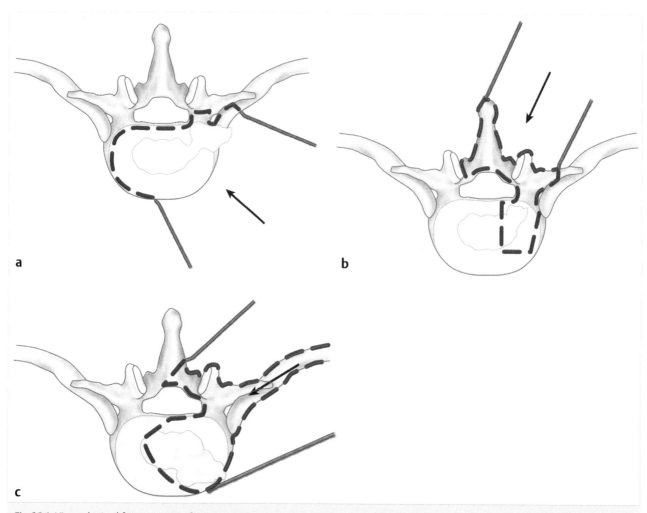

Fig. 36.1 Views obtained from a variety of access corridors to herniated thoracic disks. **(a)** Anterolateral approaches, including endoscopic thoracic approaches, provide a circumferential view of the thoracic disk. **(b)** Posterior transpedicular approaches provide view of the lateral segment of the thoracic disk. **(c)** Posterolateral costotransversectomies provide a view of the majority of the thoracic disk. (Courtesy of J. Patrick Johnson, MD; from Johnson JP, Rogers CD. Thoracoscopic diskectomy. In: Kim DH, Fessler RG, Regan JJ, eds. Endoscopic Spine Surgery and Instrumentation. New York, NY: Thieme; 2005.)

36.1.6 Evolution of Surgical Treatment Options

Thoracic disk surgery in the modern era can be dated to 1969 when Drs. Perot and Ransohoff described, in separate articles, a transthoracic procedure to treat symptomatic thoracic disk herniations. This was considered a significant advance in the ability to treat ventral compression of the thoracic spinal cord. It became clear over the ensuing decades of the 1970s and 1980s, however, that thoracic laminectomy for ventral spinal cord compression may not be optimal and could possibly lead to a worsened outcome. Anterior and/or anterolateral approaches (i.e., thoracotomy, costotransversectomy) became the gold standard of treatment for many years for primarily ventral disk herniations that required an anterior surgical approach. More recently, more novel approaches have been studied and performed with excellent outcomes, such as thoracoscopic video-assisted surgical techniques using the endoscope. Such minimally invasive techniques have allowed multiple advantages including small incisions, less postoperative patient pain, and a shorter hospital stay for patients.

Thoracic disk pathology is quite diverse and therefore surgical treatments should be tailored to the individual patient's clinical and radiographic appearances. For example, there are selected cases that could safely, and more efficiently, be treated from a posterolateral and on occasion direct posterior approaches. For instance, a patient who presents with a large **lateral soft** disk herniation that may present up to the dorsal surface of the spinal canal that has **gradually** displaced the spinal cord may be more amenable to a posterior approach. In this particular case, there is a newly created avenue for access to the herniated thoracic disks with a standard direct posterior bilateral decompressive procedure, such as a laminectomy. These cases would require that the gradual retraction of the spinal cord occurred over a period of time from the disk herniation and no additional retraction of the spinal cord would be necessary for safe removal of the compressive lesion. This would be an unusual, though not rare, case and would further illustrate the diversity of thoracic disk herniation that still could be treated from a posterior laminectomy approach.

A number of other surgical procedures with posterolateral approaches to the spinal canal have been well studied and published in the literature. These include the transpedicular approach and transpedicular costotransversectomy approaches, which are commonly performed open surgical techniques that have been proven to be quite effective and safe. These procedures are very useful for accessing thoracic disk herniation that require a more direct lateral view of the disk herniation and thereby reducing any spinal cord retraction when performing the diskectomy. Such pathology would include central calcified or soft disk herniation and large calcified disk herniation with draping of the spinal cord along the posterior aspect of the disk.

There have also been posterolateral minimally invasive surgery (MIS) procedures reported to be applied to selective cases with success (Jho and Fessler). Such techniques allow for smaller incisions and shorter hospital stays, but are technically more challenging and require a larger learning curve and the purchase of MIS instrumentation and video equipment trays.

Anterior approaches to treat thoracic disk herniation with a thoracotomy evolved to become the "gold standard" when it was clear that a direct anterior approach through the chest cavity was needed for certain difficult disk herniations that could not otherwise be safely approached through the more common posterior and posterolateral approaches. This approach, though considered a more complex surgery given the need for lung deflation and chest tube placement along with possible vascular injury and sympathetic ganglia injury, proved to be quite successful and allowed a clear direct view of the offending disk. In this manner, very gentle clear diskectomy with partial corpectomy of the levels above and below the disk space allowed for no significant neural disruption.

Subsequently, a natural progression of procedures has been developed with less invasive methodologies for the treatment of thoracic disk herniation. The development of less invasive procedures in other surgical disciplines often involving endoscopy and related percutaneous and/or small portal surgical procedures into various body cavities has successfully occurred in general surgery, orthopaedics, obstetrics and gynecology, otolaryngology, and thoracic surgery. The adaptation of some aspects of those procedures has led spine surgeons to develop techniques applicable to the treatment of thoracic disks with procedures through the thorax and without an open thoracotomy procedure.

Endoscopic thoracic diskectomy is a unique adaptation of thoracic endoscopy, also known as VATS, that was developed in thoracic surgery to treat other intrathoracic pathologies usually related to the lung, mediastinal, and cardiopulmonary systems. The use of VATS was adapted to treat spinal column problems primarily causing spinal cord compression that would otherwise require an anterior approach to the spine and in the past required an open thoracotomy. There was great interest in VATS procedures when they were initially introduced in the early 1990s and some centers and surgeons continue to perform these procedures on a regular basis. These procedures are typically performed by surgeons who have specific advanced training in such techniques and are not therefore performed by most spine surgeons.

36.1.7 Decision-Making Algorithm for Symptomatic Thoracic Disk Disease

There are a wide variety of factors that play a role in determining the most efficient and safe treatment in patients with symptomatic thoracic disk disease. These factors all reunite on the main surgical strategy in such patients: minimize or avoid any spinal cord retraction. Preoperative imaging with CT and MRI is key in determining surgical approach. For example, the most important indication to use an anterior approach, either open or endoscopic, is when a disk herniation is directly midline and causing severe compression of the spinal cord with draping of the spinal cord over the disk herniation. In this manner, there will be a direct lateral view of the offending disk without the need for spinal cord manipulation. If a disk herniation is lateral and soft and extends to the surface of the spinal canal on one, a focused posterior or posterolateral approach without costotransversectomy may be used safely.

In addition, the level of the thoracic disk herniation is also a factor as to whether an endoscopic procedure should be utilized safely. Thoracic disk herniations occurring at the extreme ends of the thoracic spinal column are not ideally treated with a VATS diskectomy. Spinal cord compression at the upper end of the spinal column (i.e., T1–T2 and T2–T3) is not easily treated with an endoscopic procedure and may be preferably treated with an anterior transcervical approach or if needed a transsternal approach by splitting the manubrium if the disk herniation is not readily accessed from an inferiorly extended standard anterior cervical diskectomy approach. At the lowest levels of the thoracic spine (i.e., T10–T11, T11–T12, or T12–L1), these disk lesions can still be treated with a VATS procedure, but difficulties of access due to a need for diaphragm retraction and possibly larger girth of the patient often make the VATS procedure more difficult, but not impossible, needing additional retraction ports and retraction instruments. These patients also tend to be older and have circumferential spinal stenosis in lower thoracic levels, and if treated from an anterior approach may be considered for an open thoracotomy rather than an endoscopic procedure in our experience.

36.1.8 Endoscopic Surgical Management for Herniated Thoracic Disk Disease

We present the medical history and clinical findings of two patients who had a VATS diskectomy procedure.

Case 1

A 56-year-old male who had an onset of severe gait imbalance over 2 months was found to have a large ventral lateral disk herniation at the T8–T9 level and had a rapid course of clinical decline in neurological function (▶ Fig. 36.2). The disk appeared to be calcified on CT and a VATS procedure was considered the ideal procedure. The procedure was successfully performed and a soft disk herniation was encountered despite the radiographic

finding on CT. Postoperative imaging showed a complete removal of the herniated disk.

Case 2

A 64-year-old male had undergone surgery for a cervical–thoracic junction stenosis causing myelopathy last year with a very lengthy postoperative course in the hospital due to multiple medical comorbidities. He had significant continued gait disturbance from known thoracic disk herniation at both T7–T8 and T8–T9 with a contiguous mass in the midline consistent with an evolving ossification of the posterior longitudinal ligament (▶ Fig. 36.3). There was signal change in the spinal cord at both levels and an anterior decompression was advised. A thoracic endoscopic procedure with a VATS image-guided surgery (IGS) appeared to be the ideal procedure to treat his two-level spinal cord compression. The procedure was successfully performed and the postoperative course was uneventful, presumably due to use of an MIS procedure.

36.1.9 Disadvantages/Advantages of the Endoscopic and Open Approaches

Unfortunately, endoscopic or VATS procedures require a steep learning curve. Thoracic disk herniation is relatively rare, and many surgeons have limited exposure to them. This is a major limiting factor for utilization of the VATS procedure. Moreover, the specialized equipment required for these procedures require advanced specialized training for most spine surgeons, who are typically not closely familiar with endoscopic instruments, and can be quite expensive to purchase. The longer instruments mandatory for thoracoscopic procedures include a power drill/burr, suction and bone dissection tools such as various curettes, Kerrison rongeurs, Penfield, and Woodson dissectors. We usually employ three portals with the assistant

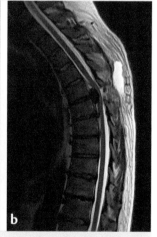

Fig. 36.2 A 56-year-old male presented with severe gait imbalance over 2 months was found on (a) axial and (b) sagittal magnetic resonance imaging (MRI) to have a large ventral lateral disk herniation at the T8–T9 level. Intraoperatively, a soft disk herniation was encountered despite the radiographic finding of calcifications on preoperative imaging.

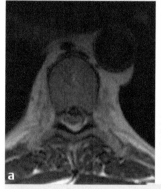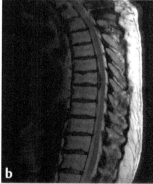

Fig. 36.3 A 64-year-old male had undergone surgery for a cervical–thoracic junction stenosis causing myelopathy in the previous year with a very lengthy postoperative course in the hospital due to multiple medical comorbidities. He had significant continued gait disturbance from known thoracic disk herniation at both T7–T8 and T8–T9 with a contiguous mass in the midline consistent with an evolving ossification of the posterior longitudinal ligament, as demonstrated on (a) axial and (b) sagittal magnetic resonance imaging. A thoracic endoscopic procedure with a video-assisted thoracoscopic surgery image-guided surgery was successfully performed and the postoperative course was uneventful.

surgeon often handling the endoscope. Sometimes, a fourth instrument can be used if another portal is placed, which allows the assistant to participate in the procedure such as using a suction or retraction of the lung. It is not uncommon during these procedures to find the lung in the way of the operative field, and keeping it retracted can be a challenge requiring the fourth portal. These maneuvers are often much less cumbersome in the open surgical routes. The basic procedures that are easily accomplished with open procedures such as using a suction and bipolar electrocautery can be difficult because of the longer instruments that are manipulated through a portal with a cantilevered or fulcrum technique as the portal is manipulated along the chest wall. In addition, imaging with a 2D endoscope may be unfamiliar to surgeons who do only open procedures, use an operative microscope, or utilize 3D imaging. Endoscopic visualization also has other logistical challenges including frequent lens cleaning to maintain good visualization that can interrupt the flow of the procedure.

In terms of minimally invasive surgical advantages, a major advantage is the small incision(s) that are performed, as opposed to the large incisions performed in open surgeries. There are usually only three small incisions to insert the portals that measure 2 to 3 cm each. This avoids the large incision associated with thoracotomies, making it less likely to experience "postthoracotomy" pain syndrome. Another advantage is the available option to add IGS that requires all the known logistics of that technology and placing a reference frame on the spinous process with another small incision. IGS with the VATS procedure provides invaluable information to the surgeon with known spatial orientation, confirmation of the spinal level, depth perception that is absent with 2D endoscopy and provides an understanding of the relationship of the surgical procedure with the spinal canal. IGS provides a precise understanding of the location of the pathology intended for resection with added safety that was not previously available. The surgical exposure in the spinal column is often smaller and less destabilizing to the integrity of the spine, making it unlikely to require a spinal fusion, which in itself is another major distinct advantage.

The disadvantages of the open approach include a larger thoracotomy incision that can result in complications common to any major surgery, such as infection. Blood loss may be greater when compared to the more minimally invasive VATS technique. Large incisions associated with thoracotomy may be quite painful with or without removal of a rib. Another disadvantage is the need of a chest tube for longer time; this may result in increased length of stay, decreased patient satisfaction, higher doses of narcotics, wound infection, pneumonia, chylothorax (albeit rare), and other cardiopulmonary complications.

Finally, advantages of the open approach relates to the incredible access and exposure that is provided, allowing the surgeons and team to have consistent clear views of the surgical pathology and surrounding structures. In addition, the open approach is always entertained as a backup procedure when performing a minimally invasive operation, in the event an unexpected complicating factor is encountered during the MIS procedures. The open approach is able to consistently provide the surgeon with the maximum exposure and visualization of the entire intrathoracic anatomy and of the spinal column,

along with visualization of sources of bleeding that can be controlled more efficiently. A microscope is routinely needed for open procedures where the surgeon has 3D visualization of the spinal anatomy and the assistant surgeon can easily participate to complete the procedure. Much of the open surgical procedure can be performed with standard familiar operative instruments that most hospitals already have in the trays.

36.1.10 Patient Selection for an Endoscopic Spinal Procedure and the Role of Instrumentation

General medical and pulmonary disease that would preclude double lumen intubation and single lung ventilation during the surgical procedure would deem the patient not to be a candidate for a VATS endoscopic procedure.

The side of surgical approach requires careful thought and attention. The location of the herniated disk is important, but other intrathoracic anatomy may dictate otherwise. Any previous thoracic surgical procedures would usually preclude a VATS procedure, because significant pleural adhesions would make retraction of the lung difficult. The location of the aorta can be a deciding factor as well. If the aorta is large and located posteriorly, that will necessitate retraction and thus make VATS a less attractive option.

Patient selection based on the location of the disk herniation is a significant factor in the author's experience. For example, the level of disk herniation and the laterality of the disk are critical. The ideal case of thoracic disk herniation treated with a VATS endoscopic procedure is one that is located in the T3–T10 levels and is centrally located ventral to the spinal cord, making it difficult to safely resect it with a posterolateral approach. Disk herniations at the T3–T10 levels are relatively easy to visualize with a thoracic endoscope and the longer surgical instruments used for these procedures work well at these levels.

Patients with disk herniations located at the extreme ends of the spinal column, that is, T1–T2, T2–T3, T10–T11, and T11–T12, are less easily treated with endoscopic procedures. Fortunately, lesions at the upper disk levels are rare. Disk herniations at upper levels, T1–T2 and T2–T3, which are located centrally with compression on the spinal cord, may require a transsternal thoracotomy. These are indeed uncommon procedures and require a large open exposure, which requires the assistance of a cardiothoracic surgeon to provide a midline sternotomy incision to access and treat the disk herniation. The lower thoracic levels can be surgically treated with thoracoscopic techniques, but the inconvenience of retracting the diaphragm and possibly the lung makes this a relatively more difficult procedure. For obese patients, the senior author (J.P.J.) prefers a small open thoracotomy that allows a direct lateral approach for lower thoracic and thoracolumbar junction that can address anterior spinal lesions, including disks. This avoids the struggles associated with retraction of the diaphragm. Another advantage of the small open thoracotomy is related to the large intercostal interspaces between the ribs that readily allow access into the chest cavity with a small thoracotomy incision. The microscope is then used, allowing high-magnification visualization for the decompression of the spinal cord.

36.1.11 Complication Avoidance

Surgical treatment for thoracic spine disk disease is fraught with the possibility of a wide variety of intraoperative and postoperative complications. Knowledge of these potential complications preoperatively is critical to performing the surgery safely and carefully. One must maintain hemostasis by continuously controlling any and all bleeding. Failure to do so may compromise adequate visualization of the surgical field, making the surgery much more challenging.

Cerebrospinal fluid (CSF) leak may be lessened by identifying calcified disks preoperatively and employing careful and precise surgical technique next to the dura, such as careful dissection of disk off the dura or even leaving a small portion of disk attached to the dura after decompression.

Neurologic injury is circumvented by avoiding any retraction of the spinal cord. Lesions are preferably gently pulled away from the spinal cord. Hence, it is important to drill into the posterior vertebrae above and below the disks to create a hole large enough to pull the herniated disk fragments into it.

Chylothorax can be avoided by knowledge of the anatomy, and utilization of clips when necessary.

36.1.12 Technical Nuances for Symptomatic Thoracic Disk Herniation

The following factors are important technical nuances for surgical treatment of symptomatic thoracic disk herniation via an open or endoscopic route:

- Localization and confirmation of the accurate spinal level in the thoracic spine is critical and can be quite difficult. Use of preoperative CT-guided coils into the appropriate pedicle and/or use of intraoperative X-ray/C-arm or image guidance help provide additional confirmation. Use of intraoperative CT is helpful for accurate localization of calcified disk herniations and can also help visualize most large soft disk herniations. Intraoperative CT combined with stereotactic navigation has enhanced the surgeon's comfort level in performing these procedures as it allows tracking of the different surgical instruments including the pneumatic drill all the way down to the level of the disk.
- Meticulous positioning of the patient on the operating room table aids in intraoperative localization as well (▶ Fig. 36.4). The portals in a VATS thoracoscopic procedure are positioned in a triangle over the level of the surgical site. A localizing intraoperative radiograph after the patient is positioned can facilitate the localization of portal placement.
- Hemostasis is very important to continuously accomplish with open and VATS procedures, but especially in VATS given the smaller endoscopic exposures. Sometimes, even a small amount of bleeding from the pleura during the start of the case can be problematic and meticulous bipolar cautery is

advised. Bone bleeding during the drilling procedure is controlled with a suction used continuously in the surgical site. Bone wax on a large cotton tip applicator is frequently used. Epidural bleeding once the spinal canal is exposed is sometimes difficult as small amounts of bleeding obstruct key anatomy visualization. Packing gently Gelfoam in the epidural space may help control bleeding.

- Drilling is the key part of the thoracoscopic procedure (▶ Fig. 36.5). Removal of the rib head overlying the pedicle and exposing the lateral aspect of the disk are the initial steps to start the procedure. The foramen can also be identified at this stage. The decompression of the ventral part of the spinal canal is the major part of the procedure, and taking the decompression across to the opposite side of the spinal canal is very important. The authors recommend drilling the posterior part of the vertebrae above and below the disk, going across to the contralateral side. Once this is done, the floor of the spinal canal can be pulled into the created surgical hole in a controlled and safe manner. Endoscopic procedures for treatment of thoracic disk herniation and spinal cord compression are demanding procedures. Experience with thoracoscopic procedures can be gained when treating other disorders. Performing sympathectomy procedures for hyperhidrosis or vertebral biopsy procedures, for example, can be useful experiences for spinal surgeons. Since three portals are often used in a thoracoscopy procedure, another skill set that must be mastered is the use of very long instruments with limited availability of an assistant. To gain a comfortable understanding of 3D anatomy and orientation using 2D imaging, the endoscopic procedures of other disciplines, such as joint arthroscopy, can be observed.

36.1.13 Clinical Pearls

In this chapter, we have discussed a wide variety of factors that are crucial in providing the best care possible to patients with symptomatic thoracic disk pathology. These factors include the following: patient history and physical examination, particular analysis of imaging characteristics, preoperative and intraoperative localization techniques, and pros and cons of open versus endoscopic surgical approaches to patients with symptomatic thoracic disk disease. Each patient has a unique presentation and set of circumstances that may favor one approach over the other. More novel and well-studied endoscopic approaches have been shown to be safe and effective, but require a steep learning curve that can be fostered by collaborating with a thoracic surgeon with thoracoscopic experience. Thoracoscopy is a safe newer technique that can be added to the spine surgeon's armamentarium when appropriately performed on the appropriate patients. Open surgical approaches must remain present as a safe backup in such cases when endoscopic procedures remain complicated or difficult.

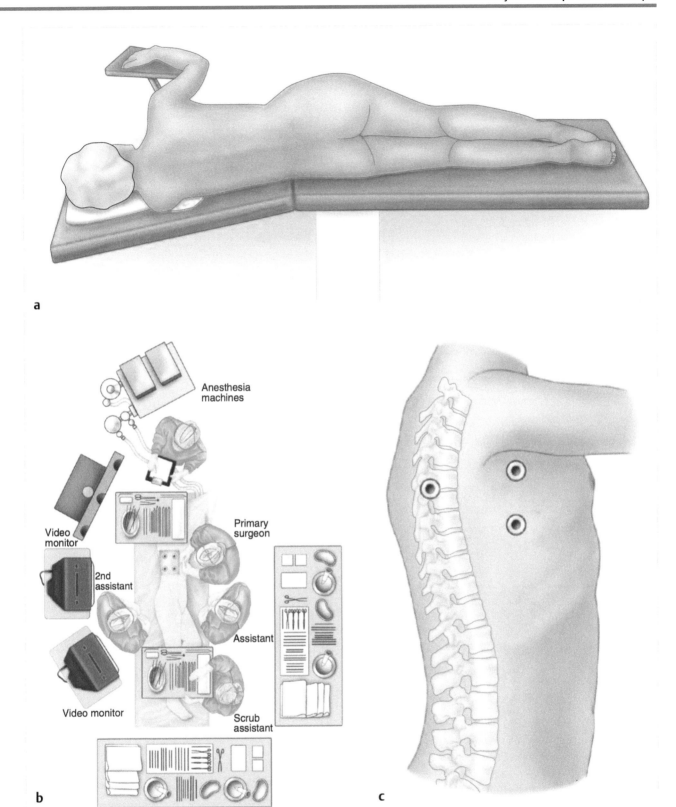

a

b

c

Fig. 36.4 Positioning is a critical component to endoscopic thoracic diskectomies. **(a)** The patient is ideally positioned in the lateral decubitus position, with the ipsilateral lung superficially and the ventilated lung down. And the arm his held in special positioning in order to expose the lateral chest wall. **(b)** The primary surgeon as well as the surgical team stands at the abdominal side of the patient A second assistant stands on the back side of the patient. Several access ports are then placed depending on the location of the herniated disk **(c)** superiorly. *(cont.)*

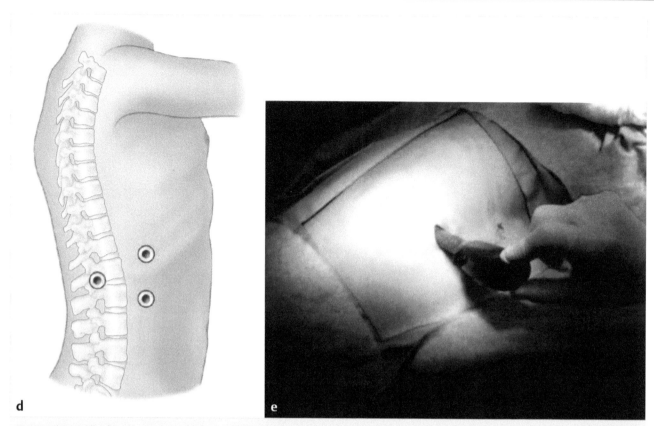

d

e

Fig 36.4 (*cont.*) (**d**) inferiorly oriented and (**e**) a variety of instruments are inserted. (Courtesy of J. Patrick Johnson, MD; from Johnson JP, Rogers CD. Thoracoscopic diskectomy. In: Kim DH, Fessler RG, Regan JJ, eds. Endoscopic Spine Surgery and Instrumentation. New York, NY: Thieme; 2005.)

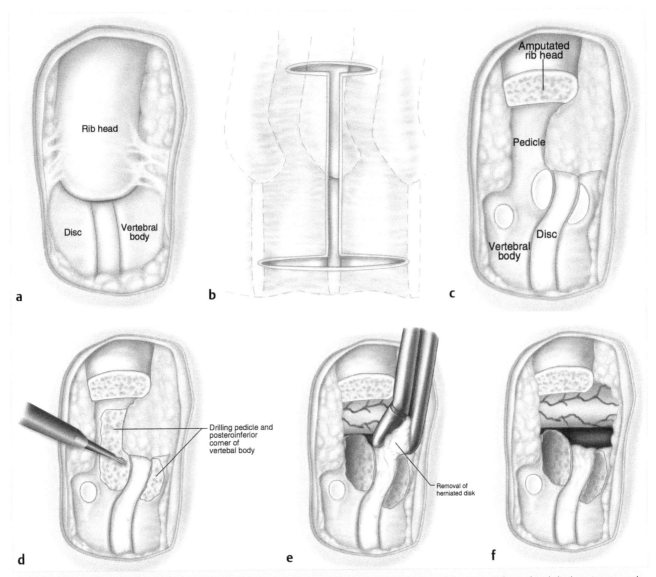

Fig. 36.5 Diagrams demonstrating the step-by-step approach to endoscopic thoracic disks. **(a)** Portal access is performed and the lung is retracted, allowing the surgeon access to the disk space by tracing the rib to the spine. **(b)** Full exposure is gained by widely dissecting the parietal pleura off the rib head. **(c)** The proximal 2 cm of the rib head is amputated using a high-speed pneumatic drill, exposing the lateral wall of the pedicle as well as the neural foramen. **(d)** The pedicle is then drilled, and after palpating the posterior margin of the vertebral body, and the superior and inferior endplates are also drilled. This allows for exposure of the dura of the spinal cord and creates a window to allow the surgeon to manipulate the disk without mobilizing the spinal cord. **(e)** An opening in the posterior longitudinal ligament and carefully removed exposing the herniated disk. Disk material is then mobilized into the bony defect created, away from the spinal cord. **(f)** The surgical resection cavity is then carefully inspected in order to confirm decompression of the spinal cord. (Courtesy of J. Patrick Johnson, MD; from Johnson JP, Rogers CD. Thoracoscopic diskectomy. In: Kim DH, Fessler RG, Regan JJ, eds. Endoscopic Spine Surgery and Instrumentation. New York, NY: Thieme; 2005.)

Suggested Readings

[1] Perot PL, Jr, Munro DD. Transthoracic removal of midline thoracic disc protrusions causing spinal cord compression. J Neurosurg. 1969; 31(4):452–458

[2] Ransohoff J, Spencer F, Siew F, Gage L, Jr. Transthoracic removal of thoracic disc. Report of three cases. J Neurosurg. 1969; 31(4):459–461

[3] Mack MJ, Regan JJ, Bobechko WP, Acuff TE. Application of thoracoscopy for diseases of the spine. Ann Thorac Surg. 1993; 56(3):736–738

[4] Regan JJ, Ben-Yishay A, Mack MJ. Video-assisted thoracoscopic excision of herniated thoracic disc: description of technique and preliminary experience in the first 29 cases. J Spinal Disord. 1998; 11(3):183–191

[5] Rosenthal D, Dickman CA. Thoracoscopic microsurgical excision of herniated thoracic discs. J Neurosurg. 1998; 89(2):224–235

[6] Anderson TM, Mansour KA, Miller JI, Jr. Thoracic approaches to anterior spinal operations: anterior thoracic approaches. Ann Thorac Surg. 1993; 55(6):1447–1451, discussion 1451–1452

[7] Jho HD. Endoscopic microscopic transpedicular thoracic discectomy. Technical note. J Neurosurg. 1997; 87(1):125–129

[8] Vollmer DG, Simmons NE. Transthoracic approaches to thoracic disc herniations. Neurosurg Focus. 2000; 9(4):e8

[9] Burke TG, Caputy AJ. Treatment of thoracic disc herniation: evolution toward the minimally invasive thoracoscopic technique. Neurosurg Focus. 2000; 9(4):e9

[10] Johnson JP, Filler AG. McBrideDQ. Endoscopic thoracic discectomy. Neurosurg Focus. 2000; 9:1–8

[11] Angevin PD, McCormick PC. Retropleural thoracotomy. Technical note. Neurosurg Focus. 2001; 10(1):ecp1

[12] Wakefield AE, Steinmetz MP, Benzel EC. Biomechanics of thoracic discectomy. Neurosurg Focus. 2001; 11(3):E6

[13] Johnson JP, Stokes JK, Oskouian RJ, Choi WW, King WA. Image-guided thoracoscopic spinal surgery: a merging of 2 technologies. Spine. 2005; 30(19): E572–E578

[14] Isaacs RE, Podichetty VK, Sandhu FA, et al. Thoracic microendoscopic discectomy: a human cadaver study. Spine. 2005; 30(10):1226–1231

[15] Hott JS, Feiz-Erfan I, Kenny K, Dickman CA. Surgical management of giant herniated thoracic discs: analysis of 20 cases. J Neurosurg Spine. 2005; 3(3):191–197

[16] Currier BL, Eismont EJC, Green BA. Thoracic disc disease. In: Rothman-Simeone: The Spine. Philadelphia, PA: Saunders; 2011:828–845

[17] Moran C, Ali Z, McEvoy L, Bolger C. Mini-open retropleural transthoracic approach for the treatment of giant thoracic disc herniation. Spine. 2012; 37 (17):E1079–E1084

[18] Lubelski D, Abdullah KG, Steinmetz MP, et al. Lateral extracavitary, costo-transversectomy, and transthoracic thoracotomy approaches to the thoracic spine: review of techniques and complications. J Spinal Disord Tech. 2013; 26 (4):222–232

[19] Oppenlander ME, Clark JC, Kalyvas J, Dickman CA. Surgical management and clinical outcomes of multiple-level symptomatic herniated thoracic discs. J Neurosurg Spine. 2013; 19(6):774–783

[20] Roelz R, Scholz C, Klingler JH, Scheiwe C, Sircar R, Hubbe U. Giant central thoracic disc herniations: surgical outcome in 17 consecutive patients treated by mini-thoracotomy. Eur Spine J. 2016; 25(5):1443–1451

37 Spinal Lumbar Diskectomy: Open versus Endoscopic

Hsuan-Kan Chang, Peng-Yuan Chang, Brandon Burroway, and Michael Y. Wang

Summary

Lumbar microdiskectomy was originally described in the 1930s, and the surgical techniques have remained relatively standard over the following century. Approach-related morbidity of this technique necessitated the development of minimally invasive techniques to access the lumbar spine. In the last two decades, tubular retractors with paramedian incisions have become popular within the community. However, the narrow surgical corridor with poor light penetration and visualization has been cited as limiting factors in the efficacy of surgery. Recently, endoscopic approaches to lumbar diskectomy have been described. In this chapter, we discuss the advantages and disadvantages of endoscopic versus traditional microsurgical approaches to herniated lumbar disks.

Keywords: lumbar, microdiskectomy, endoscopic, discectomy, laminotomy

37.1 Introduction

Similar to the evolution in many other surgical fields, like laparoscopy in general surgery or arthroscopy in sports medicine, the advancement from open surgery to more minimally invasive procedures has created revolutions in modern neurosurgical practice. The patients' increasing demand for enhanced recovery after surgery (ERAS) has become an irresistible trend. Moreover, modern surgery is changing from the era of direct visualization to image-assisted surgery that allows surgeons to operate with the aid of high-resolution image modalities. One pertinent example of surgical evolution is the way the da Vinci surgical system has gradually gained popularity for general, cardiac, urologic, and gynecologic surgeries.

In today's world, the public demands continuously improving technology. This ideology has influenced the way people think about the health care they receive. As a result, the public now demands more from their health care provider. They no longer simply expect symptom relief, but faster recovery and minimal trauma possible. The world of health care must continue working to meet their challenge. Evidence of this effect and demand can be seen in the constantly changing and improving world of spinal surgery. Endoscopic diskectomy might be the next step in the evolution of lumbar disk surgery, which has transitioned from open diskectomy to microdiskectomy (microscope-assisted diskectomy) and now to endoscopic diskectomy.[1] Endoscopic spine surgery's potential advantages over open and microscopic spinal surgery stem from two main attributes. Endoscopic surgery allows for enhanced visualization and minimal invasiveness among these three techniques. These two characteristics allow endoscopic spinal surgery advantages over its open and microscopic counterparts.

Along with the identified advantages and rapidly expanding interest, several experts have made criticisms toward endoscopic lumbar diskectomy. The clinical outcome, recurrence/reoperation rate, surgical complications, and the limitation by anatomic factors have been the major concerns regarding the endoscopic procedure. Its effectiveness, efficacy, indications, and contraindications are now the main subjects of debate. Controversy between open/microdiskectomy and endoscopic diskectomy exists and will be extensively discussed in this chapter.

37.2 Evolution of Surgical Treatment Options for the Given Pathology

Mixter and Barr reported the first lumbar intervertebral disk operation in the 1930s.[2] They performed an open laminectomy and diskectomy to resolve lumbar radiculopathy. Ever since this successful operation, spinal surgery has started its amazing development and progression. Decades later, with the introduction of microscope in surgery, Imhof et al and Iwah and Caspar both reported the first microscope-assisted diskectomies in 1977.[3,4] The technique was then refined into one of the most widely practiced procedures, microdiskectomy, performed by numerous spinal surgeons throughout the world. Microdiskectomy is composed of an interlaminar approach with partial bone resection and a small laminotomy with the assistance of a microscope. Microdiskectomy holds many advantages over open diskectomy including a smaller incision, diminished soft-tissue destruction by dilating and spreading tissue with tubular retractor rather than destroying it, and using a paramedian approach to avoid the midline tension band (▶ Fig. 37.1). In 1999, Foley and Smith published a paper describing the use of an endoscope through a tubular retractor for visualization instead of microscope.[5]

Parvis Kambin took the credit for being the very first surgeon treating lumbar disk herniation (LDH) with an endoscope. Kambin started with nonvisualized percutaneous nucleotomy for lumbar disk using a posterolateral approach in 1973. Then with the advancement of the illumination and camera systems, the first endoscopic visualization of a herniated lumbar disk and disk removal technique was published by Kambin in 1988.[6] Kambin then described a safe working "triangle"—medially bordered by traversing the nerve root, anteriorly bordered by the exiting root, and inferiorly bordered by the superior endplate of the lower lumbar vertebra—named "Kambin's triangle" (▶ Fig. 37.2), that serves as a safe corridor for endoscopic instruments to work in lumbar disk pathology.[7] As time has progressed, with the aid of advancing endoscopic instruments, such as the angled lens scope, flexible forceps, and reamers, the novel technique has advanced further toward a more extensive application and capability.

37.3 Decision-Making Algorithm

Patients usually start with nonsurgical treatment for the initial 5 to 8 weeks after specific diagnosis of LDH is made. However, there are several circumstances under which surgical intervention

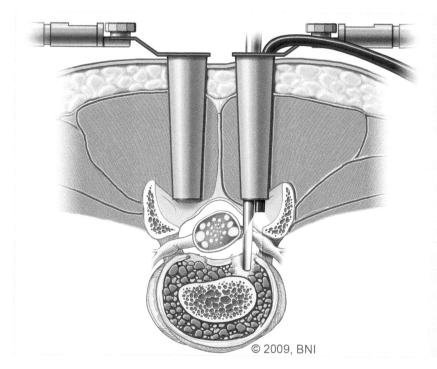

Fig. 37.1 Paramedian incision with sequential tubular dilation has improved outcomes over the traditional open microdiskectomy. Endoscopic or microscopic visualization can be employed using this technique. In this illustration, an endoscope is placed within the tubular retractor in order to provide illumination and visualization during lumbar diskectomy. (Used with permission from Barrow Neurological Institute, Phoenix, AZ.)

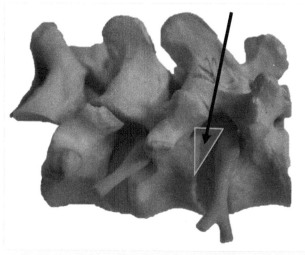

Fig. 37.2 Kambin's triangle (*blue triangle*), medially bordered by the traversing nerve root, anteriorly bordered by the exiting root, and inferiorly bordered by the superior endplate of the lower lumbar vertebra.

would likely need to take place in an emergency condition, including cauda equina syndrome (CES), progressive motor deficit (e.g., drop foot), or intolerable pain in spite of adequate pain medicine.

Nonsurgical management, often referred to as conservative management, consists of several options. Some of these management options are not derived from strong clinical evidence but are nonetheless considered useful in clinical practice by many physicians. Activity modification is one of the options, including bed rest, limitation of heavy lifting, exercise, and prolonged sitting. Bed rest should be no more than 2 to 3 days; longer periods may worsen symptoms.[8] Exercise may include walking, biking, and swimming to minimize stress to the low back.

Analgesics such as acetaminophen, nonsteroidal anti-inflammatory drugs (NSAIDs), can be useful for the initial period. More powerful pain medication like opioids is usually reserved for severe pain. Muscle relaxants are commonly used for low back pathology but have not yet shown any solid evidence. Oral steroids and antidepressants are sometimes used for low back problems. Antidepressants are often considered for chronic low back pain rather than for an acute condition.

Epidural steroid injections (ESI) serve as an option in conservative management; however, there is controversy regarding the effectiveness of ESI. Epidural injections may provide short-term relief for acute pain, but may not change the need for surgery since LDH is a structural problem.[9]

Physical therapy such as traction, heat, ice, or ultrasound are often prescribed before surgical intervention, but no benefit has been proven clinically. Many patients may go for physical therapy as a means to avoid surgical intervention. Spinal manipulation therapy (may be a part of physical therapy) and lumbar corset also have insufficient evidence to support their effectiveness.

Approximate 70% of the patients with acute LDH improve in 4 weeks after conservative treatment, and 85% do so in an average of 6 weeks.[10] The symptoms are not likely to resolve spontaneously after 5 to 8 weeks of conservative management; therefore, the surgical indication for LDH is symptomatic patients with compatible radiographic finding on magnetic resonance imaging (MRI) or computed tomography (CT) scan after 5 to 8 weeks of failed conservative management. Under certain circumstances (CES, progress motor deficit, or intolerable pain), emergency surgery should be considered regardless of conservative treatment.

Common surgical options for LDH include open standard diskectomy, microdiskectomy, and percutaneous endoscopic lumbar diskectomy (PELD). Other options include chemonucleolysis,[11] nucleoplasty, laser disk decompression,[12] and intra-diskal endothermal therapy. Standard open diskectomy and microdiskectomy are the two most widely practiced surgical techniques for LDH. Microdiskectomy has advantages over open diskectomy including reduced incision size, shorter hospital stay, expedited recovery, shorter hospital stay, and diminished blood loss. The exact indications for endoscopic lumbar diskectomy are still controversial.

With the existence of several variations, endoscopic lumbar diskectomy mainly includes two specific approaches: transforaminal and interlaminar approaches.[13] The indications for the transforaminal approach are intraforaminal disk herniations, extreme lateral, far lateral, extracanalar disk herniations, and lateral disk herniations in selected cases. The contraindications for transforaminal approach are (1) L5–S1 disk herniation in which the iliac crest and/or the L5 transverse process are roadblocks, (2) anatomical variations, (3) median and paramedian disk herniations, (4) CES that require complete decompression that can hardly be achieved through this approach, (5) disk migration caudally or cranially, and (6) degenerative lumbar spinal stenosis that causes circumferential dura and nerve root compression not only by degenerative disk herniation but also by spur, hypertrophic facet, and the ligamentum flavum.[14] L5–S1 disk herniations are better indicators for an interlaminar approach than for a transforaminal approach. One of the contraindications reported in the literature for using the endoscopic procedure may be an age of about 60 years or older.[15,16] An age cutoff of 57[15] or 60[16] years may be indicated when determining whether or not to perform the PELD procedure. Some data indicate that patients above the cutoff age have a higher risk for needing surgical revision following endoscopic procedure compared to patients undergoing open lumbar diskectomy, but patients younger than the cutoff age show no such increased reoperation risk.[15,16] This information suggests that endoscopic diskectomy should only be performed in older patients following careful consideration.[15,16] One possible rational is that the endoscopic procedure seems to have longer operation time compared with the open/microscopic procedures.[17] Longer operation time could cause adverse effects in the elderly patients. However, in a great number of surgeons' clinical practices, the endoscopic procedure is thought to provide benefit for elderly patients and those with medical morbidity to avoid complications from its nongeneral anesthetic protocol and extremely minimal invasiveness. Aside from age, diabetes has also been indicated as a cause of increased failure in endoscopic procedures.[16] The endoscopic procedure has been considered as contraindicated for treatment of recurrent LDH; nevertheless, a variation of the endoscopic procedure reported in the literature calling for a transosseous approach has shown results that can be useful in treating recurrent LDH.[18] However, the indication and contraindication for lumbar endoscopic procedure may evolve over time alongside technique and technology development.

37.4 Case Demonstration of Endoscopic Surgical Management

37.4.1 Case 1

This patient is an 83-year-old male with severe comorbidities of hypertension, heart disease, and chronic kidney disease. He had severe left leg pain primarily over the distribution of the L2–L3 dermatome with only mild back pain and no bladder or bowel problems. The patient presented with difficulty walking and standing. The patient failed pain medication, physical therapy, radiofrequency ablation, and ESI. MR image showed an obvious nerve compression by lateral disk herniation at the L2/L3 level on the left foramen (▶ Fig. 37.3). A left L2/L3 endoscopic lumbar diskectomy was performed for this old patient and the pain level significantly decreased after surgery.

Given his complicated comorbidity as well as the advanced age, general anesthesia could cause great medical risk for this patient, which was the major concern from the patient and his family. Therefore, the endoscopic procedure with only local anesthesia may be a good option that is most likely to improve

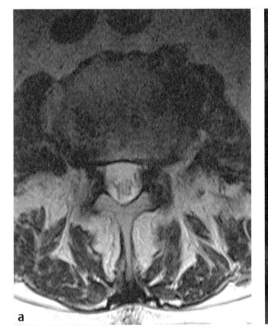
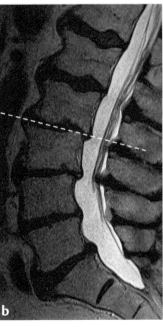

Fig. 37.3 The preoperative **(a)** axial and **(b)** sagittal magnetic resonance images of a patient with left lateral lumbar disk herniation at L2/L3.

the pain and also minimize the risk owing to his unfavorable medical condition.

37.4.2 Case 2

This patient is a 63-year-old male with a medical history of severe Parkinson's disease. He had one previous spinal surgery of L3/L4 minimally invasive transforaminal lumbar interbody fusion (MIS-TLIF) with posterior instrumentation 3 years ago. He showed great improvement after MIS-TLIF but developed new left side pain radiating from the buttock to the leg at the L4 dermatome later on. His intractable pain prevented him from sleeping, exercising, or even performing daily activities. He failed ESI and physical therapy. His symptoms were exacerbated by Parkinson's disease. The neurologic examination was intact. The preoperative MR image showed left side L4/L5 nerve root compression adjacent to the L3/L4 fusion (▶ Fig. 37.4). L4/L5 left-sided endoscopic foraminotomy and diskectomy were performed and he has gained significant pain relief following surgery.

Given the possibility that general anesthesia might make the patient's Parkinson's disease worse,[19,20,21,22] and his Parkinson's disease actually became worse after his last surgery, it is beneficial for this patient to undergo surgery without general anesthesia. Thus, the endoscopic procedure, which can be done under sedation and local anesthesia, would be beneficial for this patient. In addition, it would have been difficult to approach with a midline posterior route due to adhesive epidural scar formation from the last TLIF surgery even though the TLIF surgery utilized a minimally invasive method. Even if the endoscopic diskectomy did not result in sufficient improvement this time, it would be easier to perform further interbody fusion surgery after endoscopic diskectomy rather than microdiskectomy or standard open diskectomy.

37.5 Case Demonstration of Open/Traditional MIS Surgical Management

The demonstrated patient is a 44-year-old male with history of low back pain on and off for 3 to 4 years. He has had no previous surgeries. He started to have severe bilateral leg pain and numbness 8 weeks before surgery. It was initially on his left leg, then it moved to the right leg as well. The visual analog scale (VAS) score of leg pain was 10 out of 10. He could barely walk 10 ft. The symptoms aggravated with walking and standing but relieved with sitting. He had right leg tingling, and he felt like there was weakness of his leg. He had one trigger point injection and two ESI by a physiatrist without any relieve. Physical therapy failed to improve his condition as well. He took NSAIDs, muscle relaxants, and oral steroids for pain management but all failed to reduce pain. There was neither focal neurological deficit nor motor weakness upon physical examination. He had sensory deficits in both legs over the L5 dermatome. He denied any bladder or bowel problems at that point. The preoperative MR image showed a large central intervertebral disk herniation present at L4/L5. Significant disk height collapse was noted on preoperative lateral X-ray film (▶ Fig. 37.5). Part of the herniated disk migrated caudally behind the L5 vertebral

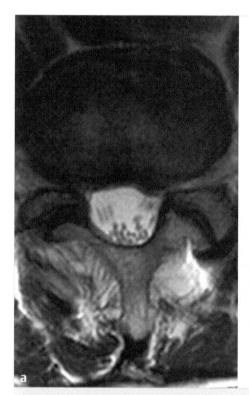
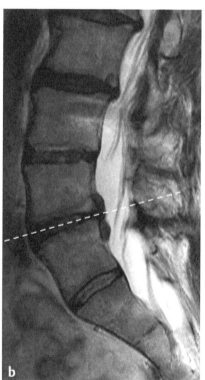
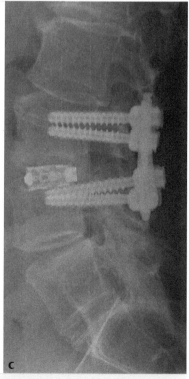

Fig. 37.4 The preoperative **(a)** axial and **(b)** sagittal magnetic resonance images as well as **(c)** X-ray film of the patient with the L4/L5 nerve root compression adjacent to the L3/L4 fusion.

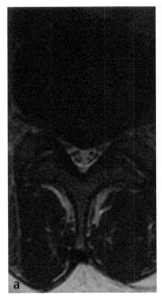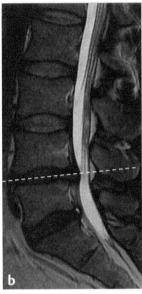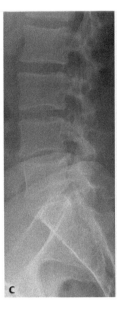

Fig. 37.5 The preoperative (**a**) axial and (**b**) sagittal magnetic resonance images showed a large central intervertebral disk herniation present at L4/L5. Significant disk height collapse was noted on (**c**) preoperative lateral X-ray film.

body causing remarkable nerve compression (▶ Fig. 37.6). The patient was severely crippled and incapacitated. An elective surgery of L4/L5 microdiskectomy was performed and the migrated disk was removed. The surgical result turned out to be excellent, and his symptoms had significant relief with only residual trivial leg discomfort. The VAS score of postoperative leg pain dropped significantly to 2 out of 10.

In most of the authors' experience and on the basis of literature review, the endoscopic technique should be reserved for patients with fresh disk fragments, small contained disk herniations, or lateral disk herniations. The endoscopic technique may not be suitable for central disk herniations, migrated disk herniations, the L5/S1 disk, cauda equine syndrome, and diffuse stenotic spinal canal resulting from not only disk degeneration but also spur, hypertrophic facet, or ligamentum flavum. One large patient series including 10,228 cases reported remarkably high rates of incomplete removal for central disk herniations, migrated disk herniations, and axillary-type disk herniations.[23] For the case demonstrated with a central disk herniation with migrated fragment, microdiskectomy may be a smart choice to deal with this kind of LDH. However, with more advanced surgical skills, a patient with a migrated disk can now be operated on with the assistance of an endoscope in experienced hands.[24] The indications of endoscopic procedures are evolving and expanding with increasing experience.

37.6 Patient Selection

A true endoscopic lumbar diskectomy typically creates access to the disk through one of two routes. The majority of procedures are done through an oblique transforaminal approach, entering through Kambin's triangle from lateral to the facet. L4/L5 and L5/S1 central and paracentral disk herniations can also be accessed through an interlaminar approach that involves approaching through the ligamentum flavum and accessing the disk just lateral to the thecal sac but medial to the facet joint, like the traditional route of microdiskectomy.

The transforaminal approach offers a complimentary approach to traditional microdiskectomy. It provides a better

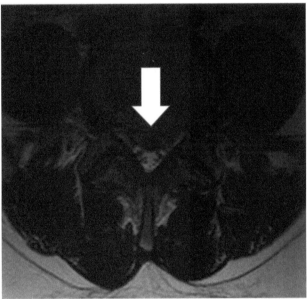

Fig. 37.6 The same patient as shown in ▶ Fig. 37.3. Part of the herniated disk migrated caudally behind the L5 vertebral body, causing remarkable nerve compression.

approach to lateral, far lateral, and foraminal disk herniation and can also be used for revision cases where epidural scar tissue from previous surgeries may be problematic. However, it is reasonable to imagine that this approach, using a posterolateral trajectory, would make removal of central disk herniations very challenging because the dural sac would be an obstacle and it would be impossible to retract the dural sac using an endoscopic approach.

There are some important drawbacks to the endoscopic procedure. The first is that recurrence may be more likely after endoscopic diskectomy. The second is that there is more risk of damaging or compressing the exiting nerve root at the time of endoscopic diskectomy. In a study by Choi et al, 20 (8.6%) out of 233 patients treated in this manner presented with a postoperative exiting root injury, such as postoperative dysesthesia or motor weakness.[25] This study suggested that exiting nerve injury was more likely to develop in patients with shorter distance between the exiting root and the lower facet measured on preoperative MR image and longer operation time. Thus, this complication may likely be avoided by (1) proper working-channel placement near the lower pedicle, away from the exiting nerve root; (2) minimizing operative time; (3) reducing moving around the working channel, which may compress the nerve root; and (4) minimizing heat coagulation and subsequent thermal damage to the nerve root.

37.7 Complication Avoidance

Complications that can result from endoscopic lumbar decompression surgery include dural tears, epidural hematomas, neural injury, inferior facet fracture,[26] and surgical site infection (SSI).[27] Although endoscopic surgery is associated with its own complications, it is thought to reduce complications in comparison to open surgery.[28] Dural tears are thought to be one of the most common complications of the endoscopic procedure to treat LDH. They have been shown to occur at rates of between 3[27] and 5%.[29] Age and bilateral decompression using a unilateral approach have been identified as independent risk factors for dural tear.[29] Although dural tear is a relatively common complication in the endoscopic procedure, it is generally small and does not require extensive repair and only necessitates care for symptoms caused by the resultant low CSF pressure.[29] The Japanese Orthopaedic Association (JOA) score for patients with dural tears is significantly worse than their peers that did not suffer the same complication; however, the Oswestry Disability Index (ODI) did not significantly vary between the two groups of patients.[29]

Several case series have reported higher prevalence of nerve root injury in endoscopic diskectomy.[30,31] The poor perception of deep structures and unfamiliarity to the technique were probably the main reason for this risk profile.[31] But there were inconsistent results in other studies that reported that the prevalence of nerve root injury with endoscopic procedure was only 1.1 to 2%.[32,33] And it was similar to those with microdiskectomy.[34] However, the risk of nerve root injury of endoscopic diskectomy was still a conflict. And with increased experience and familiarity with the procedure, the risk may be minimized.

In addition to dural tears and nerve root injury, SSIs are one of the most common complications of spinal surgery. SSIs following endoscopic procedure have been found to be relatively rare for the endoscopic procedure.[35] The endoscopic technique has been heralded as a way to decrease SSI rate by as much as 10 times when compared to open spinal surgery techniques.[35]

One drawback of abstaining from using general anesthesia when performing the endoscopic decompression is that many anesthesiologists are apprehensive to allow surgeons to put patients in the prone position without intubation.[36] To avoid any potential airway complications, an operation cutoff time of 120 minutes has been suggested, which has been shown to be more than attainable.[36] Also, since the incision size is minimal, the surgeon can rapidly close in case of emergency and move the patient to the supine position.[36]

37.8 Technical Nuances and Clinical Pearls

37.8.1 Anesthesia

As a form of minimally invasive procedure, PELD offers several advantages over traditional open lumbar diskectomy and even microscopic diskectomy. First and foremost, PELD can be performed under local anesthesia. Along with the establishment of the surgical port by introducing a series of dilators from an 18-gauge needle, the avoidance of general anesthesia provides better interactive feedback from the patient and decreased risk of nerve root injury during the surgery. Open diskectomy is usually carried out under general anesthesia. *The aforementioned advantages are counteracted by the superior airway protection and less restricted operative time, on top of the anesthetic risks that comes with the anesthesia.*

37.8.2 Skin Incision and Surgical Access

In PELD, skin incision is usually marked 6 to 12 cm paramedian to the midline, depending on the indicated segment and relative anatomical location of the pathology. The length of incision is usually 7 to 8 mm, just large enough to pass the endoscopic working port. The angle of trajectory ranges from 25 to 35 degrees on the coronal plane. The idea is to get to the disk through Kambin's triangle without negotiation with the bony structures, such as the facet, although it may be unavoidable in some patients with severely deformed structures or advanced degeneration. In that case, tools such as reamers, drills, or osteotomes can be useful to establish a proper surgical access.

An 18-gauge needle is then used for localization and estimation of the trajectory. On the anteroposterior image, the final target point of the spinal needle is the medial pedicular line, and on lateral fluoroscopic view, it is the posterior vertebral line (▶ Fig. 37.7a). At this point, some surgeons advocated the use of indigo carmine to stain the nucleus pulposus to ensure that no nervous structures are injured during the removal of the disk. The contingent precaution to compensate for the 2D surgical view provided by the endoscope is not usually done in the setting of an open diskectomy, with or without the assistance of microscope. Once the needle tip is in the desired position, a Nitinol wire stylet is passed through the needle, followed by replacement of the needle with tapered cannulated

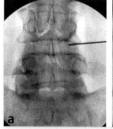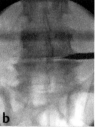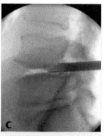

Fig. 37.7 (a) Localization and estimation of the trajectory for percutaneous endoscopic diskectomy using spinal needle. (b,c) Once the needle tip is in the desired position, a Nitinol wire stylet is passed through the needle, followed by replacement of the needle with tapered cannulated obturator and finalized by the insertion of the a bevel-ended oval-shaped endoscopic cannula.

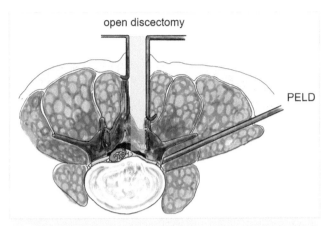

Fig. 37.8 Demonstration of working access to the disk by endoscopic technique (percutaneous endoscopic lumbar diskectomy) or open/microdiskectomy.

obturator, and finalized by the insertion of a bevel-ended oval-shaped endoscopic cannula (▶ Fig. 37.7**b, c**).

In the setting of an open diskectomy, the incision is usually 2 to 3 cm for a single-level diskectomy. Various types of retractors, most commonly the Taylor retractor and Caspar speculum, are used based on personal preference of the surgeon. The surgical access is established by exposing the spinous process, the lamina, and/or part of the facet joint, and the route is usually in the midline. With the evolution of minimally invasive concepts of treatment, more surgeons prefer to use the tubular retractor and gain access to the disk through a paramedian approach. On that occasion, the incision is made 1.5 to 2.5 cm lateral to the midline, and the tubular retractor is set directed to the inferolateral aspect of the lamina. Either way, bony structures (i.e., the inferolateral part of the lamina and/or medial part of the facet) have to be removed to establish a working access to the disk (▶ Fig. 37.8). Compared to the bony removal in PELD, which is infrequent, the amount of removed bone in open diskectomy is markedly larger to an extent that instability may be a concern after such procedure.[37,38] On top of the muscular damage, it is apparent that open diskectomy accounts for more tissue trauma before the neural decompression part of the surgery.

37.9 Neural Decompression

Removal of the disk material during PELD is quite different from the procedure in open diskectomy. Most of the discrepancies come from the conversion of a 3D surgical vision (as in open diskectomy) to a 2D view in PELD. In PELD, due to the limitation of the surgical field and instruments, the procedure is done by rotation of the scope as well as the instruments, such as micropituitary rongeurs. The angle of the endoscope ranges from 30 to 60 degrees. Along with rotatory movement, the endoscope offers a panoramic view of the surroundings. Several tricks and special instruments can be applied during the removal of disk material, such as cauterizing the cartilage to reduce the volume, backbiting disk rongeurs, and sharpers with expanding blades, which are especially useful when interbody fusion is needed.

Another hallmark difference between PELD and open diskectomy is the volume and extent of diskectomy. In PELD, the majority of decompression comes from removal of the herniated disk itself instead of a more radical diskectomy, which is commonly seen in an open diskectomy. One usually does not find trouble determining whether the decompression is sufficient enough in the setting of an open procedure; however, it can be very challenging if it is performed with an endoscope. A general rule for this is by observing the dural sac in the surroundings; regaining of pulsation of the dural sac is indicative of sufficient decompression. It is agreed that the amount of removed disk material is far less in PELD than in an open diskectomy.

The removal of lamina, facet, and ligamentum flavum tends to be more challenging in the setting of PELD, and requires more experience, techniques, and the assistance from special instruments, partly due to difficulties of surgical maneuvers in multiple planes and the difficulty in neural retraction. In other words, in patients who require interbody fusion, indirect decompression by the placement of a properly sized cage can largely attribute to the enhancement of neural decompression.

37.10 Literature Review/Evidence of Endoscopic Approach

The reduced invasiveness of endoscopic spinal surgery allows for a number of perioperative benefits and some drawbacks. One drawback that is often discussed is the reported increase in operative time in comparison to open and microscopic methods.[39,40,41] Although operative time has been shown to increase, the perioperative benefits may outweigh the cons. One of the most widely attributed benefits of endoscopic surgery is reduced blood loss associated with the technique.[39,40,42,43] Reduced blood loss is an important benefit as it can help reduce the need for intraoperative transfusions. In addition, the less invasive endoscopic approach allows surgeons to avoid epidural scar tissue formation, which may result in scar tissue–related nerve entrapment or increase the difficulty for follow-up surgery.[28]

Benefits of the procedure extend well beyond the OR and also include expedited discharge from the hospital[39,40,41,44] and return to normal daily activities and work[1,28,40,43] compared to patients undergoing the open counterpart. Postoperative discharge from the hospital following endoscopic procedure has been reported to range anywhere from the same day[42] to 11[44] or even 18 days.[43] Scarring has also been shown to be diminished in patients undergoing the minimally invasive endoscopic procedure to treat LDH.[45]

The decreased iatrogenic muscle damage also leads to a reduction in immediate postoperative back pain.[39] Using the endoscopic technique allows for reduced use of narcotics over a shorter time frame postoperatively compared to an open procedure. This is likely due to the decreased back pain and improved recovery time associated with the less invasive method.[43]

Postoperative infections[35,43,44] and perioperative complications[1,43,44] have been shown to occur in lower numbers when using endoscopy instead of an open method. Other studies, however, have shown that the complication rate does not vary between the two procedures.[40] The complication rate is still a matter of debate.

In addition to the short-term benefits of opting for the endoscopic procedure over the traditional open procedure, long-term results also favor the use of the endoscope for LDHs according to a 5-year retrospective study comparing the clinical results of the two techniques.[46]

Many of the same advantages that the endoscopic technique has over the open procedure can be seen when it is compared to a microscopic approach. The use of the endoscopic procedure to treat LDH showed equivalent or even better results than the use of microscopic procedure.[14,17,34,47] The endoscopic group showed better ODI, MacNab criteria, JOA, and VAS scores for lower leg pain in addition to reduced estimated blood loss, more rapid postoperative discharge, decreased C-reactive protein (CRP) and white blood cell (WBC)levels, reduced NSAID dosage, and fewer surgical complications.[14,47] Like the open procedure, the only statistic that favored the microscopic group was operative time.[47] In addition although endoscopic interlaminar and transforaminal diskectomy shows similar clinical results as the traditional microsurgical approach,[48] the endoscopic technique allows for reduced back pain, improves rehabilitation, decreases complications, and diminishes iatrogenic traumatization.[48]

Although the endoscopic approach has been shown to be the least invasive surgical approach to date, surgeons continue to work to satisfy the public demand for less invasive procedures. Recent advances have allowed surgeons to repair LDHs and perform lumbar spinal fusions and foraminotomies without the use of general anesthesia. The use of endoscopy and percutaneous screws allows for such minimal tissue disruption that the procedure can be performed without the use of general anesthesia.[36,45] Using local anesthesia alone allows for more rapid discharge from the hospital[45] after surgery and obviously fewer complications related to general anesthesia.[36] Patients undergoing percutaneous transforaminal endoscopic diskectomy to treat LDH have been discharged from the hospital just 2[45] to 7 hours[1] after surgery thanks to the procedure's reported 8-mm incision[45] and lack of general anesthesia. When treating patients with severe disk height collapse, patients have been discharged an average of 1.3 days after surgery.[36] The swift hospital discharge is quicker than its open and microscopic counterparts, which have been reported as 7 and 2 days,

respectively.[49] In order to avoid using general anesthetics and minimize pain, incision size is kept to a minimum and liposomal bupivacaine is utilized (off-label) to provide local analgesia.[36]

L5/S1 disk herniations have previously been reported as difficult to remove using the transforaminal endoscopic procedure[1]; thus, the interlaminar endoscopic approach was developed for L5/S1 paracentral disk herniation. Recently, there was a study reporting that transforaminal approach has been shown to help reduce surgical morbidity when used to treat patients with far lateral disk herniation at L5/S1 with foot drop as opposed to the conventional open procedure.[50] The technique calls for placing the endoscope in the anterior epidural space outside of the disk and often requires a foraminoplasty or foraminectomy.[50] The patient described in the case report indicated 90% pain relief 30 minutes after surgery and continued to report compete pain relief 6 months after surgery.[50] This incredibly rapid result is a testament to the endoscopic technique's extremely minimally invasive nature and it also demonstrates the rapidly expanding application of the endoscopic procedure in recent years.

Today the endoscopic procedure can be further utilized to treat spondylolisthesis (▶ Fig. 37.9) with additional lumbar interbody fusion and posterior instrumentation (▶ Fig. 37.10).[36] This procedure can be done without general anesthesia but only conscious sedation with local anesthesia. This novel procedure, which lasts an average of 110 minutes, shows significant improvements in postoperative outcome and rapid return to their normal life activities. Remarkable relief of leg pain and lower back disability were demonstrated after endoscopic interbody fusion. Pain dropped significantly postoperatively, with improvement of VAS and ODI scores after surgery. Eighty-seven percent of patients were able resume their daily routine after 2 weeks or less. Postoperatively, patients reported a dramatically improved quality of life. Intraoperative findings included minimal blood loss, less operative time, and a short hospital stay. The majority of patients were discharged from hospital after 1 day, despite the potential extension of hospital stay with additional number of levels fused.[36] Radiographic outcomes also demonstrated excellent results (▶ Fig. 37.11). Solid fusion was achieved in 95.8 to 100% of the cases.[36,51,52,53]

A major disadvantage of endoscopic spine surgery is the widely reported difficulty in initially mastering the techniques

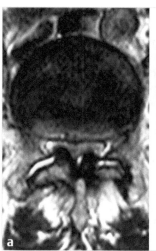
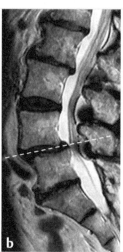
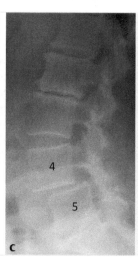

Fig. 37.9 Preoperative image of a patient with L4/L5 spondylolisthesis and nerve compression. Endoscope-assisted L4/L5 lumbar diskectomy and interbody fusion were performed for this patient. **(a)** Axial magnetic resonance (MR) image. **(b)** Sagittal MR image. **(c)** Lateral X-ray film.

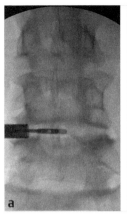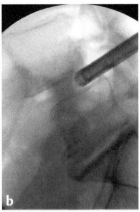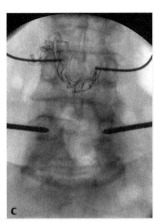

Fig. 37.10 Intraoperative image of a patient who underwent endoscope-assisted L4/L5 lumbar diskectomy and interbody fusion. **(a)** Endoscopic diskectomy. **(b)** Interbody fusion with expandable mesh cage and allograft. **(c)** Posterior instrumentation with percutaneous screws.

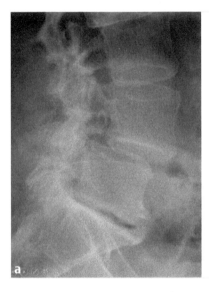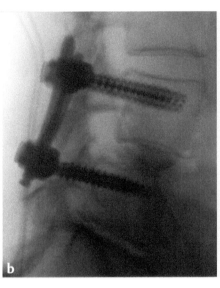

Fig. 37.11 Preoperative **(a)** and postoperative **(b)** images of a patient who received L4/L5 endoscope-assisted lumbar diskectomy and interbody fusion. The postoperative image showed solid fusion and nearly reduction of L4/L5.

required to perform the surgery.[41] One study indicates that the results of endoscopic diskectomy to treat LDH improved from a 17% failure rate during the surgeon's initial cases to a 6 to 10% failure rate after the first 70 cases.[16] Another study indicates decreasing complications with increased experience from about 11 to 5% with an especially large improvement with increased experience when using endoscope to treat lumbar degenerative diseases.[26] Even with the many advantages of endoscopic surgery, open and microscopic surgeries still remain the standard therapies for many spinal surgeries including LDH diskectomy due to the difficulty in learning the techniques required as well as the relative novelty of the endoscopic procedure.[54] The learning curve associated with the endoscopic surgery has been labeled a major concern for surgeons when they are beginning to use the technique.[55] One study reported that junior residents showed decreased acuity with the endoscope compared to the microscope in a skills lab setting.[56] The difference in dexterity when using the two tools disappeared with increased experience; however, both novice residents and experienced senior surgeons show slower execution of tasks with endoscopic visualization compared to microscopic visualization.[56] Surgical tool guidance and orientation are two aspects of endoscopic surgery that are especially difficult to master and are major reasons for the associated learning curve.[55] Surgeon experience has been reported to lead to decreased hospitalization time,[57] decreased failure and complication rate,[16,55]

decreased operative time,[55,57] and decreased radiation exposure.[58] Although inexperienced surgeons tend to expose their patients and themselves to additional radiation, the levels of radiation are not sufficiently high to cause concern.[58] In order to expedite the surgeon's learning experience and improve patient results, it is recommended that surgeons participate in surgical workshops and carefully select their patients.[55] Thus, with the steep learning curve, a potential drawback of the endoscopic procedure is the lack of surgeons who are actually capable of performing the procedure. In Japan, it has been reported that only about 20 surgeons are sufficiently handy with the percutaneous endoscopic diskectomy.[26] Although some studies indicate that increased experience improves patient outcome, another study shared a different opinion and indicated that only operation duration and hospitalization time decreased with surgeon experience, while estimated blood loss, pain scores, complication rates, recurrent herniation rates, and reoperation rates remained constant.[57] The study indicates that surgeon experience does not improve patients' long-term outcome and thus can be performed safely even by inexperienced surgeons.[57] However, with inconsistent study results, surgeons' learning curves and experience remain an important issue surrounding the endoscopic procedure.

The recurrence/residual rate after endoscopic diskectomy is one of the most debated concerns. Most of the reports consist of a comparable recurrence rate to open/microdiskectomy. But the actual statistics are highly variable ranging from 0.2 to 10 and even 20%.[59,60,61] Recurrence/residual rate may also be correlated to the surgeon's learning curve and inappropriate positioning of instruments.[23] Two recent articles revealed higher recurrence/residual rate at the earlier stage of the surgeons' learning curve.[55,62] One large series containing 10,228 patients suggested that inappropriate positioning of the working channel resulted in 33.6% of cases of incomplete removal.[23] However, the majority of the largest case series in the last 6 years showed results noninferior to microdiskectomy, with a growing number of articles describing even better results.[63]

37.11 Conclusion

This chapter has spent considerable time discussing the advantages of using one surgical technique over another and arguing which procedure is superior; however, the real answer may be that endoscopic surgery should not be seen as a replacement for microscopic or open surgery but rather as a compliment that can be used to improve the results under proper case selection, or be used under certain specific patients' condition.[64] One way to make the endoscopic procedure and others safer is for surgeons to know the indications and contraindications of using an approach instead of its counterparts.[36,40] In fact, there are still difficulties to reach a consensus due to the inconsistent evidence that may be related to different indications and experiences from the reporting surgeons. Thus, the lack of well-designed multicenter randomized controlled trial with large patient numbers and similar indications should clarify the actual efficacy of endoscopic lumbar diskectomy and whether it is superior to microdiskectomy and open diskectomy.

Despite the lack of conclusive evidence, we can still summarize the following:

- The endoscopic lumbar procedure is becoming a more popular technique and is still rapidly developing to extend its application in lumbar disease, like spondylolithesis,[36,51,52,53,65,66,67,68] multilevel,[69] and spinal stenosis.[63,70]
- Current literature suggests that lumbar endoscopic diskectomy shows slightly superior results to microdiskectomy and open diskectomy in regard to blood loss, hospital stay, tissue trauma, and patient recovery. However, further solid evidence is required to clarify its effectiveness.
- Indications, complication, recurrence/residual rate, and surgeon's learning curve are still controversial for endoscopic diskectomy. The indications of endoscopic diskectomy may extend with further advancement of technology, technique, and experience. More studies are required to firmly establish the safety and efficacy of the endoscopic diskectomy.

References

[1] Sanusi T, Davis J, Nicassio N, Malik I. Endoscopic lumbar discectomy under local anesthesia may be an alternative to microdiscectomy: a single centre's experience using the far lateral approach. Clin Neurol Neurosurg. 2015; 139:324–327

[2] Mixter WJ. Rupture of the lumbar intervertebral disk: an etiologic factor for so-called "sciatic" pain. Ann Surg. 1937; 106(4):777–787

[3] Imhof HG, von Ammon K, Yasargil MG. Use of the microscope in surgery of lumbar disk hernia. Aktuelle Probl Chir Orthop. 1994; 44:15–20

[4] Iwa H, Caspar W. A microsurgery operation for lumbar disc herniation (author's transl). No Shinkei Geka. 1978; 6(7):657–662

[5] Foley KT, Smith MM, Rampersaud YR. Microendoscopic approach to far-lateral lumbar disc herniation. Neurosurg Focus. 1999; 7(5):e5

[6] Kambin P, Nixon JE, Chait A, Schaffer JL. Annular protrusion: pathophysiology and roentgenographic appearance. Spine. 1988; 13(6):671–675

[7] Hardenbrook M, Lombardo S, Wilson MC, Telfeian AE. The anatomic rationale for transforaminal endoscopic interbody fusion: a cadaveric analysis. Neurosurg Focus. 2016; 40(2):E12

[8] Deyo RA, Diehl AK, Rosenthal M. How many days of bed rest for acute low back pain? A randomized clinical trial. N Engl J Med. 1986; 315(17):1064–1070

[9] Carette S, Leclaire R, Marcoux S, et al. Epidural corticosteroid injections for sciatica due to herniated nucleus pulposus. N Engl J Med. 1997; 336 (23):1634–1640

[10] Weber H, Holme I, Amlie E. The natural course of acute sciatica with nerve root symptoms in a double-blind placebo-controlled trial evaluating the effect of piroxicam. Spine. 1993; 18(11):1433–1438

[11] Javid MJ, Nordby EJ, Ford LT, et al. Safety and efficacy of chymopapain (Chymodiactin) in herniated nucleus pulposus with sciatica. Results of a randomized, double-blind study. JAMA. 1983; 249(18):2489–2494

[12] Choy DS, Ascher PW, Ranu HS, et al. Percutaneous laser disc decompression. A new therapeutic modality. Spine. 1992; 17(8):949–956

[13] Ruetten S, Komp M, Merk H, Godolias G. Use of newly developed instruments and endoscopes: full-endoscopic resection of lumbar disc herniations via the interlaminar and lateral transforaminal approach. J Neurosurg Spine. 2007; 6 (6):521–530

[14] Anichini G, Landi A, Caporlingua F, et al. Lumbar endoscopic microdiscectomy: where are we now? An updated literature review focused on clinical outcome, complications, and rate of recurrence. BioMed Res Int. 2015; 2015:417801

[15] Kim CH, Chung CK, Choi Y, et al. The selection of open or percutaneous endoscopic lumbar discectomy according to an age cut-off point: nationwide cohort study. Spine. 2015; 40(19):E1063–E1070

[16] Wang H, Zhou Y, Li C, Liu J, Xiang L. Risk factors for failure of single-level percutaneous endoscopic lumbar discectomy. J Neurosurg Spine. 2015; 23 (3):320–325

[17] He J, Xiao S, Wu Z, Yuan Z. Microendoscopic discectomy versus open discectomy for lumbar disc herniation: a meta-analysis. Eur Spine J. 2016; 25 (5):1373–1381

[18] Nomura K, Yoshida M, Kawai M, Okada M, Nakao S. A novel microendoscopically assisted approach for the treatment of recurrent lumbar disc herniation: transosseous discectomy surgery. J Neurol Surg A Cent Eur Neurosurg. 2014; 75(3):183–188

[19] Mantz J, Varlet C, Lecharny JB, Henzel D, Lenot P, Desmonts JM. Effects of volatile anesthetics, thiopental, and ketamine on spontaneous and depolarization-evoked dopamine release from striatal synaptosomes in the rat. Anesthesiology. 1994; 80(2):352–363

[20] Hetherington A, Rosenblatt RM. Ketamine and paralysis agitans. Anesthesiology. 1980; 52(6):527

[21] Klausner JM, Caspi J, Lelcuk S, et al. Delayed muscular rigidity and respiratory depression following fentanyl anesthesia. Arch Surg. 1988; 123(1):66–67

[22] Mets B. Acute dystonia after alfentanil in untreated Parkinson's disease. Anesth Analg. 1991; 72(4):557–558

[23] Choi KC, Lee JH, Kim JS, et al. Unsuccessful percutaneous endoscopic lumbar discectomy: a single-center experience of 10,228 cases. Neurosurgery. 2015; 76(4):372–380, discussion 380–381, quiz 381

[24] Hussein M, Abdeldayem A, Mattar MM. Surgical technique and effectiveness of microendoscopic discectomy for large uncontained lumbar disc herniations: a prospective, randomized, controlled study with 8 years of follow-up. Eur Spine J. 2014; 23(9):1992–1999

[25] Choi I, Ahn JO, So WS, Lee SJ, Choi IJ, Kim H. Exiting root injury in transforaminal endoscopic discectomy: preoperative image considerations for safety. Eur Spine J. 2013; 22(11):2481–2487

[26] Sairyo K, Egawa H, Matsuura T, et al. State of the art: transforaminal approach for percutaneous endoscopic lumbar discectomy under local anesthesia. J Med Invest. 2014; 61(3–4):217–225

[27] Zhou Y, Wang M, Wang J, Chu TW, Zhang ZF, Li CQ. Clinical experience and results of lumbar microendoscopic discectomy: a study with a five-year follow-up. Orthop Surg. 2009; 1(3):171–175

[28] Li Z, Zeng J, Song Y, et al. Effectiveness of percutaneous endoscopic transforaminal discectomy for recurrent lumbar disc herniation. Zhongguo Xiu Fu Chong Jian Wai Ke Za Zhi. 2015; 29(1):43–47

[29] Tsutsumimoto T, Yui M, Uehara M, Ohta H, Kosaku H, Misawa H. A prospective study of the incidence and outcomes of incidental dural tears in

microendoscopic lumbar decompressive surgery. Bone Joint J. 2014; 96-B (5):641–645

[30] Righesso O, Falavigna A, Avanzi O. Comparison of open discectomy with microendoscopic discectomy in lumbar disc herniations: results of a randomized controlled trial. Neurosurgery. 2007; 61(3):545–549, discussion 549

[31] Teli M, Lovi A, Brayda-Bruno M, et al. Higher risk of dural tears and recurrent herniation with lumbar micro-endoscopic discectomy. Eur Spine J. 2010; 19 (3):443–450

[32] Gotfryd A, Avanzi O. A systematic review of randomised clinical trials using posterior discectomy to treat lumbar disc herniations. Int Orthop. 2009; 33 (1):11–17

[33] Ahn Y, Lee HY, Lee SH, Lee JH. Dural tears in percutaneous endoscopic lumbar discectomy. Eur Spine J. 2011; 20(1):58–64

[34] Li M, Yang H, Yang Q. Full-endoscopic technique discectomy versus microendoscopic discectomy for the surgical treatment of lumbar disc herniation. Pain Physician. 2015; 18(4):359–363

[35] O'Toole JE, Eichholz KM, Fessler RG. Surgical site infection rates after minimally invasive spinal surgery. J Neurosurg Spine. 2009; 11(4):471–476

[36] Wang MY, Grossman J. Endoscopic minimally invasive transforaminal interbody fusion without general anesthesia: initial clinical experience with 1-year follow-up. Neurosurg Focus. 2016; 40(2):E13

[37] Chang HK, Chang HC, Wu JC, et al. Scoliosis may increase the risk of recurrence of lumbar disc herniation after microdiscectomy. J Neurosurg Spine. 2016; 24(4):586–591

[38] Lee SH, Bae JS. Comparison of clinical and radiological outcomes after automated open lumbar discectomy and conventional microdiscectomy: a prospective randomized trial. Int J Clin Exp Med. 2015; 8(8):12135–12148

[39] Shih P, Wong AP, Smith TR, Lee AI, Fessler RG. Complications of open compared to minimally invasive lumbar spine decompression. J Clin Neurosci. 2011; 18(10):1360–1364

[40] Mu X, Wei J, Li P. What were the advantages of microendoscopic discectomy for lumbar disc herniation comparing with open discectomy: a meta-analysis? Int J Clin Exp Med. 2015; 8(10):17498–17506

[41] Telfeian AE, Veeravagu A, Oyelese AA, Gokaslan ZL. A brief history of endoscopic spine surgery. Neurosurg Focus. 2016; 40(2):E2

[42] Polikandriotis JA, Hudak EM, Perry MW. Minimally invasive surgery through endoscopic laminotomy and foraminotomy for the treatment of lumbar spinal stenosis. J Orthop. 2013; 10(1):13–16

[43] Wong AP, Smith ZA, Lall RR, Bresnahan LE, Fessler RG. The microendoscopic decompression of lumbar stenosis: a review of the current literature and clinical results. Minim Invasive Surg. 2012; 2012:325095

[44] Ohya J, Oshima Y, Chikuda H, et al. Does the microendoscopic technique reduce mortality and major complications in patients undergoing lumbar discectomy? A propensity score-matched analysis using a nationwide administrative database. Neurosurg Focus. 2016; 40(2):E5

[45] Gadjradj PS, Harhangi BS. Percutaneous transforaminal endoscopic discectomy for lumbar disk herniation. Clin Spine Surg. 2016; 29(9):368–371

[46] Wang M, Zhou Y, Wang J, Zhang Z, Li C. A 10-year follow-up study on long-term clinical outcomes of lumbar microendoscopic discectomy. J Neurol Surg A Cent Eur Neurosurg. 2012; 73(4):195–198

[47] Fujimoto T, Taniwaki T, Tahata S, Nakamura T, Mizuta H. Patient outcomes for a minimally invasive approach to treat lumbar spinal canal stenosis: is microendoscopic or microscopic decompressive laminotomy the less invasive surgery? Clin Neurol Neurosurg. 2015; 131:21–25

[48] Ruetten S, Komp M, Merk H, Godolias G. Full-endoscopic interlaminar and transforaminal lumbar discectomy versus conventional microsurgical technique: a prospective, randomized, controlled study. Spine. 2008; 33(9):931–939

[49] Kahanovitz N, Viola K, Muculloch J. Limited surgical discectomy and microdiscectomy. A clinical comparison. Spine. 1989; 14(1):79–81

[50] Chun EH, Park HS. A modified approach of percutaneous endoscopic lumbar discectomy (PELD) for far lateral disc herniation at L5-S1 with foot drop. Korean J Pain. 2016; 29(1):57–61

[51] Morgenstern R, Morgenstern C. Percutaneous transforaminal lumbar interbody fusion (pTLIF) with a posterolateral approach for the treatment of denegerative disk disease: feasibility and preliminary results. Int J Spine Surg. 2015; 9:41

[52] Osman SG. Endoscopic transforaminal decompression, interbody fusion, and percutaneous pedicle screw implantation of the lumbar spine: a case series report. Int J Spine Surg. 2012; 6:157–166

[53] Yao N, Wang W, Liu Y. Percutaneous endoscopic lumbar discectomy and interbody fusion with B-Twin expandable spinal spacer. Arch Orthop Trauma Surg. 2011; 131(6):791–796

[54] Gadjradj PS, van Tulder MW, Dirven CM, Peul WC, Harhangi BS. Clinical outcomes after percutaneous transforaminal endoscopic discectomy for lumbar disc herniation: a prospective case series. Neurosurg Focus. 2016; 40(2):E3

[55] Wang B, Lü G, Patel AA, Ren P, Cheng I. An evaluation of the learning curve for a complex surgical technique: the full endoscopic interlaminar approach for lumbar disc herniations. Spine J. 2011; 11(2):122–130

[56] Cote M, Kalra R, Wilson T, Orlandi RR, Couldwell WT. Surgical fidelity: comparing the microscope and the endoscope. Acta Neurochir (Wien). 2013; 155 (12):2299–2303

[57] Ahn J, Iqbal A, Manning BT, et al. Minimally invasive lumbar decompression-the surgical learning curve. Spine J. 2015

[58] Iprenburg M, Wagner R, Godschalx A, Telfeian AE. Patient radiation exposure during transforaminal lumbar endoscopic spine surgery: a prospective study. Neurosurg Focus. 2016; 40(2):E7

[59] Yadav YR, Parihar V, Namdev H, Agarwal M, Bhatele PR. Endoscopic interlaminar management of lumbar disc disease. J Neurol Surg A Cent Eur Neurosurg. 2013; 74(2):77–81

[60] Matsumoto M, Watanabe K, Hosogane N, et al. Recurrence of lumbar disc herniation after microendoscopic discectomy. J Neurol Surg A Cent Eur Neurosurg. 2013; 74(4):222–227

[61] Tenenbaum S, Arzi H, Herman A, et al. Percutaneous posterolateral transforaminal endoscopic discectomy: clinical outcome, complications, and learning curve evaluation. Surg Technol Int. 2011; 21:278–283

[62] Chaichankul C, Poopitaya S, Tassanawipas W. The effect of learning curve on the results of percutaneous transforaminal endoscopic lumbar discectomy. J Med Assoc Thai. 2012; 95 Suppl 10:S206–S212

[63] Ahn Y. Percutaneous endoscopic decompression for lumbar spinal stenosis. Expert Rev Med Devices. 2014; 11(6):605–616

[64] Solari D, de Angelis M, Cappabianca P. Bury the hatchet: microscope and endoscope blink together to the future. World Neurosurg. 2015; 83(5):750–751

[65] Jacquot F, Gastambide D. Percutaneous endoscopic transforaminal lumbar interbody fusion: is it worth it? Int Orthop. 2013; 37(8):1507–1510

[66] Morgenstern R, Morgenstern C, Jané R, Lee SH. Usefulness of an expandable interbody spacer for the treatment of foraminal stenosis in extremely collapsed disks: preliminary clinical experience with endoscopic posterolateral transforaminal approach. J Spinal Disord Tech. 2011; 24(8):485–491

[67] Zhang X, Wang Y, Xiao S, et al. Preliminary clinical results of endoscopic discectomy followed by interbody fusion using B-twin expandable spinal spacer. Zhongguo Xiu Fu Chong Jian Wai Ke Za Zhi. 2011; 25(10):1153–1157

[68] Zhou Y, Zhang C, Wang J, et al. Endoscopic transforaminal lumbar decompression, interbody fusion and pedicle screw fixation-a report of 42 cases. Chin J Traumatol. 2008; 11(4):225–231

[69] Hur JW, Kim JS, Shin MH, Ryu KS, Park CK, Lee SH. Percutaneous endoscopic lumbar discectomy and annuloplasty for lumbar disc herniation at the low two contiguous levels: single-portal, double surgeries. J Neurol Surg A Cent Eur Neurosurg. 2014; 75(5):381–385

[70] Xu BS, Tan QS, Xia Q, Ji N, Hu YC. Bilateral decompression via unilateral fenestration using mobile microendoscopic discectomy technique for lumbar spinal stenosis. Orthop Surg. 2010; 2(2):106–110

38 Endoscopic versus Open Carpal Tunnel Release: Moderator

Hussam Abou-Al-Shaar and Mark A. Mahan

Summary

Carpal tunnel syndrome results from compression of the median nerve by the flexor retinaculum. Pain from this nerve compression can be debilitating and can result in specific sensory and motor symptoms. Surgical decompression of the median nerve has been approached traditionally using an open technique, which necessitates a larger incision with potentially larger approach-related morbidity. In recent decades, endoscopic techniques have been described to reduce approach-related morbidity. We describe here the advantages and disadvantages of the traditional open versus endoscopic carpal tunnel release surgery.

Keywords: carpal tunnel, median nerve, compression, peripheral nerve, decompression

38.1 Open Surgical Management

38.1.1 Case Example

History and Physical Examination

A 54-year-old right-handed female office worker complained of a 6-year history of progressive numbness of her right radial digits (thumb, index, and middle fingers). She reported worsening of her symptoms on manual activities associated with work. The patient experienced classic nocturnal paresthesias with awakenings. Her hypoesthesias improved mildly while wearing a brace; however, she could not maintain the brace for prolonged periods. Her symptoms affected her life significantly as evident by her low Oswestry Disability Index and percentage scores. The patient had no history of trauma or degenerative diseases of the wrist.

Physical examination revealed mild reduction in the grip strength and key pinch in the right hand compared with the left (50 vs. 57 ft/lb and 14 vs. 16 ft/lb, respectively), despite being right handed. She did not have any weakness or atrophy of her thenar muscles. She had positive radiating paresthesias on percussion of the transverse carpal ligament and Phalen's tests in the right wrist.

Electrodiagnostic studies of the median nerve demonstrated severe carpal tunnel syndrome (CTS) at the wrist (▶ Fig. 38.1). Median sensory and median motor nerves demonstrated reduced amplitude (right sensory 15 mV vs. left sensory 17 mV, with normal values > 20 mV), prolonged latency (right sensory 6 ms and motor 7.5 ms vs. left sensory 4.1 ms, with normal values < 4.5 ms), and reduced conduction velocity of the right median sensory and median motor nerves compared with the left across the wrist. Conduction within the right and left ulnar nerves was normal and without evidence of a generalized polyneuropathy. Needle electromyography demonstrated insertional activities in the right abductor pollicis brevis with chronic neurogenic changes in recruitment.

On the basis of the aforementioned findings, a diagnosis of moderate to severe right-handed CTS and mild left-handed CTS was established. The patient's condition warranted surgical intervention because no symptomatic improvement was achieved with conservative management.

Intraoperative Management

At our department, we perform both open and endoscopic carpal tunnel release surgeries under local anesthesia with sedation, according to the patient's preference. All patients are hemodynamically monitored and a venous line is standardly set. All patients receive perioperative intravenous antibiotics. The patient's arm is sterilely prepped and draped in typical surgical manner using alcohol skin scrub followed by chlorhexidine skin preparation. A 50:50 mix of 0.25% bupivacaine with epinephrine and 0.5% lidocaine with epinephrine is injected in the skin and subcutaneous tissues at the planned procedural sites for periprocedural anesthesia and hemostasis. Before the surgical incision is made, a tweezer test is performed to confirm anesthesia at the planned skin incision site. We do not commonly use a tourniquet in open carpal tunnel release surgeries, in contrast to endoscopic carpal tunnel release surgeries.

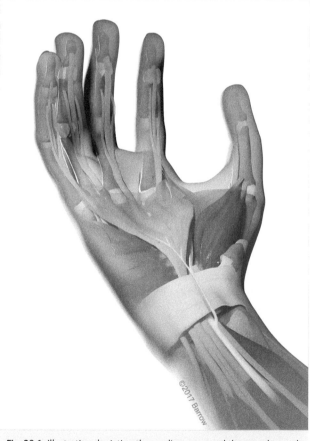

Fig. 38.1 Illustration depicting the median nerve and the carpal tunnel. (Used with permission from Barrow Neurological Institute, Phoenix, AZ.)

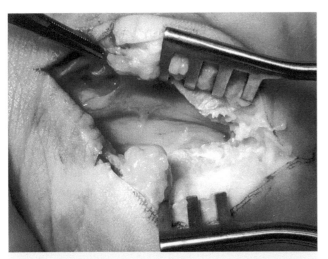

Fig. 38.2 Intraoperative photograph of the left wrist during extensile open carpal tunnel release. The patient had previously undergone an endoscopic carpal tunnel release with persistent symptoms and magnetic resonance imaging (MRI) evidence of an intact transverse carpal ligament. Scar tissue was identified below the aponeurosis of the palmaris, and above an intact transverse carpal ligament. Given the prior scar at the distal wrist crease and significant proximal swelling of the median nerve at this incision on MRI, the open carpal tunnel approach was extended into the distal forearm. Asterisk identifies severe swelling of the median nerve proximal to the transverse carpal ligament. Pound denotes both sides of the divided transverse carpal ligament.

We then create a 2-cm incision in the mid-thenar crease (▶ Fig. 38.2). Bipolar cautery is used exclusively to maintain hemostasis throughout the procedure. In the presented case, there was no significantly sized transverse palmar nerve. The dissection is carried down to the palmar aponeurosis, which is usually mobilized radially. The transverse carpal ligament can be easily identified deep to the aponeurosis and then cut with a blade until the nerve is exposed. The transverse carpal ligament is then divided both proximally and distally with tenotomy scissors. Distal decompression is confirmed with visualization of the palmar fat, while proximal decompression is carried out into the distal third of the forearm. The median nerve is then inspected for masses, none of which were found in the present case. Bipolar cautery is again used to cauterize the cut ends of the transverse carpal ligament and to assist in its retraction.

The hand is then flexed and extended to assess the gliding of the median nerve through the carpal tunnel. If there is evidence of impaired gliding, a source for stricture or tethering is sought. Impaired movement of the median nerve on flexion and extension of the wrist is rare; however, dynamic assessment of the nerve adds to the completeness of the evaluation of the surgical decompression.

After the completion of carpal tunnel release, the operative field is lavaged with copious normal saline and bacitracin. Finally, the skin is reapproximated at both sites of the incision with 3–0 nylon in a horizontal mattress fashion.

Postoperatively, the wrist is bandaged with an adhesive bandage, and patients are advised to avoid wrist immobilization. The patient in the presented case tolerated the procedure very well with no perioperative complications.

Various other minimally invasive nonendoscopic approaches, including the mini-incision midpalmar technique, have been developed to enhance the cosmetic outcomes and reduce the incidence of scar tenderness and pillar pain. The mini-incision midpalmar technique is the most widely used minimally invasive open technique. A 3-cm incision is made in the mid-palm distal to the flexion crease of the wrist to expose, visualize, and release the distal portion of the flexor retinaculum. The proximal portion of the flexor retinaculum and antebrachial fascia can then be dissected and cut using scissors in a plane deep to the subcutaneous fat and skin.

Surgical Outcome

Postoperatively, the patient in the presented case took 3 days off work. She demonstrated anticipated acute handgrip strength reduction in the right hand compared with the left (31 vs. 53 ft/lb) at her suture removal appointment. At her 3-month follow-up, the patient reported complete resolution of her nocturnal symptoms and improvement in her functionality with return of handgrip strength to normal. There was no scar tenderness or pillar pain.

After surgical management, all patients should be monitored with a questionnaire about their symptoms and examinations at regular intervals after surgery. Sutures are usually removed after 1 week. All patients are encouraged to mobilize their hands and return to their baseline functionality. A follow-up neurophysiologic evaluation may be of value but is often refused by the patient when significant clinical benefit is noticed.

The open surgical release of CTS results in high success rates in the majority of patients. It improves functionality and motor function and reduces pain and hypoesthesia. In one study of 113 patients with CTS who were followed for a minimum of 10 years after surgery, 72% reported complete abolishment of their symptoms within the first year after surgery, which increased to 74% at a minimum of 10 years. Satisfaction with the outcome was reported by 88% of patients, with 81% reporting great improvement in their quality of life. Only two patients (1.8%) required revision surgery for carpal tunnel decompression. The complications of open release of CTS are usually minimal and rarely encountered.[1] Scar tenderness and pillar pain are the most frequently encountered complications after open/tradition carpal tunnel release. In one series of 55 hands with CTS, scar tenderness and pillar pain were reported in 4 (7.3%) and 7 (12.7%) hands, respectively.[2] Such results are in concordance with other studies in regard to success, reoperation, and complication rates.

38.1.2 Advantages of Open Approach

The advantages of the open approach, in comparison with the endoscopic approach, in the present case are many. First, although there were no contraindications to the endoscopic approach in the present case, the severity of the patient's condition as evident by her physical and electrophysiological examinations and the need for a rapid cost-effective technique to relieve the patient's complaints with lower reoperation/recurrence rates made the open approach more favorable. From an economical point of view, the open approach is less expensive than the endoscopic approach, making it a more cost-effective modality. Additionally, we believe that all patients should be given transparent and adequate information about both open and endoscopic approaches in terms of success, reoperation, and complication rates in order to allow them to make an optimal decision. As reviewed in the literature section below, there is an assumed greater risk of recurrence in endoscopic carpal tunnel release, whereas there is the expectation of greater short-term pain associated with open carpal tunnel release. When reviewing options for individual patients, we consider these data in view of patient symptoms and demands. For example, in patients who perform manual labor with thickened palmar skin and greater need for grip strength, we often recommend endoscopic carpal tunnel release because the wound healing from open surgery is often challenging in these patients. In patients with severe CTS, recurrent or persistent CTS after prior release, and/or desire for lower risk for reoperation, we recommend open carpal tunnel release. In the present case, the patient requested the open surgical approach to avoid revision surgery at a later date. The long- and short-term risks and expectations should be addressed when establishing informed consent.

The open surgical approach allows for greater opening of the carpal tunnel. This has been established by postoperative computed tomography evaluation of the carpal arch, wherein open carpal tunnel release demonstrated greater than twofold increase in the angles between the pisiform and scaphoid bones and between the hamate and trapezium bones as compared with endoscopic surgery.[3] The greater increase in carpal angle is presumably due to division of the musculotendinous structures superficial to the transverse carpal ligament, such as the palmaris aponeurosis and palmaris brevis. In addition, open approaches allow for complete inspection of the median nerve for any inherent pathologies, such as peripheral nerve sheath tumors and wrist ganglion cysts, among others. We do not perform epineurotomy of the median nerve.

Postoperatively, the patient in this case reported relief of her symptoms and improvement in her functionality and quality of life with anticipated transient acute handgrip strength weakness, which returned to baseline by her 3-month follow-up appointment.

Although the larger incision in the open approach compared with the endoscopic approach might be associated with a greater incidence of scar tenderness and pillar pain, none were experienced by the presented patient. In fact, the patient reported complete satisfaction with the outcome including the aesthetic aspect. Furthermore, the reported advantage of the endoscopic technique in regard to a quicker return to work was not evident in this case, as the patient returned to work 3 days after the procedure.

38.1.3 Disadvantage of the Endoscope

The primary surgical disadvantage of the endoscopic approach is the limited approach, resulting in incomplete release of the carpal tunnel. Specifically, surgical division of the transverse carpal ligament does not release the entire carpal tunnel anatomy. Thus, all endoscopic carpal tunnel releases are, by nature of their approach, incomplete. The overlying palmaris brevis

and fascia of the palmaris longus retain tension, despite cutting of the transverse carpal ligament. Furthermore, the degree of transverse carpal ligament release in endoscopic approaches is limited to the resting tension of the ligament. The ligament cannot be opened larger than elastic recoil unless larger surgical tools are introduced into the carpal tunnel, with increased pressure on the median nerve. The incomplete release is an essential consideration, as evidenced by the slightly higher recurrence/reoperation rates in the endoscopic approach compared with the open approach.

Moreover, it is not uncommon for patients with CTS to have concomitant pathologies in the wrist joint (e.g., ganglion cyst), finger flexor tendons (e.g., anomalous palmaris longus, palmaris profundus, hypertrophied or anomalous flexor digitorum superficialis, hypertrophied anomalous lumbricals, flexor carpi radialis brevis, or accessory flexor pollicis longus, also known as Gantzer's muscle), or median nerve itself (e.g., median nerve tumor or unusual course). Visualization of these concomitant pathologies is valuable to avoid surgical failure.

Furthermore, history of wrist trauma, limited wrist extension (contraindication for endoscopic approaches), or recurrent CTS are also indications for open surgical release, limiting the efficacy of the endoscopic approach in those patients, who are more prone to iatrogenic injury during endoscopic carpal tunnel release because complete visualization of the anatomical structures in the wrist is of paramount importance to avoid any unintentional injury.

Additionally, endoscopic approaches require more surgical equipment and often expensive surgical disposable items. Thus, the open approach is less expensive per case and might be more cost-effective than the endoscopic surgery, although appraisal of cost-effectiveness remains biased by short-term data.[4,5]

38.1.4 Patient Selection

The optimal selection of CTS patients for surgical management involves multiple steps. At our institution, we discuss the relevant options for management of CTS, including (1) benign neglect, wherein we describe the natural history of progressive CTS; (2) nonsurgical treatments, such as wrist splints and physical therapy, among others; (3) steroid injections into the carpal tunnel; and (4) surgical decompression. Appropriate recognition and possible treatment of comorbid conditions that may lead to spontaneous resolution of CTS, such as acute flexor tenosynovitis, pregnancy, and pyogenic infections, among others, is essential. Management of chronic conditions that may exacerbate CTS (e.g., poorly controlled diabetes mellitus, rheumatoid disease, globulinemia) is also valuable in ensuring appropriate therapy. In addition, thorough evaluation for cervical radiculopathy is essential. For example, the presence of pain in a median distribution should prompt evaluation for a C6 or C7 radiculopathy.

To warrant surgical decompression, first, a patient's symptoms of CTS must be significantly interfering with the patient's functionality and quality of life (most commonly by disturbed sleep from nocturnal paresthesias). Second, the presence of severe neurologic loss, such as thenar muscle weakness, numbness, and atrophy, may prompt consideration of surgical intervention. As such, electrophysiological studies documenting altered/reduced median nerve sensory and/or motor functions are of paramount importance.

Because there is no clear superiority of endoscopic or open surgical approach, an individualized approach, taking into consideration each patient's unique characteristics, should be maintained. As mentioned earlier, the presence of concomitant pathologies in the wrist joint, finger flexor variations, or median nerve favors open surgical intervention. One could argue that radiologic evaluation, either by ultrasound or magnetic resonance imaging, is essential for recommending endoscopic carpal tunnel release, but optional for open release since other pathologies can be visualized during surgery. Whereas there are contraindications for endoscopic approaches, such as limited range of motion at the wrist, history of wrist trauma, or recurrent/persistent CTS after prior release, there are no strict contraindications for open release. However, we consider the following conditions that strongly favor endoscopic surgery:

- Thickened palmar skin, such as frequently occurs in manual laborers.
- Need for rapid return to work.
- Pain from prior open carpal tunnel release on the contralateral hand.

As part of informed consent, we review the surgical approach, risks, expectations, and postoperative care of both approaches, describing the differential considerations between open and endoscopic surgeries. We then provide our recommendation, based on reflection of the specific considerations of the individual patient. However, we ultimately allow the patient to make the decision if there are no contraindications and there is clinical equipoise between the surgical approaches. Notably, in our experience, most patients prefer to have the approach decided by the surgeon.

38.1.5 Complication Avoidance

A prerequisite to avoiding complications from open surgical carpal tunnel release is thoughtful patient selection as well as thorough knowledge of the anatomic structures and variations at the wrist. Patient cooperation during surgical intervention is of paramount importance to prevent any unintentional injury.

One advantage of the open approach over the endoscopic approach is the visualization of the other anatomic structures of the wrist, allowing for evaluation and treatment of other pathologies. With any surgery, meticulous dissection of the skin and soft tissues is essential to prevent any unintentional neurovascular injury. Bipolar cautery along with local pressure should be exclusively used to maintain hemostasis throughout the procedure. Complete visualization of the median nerve along with meticulous dissection of its branches is important to reduce the incidence of recurrence or median nerve injury. Finally, optimal closure of the incision wound along with early mobilization might decrease the risk of restricted gliding of the median nerve and recurrence of CTS.

38.1.6 Technical Nuances

Most experts agree that Marie and Foix[6] provided the first clear description of CTS and that Learmonth[7] published the first report of a carpal tunnel release in 1933. We do not commonly use a tourniquet in open carpal tunnel release, in contrast to endoscopic release. The tourniquet increases the surgical duration, and we prefer to visualize the microvasculature of the median nerve during surgery. Although some surgeons have strong preferences on the location of the skin incision (e.g., the ulnar side of the nail bed of the fourth digit when flexed to the wrist), we prefer to use the mid-thenar crease and carry dissection ulnarly. This reduces postoperative scar prominence in our experience. At that point, the subcutaneous tissue, palmar fascia, flexor retinaculum, and antebrachial fascia can be visualized and dissected. We utilize spreading dissection of the subcutaneous adipose, rather than sharp dissection, as the transverse palmar nerve can be readily preserved with horizontal/transverse spreading. Similarly, we prefer to spread or mobilize the palmar fascia, rather than sharply divide the aponeurosis. We find it unnecessary to protect the median nerve with an instrument inserted underneath the transverse carpal ligament. The transverse carpal ligament will retract when a full-thickness cut is achieved, creating a window in the transverse carpal ligament; however, many surgeons advocate placing a Freer elevator or Woodson elevator below the transverse carpal ligament. We split the distal forearm fascia with tenotomy scissor while retracting the proximal limb of the incision with a Ragnell retractor. Retraction provides appropriate visualization of this maneuver, which we consider essential because of the proximal swelling of the median nerve. Complete visualization of the median nerve and inspection should be carried out in every procedure, as inherent pathologies and anatomical variations are not uncommonly encountered. As described earlier, we flex and extend the wrist after completion of the decompression to ensure that the median nerve is gliding and that no tethering exists at the conclusion of surgery. Absorbable sutures, such as Vicryl (Ethicon), should be avoided because there is often an inflammatory reaction to these sutures. A dressing can be applied at the surgical site; however, we avoid dressings that limit mobility. We advocate early active wrist movement for all patients to avoid tendon or median nerve tethering from postoperative scar.

38.1.7 Literature Review/Evidence in Favor of Microscopic Approach

The issue of the superiority of the open approach over the endoscopic approach, or vice versa, has been a subject of debate for the past two decades. Multiple studies including various randomized clinical trials have shown contradictory results and outcomes in this regard. Although many surgeons still favor the open approach, some studies have shown superiority of the endoscopic approach in short-term follow-up. Generally, analyses of multiple randomized clinical trials that followed patients over long periods have concluded that both techniques are associated with similar success, satisfaction, and complication rates.[8,9,10,11,12,13] While nuances vary between studies, the message of years of comparative trials is that the procedures are essentially equivalent in long-term follow-up.[12,14]

The open approach is the primary and default approach that was developed for the purpose of carpal tunnel decompression. It allows complete visualization of the structures in the wrist. Also, it provides for inspection of the median nerve for any inherent pathology or unusual course and anatomical variations. In 2011, a survey among hand surgeons reported that 52% of them used only open release technique, 36% used mostly endoscopic release technique, and 12% regularly utilized both techniques.[15] The open technique is the de facto approach for recurrent/revision carpal tunnel release, since these are more difficult cases because of the postoperative scar. It is also the technique of choice for complex cases (e.g., rheumatoid arthritis and dialysis cases) and in the presence of inherent median nerve pathology (e.g., tumor) or anatomical variations. Therefore, it is not uncommon for endoscopic surgeons to switch intraoperatively to the open approach because of the presence of the aforementioned factors or in the cases with a narrow carpal canal.[16] The open approach is associated with a shorter operative time compared with the endoscopic approach.[13] Moreover, the open technique is associated with less financial burden compared with the endoscopic technique.[17,18,19] Thus, many surgeons consider the open approach more cost-effective than the endoscopic approach.[19,20] Interestingly, a randomized study comparing two-portal endoscopic release with open release reported patient satisfaction of 85% in the endoscopic group and 93% in the open group. The repeat surgery rate due to symptom recurrence was 5% in the endoscopic group and none in the open approach group.[21]

The short-term outcomes of a few randomized trials found a small benefit of the endoscopic approach over the open approach regarding postoperative pain, time to return to work, and postoperative handgrip strength.[8,11,22] However, various randomized clinical trials and meta-analyses failed to show a statistically significant difference regarding postoperative pain, time to return to work, and postoperative hand strength between the two techniques.[9,10,13,23,24] Those presumed short-term benefits from the endoscopic approach (which are relatively small and short lasting) are eliminated by the increased risks of recurrence and reoperation. Multiple studies have demonstrated recurrence rates that range from 0 to 10% with the endoscopic approach.[25] This is presumably due to the incomplete release of the carpal tunnel, as only the transverse carpal ligament is divided and minimal shift of the carpal bones after endoscopic surgery.[3,26] The long-term recurrence rate appears lower in the open approach, which, given the short-term results of the trials, probably is a greater effect than currently understood.

Aslani et al[23] reported a significantly longer ($p < 0.05$) return-to-work time with the open approach compared with the endoscopic approach. Moreover, they found a significantly increased risk of pillar pain in the open approach in early follow-up; however, such difference was eliminated in the fourth month of follow-up with statistically similar results. Atroshi et al[8] found less postoperative pain with the endoscopic approach but a similar length of postoperative work absence. They also noticed no differences in the CTS symptom severity and functional status scores up to 1 year after surgery between the two techniques. The same group reported their outcomes at 5-year follow-up with similar improvement in the symptoms severity score in both groups, and similar functional status, satisfaction, reoperation rate, and time to return to work.[9] In a report of their 11- to 16-year follow-up, they found that the improvements in symptoms severity score, functionality, satisfaction,

and reoperation rates were maintained with no statistically significant difference between the two groups.[10]

Although the complication rate has been shown to be statistically insignificant between the two techniques in multiple studies,[13,14,27] the complications encountered with the endoscopic technique are slightly more severe than those associated with the open approach and the incidence rate ranges from 2 to 35%.[14,16] Gümüştaş et al[27] reported a complication rate of 15.52% in the endoscopic group compared with 5.26% in the open group. In a review of 22,327 CTS cases treated via the endoscopic approach, Benson et al[28] reported major nerve injuries in 0.13%, digital nerve injuries in 0.03%, arterial arch injuries in 0.02%, and transient neurapraxias in 1.45%. Other reported complications of the endoscopic technique include tendon, vessel, and nerve injury, wound infection, and reflex sympathetic dystrophy.[13,27,29] Such complications may be higher during the surgeon's learning curve for the endoscopic approach.

Finally, it is important to keep in mind various factors and latent design biases that can influence the outcomes of an approach over another. In fact, many of those randomized clinical trials fail to address many factors related to their study designs and follow-up methodologies. In the most recent Cochrane review, the authors concluded: "overall risk of bias in studies that contribute data to these results is rather high … the quality of evidence in this review may be considered as generally low."[12] Even more importantly, the results of the trials reflect the selection criteria of the trial, not the real-world variability. Broad application of a trial and its results, without consideration of the exclusion criteria, is therefore not advised.

References

[1] Louie DL, Earp BE, Collins JE, et al. Outcomes of open carpal tunnel release at a minimum of ten years. J Bone Joint Surg Am. 2013; 95(12):1067–1073

[2] Boya H, Özcan Ö, Özteki N HH. Long-term complications of open carpal tunnel release. Muscle Nerve. 2008; 38(5):1443–1446

[3] Nazzi V, Franzini A, Messina G, Broggi G. Carpal tunnel syndrome: matching minimally invasive surgical techniques. Technical note. J Neurosurg. 2008; 108(5):1033–1036

[4] Chung KC, Walters MR, Greenfield ML, Chernew ME. Endoscopic versus open carpal tunnel release: a cost-effectiveness analysis. Plast Reconstr Surg. 1998; 102(4):1089–1099

[5] Saw NL, Jones S, Shepstone L, Meyer M, Chapman PG, Logan AM. Early outcome and cost-effectiveness of endoscopic versus open carpal tunnel release: a randomized prospective trial. J Hand Surg [Br]. 2003; 28(5):444–449

[6] Marie P, Foix C. Atrophie isole de l'eminence thenar d'origine nevritique: role du ligament annulaire anterieur du carpe dans la pathologenie de la 1esion. Rev Neurol. 1913; 26:647–649

[7] Learmonth J. The principle of decompression in the treatment of certain diseases of peripheral nerves. Surg Clin North Am. 1933; 13:905–913

[8] Atroshi I, Larsson GU, Ornstein E, Hofer M, Johnsson R, Ranstam J. Outcomes of endoscopic surgery compared with open surgery for carpal tunnel syndrome among employed patients: randomised controlled trial. BMJ. 2006; 332 (7556):1473

[9] Atroshi I, Hofer M, Larsson GU, Ornstein E, Johnsson R, Ranstam J. Open compared with 2-portal endoscopic carpal tunnel release: a 5-year follow-up of a randomized controlled trial. J Hand Surg Am. 2009; 34(2):266–272

[10] Atroshi I, Hofer M, Larsson GU, Ranstam J. Extended follow-up of a randomized clinical trial of open vs endoscopic release surgery for carpal tunnel syndrome. JAMA. 2015; 314(13):1399–1401

[11] Sayegh ET, Strauch RJ. Open versus endoscopic carpal tunnel release: a meta-analysis of randomized controlled trials. Clin Orthop Relat Res. 2015; 473 (3):1120–1132

[12] Vasiliadis HS, Georgoulas P, Shrier I, Salanti G, Scholten RJ. Endoscopic release for carpal tunnel syndrome. Cochrane Database Syst Rev. 2014(1):CD008265

[13] Hu K, Zhang T, Xu W. Intraindividual comparison between open and endoscopic release in bilateral carpal tunnel syndrome: a meta-analysis of randomized controlled trials. Brain Behav. 2016; 6(3):e00439

[14] Vasiliadis HS, Nikolakopoulou A, Shrier I, et al. Endoscopic and open release similarly safe for the treatment of carpal tunnel syndrome. A systematic review and meta-analysis. PLoS One. 2015; 10(12):e0143683

[15] Leinberry CF, Rivlin M, Maltenfort M, et al. Treatment of carpal tunnel syndrome by members of the American Society for Surgery of the Hand: a 25-year perspective. J Hand Surg Am. 2012; 37(10):1997–2003.e3

[16] Keiner D, Gaab MR, Schroeder HW, Oertel J. Long-term follow-up of dual-portal endoscopic release of the transverse ligament in carpal tunnel syndrome: an analysis of 94 cases. Neurosurgery. 2009; 64(1):131–137, discussion 137–138

[17] Helm RH, Vaziri S. Evaluation of carpal tunnel release using the Knifelight instrument. J Hand Surg [Br]. 2003; 28(3):251–254

[18] Thoma A, Veltri K, Haines T, Duku E. A meta-analysis of randomized controlled trials comparing endoscopic and open carpal tunnel decompression. Plast Reconstr Surg. 2004; 114(5):1137–1146

[19] Zhang S, Vora M, Harris AH, Baker L, Curtin C, Kamal RN. Cost-minimization analysis of open and endoscopic carpal tunnel release. J Bone Joint Surg Am. 2016; 98(23):1970–1977

[20] Rab M, Grünbeck M, Beck H, et al. Intra-individual comparison between open and 2-portal endoscopic release in clinically matched bilateral carpal syndrome. J Plast Reconstr Aesthet Surg. 2006; 59(7):730–736

[21] Macdermid JC, Richards RS, Roth JH, Ross DC, King GJ. Endoscopic versus open carpal tunnel release: a randomized trial. J Hand Surg Am. 2003; 28(3):475–480

[22] Brown RA, Gelberman RH, Seiler JG, III, et al. Carpal tunnel release. A prospective, randomized assessment of open and endoscopic methods. J Bone Joint Surg Am. 1993; 75(9):1265–1275

[23] Aslani HR, Alizadeh K, Eajazi A, et al. Comparison of carpal tunnel release with three different techniques. Clin Neurol Neurosurg. 2012; 114(7):965–968

[24] Michelotti B, Romanowsky D, Hauck RM. Prospective, randomized evaluation of endoscopic versus open carpal tunnel release in bilateral carpal tunnel syndrome: an interim analysis. Ann Plast Surg. 2014; 73 Suppl 2: S157–S160

[25] Jimenez DF, Gibbs SR, Clapper AT. Endoscopic treatment of carpal tunnel syndrome: a critical review. J Neurosurg. 1998; 88(5):817–826

[26] Viegas SF, Pollard A, Kaminksi K. Carpal arch alteration and related clinical status after endoscopic carpal tunnel release. J Hand Surg Am. 1992; 17 (6):1012–1016

[27] Gümüştaş SA, Ekmekçi B, Tosun HB, Orak MM, Bekler HI. Similar effectiveness of the open versus endoscopic technique for carpal tunnel syndrome: a prospective randomized trial. Eur J Orthop Surg Traumatol. 2015; 25(8):1253–1260

[28] Benson LS, Bare AA, Nagle DJ, Harder VS, Williams CS, Visotsky JL. Complications of endoscopic and open carpal tunnel release. Arthroscopy. 2006; 22 (9):919–924, 924.e1–924.e2

[29] Larsen MB, Sørensen AI, Crone KL, Weis T, Boeckstyns ME. Carpal tunnel release: a randomized comparison of three surgical methods. J Hand Surg Eur Vol. 2013; 38(6):646–650

39 Endoscopic versus Open Carpal Tunnel Release: Endoscope

Joachim Oertel, D. Keiner, and K. Schwerdtfeger

Summary

To date, controversy regarding efficacy, safety, and success of endoscopic carpal tunnel release compared with open carpal tunnel release persists. Several endoscopic techniques for dissection of the transverse carpal ligament are applied today with successful results in a wide range of reports. Still, in different series the results of endoscopic versus open technique are divergent. Whereas some authors report significantly improved grip strength, a decreased wrist pain and scar tenderness and a comparable risk of complications by performing endoscopic carpal tunnel release, other authors observed an increased susceptibility to reversible nerve problems and pillar pain as well a higher risk of median nerve contusion and ulnar nerve transection. In the present chapter the authors present their favored techniques of endoscopic carpal tunnel release with special emphasis on the technique itself as well as the ideal patient selection and possible pitfalls of endoscopic release of the carpal ligament. A short review of the latest analyses in favor of the endoscopic approach is given.

Keywords: carpal tunnel, median nerve, compression, peripheral nerve, decompression

39.1 Endoscopic Surgical Management

39.1.1 Case Example

History and Physical

A 53-year-old male patient suffered from typical brachialgia paresthetica nocturna and hypoesthesia of the left hand since 6 months. A slight impairment of fine motor skills was noted. Physical examination did not reveal any weakness or atrophy of the thenar muscles. The patient had no history of a trauma or degenerative disease of the wrist. However, he was subjected to a successful procedure for carpal tunnel syndrome (CTS) on the contralateral side by the open technique 2 years earlier. Current electrophysiology revealed a delayed distal motor latency (dmL) with 6.6 ms on the left side compared to 4.6 ms on the right side, thus confirming the diagnosis of left-handed CTS. Conservative treatment did not result in any improvement of the symptoms. Thus, surgical therapy was indicated.

Intraoperative Management

In the authors' department, endoscopic carpal tunnel release (ECTR) is performed using Agee's monoportal technique as well as Chow's biportal technique, with a slight preference to Chow's biportal technique. Intraoperatively, all patients are monitored with electrocardiogram (ECG) and pulse oximeter and a venous line is set standardly. The presented patient was operated on with the biportal technique. Biportal ECTR is performed with a reusable set (Karl Storz Endoskope, Tuttlingen, Germany) comprising a standard endoscope camera with a rigid 30-degree optic and a cold light source, a slotted cannula with a trocar, various dilators, and hook knives for dissection of the carpal ligament. Usually, cotton swabs are used for intraoperative cleansing of the slotted cannula (▶ Fig. 39.1).

When surgery is performed with the monoportal technique, the same endoscope camera system is used. The monoportal instrument set consists of a special pistol-shaped grip, a disposable blade assembly, and several synovia dissectors as well as hamate finders of different sizes (MicroAire Surgical Instruments, Charlottesville, VA). The blade assembly is attached to the pistol-type grip that controls the elevation of the blade.

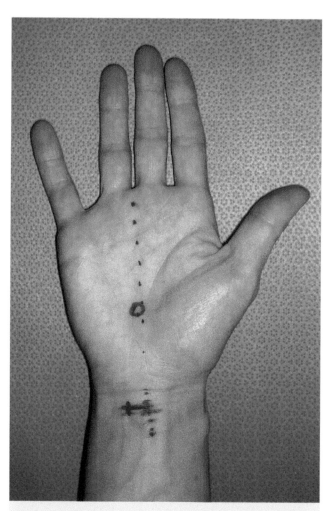

Fig. 39.1 Marking of skin incision with typical landmarks. The proximal port is located ulnar of the palmaris longus tendon; the distal port is located directly at the end of the transverse ligament in the direction of the fourth finger.

The light source and camera system are plugged to the Agee instrument for visualization of the transverse ligament.

Biportal Surgical Technique

The surgery is performed in local anesthesia. In general, using a tourniquet can be considered. However, no tourniquet is used in the authors' department for biportal ECTR since identification of the palmar arch is easier with a pulsatile vessel. The hand is positioned on an arm table. Following skin disinfection and sterile draping, the skin incisions are marked prior to local anesthesia (▶ Fig. 39.1). Local anesthesia is set in the proximal wrist crease and in the palm. A 5-mm skin incision is made directly ulnar to the palmaris longus tendon, and the palmar aponeurosis is dissected. After localization of the median nerve, the carpal canal is entered ulnar to the nerve with the dissector. The lower side of the carpal ligament with its typical rough texture should be palpated with the dissector. A small second skin incision for the exit portal is performed at the end of the transverse ligament in direction of the fourth finger (▶ Fig. 39.2). Then, the dissector is removed, and the slotted cannula with its trocar is inserted in the carpal tunnel from proximal to distal. After rotating the trocar 360 degrees in the direction of the median nerve to avoid the nerve prolapsing into the slotted cannula, the trocar is removed. The telescope with a 30-degree angled lens is inserted in the distal portal. The operating instruments are inserted in the proximal portal. The distal end of the transverse ligament is identified, and the ligament is dissected from distal to proximal with a hook knife until the ligament is dissected and fat prolapses into the canal. After that, the trocar is reinserted, and the slotted cannula is removed. The complete dissection of the ligament is controlled with the dissector. At the end of the procedure, external compression is performed for 3 to 5 minutes. The skin incisions are sutured with single stitches. Postoperatively, the wrist is bandaged with slight compression. Immobilization of the wrist is not recommended.

Monoportal Surgical Technique

Again, the surgery is performed in local anesthesia. The authors perform this procedure with the use of a tourniquet since injury to the palmar arch appears to be less likely. The preparation of the hand is performed in the same manner as described earlier. Local anesthesia is set in the proximal wrist crease. A 1-cm-long—sometimes 2-cm-long— skin incision is made in one of the wrist flexion creases between the flexor carpi ulnaris and the flexor carpi radialis muscles. After subcutaneous longitudinal dissection, the antebrachial fascia is exposed and a U-shaped incision is made on the antebrachial fascia. A synovial elevator is placed under the transverse ligament in the direction of the fourth finger. After that, a hamate finder is inserted into the carpal tunnel to create a path for the blade assembly. The blade endoscope unit is inserted into the carpal tunnel and passed distally to the end of the transverse ligament (▶ Fig. 39.3). Then, the tip of the instrument with the knife is placed distal to the edge of the ligament, and with a trigger mechanism the blade is elevated above the endoscope sheath. The instrument is withdrawn and the transverse ligament is divided from distal to proximal direction under direct visualization (▶ Fig. 39.4). Again, in case of complete dissection of the ligament, fat is prolapsing into the carpal canal. After surgery, the skin incision is sutured with single stitches and the wrist is bandaged with only slight compression. Immobilization of the wrist is not recommended.

Surgical Outcome

Postoperatively, routine follow-up examinations are performed at the first postoperative day and 2 to 3 months after surgery. Sutures are removed after 1 week. A neurophysiologic follow-up evaluation is recommended after 2 to 3 months but often refused by the patient when significant clinical benefit is seen.

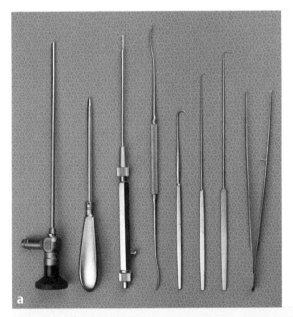
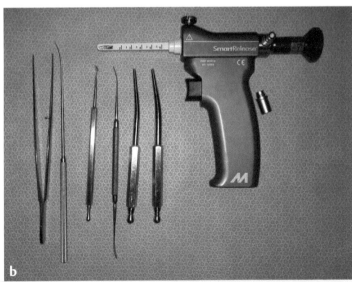

Fig. 39.2 Set for biportal endoscopic carpal tunnel surgery with 30-degree optic, slotted working cannula with trocar, hook knife, dissector and hooks, and microsurgical forceps from left to right **(a)**. Set for monoportal endoscopic surgery consisting of the pistol-shaped blade assembly (right side), various dissectors, and hamate finders, left to right **(b)**.

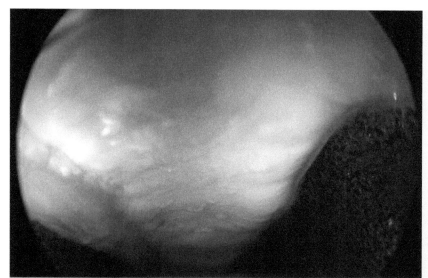

Fig. 39.3 Endoscopic view of the transverse ligament's end (*arrow*) with the 30-degree optic from the distal portal in the proximal direction.

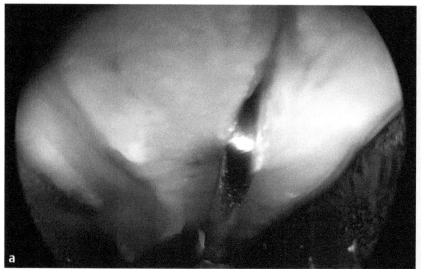

Fig. 39.4 Stepwise dissection of the transverse ligament with the hook knife inserted at the proximal port (**a**). Fat prolapsing into the working channel indicates complete dissection of the transverse ligament (**b**).

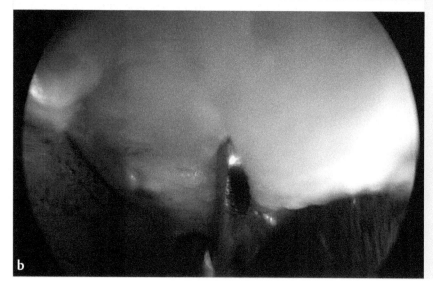

The surgical outcome is very favorable with a high success rate regarding subsidence of pain and improvement of hypoesthesia. In a series of 583 hands of 491 patients who were operated on with ECTR in the authors' former and current departments, the patients reported subsidence of the typical nocturnal pain in 558/583 (96%) cases. In 42/583 (7%) of the operated hands, the patients had pillar pain at the time of follow-up examination, which subsided thereafter. The overall complication rate was 3% (18/583). A permanent neurological deficit has not been observed so far. A transient nerve contusion of the digital nerve was observed in two patients (0.3%) and subsided in the follow-up examination. In 5/583 cases (0.8%), endoscopic surgery had to be switched to open surgery including 1 case that had to be switched due to arterial bleeding and open inspection of the surgical site. In six other cases (1.0%) of arterial bleeding, the surgery could be continued endoscopically. The postoperative course of these patients was uneventful. A revision with open carpal tunnel release (OCTR) due to incomplete dissection had to be performed in six hands (1%; ▶ Table 39.1). Two patients complained about pain in the area of the carpal tunnel and were not satisfied, although the typical clinical signs subsided. Magnetic resonance imaging (MRI) scans, X-rays, and bone scintigrams were normal and electrophysiological examination improved. In all, these results go in line with the present literature regarding the success and complication rate.

39.1.2 Advantages of Endoscopic Approach for the Case Illustration

In the present case, there were no contraindications of ECTR because the patient was fully collaborating. The extent of flexion and extension in the wrist was not reduced in spite of a large-sized hand. Thus, for a supposedly quick time of recovery biportal ECTR was planned since dissection of adjacent tissue and the total wound area can be reduced with the endoscopic approach. Although the wrist was quite sturdy, identification of the median nerve via small incision as well as insertion of the dissector and the slotted cannula was possible without any problems. The end of the transverse carpal ligament could be identified easily prior to dissection of the ligament. The postoperative course was uneventful with complete pain relief at

time of removal of the sutures and only mild residual hypoesthesia. The small skin incision of the endoscopic technique enabled a quick recovery and early return to daily activities by the time of suture removal.

39.1.3 Disadvantages of the Open Approach

If potential contraindications are excluded, ECTR is preferred to OCTR due to the supposed faster time of recovery and the earlier return to work. After standard OCTR, patients complain frequently about scar tenderness even several months after surgery, although CTS symptoms have gone completely. Reasons may lay in the extended palmar incision used in OCTR. The larger incision of the skin and subcutaneous tissue increases the risk of postoperative pain in general as well as injury to the palmar branch of the median nerve with consecutive development of a neuroma. Additionally, the use of the hand (and the wrist) might foster repetitive stress to the scar resulting in a hypersensitive or even hypertrophic scar.

39.1.4 Patient Selection

In the authors' department, the decision to perform surgical carpal tunnel release is based on several findings. The most important factor is the clinical presentation with a typical history of brachialgia paresthetica nocturna that improves by shaking, rubbing, or kneading of the hands. Permanent neurological deficits like thenar atrophy or numbness require a timely surgical therapy. Electrophysiological tests measuring dmL and/or sensory nerve velocities may be helpful to establish the diagnosis. They are mandatory to assess remaining or new complaints during the follow-up.

A period of conservative treatment may be performed in cases without permanent neurological deficits. Hormonal factors, such as pregnancy or severe unbalanced diabetes, should be taken into account prior to surgery. However, if the conservative management does not yield to an improvement of symptoms, surgery, usually ECTR, is recommended.

The majority of CTS patients presented to our outpatient clinic are successfully treated endoscopically. Basically, the patient's age or a large size of the hand (as in the presented example) is not an exclusion factor per se for ECTR. The ability of (hyper)extension of the wrist should be taken into account for the safe insertion of the endoscopic device into the carpal canal. If the extension of the wrist is impaired, OCTR should be preferred.

The patient should be able to collaborate during the surgical procedure in order to avoid complications by injuring the median nerve. For example, median nerve pain may occur if the nerve prolapses into the slotted cannula during a biportal procedure. Therefore, ECTR should be performed under local anesthesia allowing a continuous feedback by vocalizing uncommon pain.

The following are considered exclusion criteria for ECTR:
- Recurrent CTS.
- History of wrist trauma or wrist deformation (rheumatoid disease).
- Anatomic variations.
- Shunt arms.[1]

Table 39.1 The surgical outcome of endoscopic carpal tunnel release in a series of 583 hands of the authors' department shows a high success rate (a) and a similar complication rate compared to open techniques (b)

	Number (n = 583)	(%)
(a) Outcome		
Complete subsidence of nocturnal pain	558	96
Pillar pain	42	7
Switch to open surgery	5	0.8
Overall complication rate	19	3
(b) Complication		
Transient nerve contusion digital nerve	2	0.3
Switch to open surgery	5	0.8
Arterial bleeding	6	1.2
Incomplete release of the carpal tunnel	6	1

39.1.5 Complication Avoidance

Besides an appropriate selection of patients, success and failure of ECTR are highly dependent on the surgeons' experience. Thus, it is important to perform a significant number of carpal tunnel surgeries per year when using the endoscopic technique. In the authors' view, the endoscopic procedure should be reserved for surgeons with a profound experience in open as well as in endoscopic carpal tunnel surgery. If the surgeon does not perform neuroendoscopic procedures regularly, technique and function of the equipment should be trained repeatedly.

Several pitfalls can occur intraoperatively that should be borne in mind:

- If the median nerve prolapses into the working channel, the trocar often has to be reinserted and the cannula has to be turned 360 degrees in the direction of the median nerve to roll it away. In some cases, the slotted cannula and trocar have to be removed and positioned again. However, afterward it is almost always possible to proceed with the endoscopic technique.
- To avoid damage of the arterial volar arch during biportal surgical technique, the exit portal should be placed as close as possible to the distal end of the transverse ligament.
- Insertion of the trocar or the blade endoscope unit in the direction of the fourth finger is of utmost importance to avoid aiming too medially with a risk of damaging the median nerve.
- Despite the small incisions in ECTR, postoperative bleeding should be minimized by external compression at the end of the procedure.
- Modern HD camera system and Hopkins rod-lens optics provide excellent imaging and are strongly recommended.

39.1.6 Technical Nuances

Dissection of the transverse carpal ligament in an endoscopic fashion was introduced by Okutsu and colleagues in 1987.[2] They applied a self-constructed endoscope consisting of a transparent synthetic sheath and a 30-degree optic.[2,3] Since then, several different instrument sets and different surgical techniques have evolved. Today, extrabursal biportal and monoportal techniques are commonly used. A frequently used biportal—or dual-portal technique—is the Chow technique, which was introduced in 1989 as a "transbursal" procedure. Due to the frequent occurrence of transient ulnar nerve lesion, the transbursal approach has been abandoned. Since 1991, extrabursal dissection of the transverse carpal ligament has been performed commonly with no significant risk of ulnar nerve lesion.[4] In the past years, numerous studies have shown excellent results with different endoscopic techniques.[5,6,7,8,9,10,11,12,13]

Whether the mono- or biportal technique is chosen depends on the preference of the performing surgeon. The monoportal ECTR might have the advantage of an easier avoidance of volar arch damage because the volar arch is distal to the ligament. Additionally, it has been stated that the monoportal technique is easier to learn compared to the biportal technique due to the fixed-blade endoscope unit that leads to an easy handling compared to the "bimanual" dual-portal technique. If the surgeon is used to the "bimanual" handling of the dual-portal device, the technique allows a high-quality visualization combined with a very small cannula slot.

However, so far, no evidence for the superiority of one of the endoscopic techniques has been shown.

In the authors' department, Chow's biportal endoscopic technique is preferred due to the small size of the trocar and slotted cannula, the possibility to work without a tourniquet, and the quality of the endoscopic view.

39.1.7 Literature Review/Evidence in Favor of Endoscopic Approach

In the past years, a large number of studies regarding effectiveness, safety, patient satisfaction, and cost-effectiveness for ECTR have been published.[4,5,6,7,14,15] To date, there is no consensus regarding the optimal surgical treatment for CTS. The main reason is the marked heterogeneity of studies having different study designs, different outcome assessments, and surgical techniques varying in details according to the surgeon's background and experience, especially in using endoscopic armamentarium. Thus, conclusions drawn from studies and reviews are limited by the high risk of bias.

Successful results of ECTR have been presented in numerous reports.[4,8,14,16,17,18] Depending on the study, the success rates range from 92 to 98%, including follow-up periods of up to 8 years.[4,17,19] Recurrence rates vary between 0 and 10%.[19] Especially studies published before 2001 often showed better results and a lower complication rate with OCTR compared to ECTR.[20] In general, newer studies revealed no significant differences between both techniques. This was confirmed in several recently published meta-analyses and systematic reviews.

In 2015, Zuo et al published a meta-analysis including 13 randomized controlled clinical studies.[21] In 1,315 cases with CTS, endoscopic or OCTR was performed. In all, success rate in terms of symptom relief and recovery as well as the complication rate did not differ significantly. In this review, reversible postoperative nerve lesions were regarded as higher in patients operated on with ECTR compared to patients operated on with OCTR (relative risk [RR] = 2.38; $p = 0.05$). The rate of postoperative hand pain was significantly lower after ECTR compared to the open techniques (RR = 0.73; 95% CI; $p = 0.02$).

In contrast, in a meta-analysis published by Sayegh et al in 2015, 21 randomized-controlled clinical studies (1,859 hands) were analyzed. It was shown that endoscopically treated patients showed similar symptom relief, but a significantly better recovery of grip strength ($p = 0.04$) and pinch strength ($p < 0.001$) in the early postoperative period. Further, endoscopically treated patients showed a lower risk of scar tenderness ($p = 0.005$) and a similar risk of pillar pain and reoperation. Usually, these patients returned to work earlier ($p < 0.001$). Sayegh et al concluded that ECTR might appeal to patients who require an early return to work and activities.[22]

In another large review published by Vasiliadis et al in 2015, the authors included randomized controlled clinical trials comparing ECTR to standard OCTR or OCTR using a modified incision.[20] In all, 27 studies were included. Besides analysis of risks and safety of the endoscopic techniques compared to other surgical techniques, the producing functional recovery, that is, return to work and return to daily activities, was assessed.

Regarding the complication rate, ECTR resulted on average in a lower rate of minor complications when compared with OCTR.[20] The summary effect indicated that ECTR is associated with an average relative decrease in odds of minor complication of 50% compared to OCTR. Transient nerve problems in terms of numbness and paresthesia were found in endoscopic procedures more frequently, whereas open techniques resulted more often in wound problems such as infection, hypertrophic scarring, or scar tenderness, but differences did not show significance.[20] However, major complications and rates of recurrence of symptoms were comparable. Analysis of convalescence showed that return to work was on average 10 days earlier after ECTR.[20]

In all, the literature gives evidence for preference of the endoscopic technique:

• Very high success rates and low recurrence rate on long-term follow-up.[4,17,19]
• Less postoperative hand pain.[22]
• Better recovery of grip and pinch strength in the early postoperative period, less scar tenderness, and earlier return to work.[21]
• Less minor complications.[20]

Since there is no doubt that a smaller scar and a smaller wound area result in less postoperative discomfort and superior aesthetic results, the endoscopic technique shows distinct advantages even if the long-term nerve function recovery is equal with endoscopic and open techniques. The most important issue, as always, is that the surgeon has to have the knowledge and the skills to perform an endoscopic approach safely! If so, this is the preferred surgical technique!

References

[1] Okutsu I, Hamanaka I, Tanabe T, Takatori Y, Ninomiya S. Complete endoscopic carpal canal decompression. Am J Orthop. 1996; 25(5):365–368

[2] Okutsu I, Ninomiya S, Natsuyama M, et al. Subcutaneous operation and examination under the universal endoscope. Nippon Seikeigeka Gakkai Zasshi. 1987; 61(5):491–498

[3] Assmus HAG, Dombert T. Die Kompressionssyndrome des N. medianus aus Nervenkompressionssyndrome. Dresden: Steinkopff-Verlag; 1999

[4] Chow JC. Endoscopic carpal tunnel release. Clin Sports Med. 1996; 15(4):769–784

[5] Agee JM, McCarroll HR, Jr, Tortosa RD, Berry DA, Szabo RM, Peimer CA. Endoscopic release of the carpal tunnel: a randomized prospective multicenter study. J Hand Surg Am. 1992; 17(6):987–995

[6] Atroshi I, Johnsson R, Ornstein E. Endoscopic carpal tunnel release: prospective assessment of 255 consecutive cases. J Hand Surg [Br]. 1997; 22(1):42–47

[7] Boeckstyns ME, Sørensen AI. Does endoscopic carpal tunnel release have a higher rate of complications than open carpal tunnel release? An analysis of published series. J Hand Surg [Br]. 1999; 24(1):9–15

[8] Chow JC. Endoscopic release of the carpal ligament for carpal tunnel syndrome: long-term results using the Chow technique. Arthroscopy. 1999; 15(4):417–421

[9] Erhard L, Ozalp T, Citron N, Foucher G. Carpal tunnel release by the Agee endoscopic technique. Results at 4 year follow-up. J Hand Surg [Br]. 1999; 24(5):583–585

[10] Ferdinand RD, MacLean JG. Endoscopic versus open carpal tunnel release in bilateral carpal tunnel syndrome. A prospective, randomised, blinded assessment. J Bone Joint Surg Br. 2002; 84(3):375–379

[11] Mackenzie DJ, Hainer R, Wheatley MJ. Early recovery after endoscopic vs. short-incision open carpal tunnel release. Ann Plast Surg. 2000; 44(6):601–604

[12] Thoma A, Veltri K, Haines T, Duku E. A systematic review of reviews comparing the effectiveness of endoscopic and open carpal tunnel decompression. Plast Reconstr Surg. 2004; 113(4):1184–1191

[13] Trumble TE, Diao E, Abrams RA, Gilbert-Anderson MM. Single-portal endoscopic carpal tunnel release compared with open release: a prospective, randomized trial. J Bone Joint Surg Am. 2002; 84-A(7):1107–1115

[14] Brief R, Brief LP. Endoscopic carpal tunnel release: report of 146 cases. Mt Sinai J Med. 2000; 67(4):274–277

[15] Macdermid JC, Richards RS, Roth JH, Ross DC, King GJ. Endoscopic versus open carpal tunnel release: a randomized trial. J Hand Surg Am. 2003; 28(3):475–480

[16] Filippi R, Reisch R, El-Shki D, Grunert P. Uniportal endoscopic surgery of carpal tunnel syndrome: technique and clinical results. Minim Invasive Neurosurg. 2002; 45(2):78–83

[17] Keiner D, Gaab MR, Schroeder HW, Oertel J. Long-term follow-up of dual-portal endoscopic release of the transverse ligament in carpal tunnel syndrome: an analysis of 94 cases. Neurosurgery. 2009; 64(1):131–137, discussion 137–138

[18] McNally SA, Hales PF. Results of 1245 endoscopic carpal tunnel decompressions. Hand Surg. 2003; 8(1):111–116

[19] Jimenez DF, Gibbs SR, Clapper AT. Endoscopic treatment of carpal tunnel syndrome: a critical review. J Neurosurg. 1998; 88(5):817–826

[20] Vasiliadis HS, Nikolakopoulou A, Shrier I, et al. Endoscopic and open release similarly safe for the treatment of carpal tunnel syndrome. A systematic review and meta-analysis. PLoS One. 2015; 10(12):e0143683

[21] Zuo D, Zhou Z, Wang H, et al. Endoscopic versus open carpal tunnel release for idiopathic carpal tunnel syndrome: a meta-analysis of randomized controlled trials. J Orthop Surg. 2015; 10:12

[22] Sayegh ET, Strauch RJ. Open versus endoscopic carpal tunnel release: a meta-analysis of randomized controlled trials. Clin Orthop Relat Res. 2015; 473(3):1120–1132

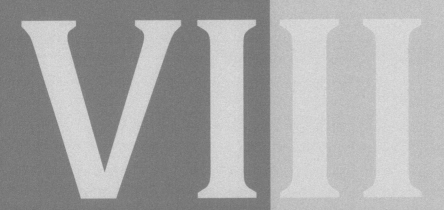

Part VIII

Technology

40 3D Endoscope versus High-Definition 2D Endoscope

Jason Chu and Nelson Oyesiku

Summary

Endoscopes have revolutionized a variety of neurosurgical sub-specialties. Early iterations of the endoscope provided minimal light illumination and higher profiles compared to today's modern endoscopes. In recent decades, improvements in chip technology have afforded the development of stereoscopic visualization via endoscopes. In this chapter, we discuss the advantages and disadvantages of 3D endoscopes versus traditional modern 2D endoscopes for neurosurgical applications.

Keywords: endoscopic, skull base, 3D, 2D, endonasal

40.1 Introduction

Since its inception, the endoscope has striven to improve surgical visualization. Although endoscopy has been incorporated into several surgical specialties, the field of neuroendoscopy is in its relative infancy. Early pioneers of the field include Walter Dandy, William Mixter, and Gerard Guiot, but it was not until the mid-1960s and the development of the modern endoscope by Harold Hopkins and Karl Storz did endoscopy become a viable, minimally invasive option for neurosurgical procedures.[1,2] Advancements of optical and video technology over the last half century have not only improved endoscopic image quality, but also led neurosurgeons to refine the endoscopic technique for skull base, intraventricular, and spinal procedures. Overall, this has resulted in excellent clinical outcomes. Within the United States, the growing popularity of neuroendoscopy is evident in a progressive shift from microscopic to endoscopic transsphenoidal approaches (TSA) for sellar lesions between 2003 and 2013.[3]

Compared to microscopy, the endoscope produces a 2D image and the lack of depth perception is considered a major disadvantage by critics of this technique.[4] The recent development of 3D endoscopes has attempted to mitigate this shortfall. Advancements in imaging technology have also led to the evolution of 2D high-definition (HD) endoscopes. One major debate among neuroendoscopists is the question: can 2D HD imaging compensate for the lack of stereoscopic vision during neuroendoscopic procedures?

40.2 The Evolution of the 3D Endoscope

Binocular vision is required for stereopsis, where differences in viewing angle between the left and right eye result in subtle disparities of the observed object (▶ Fig. 40.1). These differences are processed and interpreted by the brain to generate an appreciation of shape, size, and depth.[5] Early 3D endoscopes attempted to recreate human stereoscopy with the use of bichannel systems that delivered two slightly different images (one for each eye) to the surgeon. This was accomplished using a dual-channel optical endoscope connected to two cameras. However, the use of two different cameras often created a

discrepancy in image quality, color, brightness, and optical distortion, as well as several unwelcomed side effects, such as headache, dizziness, and eyestrain. Moreover, a large scope camera complex hindered surgical dexterity. An alternative was a "dual chip on the tip," in which two video chips are mounted at the end of an endoscope and generate two different digital images. Although this avoided optical distortion, the similar disadvantages of headache and ocular fatigue were present. Additionally, this system was unable to create a convincing 3D effect due to the close proximity of the two chips.[6]

In 1993, Becker et al reported the use of a "shutter" technique to generate a 3D image.[7] This endoscope had the advantage of being a single-channel system and utilized a rapidly alternating shutter to divide a single image into two images with slightly different angles. However, this mechanism relies on a camera in constant motion as well as an on-screen flicker that produced similar side effects as those seen with dual-channel systems.[6] Similarly, the produced 3D effect was relatively weak.

The most recent advancement in 3D endoscopy has been the development of "insect eye" technology and has been patented by Visionsense Ltd. (New York, NY) in 1996.[1,6] A 3D image is created with a dual-pupil imaging objective placed at the end of the endoscope. This objective is able to separate images into a left and a right eye channel, which are then focused onto a microarray of image sensor, similar to the compound eye of an insect. The data are then processed and digitally reconstructed. Images corresponding to the left and right channels are projected and overlaid on a display. The viewer wears polarized 3D glasses to filter the left and right channels into their respective eyes to generate a final 3D image (▶ Fig. 40.2, ▶ Fig. 40.3). The Visionsense 3D system has been approved by the U.S. Food and Drug Administration, as well as by Conformité Européenne (CE) in Europe.

The latest iteration of the Visionsense system (third generation, VSiii System; ▶ Fig. 40.4) was introduced in 2014. One of the major upgrades of this system is the ability to produce 3D images in full 1080p HD resolution (1,920 × 1,080 pixels). The 3.3-mm digital sensor is contained within a single-channel endoscope with a 4- or 5.5-mm outer diameter. The endoscope field of view (FOV) is 75 or 105 degrees with a depth of field between 15 and 70 mm. Endoscopes are available in both 0- and 30-degree viewing angles and the image quality is preserved by an autofocus mechanism within the endoscope. Images are displayed onto a 24-inch LED monitor and the viewer wears lightweight, polarized glasses for stereoscopic vision. In comparison to the previous iteration of the Visionsense endoscope (VSii), the VSiii provides a smaller endoscope, higher resolution image (standard definition [SD] [720p] vs. HD [1080p]; ▶ Fig. 40.5), and an improved console control unit for ease of use to the surgeon. Paralleling that of television technology, we anticipate the next generation of the 3D endoscope to contain ultra-HD resolution (4K/UHD, 3,840 × 2,160 pixels) to further enhance surgical visualization.

Recent systematic reviews have demonstrated the growing popularity of the 3D endoscope in clinical practice and is also reflected in the increasing number of publications over the last

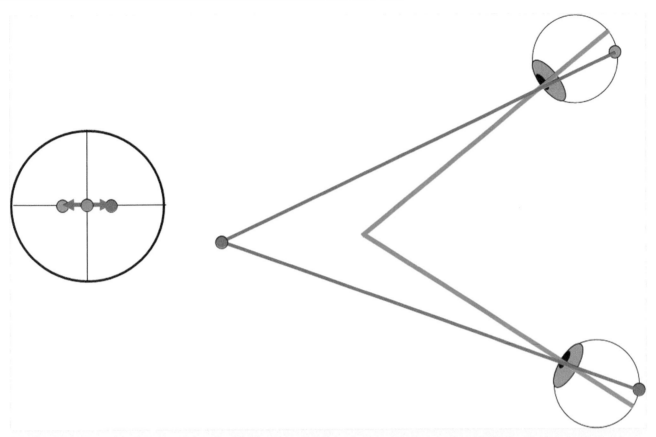

Fig. 40.1 Binocular vision is required for stereopsis. Differences in viewing angle between the left and right eye result in subtle disparities of the observed object. The interpreted differences lead to depth perception. (Adapted from http://www.visionsense.com/.)

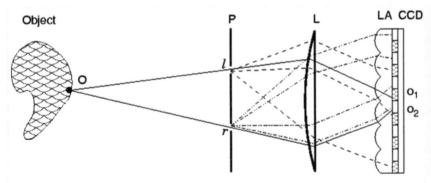

Fig. 40.2 The Visionsense Ltd. "insect eye" technology. Light from an object (O) passes through a dual-pupil imaging objective (P) and split left (l) and right (r). Light is then focused through a lens (L) onto a lenticular microarray of lenses (LA) in front of a charged coupled device (CCD) microchip. Therefore, light from the object is generated twice (O_1, left; O_2, right), and the distance between O_1 and O_2 represents the disparity between the left and right views of the object. The microchip processes these images to generate stereoscopic vision for the user. (Adapted from Tabaee et al.21)

5 years.[8,9] As the popularity of 3D endoscopy increases and becomes more widespread among clinicians, we expect this number to continue to increase.

40.3 Advantages and Disadvantages of a 3D Endoscopic Approach

The most significant and defining advantage of the 3D system is the preservation of stereoscopic vision. Several studies have demonstrated the importance of stereopsis in the understanding and interpretation of visual imagery in humans, especially when the situation becomes increasingly complex.[10] Wickens et al found that human subjects were able to more rapidly interpret an object's surface characteristics when presented

with 3D imagery compared to 2D and noted that stereopsis conferred a greater understanding of global spatial relationships.[11]

Visuomotor studies have demonstrated the importance of depth perception for tasks that require accurate hand–eye coordination. Servos et al examined the differences between binocular and monocular vision for multiple grasping tasks in human subjects. Under monocular vision, subjects not only underestimated the distance of the object, but also had significant delays in movement initiation, slower movement velocities, smaller grip apertures, and longer time to task completion when compared to binocular vision.[12] From their data, the authors also suggested that binocular vision may play a role in movement planning, programming, and accuracy of execution. Similarly, another study suggested that cues from binocular vision are

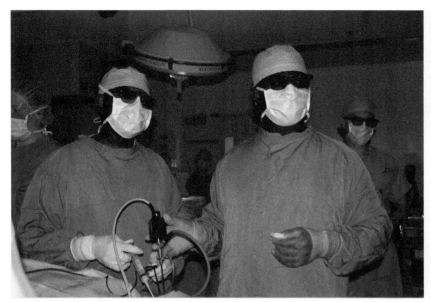

Fig. 40.3 The Visionsense VSiii in the operating room. The two surgeons are wearing polarized glasses that allow for depth perception. We typically utilize two surgeons ("2 nostrils-4 hands" technique): the endoscope is held by an assistant and is lightweight, while the primary surgeon is free for bimanual dissection.

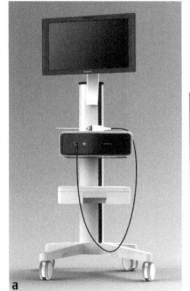

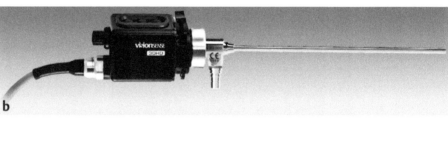

Fig. 40.4 The latest iteration of the Visionsense system: the VSiii, a full high-definition, 1080p system. **(a)** The console control unit that is made up of a 24-inch LED display, a computer, and the endoscope interface. **(b)** The VSiii endoscope. (Adapted from http://www.visionsense.com/.)

heavily utilized for visuomotor control and the placement of objects in a 3D space.[13]

From a clinical perspective, the importance of depth perception, understanding of anatomical relationships in 3D space, and accurate hand–eye coordination are paramount in neurosurgical procedures. This is especially true for those procedures that utilize the endoscope. For example, the TSA to the sella utilizes a narrow corridor that prevents the use of large instrument or excessive sweeping movements. Juxtaposed to the sella are the carotid arteries, cavernous sinus, the optic nerves, and chiasm; exact instrument placement is required to prevent injury to them. Therefore, it is imperative that the surgeon have proper visualization of the sellar anatomy, a true appreciation of the spatial relationships of critical neurovascular structures in this area, and the ability for precise instrument manipulation through the limited corridor of the nares.

Some disadvantages of the 3D systems include headaches or eye fatigue when viewing 3D images for extended periods of time, disorientation and nausea, a reduced FOV compared to traditional 2D scopes, higher equipment and maintenance costs, the need for the surgeon to wear 3D glasses, and red color saturation on the displayed image.[14]

40.4 Advantages and Disadvantages of a 2D HD Endoscopic Approach

Modern 2D endoscopes utilize HD video with superior image quality and color distinction when compared to previous generation. An image from SD endoscopes contain around 400,000 pixels, whereas an HD image contains about 2,000,000 pixels.[15,]

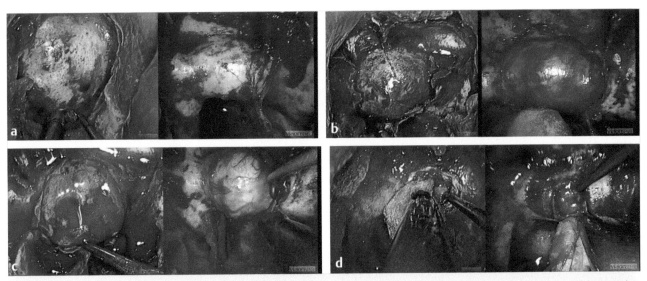

Fig. 40.5 A comparison of the Visionsense VSii (720p, left images) and VSiii (1080p, right images). **(a)** The sellar floor via a transsphenoidal approach. **(b)** Exposure of the sellar dura. **(c)** A pituitary macroadenoma. **(d)** A pituitary microadenoma. The high-definition images produced by the VSiii allow for better appreciation of the anatomy and distinction of the surgical pathology. Original images were captured in 3D and converted to 2D.

[16,17] There is also a difference in aspect ratio between HD (16:9) and SD (4:3) allowing for an expanded viewing field in HD.[17] The importance of image quality cannot be understated in endoscopic surgery and HD imaging allows the operator to better visualize and identify anatomical structures during the operation.[16] Some authors believe the resolution of HD imaging can rival the optics of the operating microscope.[17]

In the case of endoscopic pituitary surgery, Yoneoka et al investigated the effect of HD neuroendoscopy on the surgeon's ability to identify normal adenohypophysis, infundibulum, and neurohypophysis, and distinguish it from sellar pathology, including a series of pituitary adenomas and Rathke's cleft cysts.[18] The authors suggested that HD imaging allowed surgeons to better recognize the plane of dissection between normal and abnormal tissue, note the differences in color between the anterior and posterior gland, appreciate the changes in color of the entire gland after decompression, and, in conclusion, that the additive effects of advantages led to favorable results in their series of patients.

Other advantages of 2D endoscopes include angled endoscopes that allow the operator to "look around the corner." At present, the 3D endoscope is limited to 0 and 30 degrees, while 2D HD scopes are available with up to a 70-degree viewing angles (for the purposes of most neurosurgical procedures). More importantly, a recent study demonstrated that the previous generation Visionsense 3D system (VSii system) had a 52% reduction in FOV when compared to a traditional 2D HD scope (Karl Storz Hopkins II, Stryker HD camera).[19] This change in FOV is an important detail that should be recognized by practitioners who use both 2D and 3D systems and switch between the two during a single operation.

Several prototype 2D HD endoscopes have also been developed and tested. The digiCAMeleon (Karl Storz) is a multidirectional videoendoscope tested by Cavallo et al in a cadaveric model for endoscopic endonasal, intraventricular, and supraorbital approaches.[20] This unique videoendoscope contains an "all-in-one" thin cable for all electronic data and lighting and only weighs 215 g. The tip of the endoscope contains a digital sensor that can also change the direction of view between 0, 30, 45, and 70 degrees at the discretion of the operator. An autohorizon feature also enables the operator to set and maintain a viewing orientation such that rotation of the endoscope does not affect the orientation of the image on screen. Although tested in a cadaveric model, the authors concluded that this steerable, multidirectional, and ergonomic unit represents the next evolution in the HD videoendoscope technology. Along similar lines, Friedman et al[21] recently prototyped a HD flexible endoscope in a patient with a tectal mass and obstructive hydrocephalus; this unit was prototyped for a combined biopsy of the mass and endoscopic third ventriculostomy (the ETV was done using a standard, rigid endoscope). The flexible endoscope utilizes a HD camera on a chip, where there is a complementary metal oxide semiconductor (CMOS) chip at the tip of the endoscope. This chip directly converts optical images into digital images at the tip of the endoscope and minimizes the need for large, delicate fiberoptic cables. The authors believed that the increased range of motion and enhanced visualization provided by the flexible endoscope was a valuable tool, especially when combined with HD imaging, for intraventricular procedures. Given that 2D endoscopy is the current standard, it is likely that future technological innovations in endoscopy will reach the commercial market in 2D before a 3D counterpart is produced.

The main disadvantage of the 2D endoscope is that it does not provide an accurate sense of depth. With traditional 2D endoscopes, an estimate of depth perception is obtained with a combination of motion parallax and haptic feedback. Changes in object texture and shadowing as the endoscope is in motion give an indirect sense of depth. However, this requires that the endoscope be in a constant yaw, pitch, or rolling motion that can cause disorientation and difficulty with hand–eye coordination. The use of monocular cues can lead to inaccuracies in instrument placement, due to disparities between the observed instrument position on the screen and its actual location that may contribute to surgical complications during 2D endoscopic transsphenoidal surgery. In fact, some authors believe the lack of depth perception to be such a significant disadvantage that they endorse the classic microscopic approach as the "gold standard" for the TSA.[4]

40.5 Comparison of 2D HD versus 3D Endoscopy in Neurosurgery

Much of the current literature that compares 2D HD to 3D neuroendoscopy has been in transsphenoidal surgery. Tabaee et al was one of the first to report their comparative results of 2D HD to 3D endoscopy in transsphenoidal surgery for sellar lesions.[22] In their series, patients were prospectively treated with 3D SD endoscopy (Visionsense VSii) and retrospectively matched to patients who previously underwent TSA with standard 2D HD endoscopy. The authors found no difference in operative time, extent of resection, and median hospital length of stay between their two groups. Although the goal of the study was not to prove technical superiority, several operators reported improved depth perception and a "more natural feel" to surgery when utilizing the 3D endoscope. This early report suggested that 3D endoscopy was a safe technique and a viable alternative for the TSA.

A more direct comparison between the 2D HD and 3D SD endoscope (Visionsense VSii) was conducted by Fraser et al and they recruited neurosurgeons and skull-base otolaryngologists (both attending physicians and residents) to complete a simulated task in both 2D and 3D.[14] They found that 75% of their participants favored the 3D endoscope and 87.5% felt that 3D visualization assisted with their ability to complete their assigned tasks. Additionally, subjects had improved task speed and efficiency when switching from 2D to 3D. The authors suggested that 3D visualization not only allowed participants to learn the task more efficiently, but also allowed them to improve their performance after becoming familiar with the task. Similar results were seen by Kawanishi et al[23] and Shah et al.[24] Although both studies also utilized simulated TSA environments to complete a task in 2D and 3D, they independently found that users of the 3D endoscope had superior performance than with 2D. Moreover, these studies showed that novice or inexperienced users benefited the most from 3D endoscopy and suggested that it may shorten the learning curve for physicians in training.

In a clinical setting, Felisati et al recruited eight surgeons (two senior ear, nose, and throat [ENT], three junior ENT, one senior neurosurgery, two junior neurosurgery faculty) and asked them to evaluate their experience using 3D endoscopy for endonasal approaches to the anterior skull base in 52 patients.[25] They found that most surgeons, regardless of their previous skill level, were able to effectively adapt to 3D visualization in less than 10 surgical procedures. This is in contrast to the extended learning curve with 2D endoscopy that can range from 10 to 50 procedures before one becomes proficient and able to safely perform a similar procedure.[26,27] The authors reported that the junior surgeons were able to adapt more easily to the 3D system when compared to their senior counterparts. Additionally, the 3D system was also found to be more advantageous with increasing task complexity. Overall, the participants in this study favored the 3D system because of the improved precision in dissecting and a "more secure" feeling imparted by the stereoscopic vision.

An Italian group recently detailed their single-center, 3-year experience with the 3D endoscope (Visionsense VSii) in a series of 104 sellar lesions (83 macroadenomas, 7 microadenomas, 5 Rathke's cleft cysts, and 5 craniopharyngiomas, 2 solitary fibrous tumor, 1 sellar chordoma, and 1 metastasis) and 13 clival chordomas.[28,29] For their sellar lesions, 70% of their patients were noted to have achieved gross total resection at follow-up MRI; this is impressive given that 80% of their patients had a preoperative Knosp grade $\geq$ 2. Moreover, 85% of patients with a preexisting visual field deficit improved at 3-month follow-up. In their subset of functional adenomas, a biochemical remission was achieved in 70 to 80% of patients. Importantly, their complication rate was similar to that previously described with 2D endoscopy: cerebrospinal fluid (CSF) leak = 4.8%; diabetes insipidus (DI)/syndrome of inappropriate antidiuretic hormone (SIADH) = 5.7%; and vascular injury = 1.9%. In their clival chordoma series, gross total resection was achieved in 66.6% and near total resection in 11.2% of their patients. This is consistent with a previously reported complete resection rate between 50 and 80% of cases. Complications were minimal: CSF leaks were present in two patients, one case of a temporary sixth cranial nerve palsy, and no cases of vascular injury. The authors believed that the 3D system offered several advantages that allowed them to have favorable outcomes and highlighted the importance of depth perception when operating on lesions that are millimeters from critical neurovascular structures through a narrow corridor.

One of the largest clinical studies that compared the use of the 2D HD endoscopes to a 3D scope (Visionsense VSii) retrospectively analyzed the results of 160 operations over a 2-year period.[30] The authors observed no difference in overall operative time between the use of 2D and 3D endoscopy; however, one notable finding was that pituitary adenoma resection time was significantly shorter using the 3D endoscope with a difference of nearly 30 minutes when compared to the 2D counterpart. Importantly, the authors also found no differences in intraoperative CSF leak rate, extent of tumor resection, complication rate, or hospital length of stay between the 2D and 3D groups. Their data also showed that novice endoscopy users became accustomed to operating in 3D endoscope quicker than in 2D and suggested that the 3D endoscope offers less of a learning curve with spatial awareness, instrument placement, and microdissection.

These results are in accordance with recent systematic reviews that compared the efficacy of 3D endoscopy to that of 2D. Overall, the literature does not demonstrate a difference in operative factors (operative time, estimated blood loss, intraoperative CSF leak, headache, eyestrain, fatigue), clinical outcomes (extent of tumor resection, length of hospital stay), or complications (readmission rate, meningitis, postoperative CSF leak) when comparing 2D to 3D endoscopy.[8,9] Some of the main disadvantages of the 3D endoscope included poorer image quality as well as lack of an angled endoscope. Notable is that the majority of the current literature compared an older generation, SD 3D endoscope (Visionsense VSii) to a 2D HD endoscope. With the introduction of the 3D HD endoscope, a more direct comparison on the effect of 3D can be made in future studies without differences in image resolution as a confounding factor. Nonetheless, most authors agreed that even 3D SD enabled the operator to better understand the surgical anatomy, had a shorter learning curve for novice users, and was surgically efficacious when compared to 2D HD endoscopy.

At the moment, the current literature consists mainly of retrospective studies with low level of evidence. Although there appears to be no significant difference between 2D and 3D endoscopy, there are not enough data to suggest the superiority of one modality of endoscopy over the other. It is clear that prospective and randomized studies are needed in the future to better address this question.

40.6 The 3D High-Definition Endoscope

The 3D HD endoscope was developed to address one of the main disadvantages of previous 3D systems: a low image resolution. There is currently limited literature regarding the use of the 3D HD endoscope in neurosurgery given the recent implementation of this technology; for example, the HD Visionsense VSiii system was first unveiled in 2014.

One early report compared the use of 2D versus 3D and SD versus HD endoscopy in a randomized study that involved naïve surgeons in a simulated environment.[31] The authors found that 3D allowed users to complete tasks significantly faster than 2D, and HD images enabled improved accuracy compared to SD. The authors suggested that 3D and HD have differing but complementary effects and neither 3D nor HD alone could compensate for the other. Although a preclinical study, they provide convincing evidence that a 3D HD endoscope could succeed in neurosurgical procedures. Similarly, Ogino-Nishimura et al directly compared a 3D HD endoscope (Shinko Optical) to the 2D HD endoscope for endoscopic sinus and skull base surgery in cadavers.[32] In this study, 73 surgeons (63 otolaryngologists and 10 neurosurgeons, mean surgical experience between 14 and 15 years) were surveyed and nearly 90% of participants stated that the 3D HD system provided a better understanding of the anatomy over 2D HD endoscopy.

Nassimizadeh et al was the first clinical report of a 3D HD endoscope (Visionsense VSiii) in Europe.[33] In their series, the author compared the 3D HD endoscope ($n = 1$) to both a 3D SD endoscope ($n = 4$) and their previous experience with a 2D HD scope. Although they did not specifically comment on surgical outcomes, the authors noted that image quality of the 3D HD endoscope was not only comparable to conventional 2D HD endoscopy but also superior to the 3D SD system. The authors suggested that the 3D HD scope may be especially advantageous as a transitional tool for those that continue to use microscopy for TSA surgery and that the 3D HD endoscope represents the next evolution in endoscopic surgery.

40.7 Senior Author (N.O.)'s Experience

Similar to several other institutions in the United States, our group has transitioned to solely 3D endoscopy for all of our transsphenoidal surgeries. Our first experience was with the SD Visionsense VSii machine in 2009 and our initial experience

comparing the 3D to 2D systems in 58 patients (3D, $n = 26$; 2D, $n = 32$) has been reported.[34] In our hands, we found no significant differences in operative time, surgical blood loss, and mean hospital length of stay between 2D and 3D endoscopy. Additionally, we did not note any differences in postoperative complications, including CSF leaks, short-term endocrine abnormalities, and hospital readmissions. Our findings echo many of the documented advantages of using the 3D system, including stereoscopic vision and decreased learning curve for trainees. We did not experience eyestrain, nausea, disorientation, or other disadvantages reported by other authors. Wearing 3D glasses for the full stereoscopic effect was not bothersome for the surgeons or the operating room support staff.

We recently acquired the 3D HD Visionsense VSiii system in March 2014. Our experience with the VSiii has been positive and parallels the current literature with enhanced visualization and better appreciation of the anatomical relationships that accompany HD imaging. Within our first 3 months with the Visionsense VSiii, we had conducted approximately 40 transsphenoidal surgeries. When compared with our previous Visionsense VSii machine, our results suggested an improvement in operative time (mean OR time 93.4 vs. 146.5 minutes; data not published) and lower rates of intraoperative CSF leak (4.9 vs. 23%; data not published) without any difference in postoperative endocrine complications or readmission rates. As we continue to collect and analyze our data, we expect further advantages of the 3D HD to emerge. As a pituitary center of excellence and with over 2,300 of TSAs, we can confidently say that the 3D HD endoscope has become an integral tool for all of our neuroendoscopic procedures. As 3D technology continues to improve and becomes adopted at more institutions, 3D endoscopy will likely become the new standard of care for pituitary surgery.

40.8 Conclusion

In *The Pituitary Body and Its Disorders*, Harvey Cushing writes: "every step of the procedure must be conducted under the eye of the operator." The endoscope has allowed neurosurgeons to literally fulfill this dogma. The most recent advancement in endoscope technology has been the introduction of the 3D endoscope and current evidence suggests that the 3D scope is a safe tool that carries several advantages, including stereoscopic vision, a better appreciation of surgical anatomy, and a shorter learning curve. The development of the 3D HD endoscope has also addressed the poor image quality of previous 3D systems. Although there are not enough data to suggest superiority (or inferiority) of the 3D endoscope over the current 2D HD endoscope, we believe that the advantages provided by the 3D endoscope outweigh its disadvantages. Future prospective, randomized clinical studies are needed to better verify the efficacy of 3D endoscopy and address the debate between the 3D and 2D endoscopes.

References

[1] Di Ieva A, Tam M, Tschabitscher M, Cusimano MD. A journey into the technical evolution of neuroendoscopy. World Neurosurg. 2014; 82(6):e777–e789

[2] Gandhi CD, Christiano LD, Eloy JA, Prestigiacomo CJ, Post KD. The historical evolution of transsphenoidal surgery: facilitation by technological advances. Neurosurg Focus. 2009; 27(3):E8

[3] Rolston JD, Han SJ, Aghi MK. Nationwide shift from microscopic to endoscopic transsphenoidal pituitary surgery. Pituitary. 2015

[4] Mortini P. Cons: endoscopic endonasal transsphenoidal pituitary surgery is not superior to microscopic transsphenoidal surgery for pituitary adenomas. Endocrine. 2014; 47(2):415–420

[5] Freeman RD. Stereoscopic vision: which parts of the brain are involved? Curr Biol. 1999; 9(16):R610–R613

[6] Szold A. Seeing is believing: visualization systems in endoscopic surgery (video, HDTV, stereoscopy, and beyond). Surg Endosc. 2005; 19(5):730–733

[7] Becker H, Melzer A, Schurr MO, Buess G. 3-D video techniques in endoscopic surgery. Endosc Surg Allied Technol. 1993; 1(1):40–46

[8] Zaidi HA, Zehri A, Smith TR, Nakaji P, Laws ER, Jr. Efficacy of three-dimensional endoscopy for ventral skull base pathology: a systematic review of the literature. World Neurosurg. 2015

[9] Marcus H, Wan Y, Ulrich N, Reisch R. Comparative effectiveness and safety of 3D versus 2D endoscopy in skull base surgery: a systematic review. Innovative Neurosurgery.. 2015; 3(3–4):53–58

[10] Fielder AR, Moseley MJ. Does stereopsis matter in humans? Eye (Lond). 1996; 10(Pt 2):233–238

[11] Wickens CD, Merwin DH, Lin EL. Implications of graphics enhancements for the visualization of scientific data: dimensional integrality, stereopsis, motion, and mesh. Hum Factors. 1994; 36(1):44–61

[12] Servos P, Goodale MA, Jakobson LS. The role of binocular vision in prehension: a kinematic analysis. Vision Res. 1992; 32(8):1513–1521

[13] Knill DC. Reaching for visual cues to depth: the brain combines depth cues differently for motor control and perception. J Vis. 2005; 5(2):103–115

[14] Fraser JF, Allen B, Anand VK, Schwartz TH. Three-dimensional neurostereoendoscopy: subjective and objective comparison to 2D. Minim Invasive Neurosurg. 2009; 52(1):25–31

[15] Liu CY, Wang MY, Apuzzo ML. The physics of image formation in the neuroendoscope. Childs Nerv Syst. 2004; 20(11–12):777–782

[16] Conrad J, Philipps M, Oertel J. High-definition imaging in endoscopic transsphenoidal pituitary surgery. Am J Rhinol Allergy. 2011; 25(1):e13–e17

[17] Schroeder HW, Nehlsen M. Value of high-definition imaging in neuroendoscopy. Neurosurg Rev. 2009; 32(3):303–308, discussion 308

[18] Yoneoka Y, Watanabe N, Okada M, Fujii Y. Observation of the neurohypophysis, pituitary stalk, and adenohypophysis during endoscopic pituitary surgery: demonstrative findings as clues to pituitary-conserving surgery. Acta Neurochir (Wien). 2013; 155(6):1049–1055

[19] Van Gompel JJ, Tabor MH, Youssef AS, et al. Field of view comparison between two-dimensional and three-dimensional endoscopy. Laryngoscope. 2014; 124(2):387–390

[20] Cavallo LM, Di Somma A, Solari D, de Divitiis O, Bracale UM, Cappabianca P. Preliminary experience with a new multidirectional videoendoscope for neuroendoscopic surgical procedures. PLoS One. 2016; 11(1):e0147524

[21] Friedman GN, Grannan BL, Nahed BV, Codd PJ. Initial experience with high-definition camera-on-a-chip flexible endoscopy for intraventricular neurosurgery. World Neurosurg. 2015; 84(6):2053–2058

[22] Tabaee A, Anand VK, Fraser JF, Brown SM, Singh A, Schwartz TH. Three-dimensional endoscopic pituitary surgery. Neurosurgery. 2009; 64(5) Suppl 2:288–293, discussion 294–295

[23] Kawanishi Y, Fujimoto Y, Kumagai N, et al. Evaluation of two- and three-dimensional visualization for endoscopic endonasal surgery using a novel stereoendoscopic system in a novice: a comparison on a dry laboratory model. Acta Neurochir (Wien). 2013; 155(9):1621–1627

[24] Shah RN, Leight WD, Patel MR, et al. A controlled laboratory and clinical evaluation of a three-dimensional endoscope for endonasal sinus and skull base surgery. Am J Rhinol Allergy. 2011; 25(3):141–144

[25] Felisati G, Pipolo C, Maccari A, Cardia A, Revay M, Lasio GB. Transnasal 3D endoscopic skull base surgery: questionnaire-based analysis of the learning curve in 52 procedures. Eur Arch Otorhinolaryngol. 2013; 270(8):2249–2253

[26] Snyderman C, Kassam A, Carrau R, Mintz A, Gardner P, Prevedello DM. Acquisition of surgical skills for endonasal skull base surgery: a training program. Laryngoscope. 2007; 117(4):699–705

[27] O'Malley BW, Jr, Grady MS, Gabel BC, et al. Comparison of endoscopic and microscopic removal of pituitary adenomas: single-surgeon experience and the learning curve. Neurosurg Focus. 2008; 25(6):E10

[28] Pennacchietti V, Garzaro M, Grottoli S, et al. 3D Endoscopic endonasal approach and outcomes in sellar lesions: a single-center experience of 104 cases. World Neurosurg. 2016

[29] Garzaro M, Zenga F, Raimondo L, et al. Three-dimensional endoscopy in transnasal transsphenoidal approach to clival chordomas. Head Neck. 2016; 38 Suppl 1:E1814–E1819

[30] Barkhoudarian G, Del Carmen Becerra Romero A, Laws ER. Evaluation of the 3-dimensional endoscope in transsphenoidal surgery. Neurosurgery. 2013; 73(1) Suppl Operative:ons74–ons78, discussion ons78–ons79

[31] Marcus HJ, Hughes-Hallett A, Cundy TP, et al. Comparative effectiveness of 3-dimensional vs 2-dimensional and high-definition vs standard-definition neuroendoscopy: a preclinical randomized crossover study. Neurosurgery. 2014; 74(4):375–380, discussion 380–381

[32] Ogino-Nishimura E, Nakagawa T, Sakamoto T, Ito J. Efficacy of three-dimensional endoscopy in endonasal surgery. Auris Nasus Larynx. 2015; 42(3):203–207

[33] Nassimizadeh A, Muzaffar SJ, Nassimizadeh M, Beech T, Ahmed SK. Three-dimensional hand-to-gland combat: the future of endoscopic surgery? J Neurol Surg Rep. 2015; 76(2):e200–e204

[34] Kari E, Oyesiku NM, Dadashev V, Wise SK. Comparison of traditional 2-dimensional endoscopic pituitary surgery with new 3-dimensional endoscopic technology: intraoperative and early postoperative factors. Int Forum Allergy Rhinol. 2012; 2(1):2–8

41 Flexible versus Rigid Neuroendoscopy

Leonardo Rangel-Castilla

Summary

Neuroendoscopy is becoming an independent field from neurosurgery. The goals of neuroendoscope include diagnostic (direct visualization), therapeutic (fenestration, resection) and assisted (microsurgery). There are two different types of neuroendoscopes, rigid and flexible. Rigid endoscopy has been used for skull base and intraventricular pathologies, where as flexible is almost exclusively used on intraventricular diseases. Thanks to the recently developed high-definition videoscopes (chip-on-the-tip), the use of flexible neuroendoscopes is gaining more popularity. Not only the standard procedures (endoscopic third ventriculostomy) can be performed but more advanced ones can be offered (lamina terminalis fenestration, complete choroid plexus coagulation, contralateral ventricular approaches, third and fourth ventricle approaches). The use of a flexible neuroendoscope requires a learning curve. It is very different from a rigid endoscope and I advise neurosurgeons to be familiar with the equipment and practice on cadaver before attempting a procedure.

Keywords: neuroendoscopy, rigid endoscope, flexible endoscope, utility

41.1 Introduction

Modern neuroendoscopy regained momentum in the 1970s thanks to the advances in technology and the improvement in image quality and illumination. There has been a renaissance in the use of neuroendoscopic surgical procedures and the realm of neuroendoscopy has expanded far beyond the endoscopic third ventriculostomy (ETV) and choroid plexus ablation. The use of endoscopes in neurosurgery has three different purposes: *diagnostic*, *therapeutic*, and *assisting*.

Diagnostic neuroendoscopy with or without tissue biopsy has been useful in the management of patient with hydrocephalus of unknown etiology. For example, adult patients with progressive idiopathic aqueductal stenosis have been misdiagnosed with "normal pressure hydrocephalus."

Therapeutic neuroendoscopy refers to endoscopic procedures with a therapeutic goal. Over the last 30 years, intraventricular endoscopic procedures have evolved from simple (ETV, septum pellucidum [SP] fenestration) to more complex procedures (lamina terminalis fenestration, transaqueductal fourth ventricle exploration, and Magendie and Luschka foraminoplasty).

Endoscopic-assisted microsurgery refers to the use of endoscopy as an adjunct to microsurgical procedures such as skull base tumor resections or aneurysms clipping. Some procedures have evolved from endoscopic-assisted to purely endoscopic procedures, such as microvascular decompression for trigeminal neuralgia or hemifacial spasm.

41.2 Evolution of Surgical Treatment Options for the Given Pathology

In neurosurgery, there are two different types of neuroendoscopes: *the rigid and the flexible neuroendoscope* (▶ Fig. 41.1). Each type has its own indications, goals, limitations, advantages, disadvantage, complications, and contraindications (▶ Table 41.1). Although they are two completely different tools with two different learning curves, the author believes that they are complementary to each other and any endoscopic neurosurgeon should be familiar with both technologies.

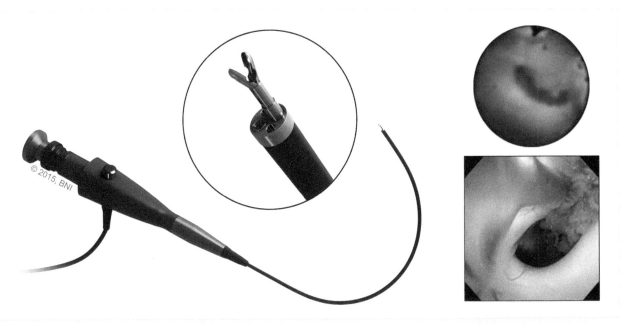

Fig. 41.1 A flexible endoscope with grasping tools inserted within ports. (Used with permission from Barrow Neurological Institute, Phoenix, AZ.)

Table 41.1 Efficacy of rigid versus flexible neuroendoscopes for a variety of pathologies

Procedure (s)	Rigid endoscope	Flexible neuroendoscope
Endoscopic third ventriculostomy	Adequate	Adequate
Septostomy	Adequate	Adequate
Monro's foraminoplasty	Adequate	Adequate
Tumor biopsy	Adequate (lateral and third ventricles)	Adequate (lateral, third, and fourth ventricles)
Tumor resection	Adequate	Not adequate
Arachnoid cyst fenestration	Adequate	Adequate
Colloid cyst resection	Adequate	Not adequate
Intraventricular neurocysticercosis	Adequate (lateral and third ventricles)	Adequate (lateral, third, fourth ventricle and basal cisterns)
Biopsy of basal cisterns	Adequate (interpeduncular, upper prepontine)	Adequate (interpeduncular, prepontine, premedullary, cisterna magna)
Lamina terminalis fenestration	Unless enlarged foramen of Monro, not adequate	Adequate
Aqueductoplasty	Adequate	Adequate
Fourth ventricle exploration	Contraindicated	Adequate
Magendie and Luschka foraminoplasty	Contraindicated	Adequate
Endoscopic-assisted shunting	Adequate	Adequate
Endoscopic-assisted microneurosurgery	Adequate	Adequate

41.2.1 Rigid Endoscope

Currently, the gold standard technology in rigid endoscopes is rod-lenses based on Hopkins patents. Numerous glass rods with optically shaped ends are self-aligning with different glass types correcting for image distortions. Improved Hopkins II endoscopes offer full HD video imaging. The large focus range and wide area of vision give the impression of "the eye at the front of the lens." Different angles of view are available; the most frequently used are 0-, 30-, and 45-degree optics that look "straight ahead"; by turning around, 45-degree optics can achieve an almost 300-degree overview. Optics with 70 and 120 degrees allow a "backward" view; this is useful when checking for complete tumor removal.

The major disadvantage is the lack of steerability and limited working area. Once the rigid endoscope is inserted in the lateral ventricle, if the entry point and the angle are appropriate, it can navigate into certain areas of the lateral and third ventricle, but no further into distal areas of the lateral ventricle (e.g., temporal horn) or cerebral aqueduct. Multiple burr holes, and possible multiple surgeries, are necessary to address intraventricular pathologies that involve more than one ventricle (e.g., infections, hemorrhage, etc.).

Types of Rigid Endoscopes

Based on imaging, irrigation, and instrumentation, rigid endoscopes can be classified into *channel scopes* or *space scopes*. *Channel scopes* have separate larger channels for instruments, smaller for irrigation, and may have an additional channel for a smaller instrument. They have a precise guidance of instruments but have a limiting main working space. *Space scopes* have a larger channel or a wide space for instrument including ultrasonic aspirator or additional flexible endoscopes. Irrigation and use of dual instruments is integrated in the large space with separate lateral nozzle.

41.2.2 Flexible Endoscope

Flexible neuroendoscopes are formed by an arrangement of fiberoptics that transmit one light point with every fiber. Each fiber has a core glass surrounded by cladding glass. The resolution of a flexible endoscope depends on the number of glass fibers (approximate diameter 7–10 μm). In a large flexible ventriculoscope with a 4-mm diameter and a 2-mm working channel, the number of fibers is around 50,000 corresponding to a resolution of 240×240 fiberoptic pixels. A 3-mm flexible endoscope is around 200×200 fiberoptic pixels.

Flexible neuroendoscopes and accessories have undergone multiple modifications aimed at improving their accuracy and safety. The first- and second-generation flexible endoscopes have outer diameters of 2.8 and 4.6 mm, respectively, and were used for observation only and simple procedures, respectively. The third-generation (currently the most commonly used) endoscopes have an outer diameter range of 2.8 to 4.8 mm with a 1- to 2-mm working channel. They accommodate a variety of forceps, needles, electrodes for cutting and coagulation, laser endoprobe for coagulation vaporization and cutting, a balloon catheter, and an endoscopic ultrasonic aspirator.

Videoendoscopes ("Distal Chip" or "Chip-on-the-Tip")

In videoscopes, the charge-coupled device (CCD) is mounted on the tip behind a lens projecting the image on the chip. The Video-Neuro-Endoscope (FLEX-X^C) is a steerable scope, with an atraumatic tip and 70 cm of length, a 2.8-mm diameter. It has a vision area of 90 degrees straightforward with a 1.5-mm chip-on-the-tip, and a 1.2-mm working channel. It has a flexion of 270 degrees (up/down) with a little loss of angulation when an instrument is inserted. An advantage is the full-screen display by quadratic imaging. This type of endoscope is also used in spinal endoscopy, from a sacral approach up to the cervical spine.

A second videoscope (VEF-V, Olympus Medical System, Tokyo, Japan) features a 120-degree field of view and 180-degree deflective tip angulation. The distal and flexible tubes have outer diameters of 5 and 4.8 mm, respectively. The 180-degree rotation of the flexible insertion tube is a unique feature of this videoendoscope. It has multiple filters that have the capacity to provide information about superficial and subependymal capillaries.

The "disadvantages" of the flexible endoscopes are low resolution and low brightness. Nowadays, this is less of a problem with the new HD flexible endoscopes or videoscopes. Glass fibers break easily, and the tiny surface cover on them may get damaged. Fiberoptics should be checked before and after use. Channels for instruments and irrigation should be immediately cleaned after the operation.

Another important disadvantage is the potential disorientation in the flexed position, particularly in patients with abnormal ventricular anatomy and no normal landmarks for orientation such as choroid plexus, foramen of Monro, SP, or mammillary bodies. Incorporation of neuronavigation to flexible endoscopy could solve this problem. Torres-Corzo and colleagues have performed the first successful cases of electromagnetic tracking of the tip of the steerable endoscope with the use of a malleable navigate wire inside of the endoscope working channel (unpublished data).

41.3 Case Illustrations

41.3.1 Endoscopic Surgical Management

History

A 16-year-old adolescent boy presented with subacute onset of nausea/vomiting, gait imbalance, diplopia, and severe headache. He also complained of headache and intermittent blurry vision over 4 to 5 months prior to his current acute symptoms. He had no past medical history of importance.

Physical Examination and Neuroimaging

On examination, the patient was awake, alert, mildly confused, and oriented to person and place. His pupils were sluggishly reactive and symmetric. Mild upper gaze palsy (Parinaud) was present. No other cranial nerve deficits were observed. Motor strength was 5/5 throughout, sensation was intact, and moderate dysmetria, nystagmus, and gait imbalance were present.

Magnetic resonance imaging (MRI) demonstrated severe hydrocephalus with subependymal edema. There was a large enhancing mass at the pineal region with mass effect on the midbrain, cerebellum, and corpus callosum. The cerebral aqueduct was occluded due to the mass ($\blacktriangleright$ Fig. 41.2).

Intraoperative Management

The patient was taken for a cerebrospinal fluid (CSF) diversion procedure. We prefer to take patients directly to a definitive and permanent procedure. In general, we perform endoscopic exploration with/without endoscopic procedure to treat hydrocephalus and address etiology, if possible. We try to avoid external ventricular drains (EVDs). In this current case of

obstructive hydrocephalus secondary to a third ventricular tumor, we believe that the patient is an excellent candidate for an ETV and tumor biopsy/resection. The patient was taken to the operating room, and under general anesthesia a burr hole was placed at the right frontal area, 2.5 cm off-midline and 1 cm in front of the coronal suture. No intraoperative neuronavigation was used. After a corticectomy was performed with bipolar electrocautery, a blunt needle was used to enter the ventricle and replaced with a peel-away sheath. The flexible neuroendoscope was inserted in the right lateral ventricle. The third ventricle was approached and inspected. First, we performed an ETV with a standard technique. Then, the flexible endoscope was steered into the posterior portion of the third ventricle, the tumor was identified, and multiple biopsies were obtained ($\blacktriangleright$ Fig. 41.2). The patient did well postoperatively, and was discharged home 48 hours later. Pathology results demonstrated germinoma.

Disadvantage/Advantages of Flexible Endoscopic Approach

The advantages of using a flexible neuroendoscope in this case included the need for only one burr hole. The steerable capabilities of the flexible neuroendoscope allowed reaching the anterior and posterior portions of the third ventricle with minimal to no manipulation of the structures around the foramen of Monro (fornix, choroid plexus, and veins). An ETV and tumor biopsy were performed during the same procedure time. With the recently developed flexible endoscopes, the quality of the image is as good as the rigid endoscope ($\blacktriangleright$ Fig. 41.2), and both procedures were performed successfully.

Disadvantage/Advantage of the Rigid Endoscopic Approach

A potential advantage of a rigid endoscope in this case would be "better" visualization of the tumor. Tumor biopsy is possible with both endoscopes. The disadvantage of the rigid endoscope is that two different burr holes would have been necessary to perform ETV and tumor biopsy. Both procedures require a different entry point and trajectory if the rigid endoscope is to be used. If one tries to perform both procedures with a single entry point, the possibility of injury to the fornix and choroid plexus is very high.

For all these reasons, we believe that the flexible endoscope is the best option for this particular patient.

41.3.2 Case Illustration 2: Endoscopic Surgical Management

History

This is a 56-year-old male who presented with severe headache, nausea/vomiting, and altered mental status. He has no past medical history of importance.

Physical Examination and Neuroimaging

On examination, the patient was awake, severely confused, and oriented to person only. Pupils were sluggishly reactive and

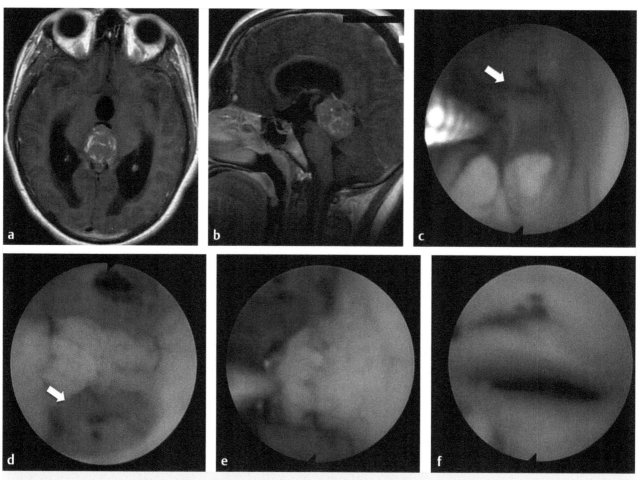

Fig. 41.2 Pineal region tumor. **(a,b)** Axial and sagittal magnetic resonance imaging with contrast demonstrating a large enhancing pineal tumor causing occlusion of the cerebral aqueductal and hydrocephalus. **(c–f)** Intraoperative endoscopic views of the procedure: **(c)** grasping forceps instrument used to perform the endoscopic third ventriculostomy (ETV); notice a thin floor of the third ventricle and the basilar artery (*arrow*). **(d)** A more posterior view of the third ventricle showing the ETV and pineal tumor (*arrow*). **(e)** Grasping forceps obtaining multiple biopsies. **(f)** Stenosis of the cerebral aqueduct due to tumor mass effect.

symmetric. No cranial nerve deficits were noticed. Motor strength was 5/5 throughout. Sensation was intact. Moderate dysmetria and nystagmus were observed.

MRI demonstrated a large heterogeneously enhancing mass arising from the corpus callosum infiltrating the roof and lateral walls of the third ventricle and extending posteriorly into the quadrigeminal plate. There is moderate hydrocephalus (▶ Fig. 41.3).

Intraoperative Management

Based on the MRI and the clinical presentation, the patient suffers from an infiltrating and possible malignancy intra-axial tumor. The patient is not a candidate for gross total resection procedure; however, diagnosis has to be made. Simultaneously, the infiltrating lesion is causing hydrocephalus secondary to the foramen of Monro stenosis/occlusion and sooner or later aqueductal stenosis. Therefore, we believe that the patient is a good candidate for endoscopic exploration, tumor biopsy, and possible CSF diversion. The patient was taken to the operating room, and under general anesthesia a burr hole was placed at the right frontal area, 2.5 cm off-midline and at the coronal suture. Intraoperative neuronavigation was used. After a burr

hole and corticectomy were performed with bipolar electrocautery, a blunt needle was used to enter the ventricle and replaced with a peel-away sheath. The rigid endoscope was inserted in the right lateral ventricle. The lateral and third ventricles were approached and inspected. The tumor was infiltrating the SP and causing stenosis of the right foramen of Monro. First, we performed a Monro foraminoplasty with a standard technique. Then, the rigid endoscope was navigated into the third ventricle and an ETV was performed. After both CSF diversion procedures were successfully performed, multiple biopsy samples were taken. An SP fenestration was considered; however, there were no areas of the septum with no tumor and we felt it was not safe to perform the procedure due to the hypervascularity of the tumor (▶ Fig. 41.3). The patient did well postoperatively, and was discharged home 48 hours later. Pathology results demonstrated glioblastoma multiforme.

41.4 Disadvantage/Advantages of Rigid Endoscopic Approach

A rigid endoscope was selected for this case because it allowed better visualization of the tumor and its hypervascular areas.

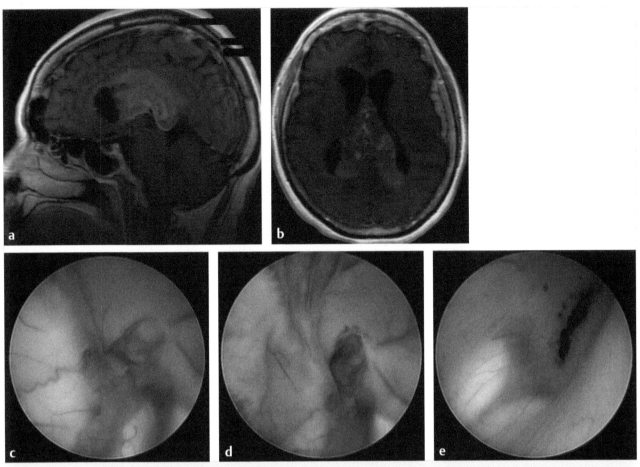

Fig. 41.3 Corpus callosum tumor. **(a)** Sagittal and **(b)** axial magnetic resonance imaging with contrast demonstrating a large infiltrating enhancing tumor mass arising from the corpus callosum infiltrating the third ventricle. **(c–e)** Intraoperative endoscopic views: **(c)** Stenosis of the foramen of Monro. **(d)** Successful Monro's foraminoplasty; observe the hypervascular tumor infiltrating the septum pellucidum. **(e)** Endoscopic third ventriculostomy.

There is the potential of significant tumor bleeding during the biopsy; therefore, a better and bigger bipolar or monopolar electrocautery instrument is needed. Also, the same burr hole and trajectory could be used for tumor biopsy and CSF diversion procedure that included the Monro foraminoplasty and ETV. Both procedures were performed successfully (▸ Fig. 41.3).

41.5 Disadvantage/Advantage of the Flexible Endoscopic Approach

A flexible neuroendoscope could be an option for this case. However, the electrocautery instrument available for the flexile endoscope is small and may not be sufficient to control bleeding from this large and hypervascular tumor.

41.6 Patient Selection

Any patient with hydrocephalus, intraventricular and/or paraventricular lesions, and basal cisterns pathologies should be considered a candidate for an endoscopic procedure.

41.6.1 Hydrocephalus

In essence, all hydrocephalus is obstructive. Differentiation between obstructive and nonobstructive hydrocephalus is based on whether the obstruction occurs in the anatomical flow pathway or at the functional level during resorption. All patients with *obstructive hydrocephalus* that requires treatment are candidates for neuroendoscopic surgery. The choice of the endoscopic procedure is made based on the level of obstruction within the ventricular system (▸ Table 41.1). *Communicating hydrocephalus* encompasses all cases in which the flow of CSF is obstructed at a point distal to the outlet of CSF from the brain. Some cases of communicating hydrocephalus are candidates for a neuroendoscopic procedure; however, patient selection could be very challenging. Patients with communicating hydrocephalus related to subarachnoid hemorrhage or infection (meningitis, ventriculitis, arachnoiditis) respond to an endoscopic procedure (third ventriculostomy, lamina terminalis fenestration) in 40 to 70% of cases. Patients with normal pressure hydrocephalus who undergo an ETV have good results in 50 to 60% of cases; however, patient selection is not yet established. Relatively younger patients whose symptoms are predominantly ataxia and urinary incontinence have better outcomes.

41.6.2 Intraventricular and Paraventricular Tumors

All patients with intraventricular and paraventricular tumors are candidates for an endoscopic procedure (▶ Table 41.1). The goal is to reestablish CSF flow in case of obstruction and tumor biopsy/resection, if possible at the same time the procedure is carried out and through the same approach. These lesions include but are not limited to primary CNS germ cell tumors (e.g., germinoma, teratoma), Langerhans cell histiocytosis, phakomatosis-related tumors (e.g., subependymal giant astrocytoma), choroid plexus tumor, ependymomas, meningiomas, pineal tumors, glial tumors, lymphoma, and metastasis. Other nontumoral lesions that are also candidates for endoscopic approach include colloid cysts, arachnoid cysts, and hypothalamic hamartoma.

41.6.3 Other Intraventricular/Basal Cistern Pathologies

Other common intraventricular clinical indications for an endoscopic procedure include *intraventricular/subarachnoid hemorrhage* (hematoma removal, SP fenestration, ETV), *arachnoid cysts* (cyst fenestration/marsupialization), *intraventricular and basal cistern neurocysticercosis* (cyst removal, SP fenestration, ETV, aqueductoplasty, Magendie and Luschka fenestration), *infection* (arachnoid biopsy ETV, SP fenestration), and *shunt malfunction* (ETV, choroid plexus cauterization; ▶ Table 41.1).

41.7 Complication Avoidance

Neuroendoscopic procedures have become quite safe because of their wide diffusion, and the large experience gathered by neurosurgeons over the last two to three decades. However, it is not free from complications, even in experienced hands. In the author's opinion, appropriate clinical indications, adequate endoscopic instrumentation (rigid, flexible, and their instruments), and adequate experience are currently the best ways to reduce the risk of neuroendoscopic complications.

41.7.1 Intraoperative Neuroendoscopic Complications

The most common complications during an endoscopic procedure include the following:

- Bradycardia, usually related to traction of the floor of the third ventricle or endoscope in the fourth ventricle or basal cisterns.
- Tachycardia, which can occur during or immediately after stretching of the third ventricle.
- Hypothermia, which could be related to wet drapes on small children or the elderly, inappropriate irrigation solution, or, less commonly, due to hypothalamic injury.
- Intraventricular hemorrhage, usually from ependymal veins, choroid plexus, and endoscope trajectory.
- Technical failure (visual obscuration, abnormal anatomy) and vascular injury (basilar artery or perforators).

41.7.2 Technical Nuances

General technical nuances during any endoscopic procedure include equipment preparation and room setup before starting the procedure, before making skin incision. Common complications such as *bradycardia* can arise from over-irrigation, irrigation with hypotonic or cold solutions, and during perforation of the third ventricle floor. Bradycardia could lead to asystole if not promptly recognized. To avoid this complication, communicate with the anesthesiologist or listen to the cardiac monitor, check outflow channels of the endoscope, and gently irrigate with isotonic solution (lactated Ringer's) only.

Intraventricular bleeding is not uncommon and the majority of the time it is related to poor technique. The most common causes include inadequate hemostasis before introducing the endoscope, inappropriate or excessive movements of the endoscope during the procedure, repeated introduction of the endoscope without peel-away sheath, the use of sharp sheaths, and the wrong removal of the endoscope (incorrect trajectory, withdrawal of the flexible endoscope in curved position). Sometimes introduction of the endoscope alone is enough to cause bleeding, especially in patients who suffered posthemorrhagic or postinfectious hydrocephalus (fragile ventricular walls) or coagulopathies. The author suggests the following: achieve adequate hemostasis before the introduction of the endoscope, plan the ideal trajectory beforehand, use neuronavigation or flexible endoscope in case of small ventricles, use blunt sheaths and peel-away sheaths if available, be familiar and perform cautious movements with the instruments, avoid stretching the floor of the third ventricle or performing the stoma too close to the pituitary infundibulum, and avoid sharp instruments or cauterization to create the stoma. Intraventricular hemorrhage is often a minor bleeding that stops spontaneously. If the bleeding source is visible, it can be cauterized. Major bleeding can cause blurry vision or complete field opacification; if that is the case, the procedure has to stop; forceful irrigation is the next step; do not panic and do not pull the endoscope because the ventricle can fill up with blood promptly and reaccess into the ventricle can be difficult or impossible. Remove the endoscope but leave the sheath in the ventricle to keep irrigation and to maintain access to the ventricle. An external drain is usually placed at the end of the procedure. Do not coagulate large veins (e.g., internal cerebral veins). Do not hesitate to convert into a craniotomy and use the microscope. Vascular injury accounts for almost all cases of intraoperatively mortality. Damage to the basilar, posterior cerebral, or anterior choroidal artery during ETV procedures or anterior communicating artery during lamina terminalis fenestration may be fatal. Patients with subarachnoid hemorrhage may have neurological deficits from vasospasm, form pseudoaneurysms, stroke, and or hydrocephalous worsening. The management is similar to aneurysmal subarachnoid hemorrhage.

Few points to avoid vascular injury include the following: know the normal and variants of neuroendoscopic anatomy, choice of proper third ventricle entry point, and avoiding sharp instruments or cauterization to open the third ventricle. Technical failure is usually associated with visual obscuration due to scope being out of focus, fogging of lenses, or incorrectly assembled equipment, unfavorable intraventricular anatomy (septa, small foramen of Monro, large massa intermedia, partial fusion of the third ventricle walls, thickening of the third ventricle), distorted anatomy due to large tumor, malformations, hemorrhages or infections, unfavorable position of the target, misplacement of the burr hole with wrong endoscope trajectory and angle, and inappropriate endoscope (rigid/flexible).

41.7.3 Early Postoperative Complications

It is not uncommon to observe *delayed awakening* after an intraventricular endoscopic procedure; it is related to transient intracranial hypertension during surgery. *Fever* is encountered as a consequence of hypothalamic irritation due to cold/excessive irrigation or stretching of the third ventricle walls. *Subdural collections* are rare (1–5%); hygroma is the most common and results as a consequence of craniocervical disproportion or CSF escape into the subdural space. Large hygromas may require surgery. *Acute subdural hematomas* occur following abrupt CSF drainage or if the dura was detached from the cortex as result of cortical bleeding. *CSF leakage or subcutaneous collections* are seen in 2% of cases and more frequent in children due to thin skin, thinner cortical mantle. CSF escapes due incorrect closure technique or increase intracranial pressure. *Neurological injuries* are seen in 3 to 4% of the cases and permanent neurological deficits in 1% of cases. Columns of the fornix are the most common site of injury, which is usually clinically silent and patients can have transient memory dysfunction or confusion. Rare neurological complications include hemiparesis and diplopia, which are seen after thalamic, brainstem, and/or cranial nerves III or IV damage; hemianopsia due to damage of the optic chiasm, Horner's syndrome, nystagmus, and peduncular hallucinosis due to diencephalic or mesencephalic injury; and psychiatric symptoms due to frontal lobe infarction. Injury to the hypothalamus, during endoscopic surgery within the third ventricle, can present with bradycardia/tachycardia, electrolyte imbalance, confusion, endocrinologic sequelae including diabetes insipidus, inappropriate secretion of antidiuretic hormone, and rarely amenorrhea. Technical nuances to prevent hypothalamic injury include adequate selection of endoscope, limited use of coagulation, avoidance of excessive movements, and not performing the procedure in unfavorable anatomical conditions.

41.7.4 Late Postoperative Complications

Infections are relatively rare (1–5%) thanks to the minimal invasive nature and the short operative times of neuroendoscopic procedures and the absence of prosthetic foreign bodies (shunts) in most of cases. Meningitis, ventriculitis, and wound infection are the main manifestations. However, infections can be complicated by the failure of the endoscopic procedure, because of intraventricular membrane formation or impaired CSF reabsorption.

Closure of ETV, a septostomy, and the recurrence of an intraventricular lesion (e.g., tumor and arachnoid cyst) are well-known problems. Sometimes, it is secondary to inadequate procedure, for example, a too small ETV, septostomy or cyst fenestration, missed visualization of secondary membranes, or misplacement of an aqueductal stent. Blockage of the

ETV, septostomy, and aqueductoplasty can occur as early complications following intraoperative bleeding with clots obstructing the stoma. Late closure of the stoma is extremely rare (0.5%) and it can occur in up to 5 to 7 years after the operation; closure of an ETV can be secondary to arachnoid and glial scarring of the floor of the third ventricle.

41.8 Clinical Pearls

When evaluating patients with intraventricular pathologies with or without hydrocephalus, the treating neurosurgeon should take into consideration multiple variables such as patient's clinical conditions, surgical anatomy, and surgeon's experience with rigid and/or flexible endoscopes, in order to offer the best surgical option: open surgery versus endoscopic surgery or shunt implantation.

All hydrocephalus is obstructive. The difference between obstructive and nonobstructive hydrocephalus is based on whether the obstruction occurs in the anatomical flow pathway or at the functional level during resorption. Endoscopic intervention can restore or bypass anatomical obstructions of CSF flow. In cases of noncommunicating hydrocephalus, endoscopic ETV may be beneficial, as it improves the compliance of ventricles that may play a critical pathophysiological role. In cases of multiloculated hydrocephalus, the aim of therapy is to reduce the morbidity of repeat procedures. Endoscopy allows this by simplifying the anatomy of the ventricular system and reducing the rate of shunt failures and the complexity of their revision.

When evaluating patients with intraventricular tumors, patient selection is of utmost importance in identifying individuals who would benefit the most from endoscopic approaches. Tumor size, location, mineralization, and vascularity should factor into this decision. *The lack of ventriculomegaly is not a contraindication to the endoscopic procedure.* Stereotactic navigation should be used to guide ventriculostomy, to direct tumor access, and to minimize torque of the endoscope on surrounding structures. For tumors causing compartmentalized hydrocephalus, simultaneous septostomy can be performed, while third ventricular and pineal region tumors causing obstructive hydrocephalus can be simultaneously treated with ETV. The number and location of burr holes and/or trajectory will vary based on the decision to perform these procedures simultaneously with resection or biopsy; however, one single burr hole is necessary if a flexible neuroendoscope is available.

Endoscopic management of intraventricular hemorrhage has gained interest among neurosurgeons. Recent studies have demonstrated faster recovery and decreased the need for permanent shunt. If it is a rigid endoscope, more than one burr hole might be necessary, whereas one burr hole is sufficient when a flexible endoscope is used. When using the flexible endoscope for the fourth ventricle hematoma evacuation, place the burr hole no more than 2 cm from the midline, since it can turn the fourth ventricle cannulation into a demanding and dangerous procedure. Before inserting the peel-away sheath, find the ventricle with a standard EVD or ventricular needle without draining the CSF. Once inside the ventricle, on first inspection with the endoscope only the reddish color

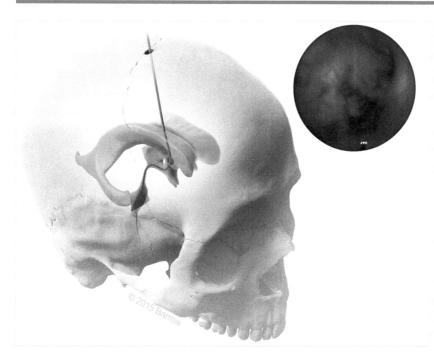

Fig. 41.4 Illustration of the transaqueductal endoscopic approach to the fourth ventricle with the flexible neuroendoscope. Intraoperative endoscopic view of the fourth ventricle. (Used with permission from Barrow Neurological Institute, Phoenix, AZ.)

of the clot in the lateral ventricle can be seen. At this stage, removing clots is to some extent done blindly, and thus it is vital to cease aspiration as soon as the reddishness begins to disappear and the white of the ventricular walls becomes visible. If the surgeon follows these simple rules and proceeds carefully and patiently, a large amount of blood can be removed. Inside the fourth ventricle, irrigation and aspiration must be rigorously isovolumetric, as clots occlude the outlets and the aqueduct is obstructed entirely by the flexible endoscope. After completion of the procedure, always leave the EVD open at 15 H_2O.

Certain patients with fourth ventricle pathologies (intraventricular hemorrhage, trapped fourth ventricle) can be managed endoscopically. The approach to the fourth ventricle is only possible with a flexible neuroendoscope (▶ Fig. 41.4). When within the cerebral aqueduct and fourth ventricle with the flexible endoscope, never lose visual contact. Inadvertent movement of the endoscope with no visualization can cause brainstem injury. Movements within the fourth ventricle should always be fine and gentle, similar to those in an aneurysm microdissection. Be very vigilant of the amount of irrigation while in the fourth ventricle. The fourth ventricle is a small compartment with minimal CSF outflow once the endoscope is in the cerebral aqueduct. Fourth ventricle hypertension can lead to bradycardia and cardiac arrest. Endoscopic anatomical knowledge is imperative. Always keep in mind the structures that have been left behind the endoscope to avoid injury to them when withdrawing the endoscope.

In pediatric patients, consider neuroendoscopic procedures as a first-line treatment in obstructive hydrocephalus and intraventricular pathologies. It is well known that patients younger than 6 months of age with hydrocephalus secondary to germinal matrix hemorrhage with basal cistern scarring managed with ETV have low success rates and may require a second procedure to treat hydrocephalus (e.g., choroid plexus cauterization, lamina terminalis fenestration, or ventriculoperitoneal shunt placement). In patients with obstructive hydrocephalus secondary to germinal matrix hemorrhage, we advocate early endoscopic surgical intervention (e.g., hematoma evacuation, ventricular lavage, ETV, and SP fenestration). In patients with hydrocephalus and an intraventricular and/or paraventricular tumor, we advocate performing ETV first and tumor biopsy and/or resection second.

The realization that the endoscope could deliver superior optic capabilities that augmented microscopic visualization in a minimally invasive fashion stirred excitement because now surgical dissections could be performed effectively in areas previously not accessible by microscopic visualization alone. Endoscopic surgery and microneurosurgery should not be exclusive. Endoscopic-assisted procedures have been applied to a large variety of extracranial and intracranial pathologies including skull base tumors of the anterior, middle, and posterior fossa, trigeminal neuralgia, intra-axial tumor resection, and clip ligation of cerebral aneurysms, among others. Surgical feats previously deemed impossible can readily be performed while maintaining minimally invasive approaches. Neuroendoscopy has expanded the capabilities afforded by conventional microscopic approaches. By using the endoscope to "look around the corner," surgery can be continued in areas not previously possible with microscopic dissection alone.

Suggested Readings

[1] Borg A, Rangel-Castilla L. Meningitis and infectious hydrocephalus. In: Torres-Corzo J, Rangel-Castilla L, Nakaji P, eds. Neuroendoscopic Surgery. New York, NY: Thieme Medical Publishers; 2016:206–213

[2] Friedman GN, Grannan BL, Nahed BV, Codd PJ. Initial experience with high-definition camera-on-a-chip flexible endoscope for intraventricular neurosurgery. World Neurosurg. 2015; 84(6):2053–2058

[3] Kawaguchi T, Nakagawa A, Endo T, Fujimura M, Sonoda Y, Tominaga T. Ventricle wall dissection and vascular preservation with the pulsed water jet device: novel tissue dissector for flexible neuroendoscopic surgery. J Neurosurg. 2016; 124(3):817–822

[4] Nishiyama K, Natori Y, Oka K. A novel three-dimensional and high-definition flexible scope. Acta Neurochir (Wien). 2014; 156(6):1245–1249

[5] Oka K. Development of a flexible neuroendoscope. In: Torres-Corzo J, Rangel-Castilla L, Nakaji P, eds. Neuroendoscopic Surgery. New York, NY: Thieme Medical Publishers; 2016:24–30

[6] Oka K. Introduction of the videoscope in neurosurgery. Neurosurgery. 2008; 62(5) Suppl 2:ONS337–ONS340, discussion ONS341

[7] Rangel-Castilla L, Nakaji P. Future of neuroendoscopy. In: Torres-Corzo J, Rangel-Castilla L, Nakaji P, eds. Neuroendoscopic Surgery. New York, NY: Thieme Medical Publishers; 2016:386–391

[8] Rodriguez-Della Vecchia R, Torres-Corzo J. Endoscopic approach to the fourth ventricle. In: Torres-Corzo J, Rangel-Castilla L, Nakaji P, eds. Neuroendoscopic Surgery. New York, NY: Thieme Medical Publishers; 2016:266–271

[9] Torres-Corzo J, Rangel-Castilla L. Lamina terminalis fenestration. In: Torres-Corzo J, Rangel-Castilla L, Nakaji P, eds. Neuroendoscopic Surgery. New York, NY: Thieme Medical Publishers; 2016:261–265

[10] Toyota T, Kageyama H, Tsuzuki N, Ishihara S, Oka K. Flexible endoscopic aspiration for intraventricular vesting hematoma. Acta Neurochir Suppl (Wien). 2016; 123:17–23

42 Endoscopic Port Surgery: Advantages and Disadvantages

William C. Newman and Johnathan A. Engh

Summary

Endoscopic port surgery is a hybrid approach to brain surgery, which combines aspects of both channel endoscopy and bimanual microsurgery for the removal of complex, deep-seated brain tumors. It is slightly more invasive than channel endoscopy and more technically challenging than standard microsurgery. It can result in a powerful and minimally invasive tool for deep-seated brain tumor resection. In this chapter, we discuss endoport surgery for intracranial intraparenchymal tumors.

Keywords: endoport, endoscopic port, endoscope, brain tumor, intraventricular tumor, colloid cyst

42.1 Introduction

The conventional technique for intracranial tumor removal is microsurgical, using either static or dynamic brain retraction to achieve tumor exposure and subsequent safe resection. Although iatrogenic surgical trauma may be limited for superficial brain tumors, this is not necessarily the case for deeper-seated lesions. For deep tumors, significant adjacent brain tissue manipulation is often necessary in order to achieve complete visualization of the tumor and to establish a dissection plane. Manipulation and dissection of the adjacent functional brain tissue may cause significant morbidity. As a result, a device that facilitates safe removal of these tumors while minimizing brain trauma is potentially attractive.

The authors will discuss endoscopic port surgery (EPS) as a potential solution for the problem of safe, minimally invasive deep tumor resection. This technique will be explored in depth through analysis of its evolution, case-based EPS discussion, and finally a broader discussion of controversies, complications, technical nuances, and clinical pearls. EPS can be a powerful tool for safe tumor resection in appropriate hands, but like any intracranial operative technique, EPS can entail substantial risk.

42.2 Evolution of Surgical Treatment Options

Endoscopy facilitates minimally invasive neurosurgery by providing a view of structures deep within the brain through an elongated tube with a light and a camera. This tube can often be inserted through a far smaller opening than would be used with conventional approaches. Initially reported by Lespinasse over a century ago, ventriculoscopic surgery has since benefited from the development of better optical devices and surgical tools, and the endoscope has been applied to other areas of neurosurgery, including skull base surgery and surgery within the cerebrospinal fluid (CSF) cisterns.[1] Hopf and Perneczky classified modern endoscopic cranial surgery into three subtypes based on the optical device used (i.e., endoscope alone vs. endoscope with microscope) and the route of surgical manipulation (i.e., through or outside the endoscope).[2] Endoscopic neurosurgery, or channel endoscopy, refers to the use of a burr hole with surgical manipulation through the endoscope using special instruments. Endoscope-assisted microsurgery is the use of the endoscope and the microscope independent of each other in the same operation. Endoscope-controlled microsurgery entails the use of a craniotomy opening with traditional microsurgical tools under endoscopic visualization. This latter definition would be the best subgroup classification for EPS, although EPS is probably best described as a hybrid between endoscopy and conventional microsurgery.

Channel endoscopy is a wonderful tool for intraventricular visualization, creation of pathways for CSF flow (e.g., third ventriculostomy, septostomy), tumoral biopsy, and potentially removal of colloid cysts or intraventricular tumors. In addition, channel endoscopy is truly minimally invasive, often requiring a cannulation only 3 to 4 mm in total diameter. However, channel endoscopy is remarkably limited in its ability to deal with large, calcified, complex or vascular lesions. Part of this limitation is that channel endoscopy is performed in a fluid medium; although this approach promotes minimal tissue disturbance, visualization is easily spoiled by a small amount of hemorrhage. In addition, both the complexity and range of motion of surgical tools are substantially limited by the shape of the endoscope itself. As a result, complex lesions are not generally amenable to resection via channel endoscopy in a fluid medium.

In contrast, endoscope-assisted microsurgery and endoscope-controlled microsurgery both allow for freedom of hand movement and visualization of tumor in the setting of hemorrhage. However, neither of these techniques addresses the issue of cortical and subcortical retraction for tumors in which a purely cisternal approach is not possible. In other words, if pial and subpial tissues need to be traversed in order to approach a tumor, then the corridor should ideally be as small as possible, while still facilitating safe tumor resection.

EPS is a hybrid approach to brain surgery that combines positive aspects of both channel endoscopy and bimanual microsurgery for the removal of complex, deep-seated brain tumors.[3] Although it is slightly more invasive than channel endoscopy and more technically challenging than standard microsurgery, the result is a powerful and minimally invasive tool for deep-seated brain tumor resection.

The technique of EPS used by the senior author (J.E.) has been extensively described.[3,4,5,6] The patient is positioned similar to a standard craniotomy, with the trajectory to the lesion of interest above the lesion itself. Image guidance, either frameless or frame based, is used to target the craniotomy, which is generally 2.5 to 3 cm in size. Following dural opening, care is taken to avoid cortical bridging veins while creating a small cortisectomy. Ideally, a trans-sulcal approach is taken to the lesion of interest. Cannulation is performed over a small needle or image-guidance probe. For ventricular lesions, the ventricle of interest is targeted. For intraparenchymal masses, the tumor itself is the cannulation target. Following removal of

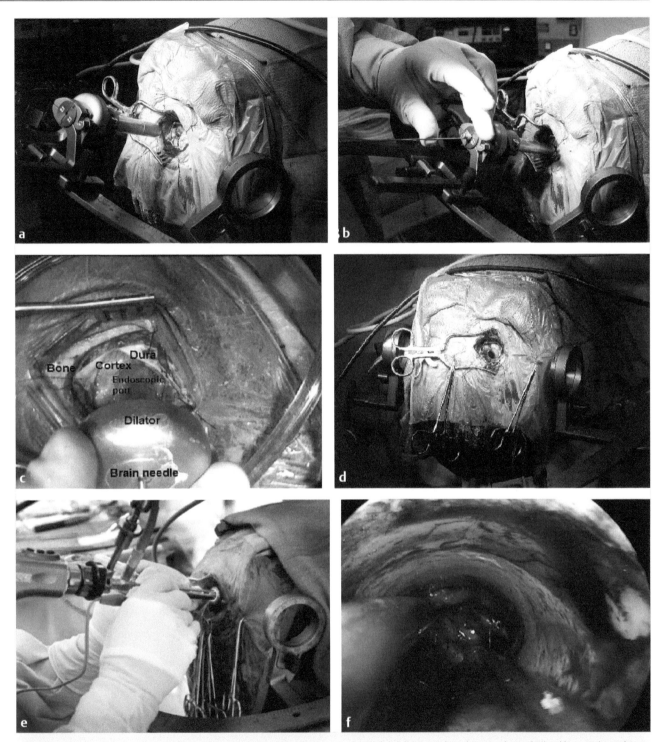

Fig. 42.1 Images depicting the setup for endoscopic port surgery. **(a)** Craniotomy and dural opening have been performed. The dilator with overlying endoscopic port is advanced just above the brain surface, and the brain needle is advanced to target depth **(b)**. **(c)** Labeled picture depicting the position of the brain needle, dilator, and endoscopic port as it penetrates the brain. **(d)** After cannulation and removal of the dilator and brain needle, the transparent port remains in place, secured by 4–0 sutures through the port and attached to the patient by hemostats. **(e)** After securing the tube, bimanual surgery takes place using the endoscope for visualization **(f)** *(cont.)*

the dilator device, the port is secured to the scalp, and the endoscope is used for visualization of the lesion while it is resected using bimanual microsurgical technique. If possible, intraoperative ultrasound or intraoperative computed tomography (CT) scanning can be used to assess the resection prior to port removal. Hemostasis is achieved, the port is carefully removed, and the wound is closed in the usual fashion (▶ Fig. 42.1).

EPS uses tubular retractors for the static and uniform distribution of displacement forces on the adjacent brain tissue. The small size of the endoscope minimizes the size of the surgical conduit with ample lighting for visualization into the corridor.

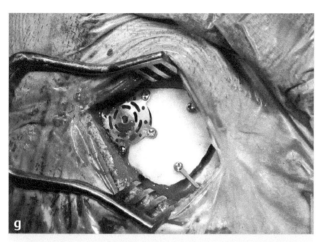

Fig 42.1 (*cont.*) After completion of resection, the bone flap is replaced and secured using titanium plating prior to closure of the incision (**g**)

The almost panoramic views generated by the endoscope provide a great degree of anatomic detail. Additionally, angled endoscopes allow the surgeon to look around a corner or behind neurovascular structures. Moreover, all of this is achieved without a need for constantly refocusing the image. Finally, the port can serve a protective role for the surrounding cortex and white matter, preventing constant manipulation and stretch injury related to bringing instruments into and out of the operative field. However, the constant application of static force from the port on the surrounding brain is a concern, especially with increased intracranial pressure (ICP). To date, despite the attractive features of port surgery, no study has definitively compared the degree of iatrogenic injury from port surgery to microsurgery for the same type of tumor.

EPS arose as a modification of techniques introduced by Dr. Patrick Kelly to deploy cylindrical retractors to approach deep brain tumors.[7,8] While Dr. Kelly's techniques were microsurgical and generally employed frame-based stereotaxy to direct a 2-cm tube, the introduction of the endoscope and modern instrumentation has facilitated openings into the brain that are generally smaller and leave even less of an impression on the surrounding brain. In addition, these systems are compatible with frameless stereotaxy. Current ports used by the senior author measure approximately 13.25 mm in diameter, with multiple lengths available. Most other ports available on the general market are similar in size. Other ports available in the general market include the NICO BrainPath (NICO Corporation, Indianapolis, IN), which has an inner diameter of 13.5 mm and lengths from 5 to 7.5 cm, and the Vycor ViewSite (Vycor Medical Inc., Boca Raton, FL), which features an ovular profile with cylinder lengths from 3 to 7 cm and distal openings of 12 to 28 mm. Of note, the latter system has a tapering shape and is usually used with the operating microscope.

42.2.1 Variations of Endoscopic Ports for Brain Surgery

A number of creative modifications of existing equipment have been performed in order to facilitate EPS. Tubular retractors have included collapsed transparent vinyl tubular retractors inflated with the finger of a latex glove[9] to silicone tubes inserted with a nasal speculum[10] to stereotactic-guided endoscopic tubular systems and beyond. In addition, physicians are adapting techniques from other fields, such as combining stereotaxy with sequentially dilating tubular retractors previously used in minimally invasive spine surgery, to create corridors to access deep-seated intracranial lesions.[11] At our institution, we are investigating balloon dilation for the creation of an operative corridor for port placement to minimize local parenchymal shear stresses transmitted by advancing ports through brain parenchyma.

These advances in endoscopic ports have been accompanied and facilitated by concurrent advances in endoscopes. Endoscopes have advanced from the 0-degree scope to a myriad of angled options with ever-improving optics, ranging from the use of fiberoptics to the advent of the rod-lens endoscope. It has been these and other advances that have paved the way for the increasing versatility of endoport and endoscope-assisted microsurgery. Due to increased interest in such techniques, commercially available systems for port surgery are now widely available on the U.S. market, including the previously described Nico Myriad (Nico Corporation) and the Vycor Viewsite (Vycor Medical Inc.).

42.3 Case Example

The following case illustrates the successful implementation of EPS for a deep-seated brain tumor. A 60-year-old right-handed woman with no significant past medical history presented with 8 months of increasingly frequent left-sided headache, word-finding difficulty, and worsening short-term memory. Her physical examination was significant for two subtle neurologic findings. First, memory testing revealed zero out of three immediate object recalls but improved to two out of three with verbal clues. In addition, the patient had developed a subtle and incomplete right visual field deficit.

A contrast-enhanced magnetic resonance imaging (MRI) of her brain (▶ Fig. 42.2) demonstrated an approximately 5 cm homogenously enhancing mass in the atrium of the left lateral ventricle with substantial surrounding edema, ventricular entrapment, and local mass effect, concerning for a meningioma. Also seen was a separate 2-cm lesion abutting the falx with no significant edema, thought to represent a second incidental tumor.

The authors believed that the larger lesion required surgical resection and that the second tumor could be addressed following recovery from the first procedure. Given the size and presentation of the tumor, radiation and observation did not appear to be viable options. A recommendation was made to attempt to remove the tumor using an endoscopic port, such that collateral injury related to tumor resection could be minimized. This was a particular concern in this case, in the light of the marked ventricular dilatation and surrounding edema, as this tumor was in the dominant hemisphere, putting not only movement and vision but also speech at risk.

The patient was taken to the operating room for a left parietal craniotomy for intraventricular tumor resection using the dilatable endoscopic port, an expandable tool used at our institution. Preoperatively, mannitol was administered at a dose of

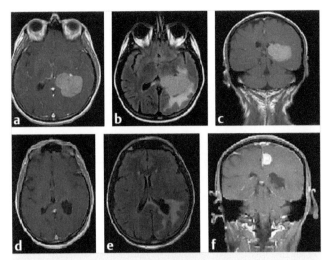

Fig. 42.2 Postcontrast T1 axial (**a**), T2 axial fluid-attenuated inversion recovery (FLAIR; **b**), and coronal postcontrast T1 (**c**) magnetic resonance imaging showing left atrial meningioma with ventricular entrapment and perilesional edema. A left-sided transparietal approach using the endoscopic port was performed with gross total resection of the left atrial lesion (**d–f**). Note the second incidental meningioma along the falx (**f**).

0.5 mg/kg to facilitate brain relaxation. She was positioned in a Mayfield head holder in the lateral position with the left side up with use of an axillary roll. A linear incision for a 3-cm craniotomy was planned with the assistance of image guidance. After completion of the craniotomy, the dura was opened in a cruciate fashion. A trans-sulcal approach was chosen through the inferior parietal lobule, in hopes of minimizing the risk of either language dysfunction or a visual field deficit. Image guidance was used to determine the trajectory of the stereotactic needle and it was placed to a depth of 3 cm. The inner stylet of the needle was replaced with a Boston Scientific XXL 14 mm × 4 cm semi-compliant balloon catheter, which, after removal of the outer cannula, was inflated slowly over 10 to 15 minutes. The balloon was deflated and removed and the endoscopic port was then placed through this corridor and secured to the scalp.

The tumor was visualized using a 0-degree endoscope. The tumor was able to be internally debulked through a combination of suction and mechanical aspiration. As the tumor collapsed, patties were placed along the ependymal surface of the ventricle and a circumferential plane was defined. The tumor capsule was then able to be removed en bloc, following coagulation and division of multiple arterial feeders from the choroidal fissure. The ventricular system was irrigated copiously and inspected for residual tumor. The port was decannulated and Surgicel was used to line the cortical edges of the cannulation entry point. A ventriculostomy drain was left in the cavity as a precaution.

Postoperatively, the patient was maintained in the intensive care unit for 2 days. She remained at her preoperative neurological baseline with some subtle paraphasic errors, which resolved by her 2-week follow-up visit. Postoperative imaging demonstrated gross total resection of the tumor with some edema around the resection site (▶ Fig. 42.2). No visual field changes were noted. Pathologic examination revealed a WHO grade 1 meningioma with a Ki-67 of 1%. At 6 months

postsurgery, there was no evidence of tumor recurrence, and the second tumor remains under observation.

42.4 Advantages and Disadvantages of Endoscopic Port Surgery

The differences between EPS and traditional microsurgery are especially apparent when comparing surgery for the removal of intraventricular lesions. Traditional microsurgical approaches to the lateral ventricles are transcortical or transcallosal, with the latter requiring at least a 10-mm callosotomy for ventricular access, but sometimes corridors of up to 20 mm to maintain binocular visualization through the operating microscope.[12] For larger intraventricular lesions, even larger corridors through subcortical white matter are necessary to achieve adequate visualization and resection. Significant morbidity after these approaches may reflect retraction or transection of underlying white matter structures, with potentially higher risks of venous infarction, neurologic deficits, and cognitive impairment.

Intraventricular use of the endoscopic port requires replacement of the normal CSF medium with an air medium, similar to microsurgery. While this does cause postoperative pneumocephalus and headache, the air medium permits the use of traditional microsurgical techniques within the ventricular system, such as bipolar coagulation or mechanical aspirators. This represents an additional benefit compared to standard working channel endoscopy, in which hemostasis can only be achieved with copious irrigation or special tools introduced through the working channel with limited mobility parallax to the endoscope. This particular benefit helps explain why a lesion such as the atrial meningioma described earlier would be almost impossible to remove using the channel endoscopy.

In the previously described case, the endoscopic port was advantageous for several reasons. First, it enabled access to the ventricular atrium using a small craniotomy and cortisectomy, minimizing exposure of brain under pressure from regional ICP elevation. Second, EPS facilitated dynamic retractor manipulation to visualize the entire tumor without substantial white matter manipulation. Third, when the tumor proved to be firm, EPS enabled bimanual technique to mechanically aspirate, cauterize, and manipulate the tumor to achieve a gross total resection. Such techniques are particularly difficult to employ via working channel endoscopy, and conventional microsurgery tends to create a larger channel into the brain for tumor resection, which can potentially lead to greater neurologic morbidity.

In general, for an atrial meningioma of substantial size, it is impossible to achieve tumoral access without some degree of cortical dissection. Clearly a transparietal approach makes the most intuitive sense in this case, given the ventricular dilatation and the long axis of both the tumor and its feeding vessels. In this particular case, with the ventricle under pressure, a small cortisectomy allows minimization of brain herniation prior to ventricular decompression. In contrast, a microsurgical approach requires substantial dissection time to reach the tumor, which can increase potential brain injury if the ICP is elevated. Using the port, cannulation can be done quickly while putting a limited portion of the brain at risk. However, care must be taken to avoid injury to superficial bridging veins during the approach to the tumor, as such an injury can be devastating.

Conversely, the most significant advantage of a microsurgical approach in this case is that it is potentially more time efficient once ventricular access has been achieved. With microsurgery, two surgeons can operate at the same time through the same cortisectomy if necessary, which can decrease operative time. In addition, although adjuvant tools for tumor resection, such as an ultrasonic aspirator or a microdebrider, are available for use with an endoscopic port, these tools are easier to deploy through a microsurgical corridor.

42.5 Patient Selection

Patient selection for EPS is based on a combination of neurologic presentation, medical comorbidities, lesion anatomy, histology, and imaging findings. In the most general sense, deep-seated lesions (i.e., those 2.5 cm or more below the cortical surface) allow for maximal utilization of the port's length without the need for a substantial craniotomy. Therefore, if a superficial lesion is accessible with minimal cortical dissection, traditional microsurgical techniques are more effective than EPS. If there is no cortical and/or subcortical cuff of tissue to preserve, then there is truly no reason to use EPS to remove a tumor.

Anatomically, lesions deep within the cerebellar hemispheres, basal ganglia, deep cerebral hemispheres, deep white matter, and intraventricular locations are most amenable to endoport surgery. If the position of eloquent white matter fibers is not clear, the authors recommend diffusion tensor imaging or high-definition fiber tracking to delineate these fibers and plan an approach that avoids their transection (▶ Fig. 42.3). For rare cases of deep-seated tumors in which speech may be at risk, awake craniotomy with EPS is a viable option.[13]

Presumed lesion histology also plays a role in patient selection. Soft and more readily suctioned tumors are more easily removed through the port. However, as our case demonstrates, firmer tumors can still be resected with a combination of internal debulking and circumferential dissection. It should be noted that hematomas are also amenable to removal using EPS; generally it is technically straightforward to aspirate the hematoma and allow the cavity to collapse around the lesion, facilitating safe clot evacuation.[14]

42.6 Anatomic and Pathologic Considerations

Supratentorial intraventricular tumors present a number of surgical challenges, with surgical approach dictated by location. Nearly all of the common pathologies are best treated with surgical excision, including colloid cysts, subependymomas, neurocytomas, and meningiomas. In the frontal horn, the transcoronal approach using the port provides direct tumor access with minimal brain manipulation. Unlike a midline callosotomy, lateral tumor extension is not an issue with this approach. In addition, by avoiding a substantial callosotomy, cognitive complications of the surgical intervention may be minimized, although this point is controversial.[15] Ventricular body tumors can be approached in a similar fashion, working posteriorly

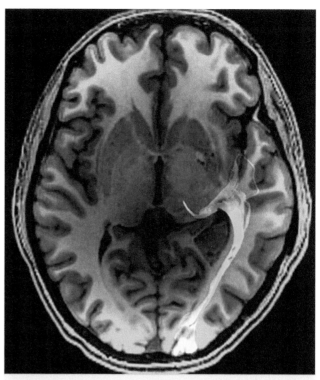

Fig. 42.3 Representative image demonstrating high-definition fiber tracking (HDFT) of the optic radiations in the axial plane wrapping around the occipital horn near an intraventricular tumor. Such images can be integrated into image guidance for trajectory planning prior to brain cannulation.

through the port, but with care to avoid excessive posterior retraction of the port to reach toward the atrium. Atrial tumors are more amenable to a transparietal approach, an approach that must be carefully tailored to avoid injury to the optic radiations or eloquent language tracts. Temporal horn tumors are generally amenable to microsurgical resection when there is substantial trapping of CSF and dilation; the port approach has limited utility here. In the anterior third ventricle, a transfrontal approach with an endoscopic port provides beautiful access, and the choroidal fissure can be opened to dilate the foramen of Monro to provide increased tumor visualization when necessary. This approach is most commonly used for the removal of colloid cysts. Posterior third ventricular tumors that require more than biopsy alone are best approached microsurgically. The fourth ventricular tumors can generally be approached microsurgically via a telovelar approach, so the port may have limited utility in these situations as well.

The port approach has been successfully used for numerous intraparenchymal brain tumors as well. The best candidates for this approach are typically deep seated, often near the ventricular system. Metastases, gliomas, cavernous malformations, and even hematomas have been successfully removed using this technique. The smaller craniotomy and decreased subcortical dissection necessitated by this technique are advantages, although there is controversy regarding the ability to obtain an equivalent degree of resection using this approach as opposed to microsurgery.

Pathologically, tumor consistency plays an important role in the ease or difficulty of resection. Soft tumors, which are discrete from the surrounding white matter, are the most ideal, as is the case with microsurgery. As the tumor becomes more solid, more vascular, or less discrete from the surrounding brain, the surgical degree of difficulty is increased. Of course, this is also the case for microsurgery. As a result, the senior author recommends adopting a learning curve for surgeons considering using EPS in their practice. Hematomas and soft subcortical intraparenchymal metastases are good early cases, with complex intraventricular tumors only to be approached after significant experience has been attained.

42.7 Complication Avoidance and Technical Nuances

The first general principle for avoidance of complications with port surgery is to consider any complications that could occur with a standard craniotomy. Every complication of a standard craniotomy can also happen with port surgery, including infection, bleeding, stroke, seizure, and wound dehiscence. Therefore, patient selection is paramount. Patients who are not a candidate for a craniotomy due to poor medical condition or extent of disease should not have port surgery as an alternative.

Because the craniotomy for port surgery is relatively small (~2.5–3 cm), care must be taken to position the patient properly and to achieve accurate registration of image guidance. The patient should be positioned in similar fashion to a standard craniotomy, with the entry trajectory into the tumor situated above the tumor itself. Improper image-guidance registration can lead to poor cannulation or brain injury. Care should be taken to avoid putting critical blood vessels at risk. This particularly applies to large bridging veins and blood vessels adjacent to tumors (▶ Fig. 42.4).

While port techniques require the creation of a small craniotomy, the brain may still try to herniate through the dural opening. In order to avoid this complication, after completion of the craniotomy and prior to opening the dura, we palpate the dura to assess how tense it is. If tense, we have the anesthesiologists decrease the patient's end tidal carbon dioxide levels and, in some cases, administer mannitol. Regional ICP elevation is best treated with tumor decompression; therefore, for soft tumors, a big advantage of port surgery is that cannulation can be performed swiftly, such that the ICP helps deliver the tumor into the port itself.

For most microsurgical approaches, a trans-sulcal trajectory to the lesion of interest is recommended over a transgyral approach, although there are exceptions to this rule. While the trans-sulcal route decreases the amount of brain tissue traversed by the port, there is a higher concentration of blood vessels within the sulcus, which can be put at risk during cannulation. However, this is not an issue in the middle of a non-eloquent gyrus, in which case a transgyral approach is not likely to increase risk. In addition, the value of a trans-sulcal approach is lost if a sizable cortical bridging vein must be sacrificed during the approach to the tumor. Careful inspection of the preoperative imaging can usually help determine the safest cannulation trajectory for a given lesion.

After resection of any lesion, hemorrhage within the resection cavity or along the cannulation tract is possible. During lesion resection, diligent placement of Cottonoid patties around

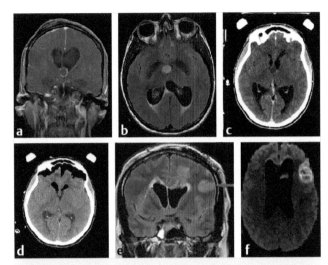

Fig. 42.4 Images of a 36-year-old female who presented in extremis with severe headaches, nausea, vomiting, and drowsiness. Magnetic resonance imaging (MRI) obtained after placement of a ventriculostomy drain demonstrates a colloid cyst in the foramen of Monro on coronal contrasted images (**a**) with hydrocephalus and transependymal flow of cerebrospinal fluid (CSF) noted on axial fluid-attenuated inversion recovery (FLAIR) sequences (**b**). Intraoperative computed tomography (CT) imaging shows patient with Leksell's frame in place with preoperative (**c**) and postoperative (**d**) imaging. Postoperative imaging demonstrates mild pneumocephalus. Postoperative coronal T2 FLAIR MRI demonstrates T2 signal change well lateral to the port cannulation site (**e**, *red arrow*). Diffusion weighted imaging (**f**) shows restriction in the same area, likely due to injury of a cortical vein during cannulation.

the tumoral edges helps catch minor bleeding and keep it in view. Following resection, the cavity must be inspected vigilantly prior to port removal. In the case of intraventricular approaches, areas of arterial bleeding are dealt with using bipolar coagulation, and venous bleeding is generally controlled using direct pressure with irrigation. For parenchymal tumors, bipolar coagulation or absorbable hemostatic agents can be used. Because the port is transparent, bleeding sites can be visualized and directly addressed during slow decannulation of the port.

Moreover, on removing the port, the tract walls should be inspected for signs of hemorrhage. If encountered, the removal should be paused and bipolar coagulation used to stop any significant bleeding. Similarly, after complete removal of the port, cortical inspection should be performed to ensure that there are no additional sites of bleeding. Routinely the authors will line the cortical entry site with Surgicel (Ethicon, Somerville, NJ) or an equivalent, absorbable hemostatic alternative.

Another concern for EPS is the possibility of postoperative obstructive hydrocephalus after resection of intraventricular tumors. While this is not a very common phenomenon in our experience, we routinely leave an external ventricular drainage catheter in the ventricular system just prior to removing the port. This drainage catheter is maintained clamped for 24 hours while ICP are recorded. If the patient tolerates this period of time with normal pressures, the drainage catheter is removed. If, however, the patient has elevated pressures or neurologic decline attributable to hydrocephalus, the drain is opened and maintained until it can be weaned or a ventriculoperitoneal shunt can be placed. As an alternative, for simpler lesions such as colloid cysts, an intraoperative CT scanner can be used to confirm that there is no substantial intraventricular hemorrhage, obviating the need to leave a ventriculostomy drain.

42.8 Clinical Pearls

The senior author is a strong advocate of the mantra "primum non nocere" as it applies to tumor surgery. Therefore, the most critical clinical pearls for port surgery involve making common sense decisions to maximize patient safety. Stroke, hemorrhage, seizures, wound infection, and neurologic deficits all can happen with port surgery just as they can with standard craniotomies. Therefore, it is important that all precautions are taken to avoid complications, mainly by applying the same considerations that are applied for standard craniotomy cases. The anesthesia team needs to be aware that the patient requires the same intravascular access and airway management that would be required for a conventional case. The intensive care unit should be used for complex cases, just as it is for conventional cases. The nursing staff should also be trained to care for these patients using essentially identical protocols to those used after a conventional craniotomy.

Having an appropriate mentor to teach the port technique is a big advantage, as it permits faster learning. Simpler cases should be attempted in early stages, followed by more complex tumors at later phases of training. For difficult cases, if bleeding obscures tumor visualization or if the tumor consistency is particularly difficult, having another set of eyes or hands in the room can help achieve an acceptable outcome.

Maximum degree of tumor removal is a common goal of most neuro-oncologic procedures, but care must be taken not to do so at the expense of morbidity. Overaggressive removal of a tumor at the expense of a substantial neurologic deficit offers the patient no benefit. Therefore, if visualization of a tumor becomes a challenge due to inability to reach around a corner or because of brain shift, it is critical to find a safe alternative to achieve tumor resection, even if that alternative is a staged approach to surgery or a subtotal resection.

Because port surgery offers a narrow corridor into tumors much larger than the tube itself, judicious use of Cottonoids is particularly helpful to achieving a safe resection. Venous bleeding from the edges of the resection cavity is inevitable, and rather than chase every small bleeder with electrocautery, patience and gentle pressure will generally preserve the operative field and allow for safe tumor removal. In addition, early and deliberate placement of patties helps delineate dissection planes between the tumor and the brain. These planes can become less discrete after hours of surgery, increasing the risk of iatrogenic brain injury.

42.9 Literature Review/Evidence in Favor of Endoscopic Approach

The strongest argument for endoscopic surgery as opposed to conventional microsurgery relates to minimizing operative time, morbidity, and recovery time. This debate has been examined for multiple pathologies, but is best shown for colloid cysts. For example, a 10-year retrospective review of patients undergoing transcallosal microsurgical versus working channel endoscopic resection of colloid cysts found that endoscopic approaches were associated with fewer infections, fewer instances of postoperative hydrocephalus requiring shunting, but more small residual cysts on follow-up imaging with similar neurological outcomes.[12] Conversely, in their systematic review and meta-analysis of the literature, Sheikh et al found that colloid cysts treated by microsurgical approach had higher rates of gross total resection, lower rates of recurrence, no difference in postoperative shunt dependency, but a higher surgical morbidity.[16] These trends toward lower complications in endoscopy and more definitive cyst removal with microsurgery are both achieved via the "hybrid approach" of EPS. At our institution, EPS for colloid cysts yielded a 96.9% total cyst resection rate with an average hospital stay of 2.7 days. In summary, the goal of EPS is to combine the best aspects of endoscopy and microsurgery and bring them together into one technique (▶ Table 42.1).

By working through the port with a fixed endoscope holder or an assistant holding the endoscope, the operator is able to utilize a bimanual surgical technique. However, this bimanual technique comes with some drawbacks. First, having the endoscope as a third instrument within the operating corridor can create a crowded working space that partially limits the surgeon's mobility. This is an argument made by proponents of using an operative microscope or the exoscope through the port. For them, improvements in the ability of the microscope to focus through a narrow corridor enable the surgeon to use bimanual technique while maximizing space within the operating corridor. However, with the light and magnification source outside of the port, visualization can be obscured by the surgeon's instruments themselves, which is a substantial issue in an already small corridor. For this reason, the senior author still prefers to have the endoscope within the port itself.

Compared to traditional open microsurgery, use of the endoscopic port allows for a smaller craniotomy, as the window need only be large enough to allow the port to be seated. Similarly, the size of the cortisectomy can be much smaller, because the port generates a cylindrical operating corridor that can be dynamically manipulated to increase the total visible area without increasing the size of the cortical opening. The firm, cylindrical nature of the port also creates a working space that has static and evenly distributed forces on the adjacent brain parenchyma.

Table 42.1 Comparison of endoscopic port surgery (EPS) with channel endoscopy and microsurgery

Channel endoscopy	EPS	Microsurgery
Smallest cortisectomy	Small cortisectomy	Larger cortisectomy
Fluid medium visualization	Air medium visualization	Air medium visualization
Instruments confined to linear trajectory along working channel	Bimanual microsurgery within cylindrical port	Bimanual microsurgery with full range of motion
Visualization easily lost with bleeding	Visualization through bleeding with direct tamponade	Visualization through bleeding with direct tamponade

While there is an increasing body of evidence supporting the role for port-based surgery for deep-seated lesions, there is a growing debate regarding whether EPS or port-based microsurgery with the use of an operative microscope achieves better outcomes. For intraventricular tumors, initial reports of EPS at our center demonstrated an 80% total or near-total resection rate.[5] For intraparenchymal tumors, initial reports of EPS for our center demonstrated 67% rates of total or near-total resection.[6] Some other groups have found the microscope to be more conducive to aggressive tumoral resection. For example, in their initial series of 20 patients undergoing port-based resection for a variety of lesions, Hong et al found the use of the endoscope to be associated with increased rates of subtotal resection.[17] However, the issue of obtaining higher rates of gross total resections may be confounded by tumor location (more than 50% of their lesions were located within the basal ganglia or thalamus) and surgeon experience. In our experience, significantly higher rates of gross total resection are possible, but there is an operative learning curve, and appropriate patient selection is paramount. In addition, the use of an ultrasound probe or intraoperative imaging is an excellent adjunct to facilitate maximal safe tumor resection, regardless of the resection technique used.

42.9.1 When Is Conventional Microsurgery Still the Ideal Approach?

While the senior author uses the EPS technique for the vast majority of supratentorial intraventricular tumor resections, this is not the case for supratentorial intraparenchymal tumors.

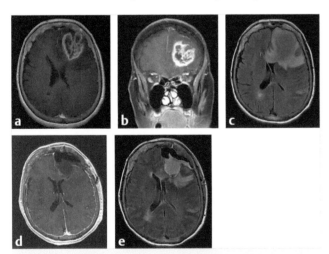

Fig. 42.5 Postcontrast magnetic resonance imaging showing a contrast-enhancing left frontal lesion **(a,b)** with significant perilesional T2 signal change **(c)** concerning for glioblastoma with significant invasion of the frontal lobe and corpus callosum. **(d,e)** Postoperative imaging showing total resection of the contrast-enhancing lesion as well as significant amount of the preoperative T2 signal change. Standard left frontal craniotomy for open microsurgical resection of the lesion was performed, because of the extensive degree of cortical involvement and the superficial presentation of the tumor.

These tumors must be carefully selected for EPS; deep tumors, which are quite discrete, are the best candidates. Conversely, superficial wide-based tumors (▶ Fig. 42.5) and tumors that invade the cortex are clearly better candidates for conventional resection, as there is no cortex or superficial white matter to protect. While the port can be used under awake conditions, most tumors for awake resection and cortical mapping are best approached conventionally.

Sometimes, port surgery does not provide an advantage for a deep subcortical tumor due to nuances related to location or size. For example, ▶ Fig. 42.6 demonstrates the case of a patient who presented with a complex seizure disorder and a tumor of the nondominant parahippocampal gyrus. Because of the patient's seizure disorder and young age, surgical resection of the small tumor was clearly indicated. However, because of the proximity of the tumor to the skull base, EPS through the inferior temporal sulcus was not going to decrease the amount of iatrogenic brain injury related to the case. Therefore, in this case, the tumor was approached microsurgically via a subtemporal approach with intraoperative ultrasound, and fluorescein dye with an integrated microscope filter was used to augment intraoperative tumoral visualization. The lesion was completely excised without complication, and histology confirmed a pilocytic astrocytoma.

42.10 Conclusion

The authors propose that EPS is an effective tool for deep brain tumor removal in appropriate hands. EPS remains a technique in evolution, but has already shown promising results for complex lesions, deep-seated lesions, and intraventricular tumors. As technological improvements continue to be made in the development of surgical instruments, endoscopes, and retractors, neurosurgeons will continue to strive to make their operations less invasive. Such innovations will hopefully provide better outcomes for the next generation of neurosurgical patients.

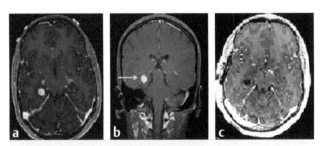

Fig. 42.6 A 25-year-old patient with new-onset partial complex seizures found to have a discrete, contrast-enhancing mass lesion in the right parahippocampal gyrus **(a,b)**. Cannulation with an endoscopic port along the inferior temporal sulcus **(b,** *yellow arrow***)** would have traversed more brain tissue than a traditional subtemporal microsurgical approach **(b,** *yellow arrow***)**. The latter approach was used with intraoperative fluorescein for complete resection of the lesion **(c)**. Proximity of the lesion to the skull base made microsurgery a more favorable option in this case.

References

[1] Grant JA. Victor Darwin Lespinasse: a biographical sketch. Neurosurgery. 1996; 39(6):1232–1233

[2] Hopf NJ, Perneczky A. Endoscopic neurosurgery and endoscope-assisted microneurosurgery for the treatment of intracranial cysts. Neurosurgery. 1998; 43(6):1330–1336, discussion 1336–1337

[3] McLaughlin N, Prevedello DM, Engh J, Kelly DF, Kassam AB. Endoneurosurgical resection of intraventricular and intraparenchymal lesions using the port technique. World Neurosurg. 2013; 79(2) Suppl:18.e1–18.e8

[4] Ochalski PG, Fernandez-Miranda JC, Prevedello DM, Pollack IF, Engh JA. Endoscopic port surgery for resection of lesions of the cerebellar peduncles: technical note. Neurosurgery. 2011; 68(5):1444–1450, discussion 1450–1451

[5] Engh JA, Lunsford LD, Amin DV, et al. Stereotactically guided endoscopic port surgery for intraventricular tumors and colloid cyst resection. Neurosurgery. 2010; 67:198–204

[6] Kassam AB, Engh JA, Mintz AH, Prevedello DM. Completely endoscopic resection of intraparenchymal brain tumors. J Neurosurg. 2009; 110(1): 116–123

[7] Kelly PJ, Goerss SJ, Kall BA. The stereotaxic retractor in computer-assisted stereotaxic microsurgery. Technical note. J Neurosurg. 1988; 69 (2):301–306

[8] Kelly PJ, Kall BA, Goerss S, Earnest F, IV. Computer-assisted stereotaxic laser resection of intra-axial brain neoplasms. J Neurosurg. 1986; 64(3): 427–439

[9] Jho HD, Alfieri A. Endoscopic removal of third ventricular tumors: a technical note. Minim Invasive Neurosurg. 2002; 45(2):114–119

[10] Yadav YR, Yadav S, Sherekar S, Parihar V. A new minimally invasive tubular brain retractor system for surgery of deep intracerebral hematoma. Neurol India. 2011; 59(1):74–77

[11] Greenfield JP, Cobb WS, Tsouris AJ, Schwartz TH. Stereotactic minimally invasive tubular retractor system for deep brain lesions. Neurosurgery. 2008; 63 (4) Suppl 2:334–339, discussion 339–340

[12] Horn EM, Feiz-Erfan I, Bristol RE, et al. Treatment options for third ventricular colloid cysts: comparison of open microsurgical versus endoscopic resection. Neurosurgery. 2007; 60(4):613–618, discussion 618–620

[13] Bodily L, Mintz AH, Engh J. Combined awake craniotomy with endoscopic port surgery for resection of a deep-seated temporal lobe glioma: a case report. Case Rep Med. 2013; 2013:401359

[14] Ochalski P, Chivukula S, Shin S, Prevedello D, Engh J. Outcomes after endoscopic port surgery for spontaneous intracerebral hematomas. J Neurol Surg A Cent Eur Neurosurg. 2014; 75(3):195–205, discussion 206

[15] Symss NP, Ramamurthi R, Kapu R, et al. Complication avoidance in transcallosal transforaminal approach to colloid cysts of the anterior third ventriclen: an analysis of 80 cases. Asian J Neurosurg. 2014; 9(2):51–57

[16] Sheikh AB, Mendelson ZS, Liu JK. Endoscopic versus microsurgical resection of colloid cysts: a systematic review and meta-analysis of 1,278 patients. World Neurosurg. 2014; 82(6):1187–1197

[17] Hong CS, Prevedello DM, Elder JB. Comparison of endoscope- versus microscope-assisted resection of deep-seated intracranial lesions using a minimally invasive port retractor system. J Neurosurg. 2016; 124(3):799–810

43 Future of Neuroendoscopy

Hasan A. Zaidi and Peter Nakaji

Summary

The future of neuroendoscopy is bright because the endoscope has recently evolved into an essential and effective neurosurgical tool with an indispensable place in the neurosurgical armamentarium. However, several obstacles remain to deter its further ascendancy. In this chapter, we describe aspects of neuroendoscopy and technology that will transform the field in the years to come. Currently, neuroendoscopy is not a panacea for all neurosurgical pathology—in certain aspects, it is inferior to traditional visualization modalities. Nonetheless, future innovations in optical physics and electronics are expected to mitigate limitations of current 3-dimensional (3D) endoscopes and to enable natural and intuitive stereoscopic endoscopic visualization. Malleable endoscopes also hold tremendous potential for innovative endoscope design that will improve surgical efficacy by improving surgeon comfort. The training of future neuroendoscopists can be improved with the use of simulation technology, such as the use of 3D printing technology to make anatomical models that are anatomically correct, to scale, and even augmented with pumps and fluid to create realistic blood and cerebrospinal fluid environments. Furthermore, future improvements in robotic technology and the use of superimposed patient-derived information on the surgical field view to create an augmented reality are likely to revolutionize minimally invasive neuroendoscopic surgery. Thus, future innovations will likely mitigate the limitations of current endoscopes. It is imperative for the field of neuroendoscopy that it continues to evolve by pushing the boundaries of minimally invasive approaches, adapting new technologies on the horizon, and redefining medical education and surgical techniques.

Keywords: development, endonasal, future, neuroendoscopy, optics, skull base, spine

43.1 Introduction

Within a few short generations, the endoscope has evolved from a novelty item into a versatile and effective neurosurgical tool. A healthy exchange of ideas among surgical subspecialties allowed the medical community as a whole to realize the potential of the endoscope. Generations of engineers toiled to refine the design of the endoscope, with each iteration decreasing its profile and improving its optical efficiency. Persistence by neurosurgical pioneers to utilize this previously untested instrument in the face of heavy criticism helped nurture their technical skills. The distribution of endoscopic knowledge through residency and fellowship training and educational courses captivated the imagination of each successive generation of surgeons, allowing endoscopic neurosurgeons to make a greater impact on the lives of their patients. The future of neuroendoscopy is bright, but several obstacles to future progress remain. Herein, we set out to elucidate various aspects of neuroendoscopy that will transform the field in the years to come.

43.2 Three-Dimensional Endoscopy

An important limitation of current-generation endoscopes is the inability to provide realistic 3-dimensional (3D) visualization of the surgical corridor. Despite steady improvements in image quality and color fidelity, the absence of stereoscopic vision can often result in a loss of visuospatial orientation that creates a steeper learning curve for the surgeon compared to that with open techniques. Trainees who are instructed to grasp objects using 2-dimensional (2D) projected images often misjudge object size and distance, which results in a longer time to move to the target, smaller peak velocities, longer deceleration phases, and smaller grip apertures.[1] Furthermore, the loss of stereoscopic visualization prevents surgeons from using their natural ability to decipher the contours of the operative corridor. In the ventral skull base, for example, the inability to recognize the opticocarotid recess can be potentially catastrophic. Critics suggest that these limitations prolong surgery and increase the risk of iatrogenic neurovascular injury.

Over the past decade, innovations in microchip arrays have led to the development of 3D endoscopes. Experts suggest that, unlike 2D endoscopes, 3D endoscopes enhance visuospatial orientation, thus improving the recognition of, and the relationship to, anatomical structures and potentially shortening the learning curve for trainees (▶ Fig. 43.1).[2] However, the 3D endoscopes currently in use are early-generation units, with several drawbacks. These endoscopes provide low image resolution with significant color distortion that results in red saturation, which can present a significant challenge to surgeons attempting to differentiate tumors from normal structures. The depth effect can result in vertigo for the primary surgeon, and some surgeons even require antiemetic treatment. Furthermore, the advantages afforded by the 3D endoscope are anecdotal, because of the lack of large-scale objective clinical trials supporting its use.[2] Future innovations in optical physics and electronics may mitigate these limitations of the current generation of 3D endoscopes. New models are in the development pipeline that will purportedly enhance resolution while maintaining color fidelity. These incremental improvements may provide enough impetus to the greater neuroendoscopic community to encourage the transition to stereoscopic endoscopic visualization.

43.3 Malleable Endoscopes

One of the many advantages provided by endoscopes is the ability to minimize approach-related trauma by reducing the size of incisions and craniotomies compared to those of conventional approaches. As a result, the surgical corridor is often narrow and crowded with instruments, resulting in increased instrument collision and surgeon frustration. Endoscopes used in modern-day neurosurgical procedures are overwhelmingly rigid, which inherently contributes to instrument conflict both within and outside the surgical cavity. The camera and cable

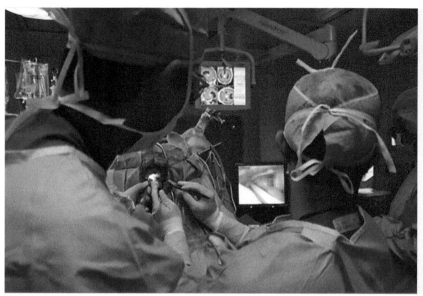

Fig. 43.1 Intraoperative image demonstrating the use of a 3D endoscope (monitor at right below neuronavigation system monitor). The surgeon and the surgery assistant both wear 3D glasses during the course of the surgery to watch the 3D video projection. (Used with permission from Barrow Neurological Institute, Phoenix, AZ.)

often collide with the hands of the primary surgeon outside the surgical cavity, and dissection tools frequently collide with the shaft of the endoscope within the surgical cavity. Frequent instrument conflict at both the front end and back end of rigid endoscopes can result in steeper learning curves, longer surgical times, and decreased safety and efficacy compared with those of open techniques. To provide additional room for surgical manipulation, surgeons often resort to removing more tissue by increasing the size of the surgical corridor, which worsens approach-related morbidity.

Over the past few years, malleable endoscopes with memory have been developed that permit the shaft of the endoscope to be bent to maintain its configuration (▶ Fig. 43.2). This malleability allows the assistant to move the camera head away from the hands of the primary surgeon outside the surgical field and to bend the rod to reduce the incidence of instrument conflict within the surgical corridor. Surgical freedom studies in cadaver models demonstrate that, unlike their rigid endoscopic counterparts, malleable endoscopes improve surgical ergonomics and reduce instrument conflict.[3] Although malleable endoscopes have not yet been approved by the U.S. Food and Drug Administration and thus have not yet been put into clinical use in the United States, they hold tremendous potential for innovations in endoscope design that will improve surgical efficacy by improving surgeon comfort. As seen historically, incremental changes to endoscope design can have profound effects on improvements in the quality, safety, and popularity of endoscopic neurosurgery.

43.4 Endoscopic Training

Technical mastery of microneurosurgery has traditionally required rigorous study of human anatomy, hours of laboratory dissection, close mentorship, and diligent oversight of trainees in the operating room. The popularity of endoscopic procedures has added an additional level of complexity to the training process for novice neurosurgeons. Trainees must be adept at using endlessly evolving navigation instruments, endoscopes, dissection tools, drills, and debridement tools, all within the confines of a narrow and crowded surgical corridor. With the

expansion of the complexities of surgical approaches and the tools associated with these procedures, the learning curve associated with effective surgical execution becomes steeper. In this dynamic environment, the traditional training process has rapidly become obsolete and ineffective in preparing future generations of endoscopic neurosurgeons. The future of endoscopic neurosurgery will depend on the development of novel surgical training curricula.

For generations, the neurosurgical community has relied primarily on the dissection of formalin-fixed cadaveric specimens to develop the technical skills of trainees. This archaic mode of training endoscopic neurosurgeons has several limitations. First, specimens are often financially and logistically difficult to obtain, and residents are often required to use the same specimen repeatedly to keep costs low. Second, the preservation of neuroanatomical structures in fixed specimens is highly variable, with key anatomical landmarks in the soft tissue often distorted during the preservation process. Being able to identify these landmarks is a critical skill for endoscopic neurosurgery novices to acquire because they will not have access to wide neuroanatomical exposures. Third, the cadaveric specimens are usually devoid of abnormal anatomical landmarks frequently encountered in the operating room. Navigating the surgical corridor and avoiding iatrogenic complications in the setting of distorted anatomy from a given surgical pathology are crucial to effective execution of neuroendoscopic surgery. Fourth, fixed specimens are often rigid and less compressible than what is typically encountered in the operating room. Endoscopic surgeons rely on the natural elasticity of the neurovascular structures to effectively execute surgical maneuvers. Surgical training using cadaveric specimens does not adequately develop the tactile feedback necessary to effectively perform neurosurgical tasks. Last, cadaveric specimens are devoid of the natural fluids of the human body, such as blood and cerebrospinal fluid. This is especially troublesome for endoscopic trainees; for example, effective execution of endoscopic third ventriculostomy requires an understanding of how to manage visual obstruction by cerebrospinal fluid within the lateral ventricles, which cannot be simulated using cadaveric specimens. These limitations of formalin-fixed cadaveric specimens often make it

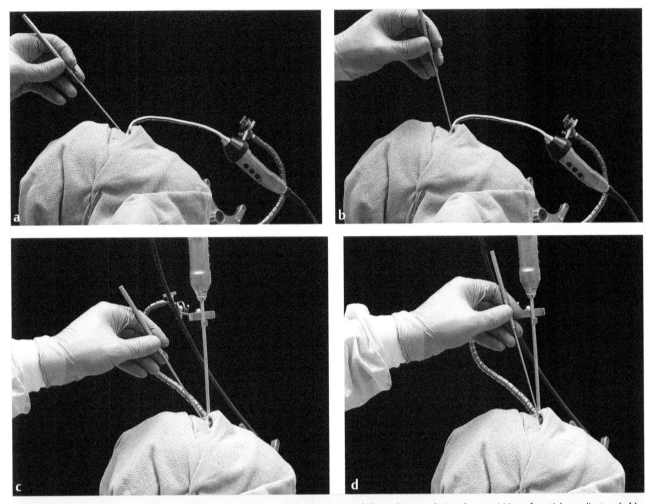

Fig. 43.2 A series of photographs demonstrating the position of the dissector and the endoscope during the acquisition of spatial coordinates. **(a,b)** Photographs illustrate how the camera of the malleable endoscope has been contoured out of the operative corridor, and how the dissector is moved **(a)** inferiorly and **(b)** superiorly. **(c,d)** Photographs demonstrate the position of the rigid endoscope as the dissector is moved **(c)** inferiorly and **(d)** superiorly, where it collides with the endoscope camera, restricting surgical freedom. (Used with permission from Barrow Neurological Institute, Phoenix, AZ.)

difficult for trainees to translate the skills developed in the laboratory to the operating room.

Given the relative rarity of endoscopic procedures in the face of increasing popularity of endoscopy, the neuroendoscopic community has been, by necessity, at the forefront of developing novel simulation tools to augment surgical training. The development of new teaching tools may help circumvent the inherent limitations of traditional cadaveric specimen dissection. Computerized simulation modules have recently gained traction as an alternative to cadaveric dissection (▶ Fig. 43.3).[4] They require little supporting staff and can create reproducible intraoperative scenarios that can be tailored to the skill level of the trainee. However, these simulators are not yet capable of replicating the delicate haptic feedback necessary to refine surgical techniques, and trainees often do not have the freedom to explore anatomy outside the regimented module. Furthermore, prohibitive costs in developing and maintaining simulators limit their widespread use.

The field of 3D printing technology has evolved rapidly over the past decade. Newer generations of printers have provided the capability to reconstruct anatomical models with incredible

fidelity at affordable prices. The latest iteration is the multimaterial printer, which simulates a range of mechanical and physical properties, from rubbery to rigid and from opaque to transparent, in a plethora of colors. These printers afford institutions the ability to print skull models with bone in hard material capable of being drilled, cartilage in softer material, a vascular tree, and tumors of different shapes and sizes. These models provide several advantages over previous surgical training modalities. They are affordable and rapidly obtainable, they do not require a full laboratory environment, they can carry a wide array of skull base pathology tailored to the skill level of the trainee, and they can be drilled and dissected to develop the haptic feedback necessary to refine intraoperative skills. Trainees use these 3D models to develop better visuospatial understanding of complex skull base vascular anatomy while also developing skills directly translatable to the operating room. Narayanan et al[5] used 3D printers to develop models of basilar invagination for endoscopic surgical dissection. This technique allows the incorporation of rare, complex pathology into simulation models to enhance the realism and tactile feedback necessary to approach these lesions. Similarly, Berhouma et al[6]

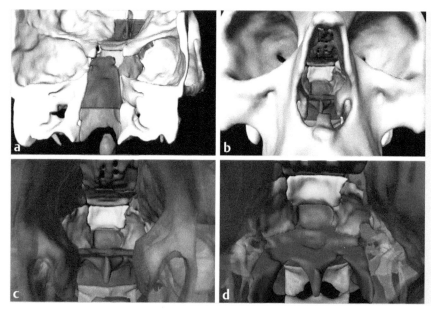

Fig. 43.3 Virtual computer-based 3D models of areas of the different endoscopic endonasal approaches to the midline skull base and cavernous sinus. Transcribriform approach (*red*); transplanum/transtuberculum approach (*pale blue*); sellar approach (*yellow*); transclival approach (*dark blue*); craniovertebral junction approach (*purple*); and cavernous sinus approach (*green*). (**a**) Posterolateral view. (**b**) Anterior view. (**c,d**) Endonasal anteroinferior perspective. (Adapted from de Notaris et al.[4])

developed a polymer-based tumor model and implanted model tumors into cadaveric embalmed heads to produce anatomical aberrations frequently encountered in neurosurgical procedures. Such models teach trainees how to avoid iatrogenic injury by recognizing how mass lesions in the ventral skull base can distort normal anatomical waypoints.

To further enhance the realism of simulation models, Winer et al[7] continuously reconstituted saline via a cervical laminectomy into cadaveric specimens and performed intraventricular neuroendoscopic approaches to better simulate working within a lake of cerebrospinal fluid. Such exercises allow trainees to gain perspective on the technical nuances associated with performing delicate neurosurgical tasks within a fluid-filled cavity. Similarly, Muto et al[8] connected cadaveric specimens to a pulsatile pump to mimic carotid artery injury during endoscopic transsphenoidal dissection. This technique provides realistic simulations of intraoperative carotid injury, with pulsatile blood and debris obscuring the surgical corridor and dirtying the endoscopic lens. As 3D printing technology improves and anatomical printouts are augmented with pumps and fluid, these constructs will ultimately supersede cadaveric specimens in realism and relevance to neurosurgical training.

43.5 Robotics

A major drawback to the use of intracranial endoscopic approaches is that they require two surgeons to work in unison to execute critical portions of the procedure. In the typical operating room setup, the primary surgeon holds instruments in both hands to perform delicate intracranial tasks, while the assistant surgeon navigates the endoscope to provide dynamic visualization. The two-surgeon approach introduces a certain level of logistical and task-based complexity. First, coordinating the schedule with an assistant surgeon can be difficult, potentially leading to delays in surgery. Second, the presence of the assistant surgeon often restricts the full range of motion in the arms and elbows of the primary surgeon, which can contribute to the loss of surgical freedom. This restriction, in combination with the presence of multiple tools within the surgical cavity,

can exacerbate instrument conflict. The surgeons themselves are also limited by the anatomical restrictions of the human body, namely, the naturally limited range of motion of their wrists and arms. Because surgical working corridors are at a premium in endoscopic neurosurgery, the field is ripe for robotic assistance in the future, which might mitigate some of these drawbacks.

Early pioneers began to address the shortcomings of the traditional two-surgeon endoscopic approach by using various mechanical devices. Pneumatic endoscopic holders were one of the earliest tools introduced in neuroendoscopy. By placing the endoscope in a static arm, which obviates the need for an additional assistant surgeon, the primary surgeon is able to exercise relatively unhindered arm movement. Doing so, however, carries its own set of drawbacks. Robotic endoscopic holders provide static visualization of the surgical corridor rather than dynamic visualization. For many surgeons, particularly those using 2D visualization, continuous movement of the endoscope provides additional visual feedback and parallax depth perception. Furthermore, the endoscopic lens frequently requires cleaning despite the use of irrigating sheaths, which requires the primary surgeon to physically remove the endoscope and clean the lens during the case, which can increase surgical time and surgeon frustration. Future development of a robotically controlled endoscopic holder that moves along with the movements of the primary surgeon may improve visualization, surgical freedom, and surgical efficiency.

Robotics assistance has steadily gained popularity in various surgical subspecialties, including gynecology, urology, obstetrics, cardiac surgery, and orthopedics. Advocates suggest that robots are particularly useful in confined spaces. Multiple pivot points and 360-degree rotation of robotic arms maximize the full use of narrow surgical corridors and provide flexibility unrivaled by manually driven instruments. Furthermore, the reduction of tremor provides precise and accurate movement of surgical instruments to the target. In a recent review, Marcus et al[9] classified surgical robots into three main categories. The first are supervisory-controlled robot systems, whereby the primary surgeon plans each step of the operation and tasks are autonomously executed by the robot under direct human supervision. The second are "master–slave" systems in which the surgeon remotely controls movements of the robotic arms. The last are shared-control systems, whereby both the surgeon and the robot share control of the primary surgical instrument, theoretically taking advantage of the natural movements of the surgeon and the precision of the robot.

Marcus et al[9] reported that more than 30 robotic systems have been developed for neurosurgical procedures. Supervisory-controlled systems represent the overwhelming majority of these robotic systems, and they have been put into clinical use for biopsy of brain lesions, intratumoral drug delivery, implantation of deep brain stimulation electrodes, and placement of pedicle screws. The surgical tasks involved in these robotic systems can be precisely defined and easily navigable with the use of computer image–guided stereotactic systems.[10,11,12,13,14] For more complex approaches, such as to reach invasive deep-seated lesions that require dynamic surgical decision-making, the ad hoc determination of surgical tasks is more difficult to define. Master–slave robotic devices, similar to the popular da Vinci robotic systems (Intuitive Surgical, Sunnyvale, CA) used for urologic operations and other surgical procedures, have been applied in a variety of cadaveric studies (▶ Fig. 43.4).[15,16] These systems typically have two or three robotic arms with multiple degrees of freedom. Several authors have demonstrated that, although these robotic systems improve surgical freedom and accuracy of tasks, they significantly increase the duration of surgery—both the preoperative setup and the length of the surgical procedure. Shared-control systems are the least used robotic systems, and few have been described in the neurosurgical literature.[17,18,19] These systems provide improved ease of use and much more natural integration into the surgical workflow.

Despite accolades from other surgical subspecialties, robotic-assisted surgery has not yet achieved the same level of commercial success within neurosurgery. Although robotic assistance has tremendous potential to produce a positive impact on neuroendoscopy in the future, current-generation robotic technology fails to provide a truly immersive environment for neurosurgeons to warrant its use. More so than in other surgical subspecialties, neurosurgical procedures are dynamic in nature and require delicate tactile feedback for effective execution of procedures. Future systems will have to overcome several challenges. Robots must be fully integrated with image-guidance systems and must provide small working channels without limiting freedom of movement to minimize approach-related trauma and maximize surgical dexterity.[9] The robot–surgeon interface will also have to be improved not only to provide high-resolution stereotactic images and improved haptic feedback but also to be integrated much more naturally into the surgical workflow to improve safety and operative time. Although current-generation robotic technology is too limited to justify its use for neuroendoscopic procedures, future improvements will indeed revolutionize minimally invasive neuroendoscopic surgery.

43.6 Augmented Reality

Computer-guided neuronavigation has also greatly revolutionized neurosurgery over the past 2 decades. It has allowed surgeons to plan surgeries more precisely to decrease incision size, reduce approach-related morbidity, and avoid iatrogenic neurovascular injury. It gives surgeons a real-time map of the operative corridor, and it can be particularly useful when traditional neuroanatomical waymarks are distorted by cranial pathology. In neuroendoscopic surgery, neuronavigation is even more critical. The minimally invasive nature of endoscopic procedures obviates the wide exposure often needed to carefully navigate to the surgical target using known anatomical landmarks. Despite its near ubiquitous application in neuroendoscopic procedures, the neuronavigation interface, as it is most often used, remains suboptimal. Surgeons are required to frequently look away from the operative corridor to a dedicated navigation workstation screen. The images on the workstations display preoperative imaging in various projections. Thus, the surgeon is required to continuously analyze these data to convert the virtual map provided by neuronavigation and project it onto the surgical landscape. For novices and experts alike, this process can result in misinterpretation and confusion because of the nonintuitive nature of navigation projections.

Advances in computer technology with ever-increasing processing speeds have allowed for the development of augmented reality for surgical navigation.[20] Augmented reality systems can take images of intracranial tumors and vascular structures obtained from preoperative scans and project these data onto endoscopic images of the surgical corridor. This type of imaging creates a more immersive, ergonomic, and seamless integration of data from the real environment with virtual information. Augmented reality can enhance the surgeon's perception of the operative corridor, allowing the surgeon to avoid important neurovascular structures en route to the surgical target. This enhanced perception is particularly useful within the confines of the narrow surgical corridor often used in neuroendoscopic procedures, when minimal exposure provides little in the way of anatomical landmarks. By superimposing patient-derived information onto the surgical field view, augmented reality can create a type of "X-ray" vision for the primary surgeon. Although the wide-scale application of augmented reality systems is currently cost prohibitive and not user friendly with regard to setup, current industrial efforts in this regard suggest that future improvements and integration into neuroendoscopes are forthcoming, which may mitigate these limitations and ultimately have considerable impact on the field.

43.7 Conclusion

The endoscope has revolutionized a variety of subspecialties in neurosurgery in a relatively short period of time. Rapidly expanding indications over the past few decades have led to the emergence of new opportunities and challenges. In its current form, neuroendoscopy does not represent a panacea for all neurosurgical pathology. Certain aspects of neuroendoscopy are inferior to traditional visualization modalities. But, as both the technology and the field evolve, innovations by future neuroendoscopists will likely mitigate the limitations of the endoscope. The survival of the endoscope as a viable alternative to traditional visualization modalities has always depended on the dynamism of neuroendoscopists. It is imperative for neuroendoscopy as a field to continue to evolve, and in so doing to push

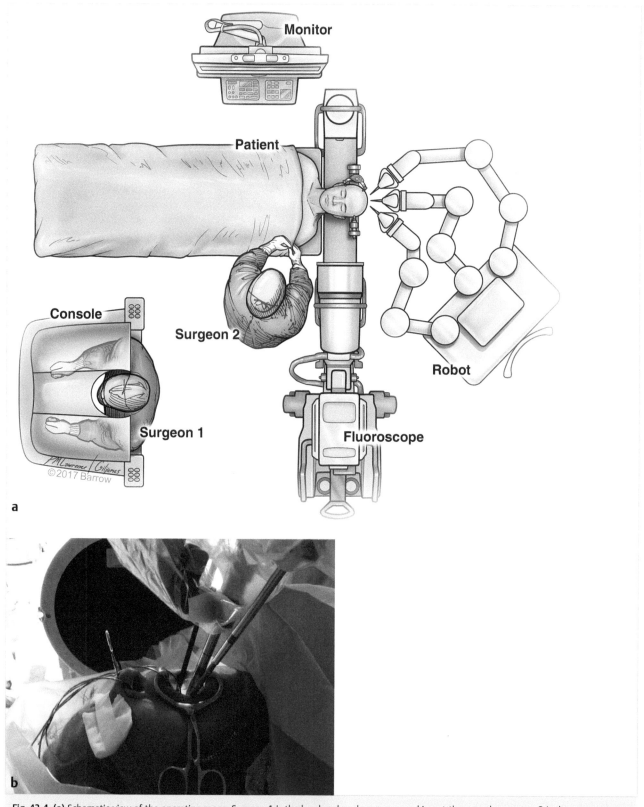

Fig. 43.4 (a) Schematic view of the operating room. Surgeon 1 is the head and neck surgeon working at the console; surgeon 2 is the neurosurgeon working at the bedside. (Used with permission from Barrow Neurological Institute, Phoenix, AZ.) (b) Lateral intraoperative view. The three robotic arms stand in the oral cavity that is opened with a mouth retractor. The retraction of the soft palate is performed by using two rubber catheters introduced through the nose and pulled out via the mouth. The C-arm fluoroscope is used for intraoperative 2D lateral control. (Adapted from Chauvet et al.[16])

the boundaries of minimally invasive approaches, to adapt new technologies on the horizon, and to redefine medical education and surgical techniques.

References

[1] Servos P, Goodale MA, Jakobson LS. The role of binocular vision in prehension: a kinematic analysis. Vision Res. 1992; 32(8):1513–1521

[2] Zaidi HA, Zehri A, Smith TR, Nakaji P, Laws ER, Jr. Efficacy of three-dimensional endoscopy for ventral skull base pathology: a systematic review of the literature. World Neurosurg. 2016; 86:419–431

[3] Elhadi AM, Zaidi HA, Hardesty DA, et al. Malleable endoscope increases surgical freedom compared with a rigid endoscope in endoscopic endonasal approaches to the parasellar region. Neurosurgery. 2014; 10 Suppl 3:393–399, discussion 399

[4] de Notaris M, Topczewski T, de Angelis M, et al. Anatomic skull base education using advanced neuroimaging techniques. World Neurosurg. 2013; 79(2) Suppl:16.e9–16.e13

[5] Narayanan V, Narayanan P, Rajagopalan R, et al. Endoscopic skull base training using 3D printed models with pre-existing pathology. Eur Arch Otorhinolaryngol. 2015; 272(3):753–757

[6] Berhouma M, Baidya NB, Ismaïl AA, Zhang J, Ammirati M. Shortening the learning curve in endoscopic endonasal skull base surgery: a reproducible polymer tumor model for the trans-sphenoidal trans-tubercular approach to retro-infundibular tumors. Clin Neurol Neurosurg. 2013; 115(9):1635–1641

[7] Winer JL, Kramer DR, Robison RA, et al. Cerebrospinal fluid reconstitution via a perfusion-based cadaveric model: feasibility study demonstrating surgical simulation of neuroendoscopic procedures. J Neurosurg. 2015; 123(5):1316–1321

[8] Muto J, Carrau RL, Oyama K, Otto BA, Prevedello DM. Training model for control of an internal carotid artery injury during transsphenoidal surgery. Laryngoscope. 2017; 127(1):38–43

[9] Marcus HJ, Seneci CA, Payne CJ, Nandi D, Darzi A, Yang GZ. Robotics in keyhole transcranial endoscope-assisted microsurgery: a critical review of existing systems and proposed specifications for new robotic platforms. Neurosurgery. 2014; 10 Suppl 1:84–95, discussion 95–96

[10] Haegelen C, Touzet G, Reyns N, Maurage CA, Ayachi M, Blond S. Stereotactic robot-guided biopsies of brain stem lesions: experience with 15 cases. Neurochirurgie. 2010; 56(5):363–367

[11] Frasson L, Ko SY, Turner A, Parittotokkaporn T, Vincent JF, Rodriguez y Baena F. STING: a soft-tissue intervention and neurosurgical guide to access deep brain lesions through curved trajectories. Proc Inst Mech Eng H. 2010; 224(6):775–788

[12] Wei J, Wang T, Liu D. A vision guided hybrid robotic prototype system for stereotactic surgery. Int J Med Robot. 2011; 7(4):475–481

[13] Lefranc M, Touzet G, Caron S, Maurage CA, Assaker R, Blond S. Are stereotactic sample biopsies still of value in the modern management of pineal region tumours? Lessons from a single-department, retrospective series. Acta Neurochir (Wien). 2011; 153(5):1111–1121, discussion 1121–1122

[14] Lieberman IH, Togawa D, Kayanja MM, et al. Bone-mounted miniature robotic guidance for pedicle screw and translaminar facet screw placement: part I—technical development and a test case result. Neurosurgery. 2006; 59(3):641–650, discussion 641–650

[15] Hong WC, Tsai JC, Chang SD, Sorger JM. Robotic skull base surgery via supraorbital keyhole approach: a cadaveric study. Neurosurgery. 2013; 72 Suppl 1:33–38

[16] Chauvet D, Missistrano A, Hivelin M, Carpentier A, Cornu P, Hans S. Transoral robotic-assisted skull base surgery to approach the sella turcica: cadaveric study. Neurosurg Rev. 2014; 37(4):609–617

[17] Matinfar M, Baird C, Batouli A, Clatterbuck R, Kazanzides P. Robot-assisted skull base surgery. IEEE International Conference on Intelligent Robots and Systems, October 29–November 2, 2007

[18] Kazanzides P, Xia T, Baird C, et al. A cooperatively-controlled image guided robot system for skull base surgery. Stud Health Technol Inform. 2008; 132:198–203

[19] Kane G, Eggers G, Boesecke R, et al. System design of a hand-held mobile robot for craniotomy. Med Image Comput Comput Assist Interv 2009;12:402–409

[20] Meola A, Cutolo F, Carbone M, Cagnazzo F, Ferrari M, Ferrari V. Augmented reality in neurosurgery: a systematic review. Neurosurg Rev. 2016

Index